CLINICAL
Nursing
PROCEDURES

BY

Barbara Kuhn Timby, RN, BSN, MA
Instructor, Medical–Surgical Nursing,
Glen Oaks Community College, Centreville, Michigan

WITH

Carol Lillis, RN, MSN
Associate Professor, Delaware County Community College, Media, Pennsylvania

Louise Gore Grose, RN, PhD
Nurse Consultant, Board of Nurse Examiners for the State of Texas; Staff Nurse,
Home Health Care Department, Holy Cross Hospital, Austin, Texas

CLINICAL
Nursing
PROCEDURES

J.B. Lippincott Company

Philadelphia

Cambridge	London
New York	Singapore
St. Louis	Sydney
San Francisco	Tokyo

Acquisitions Editor: Patricia L. Cleary
Coordinating Editorial Assistant:
  Nancy Lyons
Manuscript Editor: Helen Ewan
Indexer: Nancy Weaver
Senior Designer: Anita Curry
Production Manager: Carol A.
  Florence
Production Supervisor: Charlene
  Squibb
Compositor: Tapsco, Inc.
Printer/Binder: Murray Printing

6 5 4 3 2

Library of Congress Cataloging-in-Publication Data

Timby, Barbara Kuhn.
    Clinical nursing procedures/by Barbara Kuhn Timby with Carol
Lillis, Louise Gore Grose.
        p.   cm.
    To accompany: Fundamentals of nursing/[edited by] Carol
Taylor, Carol Lillis, Priscilla LeMone. c1989.
    Includes bibliographies and index.
    ISBN 0-397-54740-4
    1. Nursing.   I. Lillis, Carol.   II. Grose, Louise Gore.
III. Fundamentals of nursing.   IV. Title.
    [DNLM: 1. Nursing Care.   WY 100 T583c]
RT41.F882 1989 Suppl.
610.73—dc19
DNLM/DLC
for Library of Congress   88-13552
                                                                                          CIP

Any procedure or practice described in this book should be applied by the health-care practitioner under appropriate supervision in accordance with professional standards of care used with regard to the unique circumstances that apply in each practice situation. Care has been taken to confirm the accuracy of information presented and to describe generally accepted practices. However, the authors, editors and publisher cannot accept any responsibility for errors or omissions or for consequences from application of the information in this book and make no warranty, express or implied, with respect to the contents of the book.

Every effort has been made to ensure drug selections and dosages are in accordance with current recommendations and practice. Because of ongoing research, changes in government regulations and the constant flow of information on drug therapy, reactions and interactions, the reader is cautioned to check the package insert for each drug for indications, dosages, warnings and precautions, particularly if the drug is new or infrequently used.

To my students,
who have always been
the best teachers

PREFACE

Clinical Nursing Procedures has been developed to promote skills for performing a selected group of core nursing procedures that are common to most areas of nursing practice. The procedures are intended to dovetail with the conceptual areas presented in the text, *Fundamentals of Nursing*. Although there is a relationship between the textbook and this manual, the procedure manual can be used as an independent tool for learning or used collaboratively with any other theoretical text.

A great deal of thought has been given to designing a format that would support principles of learning. Since new information is best learned by relating it to past knowledge, procedures have been catalogued according to a generalized physical systems approach. The manual comprises eight units with groups of procedures that relate to general care or the structure and functioning of a particular body system. This approach builds on the learner's educational foundations in anatomy and physiology. Subdividing the content into categorized units facilitates learning by grouping information into manageable amounts. In addition, each group of procedures in a unit is arranged in an order that builds from simple to complex. Numerous line drawings and photographs enhance learning by supplementing written, abstract concepts with concrete images.

The nursing process is a universal, generic thread running throughout nursing practice. Therefore, the framework for each procedure uses the same familiar pattern.

Each procedure includes the *assessment* data that are appropriate when preparing to perform the procedure. Included are suggestions for nursing *diagnoses* that may be identified once the data have been analyzed. The taxonomy of the North American Nursing Diagnosis Association has been adopted and used in order to promote a standard for nursing communication. The etiology and defining characteristics of the diagnostic statement have been omitted in the procedures. The intent is not to suggest that this is the example to follow, but rather to indicate that these components of the diagnostic statement are unique to each client. The potential combinations of complete statements are so vast as to make any suggested list inadequate.

The discussion of *planning* proposes that the nurse consider variables that can affect the prioritized need to perform the procedure. Goals are suggested, but each nurse should strive to write a predictive statement that best documents either that the client's problem is resolved or that the procedure has accomplished its purpose. A list of equipment is provided prior to each procedure. Since each clinical facility is unique and contracts to obtain the most satisfactory supplies within its budgetary constraints, the nurse is advised to remain flexible and to adapt to using equipment that is common within the institution.

The *implementation* step of the nursing process is the described technique for performing the skill itself. To promote simplicity for the learner, each action is listed in a step-by-step progressive sequence in one column. The rationale for the action is immediately provided in an adjacent column to promote understanding of the underlying principles.

Various approaches are provided for *evaluating* the effectiveness of the procedure. Focused data, unique to reassessment, are recommended. Expected and unexpected outcomes are offered. These provide the nurse with some realistic consequences that may develop when the procedure has been performed, either successfully or unsuccessfully.

In addition to the nursing process, other components have been included in the format of each procedure. These were added to expand the student's awareness of correlated nursing responsibilities while learning to perform technical skills. For example, samples of documentation are provided to help the student learn to identify the important information that should be recorded. These samples also promote the use of appropriate terms when charting pertinent information. Variations, such as those that occur in unique situations, differences among clients at various stages in the life cycle, and modifications for home-health care, are discussed with each clinical procedure. This may help the student develop versatility when there is a need to modify a procedure in order to adapt to unusual client variables and clinical circumstances. A section on related teaching is included because nursing involves health maintenance and health promotion. The nurse can use these suggestions for discharge planning or to prepare the client to be a more knowledgeable caretaker of his own health. Restoring the client's internal locus of control promotes more active participation in health care.

Finally, there is a checklist for performing each clinical skill. Experience has shown that when a learner knows what is expected, anxiety is reduced. Therefore, the critical behaviors are identified for the benefit of the learner and the instructor. The checklist can promote independent review and practice demonstration among peers while attempting to build confidence and competence. It is hoped that the checklist will not be used to reinforce rigid, rote performance. As long as principles of nursing care are not violated, there can be some acceptable leeway during a demonstration. The checklist can serve as a record for determining that the student has met the objectives for a laboratory assignment or the partial requirements of a course.

ACKNOWLEDGMENTS

I want to thank Patricia L. Cleary, Senior Editor, for the confidence, encouragement, and creativity that she nurtures in me. The challenging task of illustrating this manual has been accomplished through the hard work and direction of Tracy Baldwin and the coordination of Eleanor Faven. The contributions of Carol Lillis and Louise Grose have been very valuable during the development of this procedure manual. Last, but not least, I need to recognize the vigilence of my husband, Ken, in holding all the loose ends of the family together until I finished this project.

Barbara Kuhn Timby, RN, BSN, MA

CONTENTS

UNIT VIII
PROCEDURES
PERTAINING
TO THE
MUSCULOSKELETAL
SYSTEM

GUIDELINES FOR USING THE PERFORMANCE CHECKLIST

Clinical performance reflects the comprehension and application of theory to practice, which is the essence of learning. Nursing requires continuous conscientious self-evaluation, peer evaluation, and evaluation by mentors. The evaluation process is intended to help identify strengths and limitations in order to develop a plan for promoting continued learning and growth.

It is suggested that the individual observing the demonstration of a procedure use the following descriptions for determining the term that best correlates with the learner's performance:

Competent (C): Indicates that the individual is prepared, organized, proceeds without hesitation, follows suggested steps in appropriate sequence, independently demonstrates safe practice, or shows manual dexterity when handling equipment.

Acceptable (A): Indicates that the individual needs more review or practice to develop competence, is somewhat disorganized, hesitates during the demonstration, partially completes one or more necessary steps, requires limited guidance or assistance, demonstrates minimal safe practice, or shows awkwardness when handling equipment.

Unsatisfactory (U): Indicates that the individual is unprepared, disorganized, lacks self-confidence, needs assistance or suggestions in order to proceed, omits necessary steps, would jeopardize the safety of a client without continued guidance or supervision, or is unsure about the use of necessary equipment.

Individuals who use the Performance Checklist are encouraged to determine the criteria for the number or percent of Competent, Acceptable, and Unsatisfactory marks that would result in passing or failing.

I

Procedures pertaining to general care

I-1   *Admitting a client to a health-care agency*

Persons are admitted to health-care agencies to receive care and treatment for acute illness; to undergo and recuperate from surgery; to acquire assistance during labor, delivery, and postpartum; to obtain diagnostic testing; and to continue recovery from long-term illness. The admission procedure is the first contact between nursing personnel and the client and the beginning of the delivery of health-care services.

PURPOSES OF PROCEDURE

The admission process is designed to

1. Establish a positive, initial relationship with the client, his relatives, or close friends.
2. Orient the client to the immediate environment and the services that are available.
3. Acquire a data base of information which generally includes a health history, comprehensive subjective and objective data related to his current health, and a physical assessment. Figure I-1-1 shows an example of a nursing admission data base form.
4. Enable the nurse to collaborate with the client to discuss his needs and expectations for care.

ASSESSMENT

OBJECTIVE DATA

- Determine the name, gender, age, admitting diagnosis or primary symptoms of the client, and the name of the attending physician.
- Estimate the expected time of arrival to the nursing unit or facility.
- Ask about special equipment that should be in readiness, such as oxygen, suction, intravenous (IV) poles, bed boards, full side rails, and so on.

SUBJECTIVE DATA

- Inquire about the relative acuity of the patient's condition.

RELEVANT NURSING DIAGNOSES

Anyone who must leave the security of his previous pattern of living for care and treatment in a health-care agency is likely to be experiencing any or all of the following nursing diagnoses:

- *Fear*
- *Anxiety*
- *Altered Family Processes*
- *Self-Care Deficit*
- *Disturbance in Self-Concept*
- *Social Isolation*

PLANNING

ESTABLISHING PRIORITIES

All clients entering a health-care agency should be provided with expedient attention and care. However, those who are experiencing difficulty breathing, have unstable vital signs, are unconscious, or are in severe pain require immediate attention.

It is imperative that all contacts with the client convey a sense of concern for his safety, comfort, and welfare. The admitting nurse's attitude toward the client is likely to be the basis for the client's first impression about the care given in the health agency. Nurses are reminded that the client is a consumer and fellow human being who deserves courtesy and protection of his legal rights. Care of other clients may need to be delegated in order to attend to the admission of a new client as expeditiously as possible.

Figure I-1-1 This hospital admission assessment record is an example of the format many health-care agencies are using to collect comprehensive baseline information on all new clients.

Doe, Jane   Age 73

1200 West Elm

Jackson, MO

00011000

(Area must be completed by RN or LPN)

PATIENT'S HEALTH HISTORY

What is reason for admission? (Patient's own words)

"I had trouble breathing and a bad cough"

Past Hospitalization and/or illnesses: (Medical, surgical, emotional problems)

1980 Heart Problems
1982 Colon Resection

NURSING ADMISSION DATA BASE
Saint Francis Medical Center

(Entire area can be completed by any patient care staff)

Date: 12-2-89   Time: 0900

ADMISSION
- ☐ Ambulatory   ☒ Wheelchair   ☐ Stretcher
- ☐ Correct identification band   ☐ Allergy band
- **Admitted From:** ☒ Home   ☐ Nursing Facility
  ☐ Emergency Room   ☐ Other _____
- **Information Given By:** ☐ Family member   ☐ Friend
  ☒ Patient   ☐ Unable to take history, patient unresponsive/ not accompanied by family or friend

Orientation to Room
- ☒ Visiting hours   ☒ Call light system (bedside/bath)
- ☒ Smoking policy   ☒ Use of phone
- ☒ Bedrails up at H.S. unless ordered otherwise
- **Valuables:** ☐ None   ☒ Sent home   ☐ To safe
- **Allergens:** (Drugs, food, tapes, dyes, other)   ☐ NKA   ☒ Allergy Bracelet Applied

Allergen	Symptoms	Treatment
Pollens	stuffy nose	none
Penicillin	rash	avoid drug

(Area must be completed by the RN or LPN)

Medications Prescribed And Non-Prescribed	Dosage	Usual Times Taken	Time Of Last Dose	Patient's Understanding Of Purpose/Problems
Aspirin	3 tabs	8-12-6	12/2 : 8 AM	for arthritis
Lanoxin	0.125 mg	8 Am	12/2 : 8 Am	for heart
Diuril	500 mg	8 - 6	12/2 : 8 Am	for heart
Milk of Magnesia	1½ oz.	bedtime	11/30/89	as needed for constipation

Medications sent ☒ To Pharmacy ☐ Home With whom? _____

FUNCTIONAL HEALTH PATTERN ASSESSMENT

(All areas of the Functional Health Pattern Assessment <u>MUST</u> be completed by the RN with the exception of #1 of Objective Data. See *)   (√) Box if data is pertinent)

SUBJECTIVE DATA:

1. **Health Perceptions/Health Management Pattern**
   General health ___Good___
   Use of: ☐ Tobacco   How much ___∅___ How long? _____
   ☐ Alcohol   How much? ___∅___ How long? _____
   Last Drink _____
   ☒ Other drugs type(s) ___see above___

2. **Nutritional/Metabolic Patterns**
   Special diet ___Low Salt___
   Meals/day ___3___   Snacks/day ___1___
   Weight: ☐ Gain   ☒ Loss   ☐ How much? ___5 pounds___
   ☐ No problems

3. **Respiration/Circulation Patterns**
   History of: ☒ Shortness of breath   ☒ With exercise
   ☐ Without exercise
   ☒ Cough   ☒ Sputum (phlegm)
   ☐ No problems   Sleeps on ___2___ pillows
   History of: ☐ Chest pain   ☒ Pedal Edema   ☐ No problems
   ☐ Pacemaker   ☐ Rate   ☐ Arrhythmias

OBJECTIVE DATA: *(#1 of objective data can be completed by any patient care staff)

1. **Clinical Data**
   Height ___64"___   Weight ___142___ ☒ Actual / approx _____
   Temperature ___99.87___ Pulse ___102___ Respirations ___30___
   Blood pressure   Right arm ___120/72___ Left arm ___124/76___
   ☐ Sitting   ☒ Lying

2. **Nutritional/Metabolic Pattern**
   Oral Mucosa: ☒ Color ___pink___ ☐ Lesions ___NO___ Moistness ___yes___
   Teeth: ☒ Dentures   ☒ Upper   ☒ Lower
   Skin integrity: ☒ Turgor normal   ☐ Other _____
   ☐ Intact   ☒ Other ___Sl. pedal edema___

3. **Respiration/Circulation Pattern**
   Breath sounds ___Rales and Rhonchi, both lower lung bases___
   Cough: ☐ Non-Productive ☒ Productive   ☒ Sputum Color ___Rusty___
   Apical Rate ___104___   Rhythm: ☒ Regular   ☐ Irregular
   Pedal edema: ☒ Present   ☐ Absent
   Right dorsalis pedal pulse: ☒ Strong   ☐ Weak   ☐ Absent
   Left dorsalis pedal pulse: ☒ Strong   ☐ Weak   ☐ Absent
   Homan's sign   Positive R ☐ L ☐   Negative R ☒ L ☒

640-009-816/0800053

SUBJECTIVE DATA (Cont'd)

4. Elimination Pattern

History of: ☐ Nausea   ☐ Vomiting   ☐ Dysphagia
☒ No Problems

Bowel Habits: Stools/Day 1/q 3 days   ☐ Soft/Formed
☒ Constipation   ☐ Diarrhea
☐ Incontinence   ☐ Melena   Last BM 12/1/89

Bladder habits: Urinates/Day 4-5X   ☒ No problem
☐ Self-Cath   ☐ Urgency   ☐ Frequency
☐ Nocturia   ☐ Dysuria   ☐ Hematuria
☐ Incontinence

5. Activity/Exercise Pattern

Energy level: ☒ Tires easily   ☐ Average
☐ High/Energy

Exercise Program: ☒ None   ☐ Other _____

Able to: ☒ Feed self   ☒ Bathe self   ☐ With assist
☒ Ambulate   ☒ Climb stairs
☒ Can do household chores

Adaptive devices: ☐ Cane   ☐ Walker   ☐ Crutches
☐ Wheelchair   ☐ Other _____ Ø

6. Sleep/Rest Pattern

Sleep problems: ☐ Trouble falling asleep
☒ Early AM waking   ☐ Other
☐ No Problems

7. Cognitive/Perceptual Pattern

Communication: Language spoken English
Understands German
Able to: ☒ Read   ☒ Write   ☐ Lip read
Cognition: ☒ No problems   ☐ Recent memory change
☐ Difficulty learning
Discomfort/pain: ☐ No   ☒ Yes   Where? L. Thorax
How do you manage your pain? use medicines,
go to bed, read Bible

8. Role/Relationship Pattern

Marital Status: ☒ Married   ☐ Single   ☐ Widowed
☐ Divorced
Children (#) 3
Occupation Housewife
Retirement activities: (Hobbies) Knits, reads

Family concerns about hospitalization? Worried about
long-term effects of illness

9. Sexuality/Reproductive Pattern (if appropriate)

Last menstrual period 20 years ago
Menstrual problems   ☐ Yes   ☒ No
Birth control measures N/A
Any sexual concerns related to illness (optional)
NO

Signature P. LeMone R.N.
Date 12/2/89

OBJECTIVE DATA (Cont'd)

4. Elimination Pattern

Abdomen: ☒ Soft   ☐ Firm
☒ Non-tender   ☐ Tender
☐ Non-distended   ☐ Distended _____ girth
☒ Bowel sounds   ☐ Bowel sounds absent
☐ Ostomies/tubes   ☐ Type _____

Urinary devices _____

5. Activity/Exercise Pattern

ROM: ☐ Full   ☒ Other Arthritic changes
Balance and gait: ☒ Steady   ☐ Unsteady
Hand grasps: ☒ Equal   ☐ Strong
Weakness/paralysis: ☐ Right   ☐ Left
Leg muscles: ☒ Equal   ☐ Strong
☐ Weakness/Paralysis ☐ Right   ☐ Left
☐ Disorientation at night
☐ Prone to falling

7. Cognitive/Perceptual Pattern

Level of consciousness: ☒ Alert   ☒ Responds to pain
☐ No response
Oriented to: ☒ Time   ☒ Place   ☒ Person
Mood: ☒ Calm   ☐ Sad   ☐ Angry   ☐ Withdrawn
☐ Other _____
Pupils: ☒ Equal   ☒ Reactive   ☐ Other _____
Cognition: ☒ Able to follow simple commands
☒ Responds appropriately to questions
☐ Unable to follow commands
☐ Other
Hearing: ☒ Normal   ☐ Impaired   ☐ Left ear
☐ Right ear   ☐ Aid
Vision: ☐ Normal   ☒ Impaired   ☒ Glasses
☐ Contact Lenses
Pain: Location and type L. lower thorax

Discharge Planning Evaluation

	A	B
1. Do you live at home alone?	Yes ☐	No ☒
2. Who lives with you? husband, Carl		
3. Do you live in a house, apartment, or trailer? house		
Do you live in a nursing home or boarding home?	Yes ☐	No ☒
4. Do you have any problems caring for yourself at home?	Yes ☐	No ☒
5. What relatives or friends are willing to help with your care if needed:		
Name: Son, Joe		
Phone: 111-2222		
6. Have you been receiving help from any person or agency while at home?	Yes ☐	No ☒
Name of person:		
Name of agency(s):		
7. Will you need any help with care to be able to return home?	Yes ☐	No ☒
8. Discharge planning coordinator or social service indicated at admission?	Yes ☐	No ☒

If yes, notify appropriate person.

SETTING GOALS
- The client will be greeted, oriented, and admitted immediately or shortly after his arrival.
- The client will provide information about his past and present health history.
- The client will be examined with minimal discomfort.
- The client will describe his perspective of his current problems, expectations for care, and problems that will need to be resolved in order to facilitate the earliest discharge possible.

PREPARATION OF EQUIPMENT

The nurse will need to gather the following equipment to complete the admission of a client to the health agency:

Thermometer
Sphygmomanometer
Stethoscope
Scales
Data base assessment form
Urine specimen container
Instruments used for physical assessment, such as an otoscope, pen-light, tongue blades, and so on

Technique for admitting a client to a health-care agency

ACTION	RATIONALE
1. Check the client's identification band. Greet the client, as the nurse in Fig. I-1-2 is doing. Introduce yourself to the client and the client to his roommate(s).	Calling the client by name, extending common courtesies, and welcoming the client and relatives often help them to feel at ease and less frightened.
2. Explain use of the bathroom and agency equipment, such as the call system, adjustable bed, television, telephone, and so on. Explain agency routines, such as meal times and visiting hours.	Explaining agency routines and how to use equipment helps put the client at ease. Knowing how to use equipment helps prevent accidents.

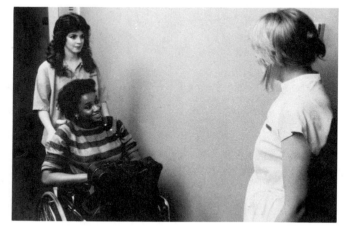

Figure I-1-2 The nurse meets and greets the client who has been escorted to the nursing unit. Sensing that she is expected and welcome will do much to relieve the client's fears and anxiety.

3. Place the signal device and other equipment so that they will be convenient for the client to use.

Being unable to call for help is unsafe and can result in accidents. When equipment is handy, accidents, such as falling, are less likely to occur.

4. Obtain the client's temperature, pulse and respiratory rates, and blood pressure. Obtain a urine specimen at a time that is convenient during the admission procedure.

It is the nurse's responsibility to obtain these signs and specimen as a basic part of the client's admission and physical assessment.

5. Provide for privacy. Ask relatives to leave unless their assistance or support is requested by the client.

Providing privacy shows respect and interest in maintaining the client's dignity.

6. Help the client to undress (Fig. I-1-3), and assist the client into a comfortable position in bed.

Assisting the client to undress and get into bed conserves the client's strength, prevents accidents, and prepares the client for physical assessment. If the client has no functional limitations, it is important to allow the client the opportunity to change alone.

7. Take care of the client's clothing and valuables. Record the inventory according to agency policy.

Losing items is upsetting to the client and can result in legal problems.

8. Indicate to relatives that they may return to the client's bedside.

Relatives have worries and fears, too. They usually feel better when they know the client is admitted, settled, and comfortable.

9. Take this time to tell the client what will be happening and what to expect (Fig. I-1-4).

It is very stressful not knowing what to expect. Explanations tend to decrease anxiety.

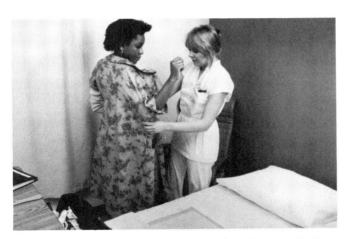

Figure I-1-3 To make the client feel comfortable and to facilitate a comprehensive physical assessment, the nurse helps the client to change into bed clothes.

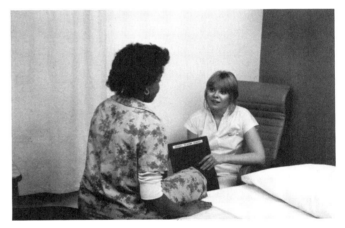

Figure I-1-4 The nurse explains the admission process and initial care activities.

10. Do necessary recording on the client's record, following agency policy. Begin the nursing history and assessment. Use judgment as to whether the information is collected with or without the family in the room.

The nursing history and assessment provide information that is unique to the client. It forms the basis for identifying his problems and care. The family's presence may inhibit the client's responses.

11. After the family has left, continue the history and assessment.

The client may divulge important information that he did not want the family to know.

SAMPLE DOCUMENTATION

Date	Time	Nurse's note
1/15	1330	60-year-old black male admitted per stretcher from the emergency room to Room 354[1] accompanied by wife. BP 150/90 right arm lying down. T-99[2] orally, P-110 and regular, R-28 and labored. Skin color is pale with cyanosis noted around mouth and nailbeds. Alert and oriented to person,

place, and time. No known allergies. Bed scale weight of 186. Placed in high Fowler's position with side rails up. Oxygen running at 4 liters per minute per nasal cannula. Clothing and valuables list completed and signed by wife. See admission assessment form for further information. 100 ml of dark amber urine obtained and sent to the laboratory for routine urinalysis. Dr. Ross's office notified of admission.

C. Foltz, RN

EVALUATION

REASSESSMENT

Each primary care nurse should make a daily head-to-toe assessment of each assigned client. Focus, or in-depth, assessments can be obtained more frequently when the client is manifesting deviations from normal in a specific body system. The continual validation and collection of information help to identify new health problems and worsening or resolution of prior health problems.

EXPECTED OUTCOMES

The client feels welcome, relaxed, and confident in the health-care agency.

The data base assessment form is completed within the first 24 hours or less of admission.

The nursing Kardex and care plan identify appropriate nursing orders specific to the client's needs.

The family feels comfortable in leaving the client in the care of the health agency's personnel.

UNEXPECTED OUTCOMES

The client demonstrates a high level of anxiety or disorientation that threatens his safety.

The client or other significant person is unable to provide information about the health history.

The client refuses to remain within the health-care agency and indicates a desire to leave against medical advice.

MODIFICATIONS IN SELECTED SITUATIONS

GENERAL VARIATIONS

Use an adult client's title and surname. A first name may be used if the client requests that the nurse do so.

When a client is critically ill, the initial collection of information may be abbreviated to include only the most pertinent data.

Extend the time over which data are collected, providing periods of rest when the client is short of breath, in severe pain, or distressed in any other way. This indicates a higher concern for the client's welfare.

If a client is unconscious or disoriented, questions concerning the health history may be obtained from the next of kin or close relative.

Allow the newly admitted person to retain or display personal items, such as bed clothing, photographs, get-well cards, and so on. This reinforces the unique identity of the client.

AGE-RELATED VARIATIONS

When infants and children are admitted to a health-care agency, both the child and the parents require emotional support. Illness and potential separation heighten anxiety.

Encourage parents to remain with a child throughout the admission process. Accommodate the parents if and when they express a desire to remain with their child. Cots and dietary trays are commonly provided parents in most health-care agencies. Hospitality homes, such as a Ronald McDonald House, may be available for temporary lodging when pediatric clients are critically ill.

Parents are the most reliable source of admission data when children are quite young. Provide privacy when answers to questions are likely to cause crying or emotions that the child may misinterpret as a potential threat to his safety.

The nurse can convey a sense of trust and respect by directing health-related questions to the older child or adolescent.

Allow young children to hold and examine equipment that will be used during a physical assessment. The nurse can reduce a child's fear by encouraging role playing with dolls or puppets.

Transport young children to a treatment area when the initial care on admission may involve obtaining blood specimens, administering injections, or starting intravenous solutions. The child is likely to understand that his room is a safe area, a place where he will not be subjected to uncomfortable or painful treatments.

Hold and gently touch a child as much as possible during admission. The child is less likely to think of hospital personnel as persons who will hurt him.

Adolescents are likely to be self-conscious about body changes. Protecting their modesty and being sensitive to their possible embarrassment during a physical examination indicate respect for this unique period during the life-cycle.

Speak slowly, clearly, and distinctly when collecting information from an elderly client. The sense of hearing can become diminished with age. It is important that the nurse not misinterpret unusual responses to questions as being due to senility.

Allow sufficient time for the elderly person to respond to questions. Hesitancy in responding can be a result of an attempt to recall events that happened many years earlier with as much accuracy as possible.

Elderly clients may experience transitional shock at the time of admission. This is characterized by confusion, disorientation, and paradoxical sleep patterns. Repetition of information, reorientation, and empathic support reduce this temporary unsettled period.

HOME-HEALTH VARIATIONS

Persons desiring home health care may be referred or may contract privately with agencies providing full-time or intermittent skilled nursing services at home.

In order for home health care to be reimbursed, there must be a written order by the physician for all services. Clients must meet certain criteria to have home care services reimbursed by Medicare and other third-party payors.

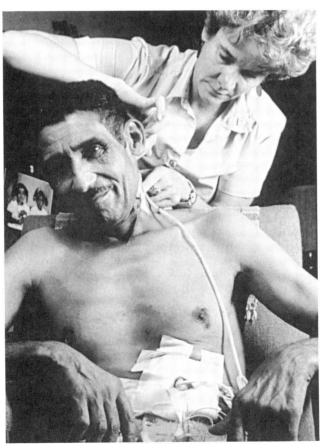

Figure 1-1-5 The nurse provides skilled nursing care within the client's home. During each visit, the nurse collects data, identifies problems that can be treated with nursing interventions, plans and provides care, and evaluates the outcomes. (Photo by Robert Coldwell, courtesy Community Home Health Services of Philadelphia)

The home health nurse, shown in Figure I-1-5, continues to carry out the nursing process of assessment, diagnosis, planning, implementation, and evaluation in relation to the needs of the client and his significant others.

When a new client is added to the home health nurse's caseload, all the persons involved in that client's care are considered. Of particular concern is the primary caregiver who often needs respite care. The nurse can assist by involving other family members, neighbors, or a home health aide to help.

Following an admission assessment, contact the physician for possible modifications of orders if the collected data suggest a need for additional services or equipment.

Insofar as possible, allow the client's routines and preferences to remain unchanged. Determine any needed modifications. Suggest strategies and adaptations as appropriate and within reason.

Discuss the goals and care plan. Explain how to notify agency personnel if an emergency or problems arise. Instructions should be simple to follow and preferably in written or printed form.

RELATED TEACHING

Explain that hospital admissions can be reduced by prophylactic medical examinations. Inform clients about community health screening fairs which are often free or inexpensive.

Educate persons about the early danger signals associated with cancer (Table I-1-1).

Identify the warning signs associated with a medical emergency (Table I-1-2). Many persons delay seeking medical treatment. The American College of Emergency Physicians (ACEP) estimates that 25% minimize the potential acuity of their symptoms.

Table I-1-1
Cancer warning signals

C	Change in bowel or bladder habits
A	A sore that does not heal
U	Unusual bleeding or discharge
T	Thickening or lump in a breast or elsewhere
I	Indigestion or difficulty in swallowing
O	Obvious change in a wart or mole
N	Nagging cough or hoarseness

(Used by permission of the American Cancer Society)

Table I-1-2
Indications of a medical emergency

1. Chest pain or upper abdominal pain or pressure
2. Difficulty breathing, shortness of breath, feeling hungry for air
3. Fainting or feeling faint
4. Dizziness, sudden weakness, or a sudden change in vision
5. Sudden severe pain anywhere in the body
6. Severe or persistent vomiting
7. Suicidal or homicidal feelings

(When to seek emergency care. In: Health Scene. Coffey Communications, Inc. November 1987, p 1)

Inform parents whose children are not under the care of a pediatrician or family practitioner that the county public health department is a resource for reduced cost immunizations and well-baby or child health care.

Refer clients to the community social and health services that are available for assisting with specific problems. Using various community services, such as home delivered meals, transportation to medical appointments, home nursing care, or assistance with home maintenance, may help to avoid subsequent admissions to an acute-care facility.

PERFORMANCE CHECKLIST

When admitting a client, the learner:

C	A	U	
[ ]	[ ]	[ ]	Checks the room to determine if it is clean and completely equipped.
[ ]	[ ]	[ ]	Collects equipment for initial assessment.
[ ]	[ ]	[ ]	Greets the client by name and introduces self, other personnel, and persons within the client's room.
[ ]	[ ]	[ ]	Demonstrates the method for adjusting the height, head, and leg positions of the bed.
[ ]	[ ]	[ ]	Explains the use of the signal light and attaches it within the client's reach.
[ ]	[ ]	[ ]	Orients the client to the location of the restroom, closet and drawer space, lounge areas, chapel, and direction of the nurses' station.
[ ]	[ ]	[ ]	Provides privacy for changing into hospital or personal bed clothing.
[ ]	[ ]	[ ]	Itemizes clothing and valuables that the client wishes to keep with him.
[ ]	[ ]	[ ]	Explains the smoking policy in the health agency if that applies.
[ ]	[ ]	[ ]	Provides the client with information on the times for meals and visiting hours.
[ ]	[ ]	[ ]	Obtains a scale weight.
[ ]	[ ]	[ ]	Positions the patient in bed for comfort.
[ ]	[ ]	[ ]	Complies with the client's wish to have his family remain or wait temporarily in a lounge area during the admission procedure.
[ ]	[ ]	[ ]	Assesses vital signs.
[ ]	[ ]	[ ]	Inquires about known allergies and current medications.
[ ]	[ ]	[ ]	Proceeds with collecting the health history based on the ability of the client to provide the information.
[ ]	[ ]	[ ]	Completes a physical assessment.
[ ]	[ ]	[ ]	Explains and collects body fluid specimens.
[ ]	[ ]	[ ]	Confers with family members to explore their concerns.
[ ]	[ ]	[ ]	Records collected information on appropriate admission forms.
[ ]	[ ]	[ ]	Notifies the physician, head nurse, or team leader reporting a summary of the significant collected data.

C = competent; A = acceptable; U = unsatisfactory

(Continued)

PERFORMANCE CHECKLIST (Continued)

C	A	U	
[ ]	[ ]	[ ]	Analyzes data and formulates an initial nursing care plan that contains a list of the client's nursing diagnoses or collaborative problems, goal statements, and nursing orders.
[ ]	[ ]	[ ]	Shares the initial data and impressions with nursing team members.
[ ]	[ ]	[ ]	Communicates with the client and his family concerning the medical and nursing orders that have been planned.

Outcome: [ ] Pass   [ ] Fail

C = competent; A = acceptable; U = unsatisfactory

Comments: _____
_____
_____

_____   _____
Student's Signature   Date

_____   _____
Instructor's Signature   Date

Assessing vital signs

The procedures that follow are subdivided into various methods for obtaining the four measurements that collectively are considered vital signs. These four include: body temperature, pulse rate, respiratory rate, and blood pressure. The term vital signs is a derivative of the Latin word *vita* which means life. The term is apropos because these four measurements reflect sensitive changes in the physiology of the body. Subtle alterations can alert the nurse to the status of a client's condition. Because these assessments can indicate minute-by-minute changes, they are often assessed frequently throughout the day. The nurse must be conscientious when repetitiously performing the procedure so that the importance of the data is not overlooked. The nurse must make critical decisions concerning the method for measuring the vital signs, the choice of equipment to use, the frequency for assessing, modifications that need to be implemented, and the significance of the data.

Assessing each respective vital sign will be discussed as a separate topic. The nurse may assess any one or combination of vital signs when gathering information about the client.

I-2   *Assessing body temperature*

Body temperature normally remains within a fairly constant range as a result of a balance between heat production and heat loss. Heat is produced primarily by exercise and the metabolism of consumed food. Heat is lost from the body primarily through the skin, the lungs, and the body's waste products. The body's temperature may change due to illness, disease, or exposure to an environment which is either extremely hot or cold.

PURPOSES OF PROCEDURE

Body temperature is assessed to

1. Determine the current level of internal body heat.
2. Evaluate the client's recovery from illness.
3. Determine if measures should be implemented to reduce a dangerously elevated body temperature.
4. Determine if measures should be implemented to conserve body heat when the body temperature is dangerously low.
5. Detect the response of a client once heat-producing or heat-reducing measures have been initiated.

ASSESSMENT

OBJECTIVE DATA

- Review the trend in previously recorded temperatures and route.
- Observe the client's ability to support a thermometer within the mouth.
- Read the client's history for any reference to recent seizures or a seizure disorder.
- Observe the ability of the client to breathe adequately through his nose with his mouth closed.
- Note if the client has had recent mouth trauma or oral surgery, rectal surgery, or a condition that affects the anus or rectum.
- Determine if the client has consumed cold or hot substances within the past 15 minutes to 30 minutes.
- Examine the color of the skin for a flushed or pale appearance.
- Feel the surface of the cheeks or forehead for warmth and moisture.

SUBJECTIVE DATA

- Ask the client if he is experiencing headache, pain, nausea, or feeling hot or cool.

RELEVANT NURSING DIAGNOSES

A person who requires the assessment of body temperature may be experiencing any of the following nursing diagnoses:

- *Potential Altered Body Temperature*
- *Hypothermia*
- *Hyperthermia*
- *Ineffective Thermoregulation*
- *Knowledge Deficit*
- *Altered Comfort*
- *Altered Oral Mucous Membranes*

PLANNING

ESTABLISHING PRIORITIES

Any time there is a sudden or unusual change in a client's condition, or the client is critically ill, the vital signs including body temperature should be assessed. Temperature measurement is indicated more often when the client has an infection, is

14

flushed and perspiring, is shaking with chills, or has a history of exposure to extremes in environmental temperatures.

SETTING GOALS

- The client's temperature will be recorded accurately using the most appropriate route.
- The client's safety and comfort will be maintained.

PREPARATION OF EQUIPMENT

To measure body temperature, the nurse may gather selected items from the following list:

Rectal or oral glass thermometer, shown in Fig. I-2-1.
Electronic thermometer (optional)
Disposable probe cover or plastic sheath
Lubricant if a rectal route is used
A watch or clock
Clean gloves (optional)

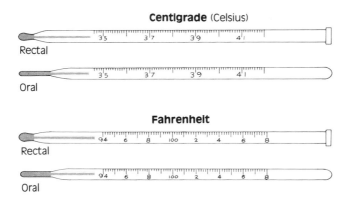

Figure I-2-1 The two glass thermometers at the top of this figure use the Celsius (Centigrade) scale to measure temperature. Each small line represents 0.1 degree. The two glass thermometers on the bottom use the Fahrenheit scale. Each small line represents 0.2 degree. Rectal thermometers have blunt bulbs; oral thermometers have long thin bulbs.

Technique for assessing body temperature by the oral method

Using a glass clinical thermometer

ACTION	RATIONALE
1. Explain the procedure to the client.	An explanation reduces apprehension and promotes cooperation.
2. Gather equipment.	Organization promotes efficient time management.
3. Wash your hands.	Handwashing deters the spread of microorganisms.
4. Wipe the thermometer with a soft tissue if it has been stored in a chemical solution, such as alcohol.	A disinfectant solution can irritate mucous membrane and produce an objectionable odor or taste. A soft tissue will conform to the surface and help to absorb any residual chemical from the thermometer.
5. Wipe the thermometer once from the bulb toward the fingers with the tissue.	Wiping from an area where there are few or no organisms to an area where organisms may be present minimizes the spread of organisms to cleaner areas.
6. Grasp the thermometer firmly with the thumb and forefinger. With strong wrist movements, shake the thermometer until the mercury line reaches at least 36°C or 95°F.	Shaking the thermometer moves the mercury back into the bulb below the previously recorded measurement.
7. Read the thermometer by holding it horizontally at eye level, and rotate it between the fingers until the mercury line can be seen clearly.	Holding the thermometer at eye level facilitates reading. Rotating the thermometer will aid in placing the mercury line in a position where it can be read best.

8. Place the mercury bulb of the thermometer well within the back of the right or left sublingual pocket, and instruct him to close his lips around the thermometer, as shown in Fig. I-2-2.

When the bulb rests deeply in the posterior sublingual pocket, it will be in contact with blood vessels lying close to the surface and will accurately measure body temperature.

9. Leave the thermometer in place for at least 3 minutes or the time interval recommended in the agency policy.

Allowing sufficient time for the mercury to expand ensures an accurate measurement.

10. Remove the thermometer, and wipe it with a tissue once from the fingers down to the mercury bulb, using a firm, twisting motion.

Cleaning from an area where there are few organisms to an area where there are numerous organisms minimizes spreading to cleaner areas. Friction helps to loosen matter from the surface.

11. Read the thermometer to the nearest tenth, as the nurse is doing in Fig. I-2-3.

Mercury may rise a bit above or below a calibration on a thermometer.

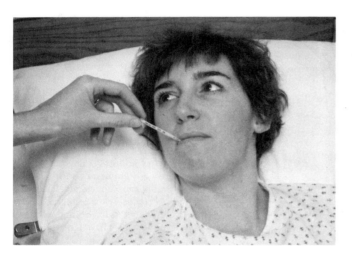

Figure I-2-2 The nurse places the thermometer to the side of the client's mouth well within the sublingual pocket.

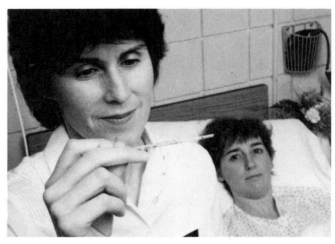

Figure I-2-3 The thermometer is held at the tip of the stem away from contact with the area held in the client's mouth. Rotating it at eye level helps the nurse to see and read accurately the calibration to which the mercury has risen.

12. Dispose of the tissue in a receptacle used for contaminated items.

Confining contaminated articles helps reduce the spread of pathogens.

13. Wash the thermometer in lukewarm soapy water. Rinse in cool water. Dry and replace the thermometer at the bedside or in the soiled utility room.

Mechanical action of washing aids in removal of organic material and organisms. All glass thermometers should be cleaned or disinfected before subsequent reuse.

14. Wash your hands.

Handwashing deters the spread of microorganisms.

15. Record the temperature on a flow sheet or paper. Report any abnormal findings to appropriate persons.

Recording provides accurate documentation for future comparisons.

Technique for assessing body temperature by the oral method

Using an electronic thermometer

ACTION	RATIONALE
1. Explain the procedure to the client.	An explanation reduces apprehension and promotes cooperation.
2. Wash your hands.	Handwashing deters the spread of microorganisms.

3. Release the electronic unit from the charging area.

Charging sustains the power of the batteries when using it as portable equipment.

4. Remove the temperature probe from within its storage compartment.

Removal of the probe automatically prepares the machine to measure and record temperature.

5. Attach a disposable cover over the probe and secure it in place.

A disposable cover acts as a barrier between organisms in the client's mouth and the probe.

6. Place the covered probe in the client's right or left sublingual pocket.

Thermometer probes placed in the middle area under the tongue have not registered as accurately as when they are placed in the areas to the sides.

7. Hold the probe in place while it is in the client's mouth, as shown in Fig. I-2-4.

If unsupported, the weight of the probe tends to fall away from the deepest areas under the tongue causing the measurement to be less accurate.

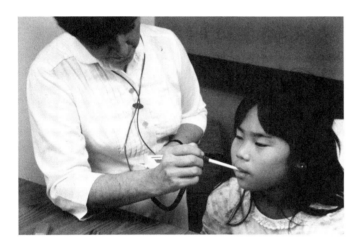

Figure I-2-4 The covered probe of an electronic thermometer weighs somewhat more than the glass counterpart. Therefore, the nurse supports the probe while it is in the client's mouth.

8. Listen for a sound or for flashing numbers to stop blinking.

Various methods are used by manufacturers to indicate when the probe ceases to sense any further change in the temperature recording.

9. Remove the probe from the client's mouth and note the numbers displayed on the electronic unit.

An electronic thermometer is not calibrated with multiple numbers. It displays one number that reflects the current measurement.

10. Press the probe release button while holding it over a receptacle.

The release button frees the disposable cover from the probe without being touched by the nurse's hands.

11. Return the probe to its storage area within the electronic unit.

The probe is protected from being broken while being transported or stored within the recording unit.

12. Wash your hands.

Handwashing deters the spread of microorganisms.

13. Record the temperature on the flow sheet or paper. Report any abnormal findings to the appropriate person.

Recording provides accurate documentation for future comparisons.

14. Return the electronic unit and reconnect it to the source for charging the batteries.

Equipment needed for other clients' use must be readily available.

Technique for assessing body temperature by the rectal method

Using a glass thermometer

ACTION	RATIONALE
1. Explain the procedure to the client.	An explanation reduces apprehension and promotes cooperation.

2. Gather equipment.

Organization promotes efficient time management.

3. Wash your hands.

Handwashing deters the spread of microorganisms.

4. Wipe, shake, and read the rectal thermometer.

A glass rectal thermometer requires the same preparation as a glass oral thermometer.

5. Don clean gloves, if desired, as shown in Fig. I-2-5. Lubricate the mercury bulb and an area approximately 2.5 cm (1 inch) above the bulb, as the nurse in Fig. I-2-6 is doing.

Gloves act as a barrier from contact with organisms in the stool or on the client's skin. Lubrication reduces friction and thereby facilitates insertion thus minimizing discomfort or injury to the mucuous membrane of the anal canal.

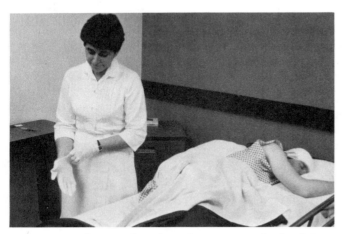

Figure I-2–5 The nurse dons clean gloves to protect her hands from stool and organisms present in the area of the anus.

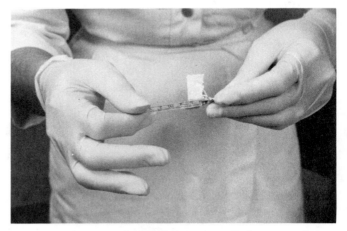

Figure I-2–6 Water-soluble lubricant is applied to a rectal thermometer in order to reduce friction and promote comfort during its insertion.

6. Provide for privacy. With the client on his side, fold back the bed linen so that the anus can be clearly seen.

If the anus is not clearly seen, the thermometer may not be placed directly into the anus. This could cause discomfort and injury.

7. Insert the thermometer, as shown in Fig. I-2-7, approximately 3.8 cm (1½ inches) in an adult, 2.5 cm (1 inch) in a child, and 1.25 cm (½ inch) in an infant.

The insertion length is adjusted according to the anatomical size of the client's rectum.

8. Permit the buttocks to fall in place while holding the thermometer in place, like the nurse in Fig. I-2-8, for 3 to 5 minutes.

The thermometer may become displaced internally or externally if it is not held in place.

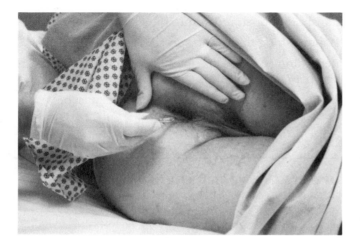

Figure I-2–7 The client has been placed onto his side so the nurse can locate the anus.

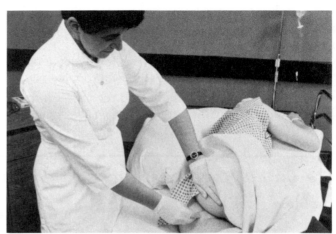

Figure I-2–8 The nurse holds the rectal thermometer in place during the entire time it is being used.

9. Remove the thermometer and wipe it once with soft tissue from the fingers to the mercury bulb, using a firm, twisting motion.

10. Wipe any residue of lubricant or stool remaining about the anus.

11. Read the thermometer and dispose of the tissue in a receptacle used for contaminated items.

12. Wash the thermometer in lukewarm soapy water. Rinse in cool water. Dry and replace the thermometer at the bedside or in the soiled utility room.

13. Wash your hands.

14. Record the temperature on a flow sheet or paper. Indicate that the rectal route was used. Report any abnormal findings to appropriate persons.

Cleaning from an area where there are few organisms to an area where there are numerous organisms minimizes the spread of organisms. Friction helps to loosen the lubricant and any fecal matter from the surface.

Removing lubricant and stool promotes the cleanliness and comfort of the patient.

Items containing organisms should be placed in containers for disposal to avoid transmitting them to other persons.

Mechanical action of washing aids in removal of organic material and organisms. All glass thermometers should be cleaned or disinfected before subsequent reuse.

Handwashing deters the spread of microorganisms.

Recording provides accurate documentation for future comparisons.

Technique for assessing body temperature by the axillary method

Using a glass thermometer

ACTION	RATIONALE
1. Explain the procedure to the client.	An explanation reduces apprehension and promotes cooperation.
2. Gather equipment.	Organization promotes efficient time management.
3. Wash your hands.	Handwashing deters the spread of microorganisms.
4. Provide privacy and move the gown to expose the axilla.	Moving the gown ensures safe and accurate placement of the thermometer.
5. Wipe the thermometer with a clean tissue if it has been stored in a chemical solution. Use a firm, twisting motion to remove the moisture.	Chemical solutions may irritate the skin. The presence of the solution may alter skin temperature. Using a soft tissue with friction helps in removing the solution.
6. Shake and read the thermometer as suggested in the procedure for obtaining an oral temperature.	The mercury must be below calibrations of the previous recording in order to assess the present temperature accurately.
7. Place the bulb of the thermometer into the center of the axilla, as shown in Fig. I-2-9.	The deepest area of the axilla will provide the most accurate measurement of the temperature.

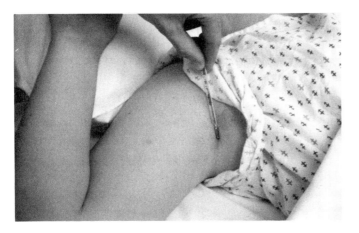

Figure I-2-9 The bulb of the thermometer is placed within the center of the axilla in order to provide the most accurate measurement of body temperature.

8. Bring the client's arm down close to his body, and place his forearm over his chest, as shown in Fig. I-2-10.

Surrounding the bulb with the skin surfaces of the axilla reduces the amount of surrounding air and ensures a reliable measurement.

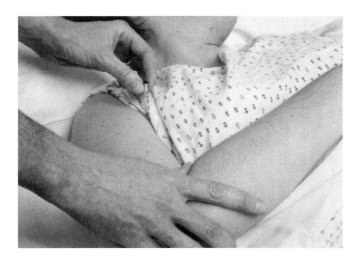

Figure I-2–10   To ensure that the thermometer records a valid measurement, the nurse positions the client's arm close to the body so that the entire bulb is in contact with skin.

9. Remain with the client, leaving the thermometer in place for 10 minutes.

Additional time is required to ensure that the mercury expands to the maximum level to record an accurate temperature.

10. Remove and read the thermometer. Clean the thermometer and replace it at the bedside or the soiled utility room.

A thermometer that has been used for an axillary temperature should be cleaned or disinfected before subsequent reuse.

11. Wash your hands.

Handwashing deters the spread of microorganisms.

12. Record the temperature on a flow sheet or paper. Indicate axillary route. Report any abnormal findings to appropriate persons.

Recording provides accurate documentation for future comparisons.

SAMPLE DOCUMENTATION

Most agencies have a schedule for assessing body temperature. A graphic sheet is a form used for charting routinely recorded measurements of body temperature as well as other vital signs. When assessing the body temperature at nonscheduled times, the nurse can record the measurements on a flow sheet or within the nurse's notes as follows:

Date	*Time*	*Nurse's note*
3/26	0800	Appears flushed and diaphoretic. T = 100° orally.
		B. Truckenmiller, RN

EVALUATION

REASSESSMENT

Each current assessment of the body temperature should be compared with the previously obtained measurements. It has been established that the temperature is generally lowest during the night and early morning. Measuring body temperature two to four times a day can reflect the diurnal rise and fall. The nurse should immediately retake any temperature that is questionable or seems inconsistent with the client's condition. A different thermometer or route may be used as alternatives for checking the validity of the measurement. More frequent measurements may be scheduled by the nurse if the client's condition changes.

EXPECTED OUTCOMES	The recorded temperature is congruent with the client's state of health.
	The integument remains intact and free of injury.

UNEXPECTED OUTCOMES	The recorded temperature is inconsistent with the client's condition.
	The recorded temperature varies significantly from the trend in recent measurements.
	The client experiences discomfort, irritation, or injury to the integument.

MODIFICATIONS IN SELECTED SITUATIONS

GENERAL VARIATIONS

Locate the anal orifice digitally while using a lubricated finger cot or glove when the client cannot be turned onto his side to obtain a rectal temperature. This technique avoids probing with the thermometer, which may injure local tissues. This technique also helps prevent placing the thermometer in a woman's vagina accidentally.

Wait for 15 minutes to 30 minutes before obtaining an oral temperature if the client has recently had hot or cold fluids, or if he has been smoking. This allows time for the temperature of the oral cavity to reflect a more accurate indication of the body's temperature.

Delay obtaining an axillary temperature if the axilla has just been washed. The water used in washing and friction created by drying the skin may influence the temperature.

Avoid taking a rectal temperature from a woman in labor. The thermometer may injure the head of the infant as it descends within the vagina.

Observe agency policy about obtaining a rectal temperature when the client has had a heart attack. It is thought by some that the thermometer may stimulate the vagus nerve causing the heart to slow to dangerous levels.

Obtain an axillary or rectal temperature on clients receiving oxygen by mask. The mask interferes with placing the thermometer in the mouth. Removing the mask may cause labored breathing due to the drop in the client's oxygen level. The effect of oxygen on oral temperature when administered by catheter or nasal cannula has been studied. The conclusion was that the effect was so small that it probably had no significance for most clinical purposes.

Avoid obtaining an axillary temperature when the client is in shock. Blood circulation to the axillary area is likely to be poor and, as a result, the axillary measurement will be inaccurate.

AGE-RELATED VARIATIONS

Obtain the first temperature on a newborn rectally if this does not contradict agency policy. This technique helps assess whether the anus is patent.

Position an infant on his side or abdomen, not on his back, while obtaining a rectal temperature. Positioning the infant on his side or abdomen reduces the danger of puncturing and injuring rectal tissues with the thermometer.

The axillary route or a temperature-sensitivity strip, shown in Fig. I-2-11, is the preferred method of evaluating the body temperature of a child under the age of 6 years. This should also be the method of choice for an adult who is confused or disoriented.

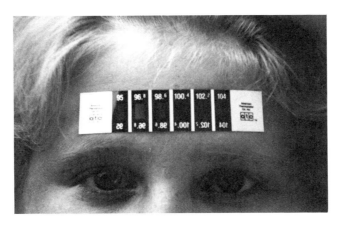

Figure I-2-11 The thermometer patch on this child's forehead contains liquid crystals which change color as the temperature changes. The scale has been adjusted to convert skin surface temperature to inner body temperature. Although the calibration is not as detailed as a glass thermometer, this type of device is simple to use for a quick assessment.

Hold an infant or young child in your arms while obtaining an axillary temperature. This technique is comforting for the child and promotes relaxation while obtaining the temperature.

HOME-HEALTH VARIATIONS

Body temperature is not generally routinely assessed. It is usually obtained only when the information is pertinent to the client's condition, such as when the client has an infection or there is a potential for infection.

Follow policy as to whether the temperature is taken with the agency's thermometer or one belonging to the client.

If an agency thermometer is used, ensure proper cleansing and disinfection between uses. Cover the thermometer with a disposable protective sheath.

If the temperature is to be obtained and recorded between visits by the nurse, teach the procedure to the client or whomever is to be responsible. Explain only one technique for assessing body temperature to avoid confusion for the learner. Provide written instructions for recording or reporting the temperatures.

RELATED TEACHING

Inform clients that a thermometer is a valuable home assessment instrument. Most pharmacies or drug stores sell inexpensive thermometers. Reusable heat-sensitive patches are also available.

Glass home thermometers should be cleaned with soap and lukewarm water and stored in a protective container between uses.

Identify the normal ranges for temperatures by various routes (Table I-2-1). Explain differences in temperature readings depending on the route used. Axillary temperature is generally a degree less than oral measurement, while a rectal temperature is usually a degree higher.

Table I-2–1
Ranges in normal body temperature

Route for measurement	Centigrade scale	Fahrenheit scale
Oral	37°C ± 0.3° to 0.6°	98.6°F ± 0.5° to 1.0°
Rectal	37.5°C ± 0.3° to 0.6°	99.6°F ± 0.5° to 1.0°
Axillary	36.5°C ± 0.3° to 0.6°	97.6°F ± 0.5° to 1.0°

Parents should be informed that a moderate fever is often a valuable defensive mechanism. Attempts to reduce a fever with aspirin should be avoided because it has been shown to be correlated with Reye's syndrome.

PERFORMANCE CHECKLIST

When assessing body temperature, the learner:

C	A	U	
[ ]	[ ]	[ ]	Analyzes data to determine the route for obtaining the body temperature and previous recordings.
[ ]	[ ]	[ ]	Washes hands and selects an appropriate thermometer.
[ ]	[ ]	[ ]	Inspects the thermometer for any cracks, chips, or defects.

C = competent; A = acceptable; U = unsatisfactory

(Continued)

PERFORMANCE CHECKLIST (Continued)

C	A	U	
[ ]	[ ]	[ ]	Explains the method for assessing body temperature to the client.
[ ]	[ ]	[ ]	Provides privacy.
[ ]	[ ]	[ ]	Helps the client to assume a position of comfort for an oral temperature, lying on his side for a rectal temperature, or supine or sitting for an axillary temperature.
[ ]	[ ]	[ ]	Shakes a glass thermometer to lower the mercury, *or* inserts the tip of an electronic thermometer into a disposable probe cover.
[ ]	[ ]	[ ]	Generously lubricates the bulb and stem of a rectal thermometer.
[ ]	[ ]	[ ]	Places the tip of the thermometer either into the posterior sublingual pocket, the rectum, or the center of the axilla.
[ ]	[ ]	[ ]	Supports the thermometer in the area of insertion.
[ ]	[ ]	[ ]	Maintains the thermometer in the mouth for at least 3 minutes, in the rectum for 3 to 5 minutes, and in the axilla for 10 minutes, or until identifying the signal from an electronic thermometer.
[ ]	[ ]	[ ]	Wipes the thermometer with soft tissue from the stem toward the bulb in order to read the calibration accurately.
[ ]	[ ]	[ ]	Disposes of probe cover or tissue within a lined receptacle.
[ ]	[ ]	[ ]	Twists the stem of a glass thermometer until the line of mercury is clearly visible at eye level.
[ ]	[ ]	[ ]	Reads the level of mercury to the nearest tenth of a degree or the digital display on an electronic thermometer.
[ ]	[ ]	[ ]	Cleans reusable thermometers.
[ ]	[ ]	[ ]	Washes hands.
[ ]	[ ]	[ ]	Evaluates the gross validity of the temperature recording; repeats and/or modifies procedure if the recorded temperature seems unusual.
[ ]	[ ]	[ ]	Writes the temperature on paper for future reference and documentation.
[ ]	[ ]	[ ]	Assists the client to a position of comfort.
[ ]	[ ]	[ ]	Replaces the thermometer in the agency's designated area.
[ ]	[ ]	[ ]	Records the temperature measurement on the appropriate agency form.
[ ]	[ ]	[ ]	Communicates unusual temperature measurements to other health care personnel.

Outcome: [ ] Pass [ ] Fail

C = competent; A = acceptable; U = unsatisfactory

Comments: _____

_____

_____

_____   _____
Student's Signature   Date

_____   _____
Instructor's Signature   Date

I-3 *Assessing the radial pulse*

Each time the heart beats, it propels oxygenated blood through arteries. The pumping action of the heart causes the walls of the arteries to expand and distend. The effect can be felt with the fingers as a wavelike sensation called the pulse. The rate of pulsations can be counted. When the radial artery is lightly compressed in the wrist area, the nurse can obtain the radial pulse rate. This site is commonly used because it is so easily accessible.

PURPOSES OF PROCEDURE

The radial pulse rate is assessed to:

1. Determine the number of heart beats occurring per minute.
2. Gather information about the heart's rhythm, the pattern of beats, and pauses between them.
3. Evaluate the amplitude, or strength, of the pulse.
4. Assess the heart's ability to deliver blood to areas of the body distant from itself, such as the fingers.
5. Assess the response of the heart to cardiac medications, activity, blood volume, gas exchange, and so on.

ASSESSMENT

OBJECTIVE DATA

- Review the trend of the pulse rate and its characteristics in previous assessments.
- Note the accessibility of the radial artery in one or the other arms.
- Count the rate of beats per minute.
- Feel the quality and rhythm of the pulsations.
- Note the temperature and color of the nearby skin which are largely results of blood flow.
- Inspect the shape, color, and texture of the nails which also are affected by the heart's ability to deliver oxygenated blood to the periphery.
- Assess the client's level of consciousness as an indication of blood flow to the cerebrum.

SUBJECTIVE DATA

- Ask the client to describe any sensations, such as palpitations or fluttering.
- Note if the client experiences chest pain, especially in relation to activity.

RELEVANT NURSING DIAGNOSES

Clients with a pulse rate that deviates from normal may be experiencing any of the following nursing diagnoses:

- *Activity Intolerance*
- *Altered Cardiac Output*
- *Altered Comfort*
- *Fluid Volume Deficit*
- *Fluid Volume Excess*
- *Altered Tissue Perfusion*

PLANNING

ESTABLISHING PRIORITIES

Nurses should always assess the client's radial pulse at the time of admission to obtain a baseline for future comparison. It is common for health agencies to routinely schedule periodic assessments of vital signs, which includes the pulse rate, on all clients within the health agency.

Assessing the radial pulse rate becomes a priority focus assessment in certain situations, such as when the client has a history of cardiac disease, is currently on medication that affects heart conduction, has had vascular surgery, or has had any injury or treatment that may alter blood volume or its circulation.

SETTING GOALS

• The pulse rate, rhythm, and amplitude will be assessed accurately.

PREPARATION OF EQUIPMENT

When assessing the radial pulse, the nurse will need:

A watch with a second hand or digital readout
Paper and pencil or pen

Technique for assessing the radial pulse rate

ACTION	RATIONALE
1. Explain the procedure to the client.	An explanation reduces apprehension and promotes cooperation.
2. Gather equipment.	Organization promotes efficient time management.
3. Wash your hands.	Handwashing deters the spread of microorganisms.
4. If the client is in a lying position, have the client rest his arm along the side of his body with the wrist extended and the palm of the hand downward. In the sitting position, have the forearm at a 90-degree angle to the body resting on a support with the wrist extended and the palm of the hand downward.	These positions are ordinarily comfortable for the client and convenient for the nurse.
5. Place your first, second, and third fingers along the radial artery, as the nurse in Fig. I-3-1 is doing, and press gently against the radius; rest the thumb in apposition to the fingers on the back of the client's wrist.	The fingertips, being sensitive to touch, will feel the pulsation of the client's radial artery. If the thumb is used for palpating the pulse, the nurse's own pulse may be felt.
6. Apply only enough pressure so that the client's pulsating artery can be felt distinctly.	Moderate pressure allows the nurse to feel the superficial radial artery expand with each heartbeat. Too much pressure will obliterate the pulse. If too little pressure is applied, the pulse will be imperceptible.

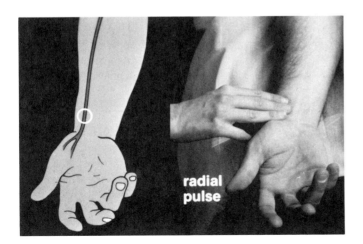

Figure I-3–1 The drawing on the left illustrates the location of the radial artery. In the photograph on the right the nurse is shown palpating a client's artery.

7. Using a watch with a second hand or digital readout, count the number of pulsations felt for 30 seconds, as the nurse in Fig. I-3-2 is doing. Multiply this number by two to obtain the rate for 1 minute.

Sufficient time is necessary to assess the rate, rhythm, and amplitude of the pulse.

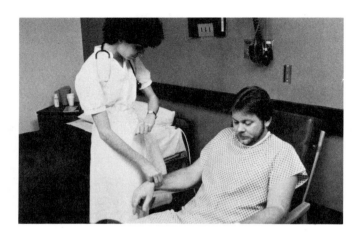

Figure I-3–2   The nurse palpates the pulsations through the radial artery and counts the rate while watching the second hand on her watch. The client's wrist is supported and comfortable.

8. If the pulse rate is abnormal in any way, palpate the pulse for a full minute or longer.

When the pulse is abnormal, longer counting and palpation are necessary to accurately identify the unusual characteristics of the pulse.

9. Assess the rhythm, amplitude, and elasticity of the vessel wall while counting the rate.

Irregularity in the heart rate affects the cardiac output. Amplitude of the pulse indicates the quality of the heart's contraction. Elasticity of the blood vessel does not affect the pulse rate but does reflect the status of the vascular system.

10. Record the pulse rate on the flow sheet or paper. Report any abnormal findings to the appropriate persons.

Recording provides accurate documentation for future comparisons.

11. Wash your hands.

Handwashing deters the spread of microorganisms.

SAMPLE DOCUMENTATION

Date	Time	Nurse's note
4/09	0955	Radial pulse 82, strong and regular. Fingers are pink and warm. Nailbeds blanch and refill immediately.
		B. Hollingsworth, LPN

EVALUATION

REASSESSMENT

The radial pulse should be recounted immediately for a full minute if any irregularities or abnormal characteristics are noted.

Each time the radial pulse is assessed, the rate should be compared with similar data previously obtained. Unusual or sudden changes in the pulse should be evaluated to determine if the client's physical condition, activity level, or emotional status has changed. Once deviations have been validated, they should be communicated to others involved in the client's care.

EXPECTED OUTCOMES

The client's pulse is strong, regular, and within the normal range for his age.

UNEXPECTED OUTCOMES

The pulse rate is below or above ranges that are normal for the client's age.
The radial pulse is not palpable.
The pulse rhythm is irregular.
The amplitude of the pulse is weak or bounding.

**MODIFICATIONS IN
SELECTED SITUATIONS**
GENERAL VARIATIONS

Allow the client to rest for 5 minutes before obtaining the radial pulse when he has been active or exercising. Activity and exercise tend to increase the pulse rate which may cause inconsistencies when compared with prior assessments.

When the client is critically ill or the pulse is weak, thready, or nonpalpable, the pulse may be detected with the use of a doppler, (Fig. I-3-3) an instrument that utilizes ultrasound to detect and amplify the sound of blood flow through the artery or other blood vessels.

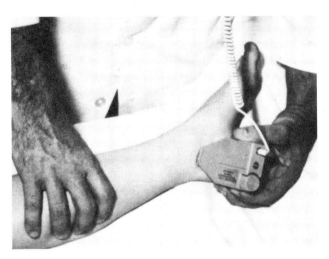

Figure I-3-3 The doppler ultrasound unit is used to assess blood flow through the lower foot.

A stethoscope may be used to listen to the heart as an alternative for assessing the heart rate when the radial pulse is inaccessible or difficult to obtain accurately. This method, referred to as counting the apical pulse rate, is discussed in Procedure I-4.

AGE-RELATED
VARIATIONS

Avoid attempts to assess the radial pulse of children under 2 years of age. The rapid rate and small area for palpation can lead to inaccurate data.

Obtain the radial pulse rate of children over age 2 when they are quiet or sleeping because it may be difficult to gain their cooperation in keeping the wrist from moving about.

Count the radial pulse rate for a full minute on a young child for the greatest accuracy.

HOME-HEALTH
VARIATIONS

Allow time for the client to rest before assessing the pulse. Getting out of bed to let the nurse in the home or other activity may temporarily increase the pulse rate.

Compare pulse rates assessed by the nurse with those measured and recorded by the client, family, or other caregivers. At periodic intervals observe and evaluate that the procedure is being performed accurately.

Provide a flow sheet and pencil so the client or caregiver can record the pulse rate and time it was taken. Indicate in writing any special instructions for withholding medication on the basis of the pulse rate. Provide the agency phone number in case clarification is needed.

RELATED TEACHING

Clients can learn to assess their own peripheral pulse rates. Use the information in Table I-3-1 for explaining the normal pulse range for a client's age.

Using the carotid pulse site in the neck is often easier than counting the radial pulse when assessing one's own pulse rate. The carotid artery can be felt at the side

Table I-3-1
Normal pulse rates per minute at various ages

Age	Approximate range	Approximate average
Newborn	120–160	140
1–12 months	80–140	120
12 months–2 years	80–130	110
2 years–6 years	75–120	100
6 years–12 years	75–110	95
Adolescent	60–100	80
Adult	60–100	80

of the neck below either ear. The client should be instructed to press lightly using the fingertips of the first, second, and third fingers when palpating a pulse.

Counting the pulse should be a daily practice when the client is taking medications to slow the heart. The client should be instructed to contact his physician as soon as possible if the pulse rate is below 60 per minute.

Inform a client of the availability of digital pulse monitoring devices if attempts to learn the palpation method are frustrating or the client demonstrates poor technique.

PERFORMANCE CHECKLIST

When assessing the radial pulse, the learner:

C	A	U	
[ ]	[ ]	[ ]	Reviews the pattern of previous assessments of the radial pulse.
[ ]	[ ]	[ ]	Gathers appropriate equipment.
[ ]	[ ]	[ ]	Explains the procedure to the client.
[ ]	[ ]	[ ]	Washes hands.
[ ]	[ ]	[ ]	Positions the client so that his arm is relaxed and supported.
[ ]	[ ]	[ ]	Allows the client to rest for at least 5 minutes following activity, unless the client's condition appears to have suddenly changed.
[ ]	[ ]	[ ]	Places the finger tips of the first, second, and third fingers on the inner surface of the wrist.
[ ]	[ ]	[ ]	Compresses the artery gently on the thumb side of the wrist against the adjacent bone.
[ ]	[ ]	[ ]	Counts the pulse for $\frac{1}{2}$ minute if regular, or a full minute if the situation indicates a need.
[ ]	[ ]	[ ]	Writes the pulse rate on paper for subsequent documentation.
[ ]	[ ]	[ ]	Makes the client comfortable before leaving the room.
[ ]	[ ]	[ ]	Washes hands.
[ ]	[ ]	[ ]	Records the rate and pulse characteristics on the graphic sheet, flow sheet, or nurses' notes.
[ ]	[ ]	[ ]	Notifies appropriate individuals concerning significant abnormalities of the pulse.

Outcome: [   ] Pass   [   ] Fail

C = competent; A = acceptable; U = unsatisfactory

Comments: _____
_____
_____

_____   _____
Student's Signature   Date

_____   _____
Instructor's Signature   Date

I-4   *Assessing the apical pulse rate*

The apical pulse rate is counted by listening at the chest rather than feeling the pulsation in an artery. The heart beats are best heard at the apex, or lower tip, of the heart as illustrated in Fig. I-4-1. The nurse places a stethoscope slightly below the level of the nipple on the chest to the left of the breastbone. The nurse listens for the "lub/dub" sound. These two sounds equal one pulsation which would be comparably felt at the radial site. It is not uncommon for the radial rate to be less than the apical due to the possibility that not all contractions of the heart may have been forceful enough to have produced a palpable wave. Therefore, an apical pulse rate is always considered the more accurate of the two rates.

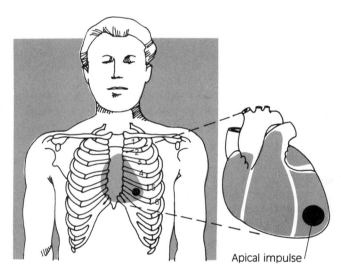

Apical impulse

Figure I-4-1 The heart is located within the thoracic cavity. The apex, or bottom, of the heart is identified by a dark circle. The point of maximum impulse can be located by identifying the fifth intercostal space and placing the stethoscope to the left of the midclavicular line.

PURPOSES OF PROCEDURE

An apical pulse rate is assessed to:

1. Determine an accurate heart rate when the radial pulse is inaccessible or difficult to assess.
2. Acquire the most accurate indication of the heart rate of clients with cardiac disease or clients who are seriously ill.
3. Assess the heart rate of children under the age of 2 years for whom radial pulse rates are not recommended.

ASSESSMENT

OBJECTIVE DATA

- Note the client's age. The apical site should be used for clients under the age of 2 years.
- Note if the client has heart or peripheral vascular disease which would indicate the need for the most accurate collection of data.
- Inspect the radial pulse site to determine its inaccessibility due to wrist restraints, casts or traction equipment, and so on.
- Scan the medication Kardex for drugs that alter the rate, rhythm, or amplitude of the heart's contractions.

- Determine if the radial pulse is abnormal. A comparison with the apical rate may provide more information with which to identify problems.
- Determine the client's ability to cooperate and refrain from speaking during the time of the assessment.
- Identify any mechanical equipment that produces noise which may interfere with accurate auscultation.

SUBJECTIVE DATA

- Ask the client to indicate if he experiences fatigue, chest pain, fainting, or palpitations.

RELEVANT NURSING DIAGNOSES

The client for whom an apical pulse is assessed may have nursing diagnoses, such as:

- *Activity Intolerance*
- *Altered Cardiac Output*
- *Altered Comfort*
- *Fluid Volume Deficit*
- *Fluid Volume Excess*
- *Altered Tissue Perfusion*

PLANNING

ESTABLISHING PRIORITIES

An apical heart rate is the preferred method for data collection when the client is critically ill or has a history of cardiac disease. The rate should be assessed daily before the administration of cardiac drugs; the drug may be withheld until the heart rate has been reported to the physician if it is dangerously high or low. The apical heart rate may be obtained as frequently as the nurse determines is necessary.

SETTING GOALS

- The apical heart rate and rhythm will be assessed accurately.

PREPARATION OF EQUIPMENT

The following equipment should be collected prior to assessing the apical heart rate:

Watch with a second hand or digital readout
Stethoscope
Paper, pencil or pen
Alcohol swab

Technique for assessing the apical pulse rate

ACTION	RATIONALE
1. Explain the procedure to the client.	An explanation reduces apprehension and promotes cooperation.
2. Gather equipment.	Organization promotes efficient time management.
3. Wash your hands.	Handwashing deters the spread of microorganisms.
4. Use an alcohol swab to cleanse the earpieces and diaphragm of the stethoscope if necessary.	Cleansing removes microorganisms and deters their transmission.
5. Assist the client to a supine or sitting position.	Proper positioning eases the identification of the anatomical site.
6. Provide privacy and move the gown to expose the upper chest area.	Moving the gown improves the ability to place the stethoscope properly and auscultate the sounds.
7. Hold the diaphragm of the stethoscope against the palm of your hand for a few seconds.	Holding the diaphragm warms the metal area that may otherwise be cold and startle the client.

8. Palpate the fifth intercostal space and move to the left of the midclavicular line over the apex of the heart as shown in Fig. I-4-2.

This anatomical location is the point of maximal impulse (PMI) where the heartbeat is easier to hear.

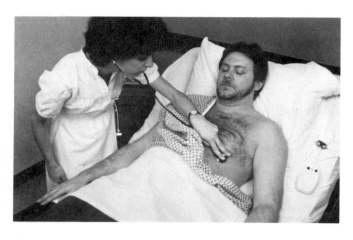

Figure I-4–2 The nurse places the stethoscope over the area where the heart beat is best heard. She watches the second hand of her watch while counting the sounds that are auscultated.

9. Listen for normal heart sounds which are identified as "lub/dub."

The sounds are made by the heart valves that separate the chambers of the heart.

10. Using a watch with a second hand, count the heartbeat for 30 seconds and multiply by two if the rhythm is regular. Count for 60 seconds if irregular rhythm is present.

Longer time interval allows for more accurate assessment of the heart rate.

11. Assess the presence of any irregularity in the heart rate and rhythm.

Normal rate and regular rhythm indicate adequate cardiac function.

12. Replace the gown and assist the client to a comfortable position.

Replacing the gown provides privacy and comfort.

13. Wash hands and reclean the earpieces and diaphragm of the stethoscope.

Cleansing deters the spread of microorganisms.

14. Record pulse on flow sheet or paper. Identify as apical rate. Report any abnormal findings to appropriate persons.

Recording provides accurate documentation for future comparisons.

SAMPLE DOCUMENTATION

Date	Time	Nurse's note
9/15	0745	Apical pulse rate 44 and regular. Lanoxin 0.125 mg held. Dr. Ragosi notified. Digoxin level ordered.
		F. Taggert, RN

EVALUATION

REASSESSMENT

The nurse should reassess any apical measurements that seem abnormal or uncharacteristic for the individual client. The nurse may wish to use another nurse's watch or stethoscope to clarify if the equipment is faulty rather than the findings. It is recommended that if the apical rate is selected for assessment that future comparisons also be obtained using this same method.

EXPECTED OUTCOMES	The heart sounds are loud and distinct.
	The apical heart rate is between 60 and 100 per minute for an adult.
	The heart sounds occur at regularly spaced intervals.

UNEXPECTED OUTCOMES	The heart sounds are soft and difficult to hear.
	The heart rate is below 60 or above 100 per minute for an adult.
	The sounds occur at irregular intervals.

MODIFICATIONS IN SELECTED SITUATIONS

GENERAL VARIATIONS

Lift a pendulous breast in order to accurately locate the fifth intercostal space on an obese female.

If possible, turn off the motors of suction machines or oxygen equipment when the noise interferes with hearing heart sounds.

Have a second nurse simultaneously count the radial pulse, both starting and stopping at the same time. When this is done, the documentation should clearly indicate which rate was obtained radially and which was obtained apically.

AGE-RELATED VARIATIONS

Obtain the apical pulse after placing a pacifier in a child's mouth or while another nurse is giving an infant a bottle in order to facilitate hearing the heart sounds.

HOME-HEALTH VARIATIONS

Note on the care plan whether the apical pulse rate is obtained. If so, assess on each visit so that the client does not become alarmed by variations in the care provided by different nurses.

Check agency policy regarding the assessment of apical and radial pulses in the home where only one registered nurse is present. Obtain the assistance of a family member or caregiver if they have been trained to assist with the procedure.

RELATED TEACHING

Explain to the client or his family the reason(s) for selecting the apical site for assessment rather than the radial.

Inform the client when his usual medications are being held without causing undue alarm.

Always provide the client with an explanation if repeated or frequent assessments are indicated.

(Performance checklist next page)

PERFORMANCE CHECKLIST

When assessing the apical heart rate, the learner:

C	A	U	
[ ]	[ ]	[ ]	Reviews the data on the client's chart concerning his medical history, drug therapy, and previously documented pulse rates.
[ ]	[ ]	[ ]	Explains the procedure to the client.
[ ]	[ ]	[ ]	Gathers equipment.
[ ]	[ ]	[ ]	Washes hands.
[ ]	[ ]	[ ]	Cleans earpieces and diaphragm of the stethoscope if using equipment shared by other personnel.
[ ]	[ ]	[ ]	Positions the client to accurately locate the area for auscultation.
[ ]	[ ]	[ ]	Identifies anatomical landmarks for appropriate placement of the stethoscope.
[ ]	[ ]	[ ]	Warms the diaphragm with the palm of the hand before placing it on the client's chest.
[ ]	[ ]	[ ]	Listens while simultaneously timing the assessment.
[ ]	[ ]	[ ]	Counts the rate for 30 seconds or a full minute when necessary.
[ ]	[ ]	[ ]	Assists the client to a comfortable position and raises side rails on a client's bed.
[ ]	[ ]	[ ]	Washes hands and recleans earpieces and diaphragm of the stethoscope.
[ ]	[ ]	[ ]	Records the rate and pulse characteristics on paper, a flow sheet, or nurses' notes.
[ ]	[ ]	[ ]	Communicates abnormalities to appropriate persons.

Outcome: [ ] Pass   [ ] Fail

C = competent; A = acceptable; U = unsatisfactory

Comments: _____

_____

_____

_____   _____
Student's Signature   Date

_____   _____
Instructor's Signature   Date

I-5

Assessing the respiratory rate

Respiration is the act of breathing. Inhalation, or inspiration, is the act of breathing in, and exhalation, or expiration, is the act of breathing out. One act of respiration consists of one inhalation and one exhalation. Respiratory rates have been observed to vary considerably in well people, although the rates in Table I-5-1 offer a good guide for evaluation.

Table I-5–1.
Normal respiratory rates at various ages

Age	Average range/minute
Newborn	30–80
Early Childhood	20–40
Late Childhood	15–25
Adulthood	
Male	14–18
Female	16–20

PURPOSES OF PROCEDURE

The respiratory rate is assessed to:

1. Determine the per minute rate on admission as a base for comparing future measurements.
2. Monitor the effect of injury, disease, or stress on the client's respiratory system.
3. Evaluate the client's response to medications or treatments that affect the respiratory system.

ASSESSMENT

OBJECTIVE DATA

- Observe the effort the client must make in order to breathe.
- Examine the color of the client's skin, nailbeds, and mucous membranes of the mouth or conjunctiva.
- Listen for any audible sounds associated with inspiration or expiration.
- Assess the effect that speaking or activity has on the client's breathing.
- Note the client's level of consciousness.
- Observe the symmetry and shape of the client's chest.
- Determine if the client prefers to sit up rather than lie down in order to breath more effectively.
- Note any increase in weight or abdominal size.
- Count each time the chest rises during a specified period of time in order to determine the rate.

SUBJECTIVE DATA

- Determine the client's need for rest in relation to activity.
- Assess the client's comfort level in relation to breathing.

RELEVANT NURSING DIAGNOSES

A person with changes in respiratory rate, effort, and volume may have any of the following nursing diagnoses:

- *Activity Intolerance*
- *Anxiety*
- *Altered Comfort*
- *Potential Alteration in Respiratory Function*
- *Ineffective Airway Clearance*
- *Ineffective Breathing Patterns*
- *Impaired Gas Exchange*

PLANNING

ESTABLISHING
PRIORITIES

The nurse should assess the respiratory rate of each newly admitted client. The respiratory rate should continue to be assessed thereafter according to the agency's policy. It is common practice to assess the respiratory rate at the same time as other vital signs. The nurse can independently assess the respiratory rate as frequently as is necessary if the client's condition changes suddenly. It is recommended that a thorough assessment of the respiratory tract be performed when the client has cardiopulmonary disease, before and after respiratory therapy, and when receiving oxygen or medications that affect the physiology of breathing.

SETTING GOALS

- The client's respiratory rate and effort will be assessed accurately.

PREPARATION OF
EQUIPMENT

When the respiratory rate is being assessed, the nurse will need:

Watch with a second hand or digital readout
Paper, pencil or pen

Technique for assessing the respiratory rate

ACTION	RATIONALE
1. Note the rise and fall of the client's chest with each inspiration and expiration while observing the time on one's watch or a wall clock. Keep the fingertips in place after counting the pulse, but observe the pattern of respirations.	It is recommended that the nurse count the respirations as subtly as possible because a client may alter his usual rate if he becomes conscious of his breathing.
2. Count the number of respirations for a minimum of 30 seconds. Multiply this number by two to obtain the client's respiratory rate per minute.	Sufficient time is necessary to observe the rate, depth, and other characteristics.
3. If respirations are abnormal in any way, count the respiratory rate for a full minute. Repeat if necessary to determine the rate and characteristics of breathing.	Full minute countings allow for the detection of unequal timing between respirations.
4. Record the respiratory rate on a flow sheet or paper. Report any abnormal findings to appropriate persons.	Recording provides accurate documentation for future comparisons.
5. Wash your hands if you touched the client or his bed linen during the assessment.	Handwashing deters the spread of microorganisms.

SAMPLE DOCUMENTATION

Date	Time	Nurse's note
2/19	0030	R-32 and shallow. States, "Raise my head up I can't seem to catch my breath." Using accessory muscles for breathing. Lips are cyanotic. Audible wheezes heard during expiration. O$_2$ at 5 L started per mask. Dr. De-

Long notified. IV of 1000 ml 5%D/W with i Gm. of aminophylline started in L wrist per dr.'s order. IV infusing well at 42 gtts./minute.

E. Calder, RN

EVALUATION

REASSESSMENT

It is always advisable to reassess the respiratory rate on a regular basis and compare the findings.

EXPECTED OUTCOMES

The rate of respirations while at rest is within normal range for the client's age.
The client's respirations are regular, noiseless, and effortless.

UNEXPECTED OUTCOMES

The rate of respirations is above or below the norm for the client's age.
The client is experiencing respiratory distress manifested by abnormal breath sounds, shortness of breath, labored breathing, pale or cyanotic color, loss of consciousness.

MODIFICATIONS IN SELECTED SITUATIONS

GENERAL VARIATIONS

Provide for at least 5 minutes to 10 minutes of rest before counting the respirations if recent activity appears to have altered the respiratory rate.
Expose the chest of a client who is breathing shallowly to obtain the most accurate assessment of the rate.

AGE-RELATED VARIATIONS

Avoid counting an infant or child's respirations during periods of crying.

HOME-HEALTH VARIATIONS

Teach the procedure for assessing and recording respiratory rate to the family members or caregiver if it must be done between visits from the nurse.
Periodically verify that the procedure is performed accurately by observing those who provide care for the client at home.
Help the home care client or his caregivers assess respiratory status by observing for shortness of breath, flaring of nostrils, and use of accessory muscles.

RELATED TEACHING

Explain to parents that children should be seen by a physician whenever they are experiencing difficulty in breathing or swallowing.
Advise clients that humidifiers or cool mist machines can add moisture to dry homes and reduce the incidence of respiratory infections.
Tell clients that running warm water in a bathtub or shower with the bathroom door closed is a quick way of adding moisture to the air.
Inform parents that apnea monitors are available for home use for premature infants or young babies who are at risk for sudden infant death syndrome (SIDS).
Advise parents to seek the advice of the family doctor when purchasing over-the-counter drugs to treat respiratory problems. Dosages are often calculated according to age or weight. Combining several over-the-counter drugs can lead to drug interactions.

(Performance checklist next page)

PERFORMANCE CHECKLIST

When assessing the respiratory rate, the learner:

C	A	U	
[ ]	[ ]	[ ]	Reviews the pattern of respiratory rates measured during prior assessments.
[ ]	[ ]	[ ]	Selects a time during which the client has been fairly inactive prior to the assessment.
[ ]	[ ]	[ ]	Unobtrusively observes the client's respirations while seeming to be involved in another activity.
[ ]	[ ]	[ ]	Counts the respiratory rate for a minimum of 30 seconds or a full minute if the pattern of respirations seems to deviate from normal.
[ ]	[ ]	[ ]	Washes hands if contact was made with the client or furnishings within the room.
[ ]	[ ]	[ ]	Records the data on note paper, a focus sheet, graphic sheet, or nurse's notes.
[ ]	[ ]	[ ]	Communicates any changes or unexplained deviations from previously collected measurements.

Outcome: [ ] Pass   [ ] Fail

C = competent; A = acceptable; U = unsatisfactory

Comments: _____

_____

_____

_____   _____
Student's Signature   Date

_____   _____
Instructor's Signature   Date

I-6

Assessing blood pressure

Blood is circulated through a loop involving the heart and blood vessels. Blood pressure is the force produced by the volume of blood pressing on the resisting walls of the arteries. Blood pressure is commonly abbreviated BP. Its measurement is expressed as a fraction. The numerator is the systolic pressure, and the denominator is the diastolic pressure. Studies of healthy persons show that blood pressure can fluctuate within a wide range and still be normal. Table I-6-1 provides a guide for average normal and upper limits of normal blood pressure measurements for persons of various ages. Because individual differences can be considerable, it is important to analyze the usual ranges and patterns of measurements for each particular person.

Table I-6–1
Average and upper limits of blood pressure according to age

Age	Average normal blood pressure	Upper limits of normal* blood pressure
1 year	95/65	Undetermined
6–9 years	100/65	119/79
10–13 years	110/65	124/84
14–17 years	120/80	134/89
18+ years	120/80	139/89

* Levels determined by the 1984 Joint National Committee on Detection, Evaluation, and Treatment of High Blood Pressure.

PURPOSES OF PROCEDURE

The blood pressure is assessed to:

1. Determine the systolic and diastolic pressure of the client during admission in order to compare his current status with normal ranges.
2. Acquire data that may be compared with subsequent changes that may occur during the care of the client.
3. Assist in evaluating the status of the client's blood volume, cardiac output, and vascular system.
4. Evaluate the client's response to changes in his medical condition as a result of treatment with fluids or medications.

ASSESSMENT

OBJECTIVE DATA

- Review previous recordings of blood pressure measurements; some persons carry wallet-sized cards on which their blood pressure readings have been recorded at a physician's office or community screening center.
- Read the chart or ask the client if he has ever been treated for high blood pressure or told he has low blood pressure.
- Scan the medication Kardex for medications that control or affect blood pressure.
- Inquire about the client's family history of heart disease, such as heart attacks or strokes.
- Observe the accessibility of the arm for applying the blood pressure cuff.

- Note the size of the arm in relation to the required size of the blood pressure cuff. Table I-6-2 provides guidelines for the recommended bladder sizes within the cuff.
- Determine the need to assess the BP in a lying, sitting, or standing position.

Table I-6–2
Recommended bladder sizes for a blood pressure cuff

Arm circumference at midpoint* (cm)†	Cuff name	Bladder width (cm)†	Bladder length (cm)†
5–7.5	Newborn	3	5
7.5–13	Infant	5	8
13–20	Child	8	13
24–32	Adult	13	24
32–42	Large Adult	17	32
42–50‡	Thigh	20	42

* Midpoint of arm is defined as half the distance from the acromion to the olecranon.
† 1 inch = 2.5 cm
‡ In persons with very large limbs, the indirect blood pressure should be measured in the leg or forearm.
(Report of a Subcommittee of the Postgraduate Education Committee, American Heart Association: Recommendations for Human Blood Pressure Determination by Sphygmomanometers. Dallas, American Heart Association ©1987. Reprinted with permission.)

SUBJECTIVE DATA

- Inquire about recent headaches, blurred vision, difficulty talking, temporary weakness on one side of the body, or chest pain.
- Ask if rings or shoes have become tight and difficult to remove.

RELEVANT NURSING DIAGNOSES

Persons whose blood pressure assessments have a repeated pattern of deviation from normal may have nursing diagnoses such as:

- *Activity Intolerance*
- *Altered Cardiac Output*
- *Fluid Volume Excess*
- *Fluid Volume Deficit*
- *Knowledge Deficit*
- *Altered Nutrition: More Than Body Requirements*
- *Altered Tissue Perfusion*
- *Altered Health Maintenance*

PLANNING

ESTABLISHING PRIORITIES

All clients should have their blood pressure assessed on admission and according to agency policy as long as the measurements are within normal ranges. Whenever there is a sudden change in the client's condition, the blood pressure is likely to reflect a relative measure of the client's state of acuity. It is not uncommon for nurses to assess the blood pressure on unstable clients every 5 minutes. Critically ill clients may have their blood pressure monitored continuously by inserting a sensor directly within an artery.

The nurse should assist the client to a position of comfort and provide a period of inactivity when preparing to establish the initial blood pressure measurement. The same conditions for measuring blood pressure should be repeated during subsequent assessments. Therefore, if the first recording is taken in the right arm while the client is sitting, other assessments should be performed similarly. If the client is prone to fainting or takes medication that will cause his blood pressure to fall when rising to an upright position, the nurse should plan to take a recording in both a lying and then a standing position. Safety precautions should be observed if there is any danger that the client may lose consciousness.

SETTING GOALS

- The client's blood pressure will be assessed accurately and as frequently as necessary to obtain sufficient data.

PREPARATION OF
EQUIPMENT

The nurse should collect the following equipment when preparing to assess the client's blood pressure:

Stethoscope
Sphygmomanometer—An aneroid or a mercury manometer, shown in Fig. I-6-1, may be available. The gauge should be inspected to validate that the needle or mercury is within the zero mark.
Blood pressure cuff of appropriate size
Paper, pencil or pen
Alcohol swab

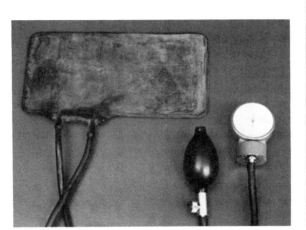
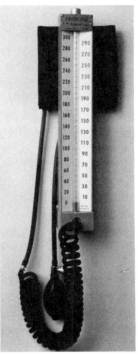

Figure I-6–1 An aneroid manometer has a round gauge. A needle moves about the numbers on the dial during blood pressure assessment. The mercury manometer has a tall column. Mercury rises and falls within the calibrated column when assessing blood pressure.

Technique for assessing blood pressure

ACTION	RATIONALE
1. Explain the procedure to the client.	An explanation reduces apprehension and promotes cooperation.
2. Gather equipment. Use an alcohol swab to clean earpieces and the metal parts of the stethoscope if necessary.	Organization promotes efficient time management. Cleaning deters the transmission of microorganisms.
3. Select a blood pressure cuff of an appropriate size for the client.	A cuff that is too large or too small will produce a false reading.
4. Wash your hands.	Handwashing deters the spread of microorganisms.
5. Delay obtaining the blood pressure if the client is emotionally upset, is in pain, or has just exercised, unless it is urgent to obtain the blood pressure.	Factors such as emotional upset, exercise, and pain will alter usual blood pressure measurements.

6. Select the appropriate arm for the application of the cuff (no IV infusion, breast or axilla surgery on that side, cast, arteriovenous shunt, injured or diseased limb).

7. Have the client assume a comfortable lying or sitting position with the forearm supported at the level of the heart and the palm of the hand upward.

8. Expose the area of the brachial artery by removing garments, or move a sleeve, if it is not too tight, above where the cuff will be placed.

9. Center the inflatable area of the cuff over the brachial artery, approximately midway on the arm, so that the lower edge of the cuff is about 2.5 to 5 cm (1 to 2 inches) above the inner aspect of the elbow, as shown in Fig. I-6-2. The tubing should extend from the edge of the cuff nearer the client's elbow.

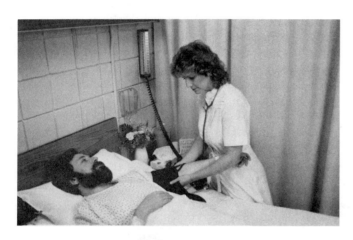

10. Wrap the cuff around the arm smoothly and snugly, and fasten it securely or tuck the end of the cuff well under the preceding wrapping. Do not allow any clothing to interfere with the proper placement of the cuff.

11. Check that a mercury manometer is in a vertical position. The mercury must be within the zero area with the gauge at eye level. If an aneroid gauge is used, the needle should be within the zero mark.

12. Palpate the brachial or radial pulse by pressing gently with the fingertips.

13. Tighten the screw valve on the air pump, as shown in Fig. I-6-3.

14. Inflate the cuff while continuing to palpate the artery, as shown in Fig. I-6-4. Note the point on the gauge at which the pulse disappears.

15. Deflate the cuff and wait 15 seconds.

Measurement of blood pressure may temporarily impede circulation to a diseased or compromised extremity.

This position places the brachial artery on the inner aspect of the elbow so that the bell or diaphragm of the stethoscope can rest on it easily.

Clothing over the artery interferes with the ability to hear sounds and may cause inaccurate blood pressure readings. Tight clothing on the arm causes congestion of blood and possibly inaccurate readings.

Pressure in the cuff applied directly to the artery will provide the most accurate readings. If the cuff gets in the way of the stethoscope, readings are likely to be inaccurate. A cuff placed upside down with the tubing toward the patient's head will give a false reading in most cases.

Figure I-6–2 The blood pressure cuff is applied to the upper arm after clothing has been moved from the area. The cuff is centered over the brachial artery.

A smooth cuff and snug wrapping produce equal pressure and help promote an accurate measurement. A cuff too loosely wrapped will result in an inaccurate reading.

Tilting a mercury manometer, inaccurate calibration, or improper height for reading the gauge can lead to errors in determining the pressure measurements.

Palpation helps identify when the cuff has been inflated enough to occlude blood flow.

The bladder within the cuff will not inflate with the valve open.

To identify the first Korotkoff sound accurately, the cuff must be inflated to a pressure above the point at which the pulse can no longer be felt.

Allowing a brief pause before continuing allows the blood to refill and circulate through the arm.

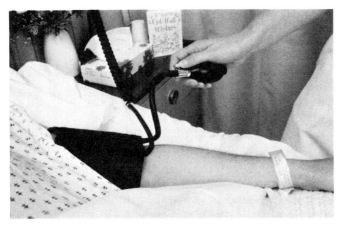

Figure I-6–3 The nurse tightens the screw valve so that air cannot escape while the bladder is inflated.

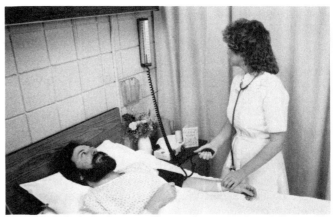

Figure I-6–4 The nurse palpates the radial pulse to determine the amount of pressure that occludes blood flow.

16. Assume a position, like the nurse in Fig. I-6-5, that is no more than 3 feet away from the gauge.

17. Place the stethoscope earpieces in the ears properly.

18. Place the bell or the diaphragm of the stethoscope, shown in Fig. I-6-6, with as little pressure as possible over the artery where the pulse is felt. Do not allow the stethoscope to touch clothing or the cuff.

A distance of more than about 3 feet can interfere with accurate readings of numbers on the gauge.

The eartips should be directed downward and forward to fit the shape of the ear canal.

Having the bell or diaphragm directly over the artery makes more accurate readings possible. Heavy pressure on the brachial artery distorts the shape of the artery and the sound. Placing the bell or the diaphragm away from clothing and the cuff prevents noise that will distract from the sounds made by blood flowing through the artery.

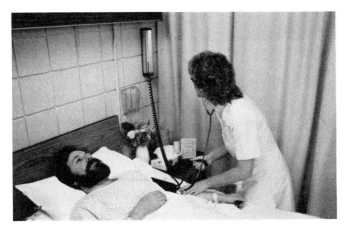

Figure I-6–5 The nurse positions herself to read accurately the meniscus formed by the mercury within the manometer.

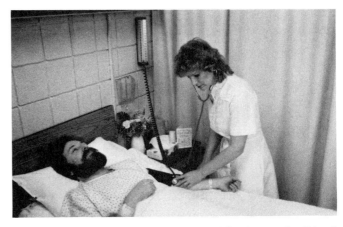

Figure I-6–6 The bell of a stethoscope amplifies the sounds of blood moving through the artery better than the diaphragm. The nurse places the bell over the artery and holds it lightly in place.

19. Pump the pressure 30 mm Hg above the point at which the pulse disappeared.

20. Note the point on the gauge at which there is an appearance of the first faint, but clear sound, which

Increasing the pressure above where the pulse disappeared ensures a period of time before hearing the first sound that corresponds with the systolic pressure. It prevents misinterpreting phase II sounds as phase I.

Systolic pressure is the point at which the blood in the artery is first able to force its way through the vessel at

slowly increases in intensity. Note this number as the systolic pressure.

21. Read the pressure to the closest even number.

22. Do not reinflate the cuff once the air is being released to recheck the systolic pressure reading.

23. Note the pressure at which the sound first becomes muffled. Also observe the point at which the last sound is heard. These may occur separately or at the same point.

24. Allow the remaining air to escape quickly. Repeat any suspicious readings but wait 30 seconds to 60 seconds between readings to allow normal circulation to return in the limb. Be sure to deflate the cuff completely between attempts to check the blood pressure.

25. If it is difficult to hear sounds when checking the blood pressure, raise the client's arm over his head for 15 seconds just before rechecking the blood pressure.

26. Inflate the cuff while the client's arm is elevated and then gently lower the arm while continuing to support it.

27. Position the stethoscope and deflate the cuff at the usual rate while listening for Korotkoff sounds.

28. Remove the cuff, clean and store the equipment.

29. Record the client's position, the arm used to obtain the blood pressure, and the readings that correspond to the systolic readings. Compare to previous readings, and report any abnormalities to appropriate persons.

a similar pressure exerted by the air bladder in the cuff. The first sound is phase I of Korotkoff sounds.

It is common practice to read blood pressure to the closest even number.

Reinflating the cuff while obtaining the blood pressure is uncomfortable for the client and may cause an inaccurate reading. Reinflating the cuff causes congestion of blood in the lower arm, which lessens the loudness of Korotkoff sounds.

The point at which the sound changes corresponds to phase IV of Korotkoff sounds and is considered the first diastolic pressure reading. According to the American Heart Association (AHA), this is used as the diastolic pressure recording in children. The last sound heard is the beginning of phase V and is the second diastolic measurement. The AHA recommends also recording the fifth Korotkoff sound as the second diastolic pressure in adults.

False readings are likely to occur if there is congestion of blood in the limb while obtaining repeated readings.

Raising the arm over the head helps relieve congestion of blood in the limb, increases the pressure differences, and makes the sounds louder and more distinct in the lower arm.

Supporting the client's arm while it is lowered prevents altering the pressure in the manometer by as much as 20 mm Hg to 30 mm Hg.

The techniques used throughout the remaining assessment of blood pressure do not require any further modification.

Equipment that must be shared among personnel should be left ready for use.

Circumstances for assessing the blood pressure should be consistent for future comparisons.

SAMPLE DOCUMENTATION

Date	Time	Nurse's note
5/01	0400	B.P. 150/82/60 in right arm while sitting.
		A. Lee, RN

EVALUATION

REASSESSMENT

The client's blood pressure should be rechecked if the readings are inconsistent with his general condition or if the measurements have changed remarkably since the last time it was assessed.

EXPECTED OUTCOMES	The client's blood pressure is within the normal range for persons his age.
UNEXPECTED OUTCOMES	The client's systolic or diastolic blood pressure is above or below the normal range for persons his age. The client's systolic or diastolic pressure has changed suddenly since the last assessment. Korotkoff sounds are not audible or distinct enough to facilitate an accurate assessment.
MODIFICATIONS IN SELECTED SITUATIONS GENERAL VARIATIONS	Assess the blood pressure using the thigh if access to the brachial artery is obscured. A wide cuff should be selected, and the client should be positioned on his abdomen for adequate palpation of the popliteal artery. Adjust the evaluation of the blood pressure recording if the thigh is used because the pressure in the lower extremities tends to be higher than in the upper extremities. Blood pressure can be determined by palpating the pulse at the time the valve is released. However, this method will only produce the systolic measurement.
AGE-RELATED VARIATIONS	Use a pediatric-sized cuff according to the size of the child.
HOME-HEALTH VARIATIONS	When a client is admitted to a home health agency, assessment of the blood pressure typically remains a responsibility of the nurse. Should readings differ significantly from baseline, review the client's medication administration routine. If appropriate, determine that the client is taking *only those medications that have been prescribed for him.* If family members request the nurse to assess their blood pressure, follow agency policy.
RELATED TEACHING	Advise adults to have their blood pressure assessed at least yearly. Inform clients about the availability of self-monitoring digital blood pressure equipment. Although costly, most provide easy-to-read systolic and diastolic measurements. If the adult client's systolic pressure is between 140 mm Hg and 199 mm Hg or the diastolic pressure is between 90 mm Hg and 104 mm Hg, the client should be seen promptly, delaying no longer than 2 months. If the adult client's systolic pressure is over 200 mm Hg or the diastolic pressure is 105 mm Hg to 114 mm Hg, the client should be seen promptly, delaying no longer than 2 weeks. Persons with higher pressures should be seen by a medical doctor immediately. Persons with confirmed hypertension should be instructed to take their medications on a regular basis, reduce their weight and salt intake, and learn stress management techniques.

(Performance checklist next page)

PERFORMANCE CHECKLIST

When assessing blood pressure, the learner:

C	A	U	
[ ]	[ ]	[ ]	Reviews the client's history, prescribed medications, and any prior assessment data.
[ ]	[ ]	[ ]	Explains the procedure to the client.
[ ]	[ ]	[ ]	Evaluates the size and accessibility of the arm for use during the assessment.
[ ]	[ ]	[ ]	Gathers appropriate equipment.
[ ]	[ ]	[ ]	Washes hands.
[ ]	[ ]	[ ]	Positions the client similarly to previous assessments, commonly either sitting or lying down.
[ ]	[ ]	[ ]	Removes or rearranges clothing to expose the area where the cuff will be applied.
[ ]	[ ]	[ ]	Extends the arm with the palm facing upward.
[ ]	[ ]	[ ]	Applies the cuff approximately 1 inch to 2 inches above the inner aspect of the elbow with the bladder over the brachial artery.
[ ]	[ ]	[ ]	Arranges the manometer gauge at eye level.
[ ]	[ ]	[ ]	Palpates the brachial artery with the fingertips.
[ ]	[ ]	[ ]	Tightens the valve on the cuff and inflates until the pulse disappears.
[ ]	[ ]	[ ]	Deflates the cuff and waits a minimum of 30 seconds.
[ ]	[ ]	[ ]	Inserts the earpieces of the stethoscope.
[ ]	[ ]	[ ]	Positions the bell or diaphragm over the point at which the artery was palpated.
[ ]	[ ]	[ ]	Reinflates the blood pressure cuff to 30 mm Hg above the point at which the palpated pulse disappeared.
[ ]	[ ]	[ ]	Releases the valve slowly, controlling the rate of descent to 2 mm Hg to 4 mm Hg per second.
[ ]	[ ]	[ ]	Notes the changes in sounds with the calibrations on the gauge as the air is released from the bladder cuff.
[ ]	[ ]	[ ]	Removes the cuff or allows 30 seconds before reinflating again.
[ ]	[ ]	[ ]	Assists the client to a position of comfort.
[ ]	[ ]	[ ]	Washes hands.
[ ]	[ ]	[ ]	Records the pressure measurements on a flow sheet, note paper, graphic sheet, or in the nurse's notes.
[ ]	[ ]	[ ]	Replaces the stethoscope and sphygmomanometer.
[ ]	[ ]	[ ]	Communicates unusual findings to appropriate persons.

Outcome: [ ] Pass   [ ] Fail

C = competent; A = acceptable; U = unsatisfactory

Comments: _____

_____

_____

_____   _____

Student's Signature   Date

_____   _____

Instructor's Signature   Date

Promoting medical asepsis

One of the nurse's primary responsibilities is to halt the spread of microorganisms and minimize the threat of infection. Activities practiced for this reason are referred to as *aseptic techniques.* When nurses perform procedures that reduce the number and transfer of pathogens, they are practicing medical asepsis, or clean technique. Some examples are: handwashing, cleaning and disinfecting a glass thermometer, and caring for a client on isolation precautions. Making an unoccupied and occupied bed will also be included because keeping the environment clean controls the potential reservoir of infection. The nurse's technique when changing and disposing of linen controls the exit of organisms from a reservoir as well as the vehicle for transmission.

I-7 *Handwashing*

Handwashing is a simple, yet most effective way to help prevent the spread of organisms. Handwashing is effective in breaking the infection process cycle, shown in Fig. I-7-1, by altering the reservoir and vehicle of transmission. Opinions differ concerning the types of cleansing agents, the frequency, and recommended length of time for handwashing. Regardless of these differences, the consensus is that handwashing is the most important procedure in the prevention of infections among clients and nurses. However, despite the most scrupulous practice of handwashing, it is not considered possible to clean the skin of all microorganisms.

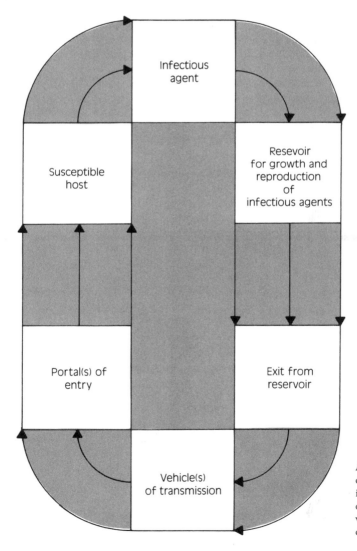

Figure I-7-1 The infection process cycle consists of a sequence of interrelated factors. Interrupting the cycle with measures such as handwashing can halt the spread of microorganisms.

PURPOSES OF PROCEDURE

Handwashing is performed to:

1. Remove the natural body oil and dirt from the skin.
2. Remove transient microbes, those normally picked up by the hands in the usual activities of daily living.
3. Reduce resident microbes, those normally found in creases of the skin.
4. Prevent the transmission of pathogens, disease-producing organisms, among susceptible persons.

ASSESSMENT

OBJECTIVE DATA

- Determine whether nursing care will involve direct contact between the nurse and the client.
- Assess the client's risk for acquiring an infection. Those at high risk include the very young, for instance a newborn or premature infant, the elderly, and those with suppressed immune systems.
- Read the client's record to obtain data that indicate an actual infection or potential for infection, such as elevated body temperature recordings. Look especially for culture reports identifying growth of specific pathogens.
- Inspect the client for drainage from the skin or other body orifice.
- Note the presence of invasive equipment or treatment that alters the skin barrier.

SUBJECTIVE DATA

- Ask if the client feels achey, tired, weak, hot, or chilled.
- Determine if the client is aware of having been exposed to another person who may have had a contagious disease.

RELEVANT NURSING DIAGNOSES

Handwashing is a basic aseptic practice involved in all aspects of providing care to persons who are sick or well. It becomes especially important when clients have nursing diagnoses, such as:

- *Potential for Infection*
- *Altered Body Temperature*
- *Impaired Skin Integrity*

PLANNING

The nurse should perform handwashing:

ESTABLISHING PRIORITIES

Before and after contact with any client.
When assisting with or performing any procedure, especially one in which the nurse could transfer pathogens through the skin or body openings.
Whenever gloves are used.
When handling blood, body fluids, secretions, or excretions, or during any contact with mucous membranes.
When there is contact with any object that is likely to be a reservoir of organisms, such as soiled dressings and bedpans.
After urinary or bowel elimination.
Before eating.

SETTING GOALS

- The number of organisms on the hands will be reduced by frequent and thorough handwashing.
- Susceptible clients will be free of infection.
- The nurse will not acquire an infection as a result of transmitting organisms from the hands to other portals of entry.

PREPARATION OF EQUIPMENT

The nurse will need the following to perform adequate handwashing:

Source of running tap water
Liquid or bar soap
Orangewood stick
Paper towels
Lotion

Technique for handwashing

ACTION	RATIONALE
1. Stand in front of the sink. Do not allow your uniform to touch the sink during the washing procedure.	The sink is considered contaminated. Uniforms may carry organisms from place to place.
2. Remove jewelry.	Removal of jewelry facilitates proper cleansing. Microorganisms may accumulate in settings of jewels.
3. Turn on water, and adjust the force. Regulate the temperature until the water is warm.	Water splashed from the contaminated sink will contaminate your uniform. Warm water is more comfortable and has less tendency to open pores and remove oils from the skin. Organisms can lodge in roughened and broken areas of chapped skin.
4. Wet the hands and wrist area. Keep hands lower than elbows to allow water to flow toward fingertips, as shown in Fig. I-7-2.	Water should flow from the cleaner area toward the more contaminated area. Hands are more contaminated than forearms.
5. Use about one teaspoon of liquid soap from dispenser or lather thoroughly with bar soap. Rinse bar, and return it to soap dish.	Rinsing the soap removes the lather which may contain microorganisms.
6. With firm rubbing and circular motions, wash the palms and backs of the hands, each finger, the areas between the fingers, the knuckles, wrists, and forearms, as shown in Fig. I-7-3. Wash up the forearms at least as high as contamination is likely to be present.	Friction caused by firm rubbing and circular motions helps to loosen dirt and organisms which can lodge between the fingers, in skin crevices of knuckles, on palms and backs of the hands, as well as the wrists and forearms. Cleaning least contaminated areas (forearms and wrists) after hands are clean prevents spreading organisms from the hands to the forearms and wrists.

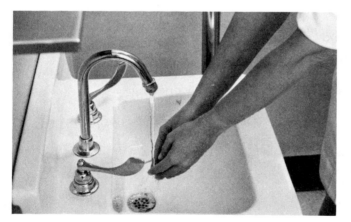

Figure I-7-2 The nurse wets his or her hands and wrists prior to using soap to work up a lather. The nurse stands away from the sink to avoid coming in contact with organisms that may be present on its surface.

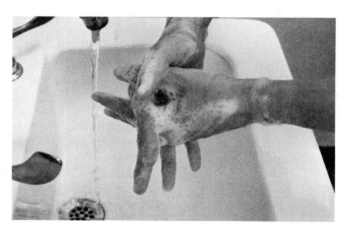

Figure I-7-3 The nurse rubs hands together creating friction while washing hands with soap.

7. Continue this friction motion for 10 seconds to 30 seconds.	Length of handwashing is determined by the degree of contamination.
8. Use fingernails of the other hand or a clean orangewood stick to clean under fingernails.	Organisms can lodge and remain under the nails where they can grow and be spread to others.
9. Rinse thoroughly, as shown in Fig. I-7-4.	Running water rinses organisms and dirt into the sink.

10. Dry hands and wrists with a paper towel, as shown in Fig. I-7-5. Use a paper towel to turn off the faucet.

Drying the skin well prevents chapping. Dry hands first because they are the cleanest and least contaminated area. Turning the faucet off with a paper towel protects the clean hands from contact with a soiled surface.

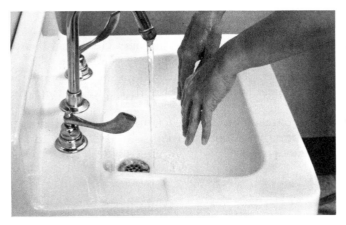

Figure I-7-4 The nurse holds hands lower than the forearms, allowing rinse water to drain from the fingertips.

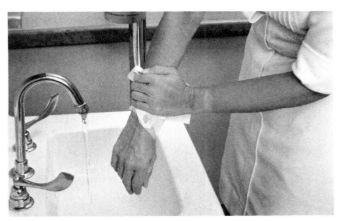

Figure I-7-5 The nurse blots each hand dry with a separate paper towel. Before disposing of the towel, the nurse will use it to touch the faucet handles to turn the water off without recontaminating the hands.

11. Use lotion on hands if desired.

Lotion helps to keep the skin soft and prevents chapping.

EVALUATION

REASSESSMENT

The nurse should continue to observe the client for infection-related symptoms. Epidemiologic data on personnel and clients should be tabulated by the infection control nurse to determine that the incidence of infection is not increasing above expected levels.

EXPECTED OUTCOMES

The nurse's hands are washed before and after each contact with the client, before preparing equipment for client care, and whenever they become obviously soiled.
The client is provided the opportunity to wash his hands during routine personal hygiene, after urinary or bowel elimination, and before eating.

UNEXPECTED OUTCOMES

The client or the nurse acquires an infection related to inadequate handwashing.

MODIFICATIONS IN SELECTED SITUATIONS

GENERAL VARIATIONS

Removal of all jewelry, except a plain wedding band, is recommended. Although rings increase the number of microbes present on the hands, increasing the time of hand washing and rinsing to 1 full minute will achieve a level of cleanliness comparable to that on the hands of non-ring wearers.

Use liquid soap supplied in a dispenser rather than bar soap when possible. Bar soap that is exposed to the skin surface is likely to collect and harbor organisms on its surface from the previous user.

If the skin becomes dry and irritated from frequent handwashing, the nurse may consider applying moisture-restoring lotion. Irritated skin harbors organisms and is difficult to clean adequately.

Adequate handwashing can be achieved with a 10-second to 30-second scrub when exposure to contamination is minimal. However, hands that are visibly soiled may take from 1 minute to 4 minutes to wash them thoroughly.

Remove nailpolish for the best control of microbial growth. Chipped nailpolish tends to collect and harbor organisms.

In addition to the more common hand faucets, knee- and foot-operated controls may be used. Sinks with elbow controls are generally used in a surgical setting.

HOME-HEALTH
VARIATIONS

Request permission to use the lavatory to wash hands before and after providing care. Setting a good example reinforces the importance of handwashing to the client.

Carry soap, preferably liquid or foam, and disposable towels. Avoid using terry or linen towels and bar soap that are present in the client's bathroom. Items used by the client and other members of the family are likely to harbor organisms that are foreign to those of the nurse.

RELATED TEACHING

The nurse can teach by example that handwashing is the simplest and most effective way to prevent the spread of infection.

Instruct children at an early age in proper handwashing techniques. Offer clients the opportunity to wash hands before eating and after elimination to reinforce the priority occasions for handwashing.

Individually dispensed paper towels or hand towels for each individual are preferred. Warm air dryers are recommended in public restrooms. Rolls of cloth towels become contaminated if a clean surface is not continuously available to each person after handwashing.

PERFORMANCE CHECKLIST

When performing handwashing, the learner:

C	A	U	
[ ]	[ ]	[ ]	Identifies at least four situations that indicate a need for handwashing.
[ ]	[ ]	[ ]	Repositions sleeves of a uniform or sweater to the mid-forearm.
[ ]	[ ]	[ ]	Removes rings with elevated stones and grooves.
[ ]	[ ]	[ ]	Removes or relocates watch from the wrist area.
[ ]	[ ]	[ ]	Stands without touching the uniform to the sink.
[ ]	[ ]	[ ]	Wets the hands, wrists, and forearms so that the flow of water drains downward from the fingertips.
[ ]	[ ]	[ ]	Dispenses soap.
[ ]	[ ]	[ ]	Uses mechanical friction to lather the soap while washing all the surfaces of the palms, backs of the hands, fingers, wrists, and forearms.
[ ]	[ ]	[ ]	Sustains handwashing for a minimum of 10 seconds to 30 seconds or 1 minute if wearing a ring.
[ ]	[ ]	[ ]	Cleans beneath fingernails.
[ ]	[ ]	[ ]	Rinses the hands under running water so that the lathered soap drains from the forearm to the fingertips. Rinses bar soap, if used, before replacing it within a soap dish.
[ ]	[ ]	[ ]	Uses a fresh paper towel, wiping toward the wrist and forearm when drying each respective hand.
[ ]	[ ]	[ ]	Disposes wet paper towels into a lined waste receptacle.
[ ]	[ ]	[ ]	Turns off the faucet using knee or elbow controls or uses a paper towel to turn off a hand-operated faucet.

Outcome: [ ] Pass   [ ] Fail

C = competent; A = acceptable; U = unsatisfactory

Comments: _____

_____

_____

_____   _____
Student's Signature   Date

_____   _____
Instructor's Signature   Date

I-8

Cleaning and disinfecting a glass thermometer

Electronic thermometers with disposable probe covers are being used instead of glass thermometers in most health agencies. However, nurses should be capable of cleaning and disinfecting glass thermometers whenever this may be necessary, such as in the care of clients in isolation. Furthermore, this type of thermometer is generally used within the home. The nurse may determine that a client will need to learn how to care for this type of thermometer during home use.

PURPOSES OF PROCEDURE

A glass thermometer is cleaned and disinfected to:

1. Remove mucus and secretions from the surface.
2. Remove lubricant when the thermometer was used to obtain a rectal temperature.
3. Remove organisms that have been deposited on the area of the thermometer placed within the body.
4. Prevent the transmission of pathogens to others when a glass thermometer is reused.

ASSESSMENT

OBJECTIVE DATA

- Inspect the thermometer for the appearance of dried mucus or other residue. If the sanitary condition of a thermometer is ever questionable, the nurse should obtain another thermometer.
- Determine the agency policy concerning the nurse's responsibilities for cleaning and disinfecting multiple-use glass thermometers. In most hospitals, nurses place soiled thermometers in a utility room, and personnel in the central supply unit clean and disinfect them.

SUBJECTIVE DATA

- Assume that the cleanliness of an uncovered and unprotected thermometer is suspect. Before its use, the nurse should prophylactically clean and disinfect the thermometer.

RELEVANT NURSING DIAGNOSIS

When cleaning and disinfecting a glass thermometer, the nurse is implementing actions related to clients with the following nursing diagnosis:

- *Potential for Infection*

PLANNING

ESTABLISHING PRIORITIES

The nurse should use a glass thermometer whenever an electronic thermometer is malfunctioning or inappropriate to use. All equipment that is reused among clients within a health agency must be cleaned and disinfected.

Glass thermometers should be used on all clients in isolation. The thermometer should be left within the room during the time of the client's care and cleaned between uses. Disinfection and removal are carried out when the client is transferred, discharged, or no longer requires communicable disease control measures.

SETTING GOALS

- Glass thermometers will be clean and stored under medically aseptic conditions.
- Glass thermometers will be disinfected according to the agency's policy before being reused for another client.

PREPARATION OF EQUIPMENT

The nurse will need the following items to clean and disinfect a glass thermometer:

Soft tissues
Soap or detergent solution
Running water
Chemical solution (if specified)

Technique for cleaning and disinfecting a glass thermometer

ACTION	RATIONALE
1. Use clean, soft tissues for wiping and cleaning the thermometer.	The texture of soft tissues facilitates contact with all surfaces of the thermometer in order to remove organic matter which interferes with disinfection.
2. Use a fresh tissue each time the thermometer must be wiped.	Using a clean surface prevents redistributing organic matter.
3. Hold the tissue at the stem end near the fingers holding the thermometer, as shown in Fig. I-8-1.	Cleaning from an area where there are few organisms to an area where there are numerous organisms minimizes the spread of organisms to cleaner areas.
4. Wipe down toward the bulb, using a twisting motion.	Friction helps to loosen mucus, lubricant, or fecal matter from the surface.
5. After the thermometer has been wiped, clean it with soap or detergent solution, again using friction.	Soap or detergent solutions loosen adhered matter.
6. Rinse the thermometer under cold, running water.	Rinsing with water helps to remove organisms and foreign material loosened by washing. Also, certain chemical solutions are rendered ineffective in the presence of soap—for example, benzalkonium chloride (Zephiran chloride).

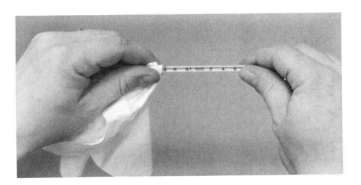

Figure I-8-1 The nurse wipes a clean tissue from the stem of the thermometer toward the bulb, which was in the client's mouth. The tissue collects and moves microorganisms from the cleaner areas of the thermometer to the area of greater contamination.

ACTION	RATIONALE
7. Dry the thermometer after it has been rinsed.	The strength of a chemical solution is diluted if a film of water covers the thermometer.
8. Immerse the thermometer in the chemical solution specified.	Chemical solutions must be used in proper strength for the proper length of time to be effective. Heat cannot be used to disinfect a glass clinical thermometer because heat sufficient to kill organisms will cause the mercury to expand beyond the column and ruin the thermometer.
9. Rinse the thermometer with water after disinfection and before reuse.	Chemical solutions may irritate the mucous membrane of the mouth or the rectum. Also, they may have an objectionable odor and taste.

10. Return the thermometer to the storage receptacle.	Covering the thermometer protects it from becoming broken and contaminated with organisms in the general environment.
11. Wash your hands.	Handwashing deters the spread of microorganisms.

EVALUATION

REASSESSMENT

Each time a thermometer is used, it should be inspected. If the sanitary condition of thermometers is found to be suspect on several occasions, the infection control nurse should be notified. The infection control nurse will investigate the possibility that the guidelines are not being followed by all personnel. Inservice programs may be planned to review the steps for cleaning and disinfecting glass thermometers.

EXPECTED OUTCOMES

The glass thermometer is free of mucus and body excretions.
The glass thermometer is stored in a holder at the bedside or in the clean utility room.

UNEXPECTED OUTCOMES

The glass thermometer appears soiled or the calibrations are difficult to read.
The glass thermometer has been left on the client's bedside cabinet or uncovered inside the client's drawer.

MODIFICATIONS IN SELECTED SITUATIONS

GENERAL VARIATIONS

Individual glass thermometers may be issued to each client on admission. It is reused by the same client throughout the time in the health agency. It is common practice to clean and store the thermometer at the bedside within a container of disinfectant, such as alcohol.
Thermometers used for clients having hepatitis may be discarded when the client is discharged because of the potential risk if organisms are not destroyed.
It is possible to avoid cleaning and disinfecting thermometers between uses by applying a thin, flexible, plastic sheath on the thermometer, as shown in Fig. I-8-2. It is important that the nurse's hands be washed after touching a soiled sheath before reapplying another.

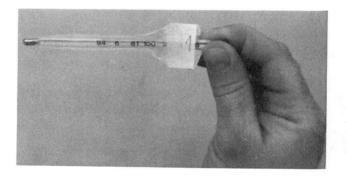

Figure I-8-2 This thermometer has been covered with a thin, plastic sheath. If the sheath ever becomes perforated during use, the thermometer must be cleaned and disinfected before a second use.

HOME-HEALTH VARIATIONS

Check agency policy regarding the use of an agency thermometer or one supplied by the client. Inspect the thermometer owned by the client. Before use, verify that appropriate cleansing and storage procedures have been followed.
Thermometers used in a home may be cleaned with soap and water and then stored for reuse if it is only being used by one person. Multiple users of a home thermometer indicate a need to also disinfect the thermometer between uses.
Strictly adhere to cleansing, disinfecting, and storing procedures of a thermometer used for multiple clients.

RELATED TEACHING

Teach clients to hold a glass thermometer securely during cleaning. Some may prefer to line the sink with a towel. Thermometers break easily when dropped on a hard surface.

Advise clients that mercury released from a broken thermometer should be collected and disposed. Heavy metals, such as mercury, can be toxic if ingested by a child or pet.

Clients should be informed when it is agency practice to cover a glass thermometer with a plastic sheath. A client may misinterpret the use of a sheath to mean that he has a contagious disease.

Persons who use protective sheaths on thermometers should be taught to inspect them carefully. Some brands are sturdier than others. It has been found that some brands may perforate before or with use.

Tell the client that any soap or detergent can be used for cleaning a thermometer as long as sufficient mechanical friction and rinsing accompany cleaning.

Explain that boiling is not an appropriate method for disinfecting a thermometer because high temperatures will expand the mercury beyond the area within the column in which it is contained.

PERFORMANCE CHECKLIST

When cleaning and disinfecting a glass thermometer, the learner:

C	A	U	
[ ]	[ ]	[ ]	Holds the thermometer at the end opposite that which was in contact with the client.
[ ]	[ ]	[ ]	Uses a clean, paper tissue and a twisting motion to wipe the thermometer toward the bulb end.
[ ]	[ ]	[ ]	Rinses the glass thermometer with cool water allowing the water to drain toward the bulb.
[ ]	[ ]	[ ]	Applies soap or detergent to a clean tissue and twists the tissue down the length of the thermometer with firm, mechanical friction.
[ ]	[ ]	[ ]	Rinses the soap from the thermometer under running water from the fingertips to the bulb.
[ ]	[ ]	[ ]	Dries the thermometer with a clean tissue.
[ ]	[ ]	[ ]	Soaks the thermometer in a chemical solution of disinfectant for the prescribed length of time.
[ ]	[ ]	[ ]	Rinses the soaked thermometer with cool running water.
[ ]	[ ]	[ ]	Stores the thermometer in an individual receptacle or in a covered container with other disinfected thermometers.
[ ]	[ ]	[ ]	Washes hands before proceeding with direct client care.

Outcome:　[ ] Pass　　[ ] Fail

C = competent; A = acceptable; U = unsatisfactory

Comments: _____

_____

_____

_____	_____
Student's Signature	Date
_____	_____
Instructor's Signature	Date

I-9 *Caring for a client on isolation precautions*

Isolation precautions are medically aseptic methods to limit the spread of infectious diseases. The primary principle underlying isolation precautions is that various barriers are used to contain pathogens and restrict their transfer to others. Not all individuals who harbor infectious organisms will require the same kinds of barriers. The precautions used are related to the method by which the disease can be transmitted.

PURPOSES OF PROCEDURE

Isolation precautions are used to:

1. Block contact with the infectious organisms by whatever manner those microbes may exit from the client.
2. Protect the nurse from self-contamination through a portal of entry.
3. Prevent the transfer of pathogens to other susceptible clients or visitors.

ASSESSMENT

OBJECTIVE DATA

- Identify the medical diagnosis.
- Review the laboratory reports that validate the diagnosis.
- Investigate the various methods by which the client's disease can be transmitted, such as droplets, blood, stool, and so on.
- Refer to the Centers for Disease Control (CDC) guidelines or the agency's infection control manual concerning the recommended method for controlling transmission of the disease.
- Consult the infection control nurse or committee when the choice of isolation precaution is unclear.

SUBJECTIVE DATA

- Interview and observe the client to acquire information about his cluster of symptoms.

RELEVANT NURSING DIAGNOSES

A client who is being cared for on isolation precautions is likely to have one or more of the following nursing diagnoses:

- *Diversional Activity Deficit related to Monotony of Confinement*
- *Social Isolation*
- *Altered Family Processes related to an Ill Family Member*
- *Powerlessness*
- *Disturbance in Self-Concept*

PLANNING

ESTABLISHING PRIORITIES

Even before a definite diagnosis of a contagious disease has been confirmed, the nurse may institute isolation precautions. Merely suspecting that the client may be infected is a legitimate basis for protecting against the potential threat of its spread. Epidemics have resulted when persons ignored or hesitated to confine infectious clients.

SETTING GOALS

- The organisms specific to the client's infection will be blocked from transfer to other susceptible hosts.

- There will be no new cases of the infectious disease among other clients within the health care agency.
- All personnel involved with the ill client's care will remain free of infection.

PREPARATION OF EQUIPMENT

The nurse will need to assemble various items when carrying out isolation precautions. Not all of the following will be required in each case. The nurse is advised to review the agency's policies. It may be anticipated that the following equipment will be needed:

A private room with toilet and sink
Soap dispenser and paper towels
Antimicrobial cleaning solution
Lined trash containers
Disposable container for contaminated needles or other sharp instruments
Linen hamper with liner
Cloth laundry bags
Supply of gowns, masks, and gloves as indicated
Labels to identify contaminated supplies, trash, and linen
Disposable personal care items, such as basin, bedpan, urinal, drinking pitcher and glass
Instruction card for door

Technique for caring for a client on isolation precautions

ACTION	RATIONALE
1. Check physician's order for type of isolation and review precautions in Infection Control Manual.	The mode of transmission of the organism determines the type and degree of precautions.
2. Plan nursing activities and gather necessary equipment prior to entering client's room. Supplies may include:	Organization facilitates performance of task and adherence to isolation precautions.

Bed linens
Gown and personal hygiene items
Equipment to measure vital signs (if not already in the room)
Medications
Water pitcher, cups, and water
Specimen collection equipment
Isolation apparel
Isolation disposal supplies

3. Provide instruction about isolation to client, family members, and visitors.	An explanation encourages cooperation of client and family and reduces apprehension about isolation procedures.
4. Wash your hands.	Handwashing deters the spread of microorganisms.
5. Put on gown, gloves, and mask if recommended as isolation precaution:	Apparel interrupts the chain of infection; it protects the client and the nurse.
a. Tie gown securely at neck and waist, as shown in Fig. I-9-1.	Gown should protect the entire uniform.
b. Use clean disposable gloves. If worn with gown, draw glove cuffs over gown sleeves.	Gloves protect hands and wrists from microorganisms.
c. Mask must be securely tied and fitted to face.	Mask protects nurse from droplet nuclei and large particle aerosols.

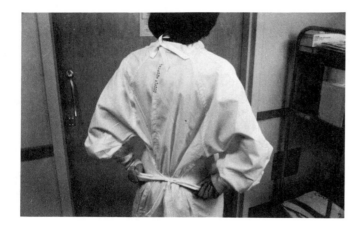

Figure I-9-1 The nurse dons a gown to protect the uniform. The gown is tied at the neck and waist to cover all areas of clothing.

6. Enter client's room with necessary equipment. Place equipment on paper towel if necessary to avoid contamination. Leave chart and flow sheets outside room on isolation cart.

Avoids direct contact with infected material.

7. Measure vital signs using client's equipment in room (thermometer, sphygmomanometer, and stethoscope). A watch should not come into contact with contaminated material. Place within a clear plastic bag or on a clean paper towel. Vital sign recording may also be noted on a clean towel.

Leaving equipment in room prevents spread of microorganisms to other clients. Alcohol may be used to cleanse nurse's equipment, such as the stethoscope, prior to removal and use for another client.

8. Assist client with care. Discard his gown and linens in isolation laundry bag and paper products in isolation waste container (Fig. I-9-2).

Identifies need for special precautions with waste disposal and laundry process.

9. Administer medications as ordered by physician. Discard syringes in disposal container kept in room.

Reduces the risk of needle stick with contaminated needle.

10. Collect specimens and label appropriately. Place in a bag held by assistant outside of room for transport to laboratory.

Outer wrap is not contaminated, and label indicates isolation precautions.

11. Dispose of linen bags and waste bags when necessary and, usually, at the end of each shift:

Double bagging and proper labeling ensure safe transporting of contaminated material. A cuffed clean bag protects the assistant from soiled items in the client's room.

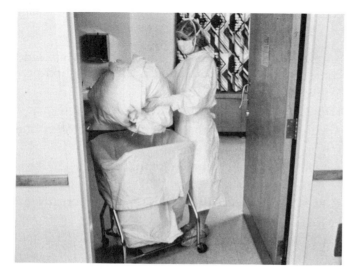

Figure I-9-2 Soiled linen is collected in a laundry hamper kept within the client's room.

a. Tie bags securely.

b. Place linen in a clean disposable bag opened and held by assistant with top edge cuffed over assistant's hands, as shown in Fig. I-9-3. Use same technique and place waste bag in duplicate container for disposal according to agency policy.

c. Label and identify the double-bagged items, as shown in Fig. I-9-4.

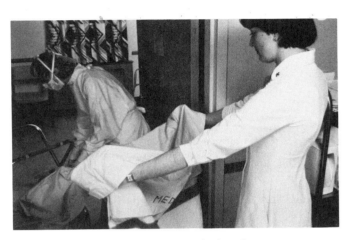

Figure I-9-3 Double-bagging is a method used to remove contaminated items from an isolated area. The assistant holds a clean laundry bag while protecting hands with a wide cuff of fabric. The nurse within the isolation room deposits a fastened bag of soiled linen. The assistant will then close and label the outer bag. Only the inside contents are considered contaminated.

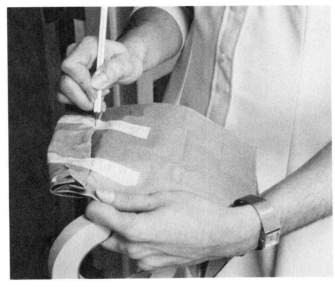

Figure I-9-4 Items removed from an isolation room are sealed and labeled so that others who must handle them are aware that they must follow infection control precautions.

12. Remove gloves, gown, and mask before leaving, and place in appropriate receptacle:

a. Untie waist strings of gown first. Grasp outside of one glove and turn inside out to remove. Drop in waste container. Repeat procedure with second glove, as shown in Fig. I-9-5.

All protective garments are considered contaminated and must not be worn outside the room.

Ungloved hand is clean and should not touch contaminated areas. Waist strings of gown are considered contaminated.

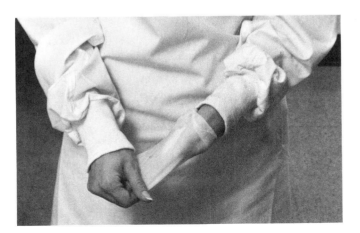

Figure I-9-5 Gloves are removed by turning them inside out. The nurse touches only the inside of the gloves to avoid coming into contact with the pathogens causing the client's infection.

b. Untie mask and drop by strings into waste container.

Center of mask is contaminated. Strings are considered clean.

c. Untie neck strings of gown. Remove gown without touching outside of gown, as shown in Fig. I-9-6. Neck band may be grasped to pull off gown. Turn gown inside out and drop in laundry bag.

Neck strings are considered clean. Outside of gown is contaminated.

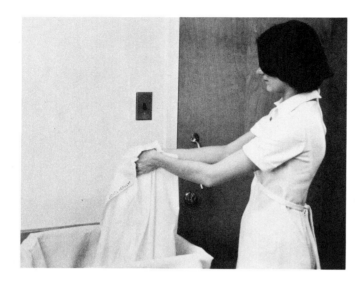

Figure I-9-6 The nurse avoids touching the outer surface of the gown while removing it. The soiled gown is deposited in the linen hamper within the client's room.

13. Wash hands thoroughly.

Prevents spread of microorganisms.

14. Retrieve watch, and check notation of vital signs.

Clean hands may touch clean equipment.

15. Close door to room when leaving.

May depend on type of isolation. Check agency policy.

16. Record maintenance of isolation precautions and client's response in chart.

Ensures adequate documentation. Clients may require additional emotional support due to sensory deprivation and feelings associated with being isolated for a disease process.

SAMPLE DOCUMENTATION

Date	Time	Nurse's note
6/09	1000	Drainage/Secretion Precautions maintained. Flank incision draining copious amts. of purulent drng. Dressing changed ×3. States, "I'm so lonely. I think my family is afraid to visit me."

J. Roth, RN

EVALUATION

REASSESSMENT

The nurse should monitor laboratory tests, such as culture reports, which may indicate that the infectious period has passed and the isolation precautions may be discontinued. Observe visitors and other personnel for compliance with the posted isolation precautions.

EXPECTED OUTCOMES

There are no additional cases of the infectious disease among personnel, other clients, or visitors.

UNEXPECTED OUTCOMES

Other confirmed cases are reported among individuals who may have had contact with the client, the client's nurse, or his contaminated equipment.

MODIFICATIONS IN SELECTED SITUATIONS

GENERAL VARIATIONS

Persons at risk, such as clients who are immunosuppressed, malnourished, or who have open skin should be assigned to personnel other than the nurse caring for the isolation client.

Use the infection control nurse for educating clients and staff about effective infection control techniques in addition to collecting statistics.

Follow either category-specific guidelines or disease-specific guidelines when planning methods to control the spread of known pathogens.

The optimum precaution would be to place the intensive care client with a communicable disease in a private room. When this is not possible, the isolation area may be marked off by cubicle curtains or tape on the floor.

A female visitor should not carry a purse into an isolation room. It may be placed within a plastic bag and then may be carried by the visitor. The plastic bag can be opened just prior to leaving. Once the hands are clean, the purse can be retrieved from the bag and carried from the room.

AGE-RELATED VARIATIONS

Separation of a child from his or her parents and contact with others can be extremely traumatic to all involved. The nurse may encourage parents to visit as frequently and as long as desired. In the interim, the nurse should make an effort to alter the stimuli and provide contact with children who may react negatively to the isolation experience.

If there are adequate personnel in a newborn nursery, opportunity for thorough handwashing, and sufficient space between each infant, a private room for a baby with a contagious disease may not be necessary.

Until the source of an infection in a nursery is identified, groups of infants born within the same 24-hour to 48-hour period may be kept in a single room. The room is then cleaned thoroughly when all the infants have been discharged.

HOME-HEALTH VARIATIONS

In the home, the client may be instructed to improvise with the resources and supplies available. The nurse needs to emphasize effective handwashing and hygiene practices to interrupt the chain of infection.

Family members should avoid use of a common drinking cup and towels in a bathroom.

Boiling contaminated items, using a steam pressure cooker, and hanging pillows and blankets in the sunshine are common home methods for destroying contagious microorganisms.

RELATED TEACHING

The client and his family should be instructed about the contagious disease, its modes of transmission, and how to carry out the required precautions.

Health agency staff should periodically review the practices involved in isolation precautions. When personnel are inconsistent, the client may question the quality of his care.

(Performance checklist next page)

PERFORMANCE CHECKLIST

When isolation precautions are performed, the learner:

C	A	U	
[ ]	[ ]	[ ]	Prepares the room with essential basic equipment.
[ ]	[ ]	[ ]	Posts an instruction card on the outside of the room door.
[ ]	[ ]	[ ]	Stocks supplies of gowns, masks, gloves, trash disposal bags, and linen bags, outside the client's room.
[ ]	[ ]	[ ]	Removes watch, if needed within the isolation room, and places it within a clear plastic bag or on a clean paper towel.
[ ]	[ ]	[ ]	Removes cap, if worn, and rings; then proceeds to wash hands.
[ ]	[ ]	[ ]	Dons a gown, if required, taking care to cover the entire front and back of the uniform.
[ ]	[ ]	[ ]	Ties a mask, if required, securing it over the nose.
[ ]	[ ]	[ ]	Applies gloves, if required, covering the cuff of the gown.
[ ]	[ ]	[ ]	Organizes several tasks that can be accomplished during one block of time within the isolation room.
[ ]	[ ]	[ ]	Disposes of soiled laundry and trash in respective containers within the client's room.
[ ]	[ ]	[ ]	Secures soiled linen and trash within bags by tying or fastening.
[ ]	[ ]	[ ]	Places secured laundry and trash bags within a clean bag held by an assistant outside the client's room.
[ ]	[ ]	[ ]	Takes care that only the inside of the clean bag is touched.
[ ]	[ ]	[ ]	Instructs assistant to seal and label bags identifying its source from an isolation room.
[ ]	[ ]	[ ]	Removes isolation garments in the following sequences: • Unties front waist strings on gown. • Removes gloves turning them inside out and disposing them within a trash receptacle. • Removes mask. • Unfastens neck strings of gown. • Removes gown without touching the outside surface.
[ ]	[ ]	[ ]	Opens plastic bag and slides watch to a clean paper towel.
[ ]	[ ]	[ ]	Performs thorough handwashing.
[ ]	[ ]	[ ]	Collects watch and other equipment that has been kept clean within the room.
[ ]	[ ]	[ ]	Uses a paper towel when opening the inside door handle of the isolation room.
[ ]	[ ]	[ ]	Discards the paper towel within a lined waste receptacle within the client's room.
[ ]	[ ]	[ ]	Closes the client's door, if required.

Outcome: [ ] Pass   [ ] Fail

C = competent; A = acceptable; U = unsatisfactory

Comments: _____
_____
_____

_____   _____
       Student's Signature   **Date**

_____   _____
      Instructor's Signature   **Date**

I-10 *Making an unoccupied bed*

The linen in a health agency is changed frequently, in some cases daily or more often if necessary. This routine practice is followed because bed linen is a reservoir of microorganisms acquired from contact with the client's skin, his excretions, and secretions. In an effort to control costs, only heavily soiled linen is changed.

The nurse must change linen in such a way that the potential for transferring microbes is reduced. Microbes must be restricted to the soiled linen by folding the soiled surface in upon itself, holding the removed linen away from the uniform, and depositing the linen in a hamper, cart, or chute without touching the floor of the client's room. The nurse must also practice appropriate handwashing because the client is both a reservoir of microbes and a susceptible host.

PURPOSES OF PROCEDURE

Bedmaking is performed to:

1. Provide comfort for the client.
2. Maintain a hygienic environment.
3. Reduce transmission of microorganisms.
4. Stimulate and refresh the client.

ASSESSMENT

OBJECTIVE DATA

- Assess the type and extent of soiling, such as urine, feces, emesis, blood, serum, food, perspiration.
- Determine the amount of soiled linen that requires replacement.
- Observe the client's activity tolerance based on his level of consciousness, stability of vital signs, muscular strength, and so on.
- Note the presence of therapeutic equipment, such as catheter drainage tubing, which may need to be unfastened from the current linen.

SUBJECTIVE DATA

- Ask the client to indicate if he is experiencing vertigo, nausea, severe pain, fatigue, or weakness.
- Inquire as to the client's preference for the amount, type, or placement of linen for comfort.

RELEVANT NURSING DIAGNOSES

Bedmaking may be especially pertinent to clients with the following nursing diagnoses:

- *Altered Comfort*
- *Potential for Infection*
- *Altered Body Temperature*
- *Altered Bowel Elimination: Incontinence*
- *Altered Patterns of Urinary Elimination*
- *Potential of Impaired Skin Integrity*

PLANNING

ESTABLISHING PRIORITIES

When linen becomes saturated with secretions and bodily excretions, there is a greater potential for skin breakdown. Therefore, wet, soiled linen should be changed immediately. Bedmaking may be temporarily deferred if the linen remains relatively clean and dry. Removing wrinkles and tightening the sheets may be all that is necessary.

SETTING GOALS

- The bed will be clean and wrinkle-free.
- The client will remain safe and comfortable while out of bed.

PREPARATION OF EQUIPMENT

The following is a list of commonly used supplies when making a bed:

Two flat sheets (or one flat sheet and one fitted sheet)
Drawsheet
Blankets
Bedspread
Pillowcase(s)
Linen hamper or bag
Bedside chair
Waterproof sheet or protective pad (optional)

Technique for making an unoccupied bed

ACTION	RATIONALE
1. Assemble equipment and place on bedside chair in order in which it will be used.	Organization promotes efficient time management.
2. Wash your hands.	Handwashing deters the spread of microorganisms.
3. Adjust bed to the high position, and drop the side rails.	Having the bed in the high position and the side rails down reduces strain on the nurse.
4. Check bed linens for client's personal items, and disconnect the call bell or any tubes from the bed linens.	It is costly and inconvenient when personal belongings are lost.
5. Loosen all linen while moving around the bed from the head of the bed on the near side to the head of the bed on the far side.	Loosening linen helps prevent tugging and tearing linen. Loosening the linen and moving around the bed systematically reduces strain caused by reaching across the bed.
6. Fold reusable linens, such as blankets or spread, in place on the bed in fourths, and then hang them over a clean chair.	Folding saves time and energy when reusable linen is replaced on the bed. Folding linens while they are on the bed reduces strain on the nurse's arms.
7. Snugly roll all of the soiled linen inside of the bottom sheet and place directly into the laundry hamper. Do not place them on the floor or on furniture. Do not hold soiled linens against the uniform, as shown in Fig. I-10-1.	Rolling soiled linens snugly and placing them directly into the hamper helps prevent the spread of organisms. The floor is heavily contaminated; soiled linen will further contaminate furniture. Soiled linen contaminates the uniform and may spread organisms to another client.

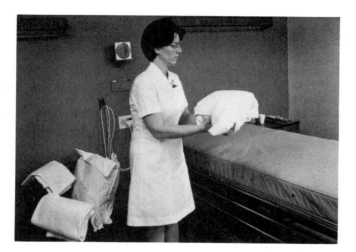

Figure I-10–1 The linen has been folded into a compact ball with the soiled areas toward the inside. The nurse carries the laundry away from her uniform so it does not become contaminated with pathogens.

8. Grasp the mattress securely and shift it up to the head of the bed.

Allows more foot room for the client and moves the mattress against the head of the bed.

9. Place the bottom sheet with its center fold in the center of the bed, as shown in Fig. I-10-2, and high enough to have a sufficient amount of sheet to tuck under the head of the mattress.

Opening linens on the bed reduces strain on the nurse's arms and diminishes the spread of organisms.

10. Tuck the bottom sheet securely under the head of the mattress on one side of the bed, making a corner according to agency policy. A mitered corner is shown in Fig. I-10-3. Tuck the sides of the bottom sheet under the mattress on the one side.

Making the bed on one side and then completing the bed on the other side saves time. Having the bottom linens free of wrinkles reduces discomfort to the bed-ridden client.

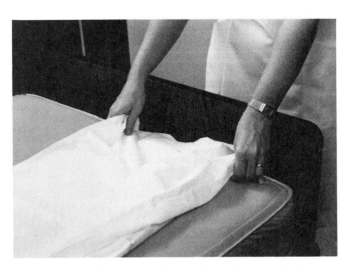

Figure I-10-2 The nurse unfolds the linen rather than shaking it in the air. The nurse uses the folds of the linen to center it on the mattress.

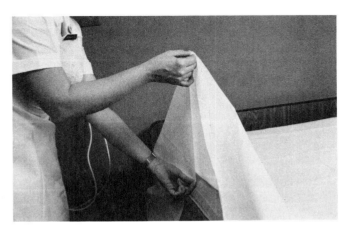

Figure I-10-3 To make a mitered corner, the nurse folds a triangular section of sheet on the corner of the bed. The flap is brought back down and folded under the mattress.

11. If a waterproof sheet or protective pad is used, place it over the bottom sheet so that it will be under the client's chest-to-knee area. Place the cotton drawsheet in the same manner, shown in Fig. I-10-4, over the waterproof covering. Not all agencies use drawsheets routinely. The nurse may decide to use one.

When a client soils his bed, drawsheets can be changed without the bottom and top linens on the bed. Having all bottom linens in place before tucking them under the mattress avoids unnecessary moving about the bed. A drawsheet also is an aid when moving the client in bed.

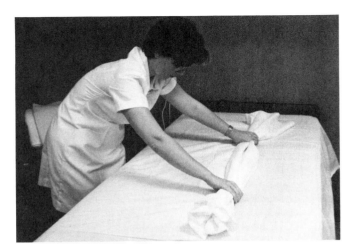

Figure I-10-4 A draw sheet is positioned so that it will be located under the middle of the client's body.

12. Move to the other side of the bed to tuck in the bottom linens on that side, as shown in Fig. I-10-5. Using a fitted bottom sheet eliminates the need to mitre corners.

Tucking all the linen on one side of the bed at one time reduces work and promotes efficiency.

13. Secure the top of the sheet under the head of the mattress, and mitre the corner. Pull the remainder of the sheet tightly and tuck under the mattress. Do the same for the drawsheet.

Rids the bottom linens of any wrinkles which can cause discomfort for the client.

14. Place the top sheet on the bed with its center fold in the center of the bed and with the top of the sheet placed so that the hem is even with the head of the mattress. Unfold the top sheet in place, as shown in Fig. I-10-6. Follow the same procedure with the top blanket or spread it placing the upper edge approximately 6 inches below the top of the sheet.

Opening linens by shaking them spreads organisms about the air. Holding linens overhead to open them causes strain on the nurse's arms.

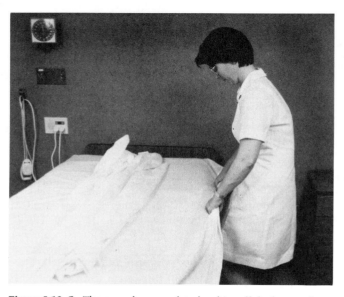

Figure I-10-5 The nurse has completed tucking all the bottom linen on one side of the bed. Once on the other side, the remaining bulk of folded linen can be pulled and tucked under the mattress.

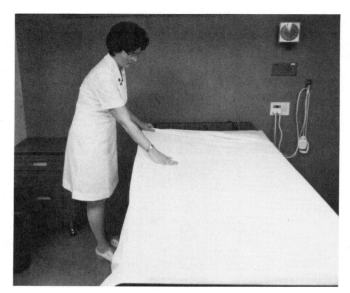

Figure I-10-6 The nurse smooths each layer of linen to ensure that the bed is free of wrinkles.

15. Tuck the top sheet and blanket under the foot of the bed on the near side. Mitre the corner.

Saves time and energy. Keeps top linen in place.

16. Fold the upper 6 inches of the top sheet down over the spread and make a cuff, as shown in Fig. I-10-7.

Makes it easier for the client to get into bed and pull the covers up.

17. Move to the other side of the bed and follow same procedure for securing the top sheets under the foot of the bed and making a cuff.

Working on one side of the bed at a time saves energy and is more efficient.

18. Place the pillows on the bed. Open each pillow case in the same manner as opening other linens. Gather the pillowcase over one hand toward the closed end. Grasp the pillow with the hand inside the pillowcase. Keeping a firm hold on the pillow, pull the cover onto the pillow.

Opening linens by shaking them causes organisms to be carried about on air currents. Covering the pillow while it rests on the bed reduces strain on the nurse's arms and back.

19. Place the pillow at the head of the bed with the open end facing toward the window.

Provides for a neater appearance.

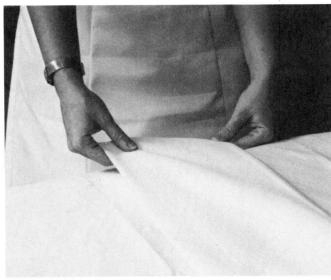

Figure I-10-7 A neat cuff is formed by folding the excess length of the top sheet over the spread or blanket.

20. Fan-fold or pie-fold the top linens.

Having linens opened makes it more convenient for the client to get into bed.

21. Secure the signal device on the bed according to agency policy.

Having the signal device handy for the client makes it possible for him to call for assistance as necessary.

22. Adjust the bed to the low position.

Having the bed in the low position makes it easier and safer for the client to get into bed.

23. Dispose of soiled linen according to agency policy. Wash your hands.

Deters the spread of microorganisms.

SAMPLE DOCUMENTATION

Date	Time	Nurse's note
2/16	1945	Perspiring profusely. Partial bath administered. Assisted to bedside chair. Bed linen changed.
		D. Moore, LVN

EVALUATION

REASSESSMENT

As the soiled linen is removed, the nurse may determine that extra linen would be appropriate. For instance, a waterproof pad may be desirable. The client's condition should be observed frequently. The nurse may wish to abandon bedmaking and return him to bed.

EXPECTED OUTCOMES

Organisms from the soiled linen are confined to the inner surfaces of the linen.
Replacement linen is applied without transferring organisms from contaminated areas within the immediate environment, such as the floor.
The nurse expends a minimum of energy and uses maximum musculoskeletal efficiency.
The client tolerates ambulating or resting in a chair during bedmaking.

UNEXPECTED OUTCOMES

The client's condition worsens, and bedmaking may be stopped in lieu of safety.
Linen drops on the floor and must be discarded.

MODIFICATIONS IN SELECTED SITUATIONS

A toe pleat, a vertical or horizontal fold of top linen shown in Fig. I-10-8, can be formed to provide ample room for the toes.

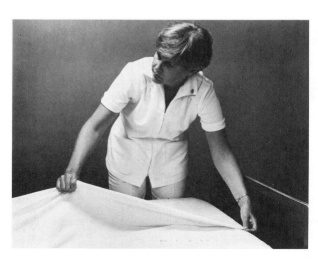

Figure I-10–8   The nurse makes a toe pleat by using a vertical fold in the top sheet near the bottom of the bed.

GENERAL VARIATIONS

A square corner is another technique for securing flat sheets beneath a mattress.

Maintain the bed in a flat but high position if the client will return to the bed from a stretcher.

Fold all top linen to the side or extreme bottom of the bed if the client will be returning from the operating room.

When an egg-crate mattress is used, the bottom linen is not pulled tightly or the purpose of the device is minimized.

AGE-RELATED VARIATIONS

Elderly persons or those with compromised circulation may desire extra blankets. A flannel bath blanket may substitute as a top or bottom sheet for absorption and warmth.

Crib mattresses are generally covered with fitted sheets. Top sheets and pillows tend to be omitted. Children are warmed and comforted by a soft blanket that is proportionate to their body size.

HOME-HEALTH VARIATIONS

When making a conventional bed that is not adjustable in the client's home, protect your back by bending your knees.

Make a drawsheet by folding a flat sheet in half crosswise.

Place soiled linen directly into the client's hamper or washing machine.

Medical supply companies are a resource for purchasing absorbent, disposable pads which will reduce the volume of laundering.

Detergent and household bleach are good antimicrobial agents for washable fabrics. Microbes can be further reduced by using hot water for washing and by drying linen outside in the sunshine.

Down pillows may be protected with waterproof plastic covers, or they may be aired and exposed to sunlight periodically. Pillows made from synthetics are generally washable; consult the manufacturer's instructions.

RELATED TEACHING

The nurse may wish to demonstrate various methods for securing corners of a flat bottom sheet.

The sides of cribs should be in safe, working order. When purchasing a new crib, parents can be advised to note if the crib meets the requirements of the Consumer Product Safety Commission.

Bottles should not be propped; infants should be positioned on the side or abdomen to avoid choking and aspiration. A receiving blanket, soft terrycloth towel, or disposable pad can be placed under the child's head to absorb any formula that may be regurgitated.

PERFORMANCE CHECKLIST

When making an unoccupied bed, the learner:

C	A	U	
[ ]	[ ]	[ ]	Washes hands.
[ ]	[ ]	[ ]	Collects assorted clean linen.
[ ]	[ ]	[ ]	Places the linen on a clean area within the room, such as a bedside chair or table.
[ ]	[ ]	[ ]	Arranges the clean linen in the order that it will be used.
[ ]	[ ]	[ ]	Provides the client with slippers and robe.
[ ]	[ ]	[ ]	Assists the client to transfer from the bed to a chair.
[ ]	[ ]	[ ]	Raises the bed so that the mattress is approximately waist high.
[ ]	[ ]	[ ]	Lowers the side rails and adjusts the bed to a flat position.
[ ]	[ ]	[ ]	Disconnects the signal cord and other equipment that may be attached to the linen, such as a catheter drainage tube.
[ ]	[ ]	[ ]	Inspects the bed for loose personal items, such as pens, eyeglasses, hearing aid, and so on.
[ ]	[ ]	[ ]	Folds and removes the linen that will be reused.
[ ]	[ ]	[ ]	Loosens linen on all sides of the bed.
[ ]	[ ]	[ ]	Rolls the linen with the soiled side inward making a small enough bundle that can be carried without touching the floor or the uniform.
[ ]	[ ]	[ ]	Deposits soiled linen within a laundry bag, hamper, cart, or chute.
[ ]	[ ]	[ ]	Adjust the position of the mattress.
[ ]	[ ]	[ ]	Centers and unfolds the bottom sheet.
[ ]	[ ]	[ ]	Applies a waterproof sheet and drawsheet, if needed.
[ ]	[ ]	[ ]	Tucks and mitres the corners on one half of the bed.
[ ]	[ ]	[ ]	Moves to the opposite side of the bed and repeats the above step.
[ ]	[ ]	[ ]	Centers and unfolds the top sheet.
[ ]	[ ]	[ ]	Unfolds and places the blanket and spread approximately 6 inches below the edge of the top sheet.
[ ]	[ ]	[ ]	Secures the top sheet, blanket, and spread under the foot of the mattress on each respective side.
[ ]	[ ]	[ ]	Folds the upper linen to the foot of the bed.
[ ]	[ ]	[ ]	Reattaches the signal cord to the bed.
[ ]	[ ]	[ ]	Removes soiled pillowcase and reapplies a clean pillowcase without shaking or touching the pillow to the uniform.
[ ]	[ ]	[ ]	Replaces the bed in a low position.
[ ]	[ ]	[ ]	Washes hands before performing other nursing care.

Outcome: [ ] Pass   [ ] Fail

C = competent; A = acceptable; U = unsatisfactory

Comments: _____

_____

_____

_____	_____
Student's Signature	Date
_____	_____
Instructor's Signature	Date

I-11 *Making an occupied bed*

Some situations and health conditions require that the client remain in bed at all times during convalescence. Clients who are unconscious, critically ill, in continuous traction, and so on, necessitate that the nurse make the bed while the client occupies the bed.

PURPOSES OF PROCEDURE

An occupied bed is made to:

1. Provide comfort for the client.
2. Maintain a hygienic environment.
3. Reduce transmission of microorganisms.
4. Refresh the client.
5. Conserve the client's energy.

ASSESSMENT

OBJECTIVE DATA

- Identify the client's current activity order.
- Note the presence and use of equipment that is not portable, such as traction.
- Review the stability of the client's recent vital signs.
- Read the most recent documentation concerning the client's response to activity.
- Observe the client's level of consciousness.
- Note any weakness or paralysis that would interfere with transferring from the bed.

SUBJECTIVE DATA

- Ask the client to indicate if he has experienced any current or recent chest pain, vertigo, severe nausea, or other symptoms which would indicate a potential for injury or discomfort with activity.

RELEVANT NURSING DIAGNOSES

Clients who must remain in bed while it is made are likely to have nursing diagnoses such as:

- *Self-Care Deficit*
- *Impaired Physical Mobility*
- *Potential for Injury*
- *Activity Intolerance*
- *Altered Cardiac Output: Decreased*
- *Altered Comfort*
- *Impaired Gas Exchange*

PLANNING

ESTABLISHING PRIORITIES

Bedmaking may be deferred if the client is in extreme pain or respiratory distress. Bottom linen may be straightened and tightened unless it is extremely soiled or wet. It may be desirable to premedicate clients who are likely to experience discomfort from turning and lifting during bedmaking. The nurse may choose to change only the most soiled pieces of linen.

SETTING GOALS

- The client will remain safe and comfortable during bedmaking.
- The remade bed will be clean and wrinkle-free.

PREPARATION OF EQUIPMENT

The following items may be gathered prior to making an occupied bed:

Two flat sheets (or one flat sheet and one fitted sheet)

Blanket (optional)
Pillowcases
Linen hamper or bag
Bedside chair
Waterproof sheet or protective pad (optional)
Bath blanket (optional)

Technique for making an occupied bed

ACTION	RATIONALE
1. Explain the procedure to the client. Check the chart for limitations on the client's physical activity.	Facilitates client cooperation and determines his level of activity.
2. Wash your hands.	Handwashing deters the spread of microorganisms.
3. Assemble equipment and place on bedside chair in the order in which it will be used.	Organization facilitates the performance of the task.
4. Close the door or curtain.	Provides privacy.
5. Adjust the bed to high position. Lower the side rail nearest you leaving the opposite side rail up. Place the bed in a flat position if the client can tolerate it.	Having the bed in high position reduces strain on the nurse. Having the mattress flat facilitates making a wrinkle-free bed.
6. Check the bed linens for the client's personal items, and disconnect the call bell or any tubes from the bed linens.	It is costly and inconvenient when personal items are lost. Disconnecting tubes from linens prevents discomfort and accidental dislodging of tubes.
7. Place the bath blanket, if available, over client. Have him hold onto the bath blanket while you reach under it and remove top linens, as the nurse in Fig. I-11-1 is doing. Leave the top sheet in place if the bath blanket is not used. Fold linen that is to be reused over the back of a chair. Discard soiled linen in a laundry bag or hamper.	Provides warmth and privacy.

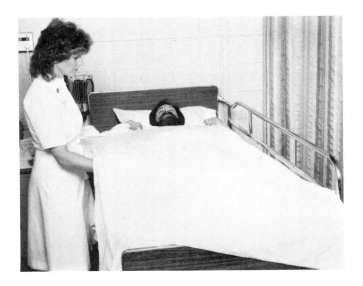

Figure I-11-1 While the client holds the bath blanket in place, the nurse removes the top linens by pulling them toward the bottom of the bed.

8. Grasp the mattress securely and shift it up to the head of the bed. (This may require the assistance of another person.)	Allows more foot room for the client and positions the mattress against the head of the bed.

9. Assist the client to turn toward the opposite side of the bed, and reposition the pillow under his head.

Allows the bed to be made on the vacant side.

10. Loosen all bottom linens from the head and side of the bed.

Facilitates removal of linens.

11. Fan-fold the soiled linens as close to the client as possible, as shown in Fig. I-11-2.

Facilitates removal of linens when the client turns to the other side.

12. Use clean linen and make the near side of the bed following steps 9, 10, and 11 in Procedure I-10, "Making an Unoccupied Bed." Fan-fold clean linen as close to the client as possible, as shown in Fig. I-11-3.

Positions clean linen to make the other side of the bed.

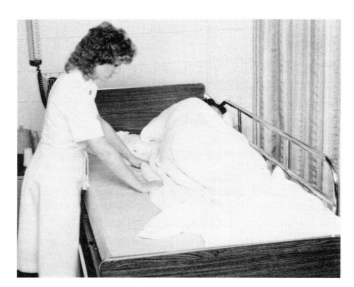

Figure I-11–2 The soiled linen is folded on itself and rolled close to the client who has been positioned to the far side of the bed.

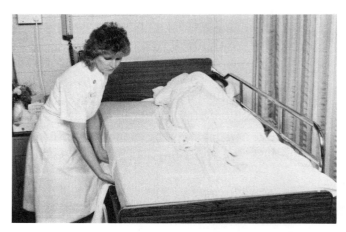

Figure I-11–3 The bottom sheets are tucked under the mattress. The nurse bends her knees to avoid injuring her back.

13. Raise the side rail. Move to the other side and lower the side rail. Assist the client to roll over the folded linen behind him and toward the other side. Reposition the pillow and bath blanket or top sheet.

Ensures client safety. Movement allows the bed to be made on the other side. The bath blanket provides warmth and privacy.

14. Loosen all bottom linen and remove it, as shown in Fig. I-11-4. Place it in the linen bag or hamper. Hold the soiled linen away from the front of the uniform.

Proper disposal of soiled linen prevents the spread of microorganisms.

15. Ease the clean linen from under the client. Pull taut and secure bottom sheet under the head of the mattress. Mitre the corner. Pull the side of the sheet taut and tuck it under the side of the mattress. Repeat with the drawsheet.

Removes wrinkles and creases in linens which are uncomfortable to lie on.

16. Assist the client to return to the center of the bed. Remove the pillow and change the pillowcase before replacing the pillow on the bed with the open end facing the window.

Provides for a neater appearance.

17. Apply the top linen so that it is centered, as shown in Fig. I-11-5, and the top hems are even with the head of the mattress. Have the client hold onto the top linen so the bath blanket can be removed.

Allows bottom hems to be tucked securely under the mattress. Provides for privacy.

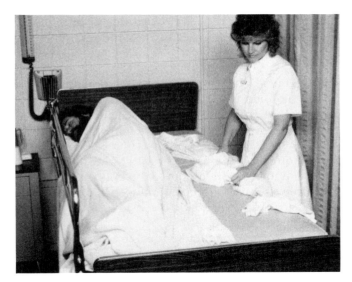

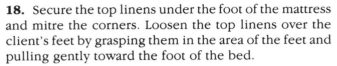

Figure I-11–4 After turning the client to the opposite side of the bed, the nurse removes the soiled linen.

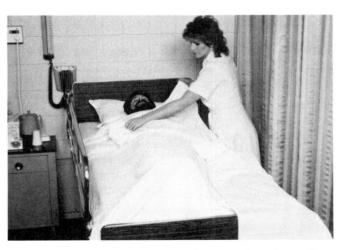

Figure I-11–5 To maintain privacy, the nurse places the top linen over the client's bath blanket.

18. Secure the top linens under the foot of the mattress and mitre the corners. Loosen the top linens over the client's feet by grasping them in the area of the feet and pulling gently toward the foot of the bed.

Provides for neat appearance. Loosening linens over the client's feet gives more room for movement.

19. Raise the side rail. Lower the bed height and adjust the head of the bed to a comfortable position. Reattach the call bell and drainage tubes.

Provides for the client's safety.

20. Dispose of soiled linens according to the agency policy. Wash your hands.

Prevents the spread of microorganisms.

SAMPLE DOCUMENTATION

Date	Time	Nurse's note
12/07	0900	Dangled on edge of bed. States, "I'm going to faint." Assisted to recline in bed. Pale color noted. BP 120/80. Alert but reluctant to sit up. Occupied bed made.
		L. Wise, LPN

EVALUATION

REASSESSMENT

The nurse should review the medical orders frequently for changes in the client's activity order. Objective and subjective assessments of the client may be shared with the physician when considering modifications for care.

EXPECTED OUTCOMES

The client's bed is remade while maintaining his privacy, safety, warmth, and comfort.
The clean laundry does not come in contact with soiled areas, such as the floor.
The soiled laundry is kept from contact with the nurse's uniform and is disposed properly.
The nurse remains free of injury through proper use of body mechanics and assistance from the client or other personnel.

UNEXPECTED OUTCOMES

The client's condition suddenly changes during the effort of turning or lifting.

The physician or other agency personnel have the need to examine the client or provide special care, such as respiratory therapy.

MODIFICATIONS IN SELECTED SITUATIONS

GENERAL VARIATIONS

A client gown may be worn over the nurse's uniform if it is likely that it will come in contact with soiled areas of the linen, the client's secretions, or excretions. The gown should be removed before providing care to other clients.

Corn starch may be sprinkled on the lower sheet to prevent friction when the client moves across the linen.

Provide the client with a trapeze and directions for assisting with lifting and turning.

Place a folded, but loose, sheet from under the shoulders to the buttocks for lifting and turning a client who is unable to assist with positioning changes.

Request hypoallergenic linen for those clients whose skin is sensitive to the agency's routine laundering procedures.

The linen may be secured by making a square corner rather than mitering the corner.

Depending on the client's condition and equipment, it may be more appropriate to make the bed from top to bottom rather than from side to side.

AGE-RELATED VARIATIONS

Very thin, elderly, and malnourished clients often have skin that can become easily broken. Skin protective aids, such as an egg crate mattress may be applied to the bed as a preventive measure.

Use of disposable diapers or waterproof pads may reduce linen changes for children who are not bowel or bladder trained or who are incontinent.

HOME-HEALTH VARIATIONS

For the client who uses a conventional bed, use extra caution to keep him from falling out of bed when turned away from the nurse.

Varying colors and designs on sheets will add a variety of stimuli for persons who suffer from the monotony of being restricted to a bed and one room.

Waterproof underwear may be used to reduce linen changes for incontinent clients.

Fitted bottom sheets help to keep the sheet taut and wrinkle free.

A hospital bed and trapeze may be rented or purchased when a client is likely to be confined to bed for an extended period of time. Clients may be referred to local, state, or federal health assistance agencies, such as the American Cancer Society, Hospice, and so on, for obtaining specialized equipment.

The extension leaf from a dining table, a hollow door, or a plywood board may be used to provide support under a home mattress.

RELATED TEACHING

A client should be taught to pull and lift his body using a trapeze and the side rails.

PERFORMANCE CHECKLIST

When an occupied bed is made, the learner:

C	A	U	
[ ]	[ ]	[ ]	Determines the need for restricting the client to bed.
[ ]	[ ]	[ ]	Assesses the type and amount of clean replacement linen.
[ ]	[ ]	[ ]	Delivers clean linen to the bedside.
[ ]	[ ]	[ ]	Washes hands.
[ ]	[ ]	[ ]	Arranges the linen in the order in which it will be used.
[ ]	[ ]	[ ]	Explains the plan for changing the bed with the client.
[ ]	[ ]	[ ]	Protects the privacy of the client by closing the room door and cubicle curtains.
[ ]	[ ]	[ ]	Elevates the bed to a high position.
[ ]	[ ]	[ ]	Places the client in a supine position if tolerated.
[ ]	[ ]	[ ]	Covers the client with a bath blanket or top sheet.
[ ]	[ ]	[ ]	Lowers the side rail and detaches all tubes and equipment that have been secured to the linen.
[ ]	[ ]	[ ]	Folds the spread and blanket for reuse, if possible.
[ ]	[ ]	[ ]	Assists the client to roll onto his side toward the far side of the bed.
[ ]	[ ]	[ ]	Loosens the linen on the near side of the bed.
[ ]	[ ]	[ ]	Rolls the bottom linen toward the center of the bed with the soiled side inward.
[ ]	[ ]	[ ]	Applies the bottom linen to the vacant side of the bed.
[ ]	[ ]	[ ]	Folds the clean unmade half of the linen at the middle of the bed.
[ ]	[ ]	[ ]	Raises the side rail.
[ ]	[ ]	[ ]	Moves to the opposite side of the bed.
[ ]	[ ]	[ ]	Assists the client to roll over the soiled and clean linen in the center of the bed and lie on the other side.
[ ]	[ ]	[ ]	Loosens the soiled linen.
[ ]	[ ]	[ ]	Removes and disposes of the linen within a linen bag or room hamper.
[ ]	[ ]	[ ]	Unrolls the folded clean linen.
[ ]	[ ]	[ ]	Pulls the linen to remove any slack that may have formed during the turning process.
[ ]	[ ]	[ ]	Secures the bottom linen as on the opposite side.
[ ]	[ ]	[ ]	Repositions the client to the center of the bed or alternative position of comfort.
[ ]	[ ]	[ ]	Removes pillow and pillowcase; changes the pillowcase and returns the pillow.
[ ]	[ ]	[ ]	Places open end of pillow opposite the door.
[ ]	[ ]	[ ]	Applies top linen.
[ ]	[ ]	[ ]	Instructs the client to grasp the clean top linen.
[ ]	[ ]	[ ]	Withdraws bath blanket or soiled top sheet from the bottom of the bed.
[ ]	[ ]	[ ]	Tucks top linen beneath the mattress.
[ ]	[ ]	[ ]	Provides adequate room for toes.
[ ]	[ ]	[ ]	Folds the hem of the top sheet to form a cuff over the blanket and spread.

C = competent; A = acceptable; U = unsatisfactory

(Continued)

PERFORMANCE CHECKLIST (Continued)

C	A	U	
[ ]	[ ]	[ ]	Reattaches the signal cord and equipment to the bed.
[ ]	[ ]	[ ]	Raises the side rail and lowers the height of the bed.
[ ]	[ ]	[ ]	Disposes of the linen from the room into a laundry cart or chute.
[ ]	[ ]	[ ]	Washes hands.

Outcome: [ ] **Pass**   [ ] **Fail**

C = competent; A = acceptable; U = unsatisfactory

Comments: _____

_____

_____

_____	_____
Student's Signature	**Date**
_____	_____
Instructor's Signature	**Date**

Maintaining surgical asepsis

Surgical asepsis, or sterile technique, includes those practices that keep objects and areas totally free of microorganisms. These conditions are regularly required in the operating room, labor and delivery areas, and during certain diagnostic tests. However, there are instances when the bedside nurse must implement sterile technique. Insertion of a catheter and sterile dressing changes are two procedures that require surgical asepsis. The nurse must become knowledgeable and proficient at donning and removing sterile gloves and donning a sterile gown in preparation for those situations in which sterile technique must be maintained.

I-12   *Donning and removing sterile gloves*

Hands should always be washed thoroughly before donning and after removing sterile gloves. Handwashing is modified in certain ways if the nurse will be participating with a surgical or obstetric procedure. All jewelry is removed. The hands and the entire length of the arm to the elbow are scrubbed with a hand brush. The length of time for scrubbing is extended, in some cases from 3 minutes to 10 minutes. The scrubbed hands are considered the cleaner area and, therefore, rinsing and draining are in the direction of the elbows.

Sterile gloves are donned so that only the inside of the gloves comes in contact with the hands. After the gloves are on, sterile items may be handled. Careful removal of the gloves reduces any hand contact with contaminated materials.

PURPOSES OF PROCEDURE

Sterile gloves are donned to:

1. Produce a microbe-free surface over the hands.
2. Facilitate using the hands when handling sterile equipment.
3. Prevent transferring organisms from the nurse's hands into a portal of entry within the client.

ASSESSMENT

OBJECTIVE DATA

- Review the procedure or care that must be implemented to determine if it must be performed using sterile technique.
- During the physical assessment, determine if the skin is intact or is likely to be compromised during the procedure.
- Determine if touching a client will introduce organisms where they are likely to grow, reproduce, and cause infection.

SUBJECTIVE DATA

- In the emergency room, doctor's office, or upon admission, inquire about the client's current health problems and medications. If the nurse suspects that the client may be immunosuppressed, sterile gloves should be worn to protect him from organisms that most other persons could resist.

RELEVANT NURSING DIAGNOSES

Donning and removing sterile gloves are especially related to clients with the following nursing diagnoses:

- *Potential for Infection*
- *Impaired Skin Integrity*
- *Impaired Tissue Integrity*

PLANNING

ESTABLISHING PRIORITIES

A basic principle of surgical asepsis is that only sterile items can come in contact with other sterile items. Therefore, whenever sterile equipment must be handled, wearing sterile gloves becomes a necessity.

Sterile gloves should always be worn when touching or caring for an open wound.

SETTING GOALS

- Sterile gloves will not contact nonsterile objects while being donned.
- Gloved hands will be held in front and above the level of the waist.
- Soiled gloves will be removed so as to enclose and contain microbes.

PREPARATION OF
EQUIPMENT

The nurse will need the following:

Package of sterile disposable gloves in the appropriate size.
Work area of sufficient space that is approximately at waist level and free of other
equipment.

Technique for donning and removing sterile gloves

ACTION	RATIONALE
1. Wash and dry hands carefully.	Handwashing deters the spread of microorganisms. Gloves are easier to don when hands are dry.
2. Place sterile glove package on clean, dry surface above your waist.	Moisture could contaminate the sterile gloves. Any sterile object held below the waist is considered contaminated.
3. Open the outside wrapper by carefully peeling the top layer back, as shown in Fig. I-12-1. Remove inner package, handling only the outside of it.	Maintains sterility of gloves in inner packet.
4. Carefully open the inner package and expose the sterile gloves with the cuff end closest to you, as shown in Fig. I-12-2.	The inner surface of the package is considered sterile.

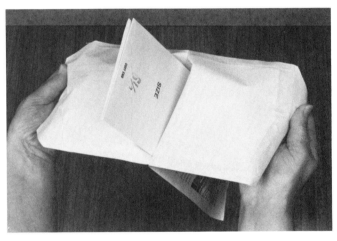

Figure I-12-1 A pair of sterile gloves are contained within this inner wrapper. The nurse peels the outer wrapper to prepare for donning the gloves.

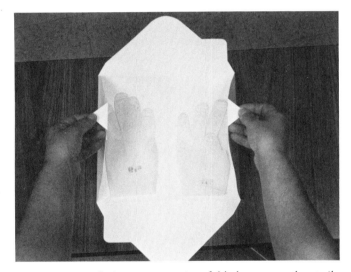

Figure I-12-2 The inner wrapper is unfolded to expose the sterile gloves. They have been carefully packaged so they are in the best position for donning without contamination.

5. With the thumb and forefinger of nondominant hand, grasp the top edge of the folded cuff of the sterile glove for the dominant hand, as shown in Fig. I-12-3.	Unsterile hand only touches inside of glove. Outside remains sterile.
6. Lift and hold glove with fingers down. Be careful it does not touch any unsterile objects.	Glove is contaminated if it touches unsterile object.
7. Carefully insert the dominant hand into the glove and pull it on, as shown in Fig. I-12-4. Leave the cuff folded down until the other hand is gloved.	An attempt to unfold the cuff with unsterile hand may result in contamination of sterile glove.
8. Holding thumb outward, slide fingers of gloved hand under cuff of remaining glove, as shown in Fig. I-12-5, and lift the glove upward.	Thumb is less likely to become contaminated if held outward.

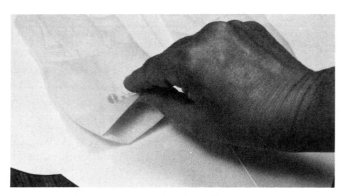

Figure I-12–3 The nurse touches the cuff of the glove that will be worn on the nondominant hand.

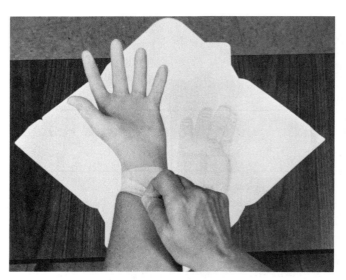

Figure I-12–4 Without touching any unsterile areas or objects, the nurse pulls the glove on while maintaining hold of the cuff of the glove.

9. Carefully insert nondominant hand into glove. Adjust gloves on both hands touching only sterile areas, as shown in Fig. I-12-6.

Sterile surface touching sterile surface prevents contamination.

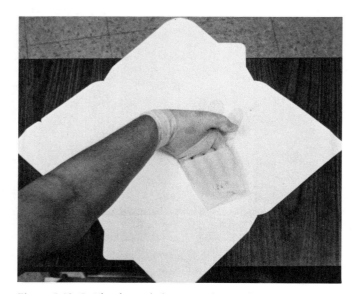

Figure I-12–5 The donned glove must be carefully inserted under the cuff so that it is not contaminated when the ungloved hand is inserted.

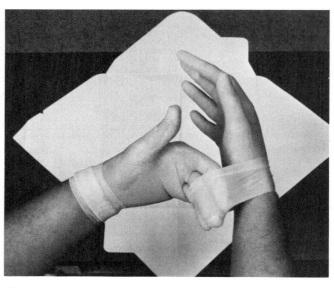

Figure I-12–6 The dominant hand is guided into the remaining glove. While the gloved hand is protected within the cuff, the second glove is stretched and pulled into place.

TO REMOVE GLOVES

1. Using dominant gloved hand, grasp other glove near cuff end and remove by inverting it, as shown in Fig. I-12-7, keeping the contaminated area on the inside.

2. Slide fingers of ungloved hand inside the remaining glove, as shown in Fig. I-12-8. Grasp the glove on the inside, and remove it by turning it inside out.

3. Discard gloves in appropriate container, and wash hands.

Contaminated area will not come in contact with hands or wrists.

Contaminated area does not come in contact with hands or wrists.

Handwashing reduces the spread of microorganisms.

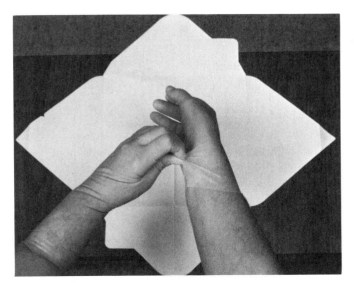

Figure I-12–7 A soiled glove is removed by pulling it inside out.

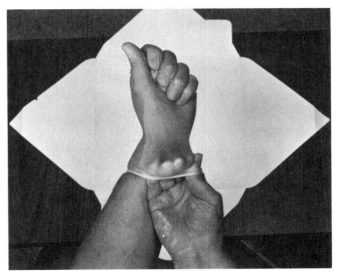

Figure I-12–8 The nurse avoids touching the contaminated surface of the remaining glove by touching only the inside surface.

EVALUATION REASSESSMENT	The nurse must develop an awareness of how gloves are applied and used. Any suspicion that the outside of the sterile gloves has been touched during application or the time of their use requires that they be removed and another sterile pair re-applied.
EXPECTED OUTCOMES	The gloves remain sterile and intact throughout their use. The client does not acquire a nosocomial infection (*i.e.,* an infection that occurs while the client is receiving health care).
UNEXPECTED OUTCOMES	One or both gloves break as a result of inadequate size or defective construction. The gloves touch an unsterile area during the time of their application or use. The gloves become lacerated with sharp equipment.
MODIFICATIONS IN SELECTED SITUATIONS GENERAL VARIATIONS	Nurses who require larger or smaller sizes than those usually purchased by the health agency may request that special sizes be obtained and stocked for their personal use. Reusable sterile gloves are available and are more sturdy. Reusable gloves must be cleaned and resterilized after each use. Discarding reusable gloves adds to an agency's expenses.
HOME-HEALTH VARIATIONS	Assure the availability of sterile gloves if they are needed. Check the expiration dates on the wrappers. Verify that the wrappers are dry and intact. If the area for handwashing is located some distance from the client's bedside, try to avoid touching objects or doorknobs between the areas before donning sterile gloves. If the used gloves are extremely soiled, temporarily dispose of the items in a waste receptacle. Transfer the soiled gloves to another waste container outside the client's residence before terminating the visit.
RELATED TEACHING	Explain that the hands can never be sterilized even with vigorous handwashing. When sterile gloves are used, it should be explained to the client that their use is for his protection.

PERFORMANCE CHECKLIST

When donning and removing sterile gloves, the learner:

C	A	U	
[ ]	[ ]	[ ]	Washes and dries hands.
[ ]	[ ]	[ ]	Obtains a package of sterile gloves in the appropriate size.
[ ]	[ ]	[ ]	Clears a workplace that allows for opening the packet without potential for contact with other articles.
[ ]	[ ]	[ ]	Opens the outer layer of the wrapped gloves.
[ ]	[ ]	[ ]	Unfolds the inner wrapper without touching the gloves.
[ ]	[ ]	[ ]	Positions the package so that the cuffs are closest.
[ ]	[ ]	[ ]	Picks up the glove for the dominant hand at the folded cuff with the nondominant thumb and index finger.
[ ]	[ ]	[ ]	Allows adequate space away from the work area for inserting the fingers.
[ ]	[ ]	[ ]	Holds the fingers of the glove downward.
[ ]	[ ]	[ ]	Inserts the dominant hand into the glove pulling at the cuff to promote adequate coverage of the hand.
[ ]	[ ]	[ ]	Inserts gloved fingers under the cuff of remaining glove resting on the package liner.
[ ]	[ ]	[ ]	Inserts nondominant hand into glove.
[ ]	[ ]	[ ]	Unfolds cuff without touching wrist.
[ ]	[ ]	[ ]	Adjusts fit and removes wrinkles while only touching the sterile surface of one gloved hand to the sterile surface of the other.

To Remove Gloves

[ ]	[ ]	[ ]	Grasps glove near outer wrist area using dominant gloved hand.
[ ]	[ ]	[ ]	Stretches the cuff pulling it inside out during removal.
[ ]	[ ]	[ ]	Holds the removed glove with the dominant hand.
[ ]	[ ]	[ ]	Slides fingers of nondominant hand under the inside of the gloved hand.
[ ]	[ ]	[ ]	Stretches the inner glove surface to facilitate inverting it over the previously removed glove.
[ ]	[ ]	[ ]	Disposes of the soiled gloves in a lined waste receptacle.
[ ]	[ ]	[ ]	Washes hands thoroughly.

Outcome: [ ] Pass   [ ] Fail

C = competent; A = acceptable; U = unsatisfactory

Comments: _____

_____

_____

_____   _____
Student's Signature   Date

_____   _____
Instructor's Signature   Date

I-13   *Donning a sterile gown*

Wearing a sterile gown is the most efficient method of preventing the transmission of organisms from the nurse's uniform to a client. Most sterile gowns are made of cotton and are reused. Once cleaned, the gown is folded to enable its application without contamination and is sterilized. The nurse must take care when unwrapping a sterile gown that only the inner surfaces are touched. Those who assist a nurse with donning a sterile gown must also understand how to provide help without contaminating the gown.

PURPOSES OF PROCEDURE

A sterile gown is donned to:

1. Provide a barrier between organisms on the nurse's uniform and the client.
2. Maintain a microbe-free covering over the nurse's uniform.
3. Prevent a nosocomial infection associated with an invasive procedure, such as surgery.

ASSESSMENT

OBJECTIVE DATA

- Review the agency's procedure manual to determine the recommendation for a sterile gown while performing a specific skill.
- Review the agency's policies concerning special garments worn by surgical, obstetric, and nursery personnel.
- Identify special policies when providing care in a burn, transplant, or oncology unit.

SUBJECTIVE DATA

- A sterile gown may be used if the nurse suspects that the client's immune system or bone marrow function may be severely compromised, but has no objective data indicating this.

RELEVANT NURSING DIAGNOSES

When a situation requires the use of a sterile gown, the nurse is likely caring for a client with one or more of the following nursing diagnoses:

- *Potential for Infection*
- *Potential (or Actual) Impaired Skin Integrity*
- *Potential (or Actual) Impaired Tissue Integrity*

PLANNING

ESTABLISHING PRIORITIES

Many nursing procedures require the nurse's knowledge of the principles of surgical asepsis. Infection control is one of the major challenges among all health-care personnel. The nurse must never take the application of sterile garments lightly. Lax or haphazard sterile technique creates a high potential for risk among clients who depend on nursing integrity for their care.

SETTING GOALS

- The upper anterior surface of the gown will remain free of microbes.
- The client will not be in direct contact with organisms on the surface of the nurse's uniform.

PREPARATION OF EQUIPMENT

The nurse will need to obtain:

A wrapped pack containing a sterile gown.
Another nurse to assist with fastening the gown.

Technique for donning a sterile gown

ACTION	RATIONALE
1. Inspect the tape used to secure the gown. Note that it confirms the sterility of the contents.	When packs are sterilized, a special tape is used which changes color or pattern with heat. Contents should not be used if the tape color remains unchanged when heated.
2. Apply a mask and hair cover, if needed.	Nonsterile garments should be applied first.
3. Perform a surgical scrub when indicated.	A surgical scrub is more effective in removing organisms than simple handwashing.
4. Open the outer wrapper of the package containing a sterile gown, as shown in Fig. I-13-1.	All sterile wraps are removed in such a way as to prevent reaching across the contents and risking contamination.
5. Pick up the sterile gown at the neck area.	The gown is wrapped so that the inside surface of the neck area is uppermost.

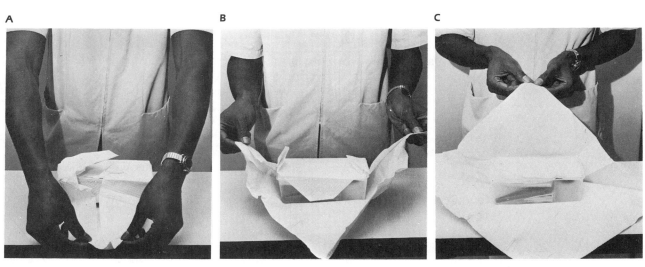

A   B   C

Figure I-13-1 (*A*) The nurse opens a sterile package by folding the top-most part of the wrapper away from the body. This leaves the sterile contents covered. (*B*) The nurse unfolds the next layer of the wrapper to the sides. The sterile contents remain covered by the last layer of wrapper. (*C*) The last layer is unfolded toward the body. The inner surface of the wrapper and the contents are sterile. At no time does the nurse reach across uncovered sterile supplies.

6. Hold the folded gown away from the front of the uniform and other unsterile areas.	The gown could become contaminated if held close to the nurse.
7. Unfold the gown while suspending it above the floor, as shown in Fig. I-13-2.	The floor is a reservoir of dirt and pathogens.
8. Insert an arm into each sleeve without touching the sterile outer surface of the gown.	The inner side of the gown is clean; the outer side must remain sterile.
9. Have an assistant, like the one in Fig. I-13-3, pull the inside of the sleeves to adjust the fit of the gown.	The fit can be adjusted without contamination if the inner surfaces are touched.
10. Using sterile gloves, the assistant may secure the fasteners on the outside of the gown.	The gown must be closed so that the entire uniform is covered. Touching the ties with bare hands would cause contamination.
11. Proceed with applying sterile gloves as described in Procedure I-12.	When a sterile gown is worn, the situation will usually also require sterile gloves.

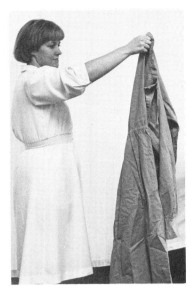

Figure I-13-2 The nurse unfolds a sterile gown while suspending it above the floor away from her uniform. The part being touched will eventually lay against her uniform. The outside of the gown remains sterile.

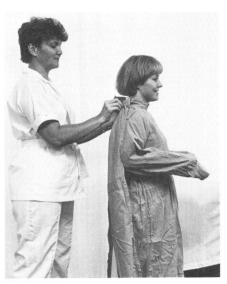

Figure I-13-3 One nurse helps the other adjust a sterile gown. To maintain the sterility of all outer surfaces of the gown, the fasteners will need to be secured while wearing sterile gloves.

EVALUATION	
REASSESSMENT	If it becomes apparent that the gown has become contaminated, the nurse must change the gown immediately.
EXPECTED OUTCOMES	The outside front of the gown remains untouched. No direct contact is made with articles in the physical environment that are likely to contain organisms.
UNEXPECTED OUTCOMES	The gown touches the floor or some other nonsterile object. The gown becomes wet from blood, irrigation solution, or other body secretions. A wet surface acts as a wick and will promote the transfer of underlying organisms to the gown's surface.
MODIFICATIONS IN SELECTED SITUATIONS	After the nurse dons sterile gloves, the assistant may use sterile forceps to hand the gown fasteners to the nurse for securing at the front of the gown.
GENERAL VARIATIONS	
HOME-HEALTH VARIATIONS	Sterile gowns used in the home health-care setting are likely to be made of paper. While they are easier to dispose of after use, paper gowns do not unfold as easily as cotton gowns. If a pack containing a sterile paper gown is transported in the car to the client's home, avoid possible contamination with moisture or sharp objects that can penetrate the pack. Following agency procedure, dispose of the used gown in a waste receptacle in the client's room. If the gown is extremely soiled, transfer the soiled gown to a waste container outside the client's residence at the conclusion of the visit.
RELATED TEACHING	All clients should be informed that sterile gowns are one method for ensuring that the potential for infection has been reduced.

PERFORMANCE CHECKLIST

When donning a sterile gown, the learner:

C	A	U	
[ ]	[ ]	[ ]	Performs thorough handwashing or a surgical scrub.
[ ]	[ ]	[ ]	Applies a cap and mask, if needed.
[ ]	[ ]	[ ]	Opens a package of sterile gloves for application after the gown.
[ ]	[ ]	[ ]	Obtains and confirms the sterility of the wrapped gown package.
[ ]	[ ]	[ ]	Requests an assistant to stand by for help.
[ ]	[ ]	[ ]	Clears sufficient space in which to work.
[ ]	[ ]	[ ]	Opens the pack without contaminating the contents.
[ ]	[ ]	[ ]	Unfolds the gown while holding the inner neck area.
[ ]	[ ]	[ ]	Inserts each arm within the gown.
[ ]	[ ]	[ ]	Pauses while the assistant adjusts the gown.
[ ]	[ ]	[ ]	Dons sterile gloves.
[ ]	[ ]	[ ]	Fastens gown without contamination.

Outcome: [ ] Pass   [ ] Fail

C = competent; A = acceptable; U = unsatisfactory

Comments: _____

_____

_____

_____

_____	_____
Student's Signature	**Date**
_____	_____
Instructor's Signature	**Date**

I-14   *Caring for the client preoperatively*

Clients who undergo surgery range from those who have preplanned, in some cases elective, procedures to those who have unplanned emergency surgery. Surgical clients represent all ages in the life cycle who may be functioning at various levels of health. Nurses must be astute at using the nursing process when caring for preoperative clients. The nurse must assess the presurgical risk factors and the potential alterations associated with the operative procedure. Identifying the client's unique nursing diagnoses forms a basis for planning to restore the client to optimal functioning.

PURPOSES OF PROCEDURE

A nurse provides preoperative care to:

1. Assess the client holistically for biopsychosocial alterations.
2. Obtain a baseline of information with which to compare the client's intraoperative and postoperative responses.
3. Plan and implement measures that prevent, reduce, or eliminate common and unique problems of the surgical client.
4. Provide preoperative teaching to avoid potential complications.
5. Respond to the client's unanswered questions or need for explanation.
6. Provide support to the client and his family during an experience that most find frightening.

ASSESSMENT

OBJECTIVE DATA

- Read the client's health history which includes the present and previous illnesses, prior surgeries, current medications, and so on.
- Examine information on the data base assessment form.
- Review the client's trend in vital signs.
- Assess the client's laboratory test results.
- Observe the client's appearance, state of nutrition, and hydration.
- Refresh one's knowledge of the scheduled surgical procedure by reviewing information in a current surgical reference.
- Determine the availability of the client's support persons.

SUBJECTIVE DATA

- Determine the client's perception and comprehension of the proposed surgical procedure.
- Ask the client questions about his life-style that relate to surgical risks, such as about alcohol and tobacco use.
- Analyze the quantity and quality of stressors in the client's recent experience.

RELEVANT NURSING DIAGNOSES

Examples of nursing diagnoses that may be applicable to clients in the preoperative phase are:

- *Anxiety*
- *Fear*
- *Ineffective Individual Coping*
- *Anticipatory Grieving*
- *Potential for Infection*
- *Knowledge Deficit*
- *Potential Ineffective Airway Clearance*
- *Potential Fluid Volume Deficit*

PLANNING

ESTABLISHING
PRIORITIES

In emergency situations it is not possible to prepare a client as extensively as one would like. The preoperative checklist, shown in Fig. I-14-1, can be used as a guideline for the essential aspects of preoperative care. The aim is to prepare the client safely so that surgery is not delayed. Time and the physical condition of the client dictate those preoperative clients who must be attended to before other nursing responsibilities.

Pre-Op Surgical Checklist

Nurse's Name: _____

O.R.		Comments or Lab Values	Nurses' Initials
	PRE OP HYPO ORDERED		
	NPO AFTER MIDNIGHT OR AS ORDERED		
	I.D. BAND ON PATIENT		
	PRE-OP TEACHING DONE		
	SURGICAL PERMIT SIGNED		
	INFORMED CONSENT SIGNED (IOL OR LASER CASES)		
	OPERATIVE AREA SHAVE PREPPED		
	HISTORY AND PHYSICAL DICTATED		
	CBC REPORT ON CHART	HGB.	
		HCT.	
	URINALYSIS REPORT ON CHART		
	PROFILE REPORT ON CHART IF ORDERED	K+	
	(NORMAL RANGE K+ 3.5 to 5)		
	BLOOD SCREENED _____ TYPED & X MATCHED	Exp. Date / # of Units Set Up	
	PT AND PTT	PT / PTT	
	CHEST X-RAY REPORT ON CHART		
	EKG		
	T _____ P _____ R _____ BP _____		
	DENTURES OR PARTIAL PLATE REMOVED		
	CONTACT LENSES OR GLASSES REMOVED		
	JEWELRY REMOVED OR SECURED		
	HAIR PINS. MAKE UP AND NAIL POLISH REMOVED		
	HEARING AID TO O.R. WITH PATIENT		
	BATHED		
	O.R. GOWN ON PATIENT		
	VOIDED OR CATHETERIZED AND FOLEY EMPTIED		
	PRE-OP ANTIBIOTIC GIVEN IF ORDERED		
	PRE-OP MEDICATION GIVEN		
	ALLERGIES		
	FAMILY O.R. WAITING ROOM		
	OLD CHART TO O.R.		
	X-RAY FILMS FROM FLOOR TO O.R.		

Floor Nurse Sending Patient to O.R.: _____ O.R. Nurse Receiving Patient: _____

Arrival Time: _____

COMMENTS:

Figure I-14-1   This preoperative checklist is an example of most that are used by hospitals. The checklist provides a quick reference on the essential preparation of the preoperative client.

SETTING GOALS

• The client will be prepared physically and emotionally without any delay in the operative schedule.

PREPARATION OF EQUIPMENT

Generally most, but possibly not all, of the following will be needed when caring for the preoperative client:

Consent form
Data base/admission assessment form
Preoperative checklist
Thermometer, stethoscope, and sphygmomanometer for vital signs
Scales for an accurate weight
Urine specimen container, if test is ordered
Denture cup for removing dentures and partial bridgework
Hospital gown, cap, and elastic stockings when required
Skin preparation kit, if required
Syringe and preoperative medications
Intravenous fluid, tubing, and venipuncture device

Technique for caring for the preoperative client

ACTION	RATIONALE
1. Identify clients for whom surgery is a greater risk:	Allows for recognition of clients who may be prone to complications after surgery.
a. Very young and elderly clients	
b. Obese or malnourished clients	
c. Clients with fluid and electrolyte imbalances	
d. Clients in poor general health from chronic diseases and infectious processes	
e. Clients taking certain medications (*i.e.,* anticoagulants, antibiotics, diuretics, depressants, steroids)	
f. Clients who are extremely anxious	
2. Review nursing data base, history, and physical examination. Check that baseline data are recorded.	Identifies clients who are surgical risks.
3. Check that diagnostic testing has been completed and that results are available.	May influence type of surgery and anesthetic as well as timing of surgery or need for additional consultation.
4. Promote optimal nutritional and hydration status.	Promotes wound healing.
5. Identify learning needs of client. Conduct preoperative teaching regarding the following:	Minimizes surgical risk and allays anxiety by preparing clients for postoperative period.
a. Coughing and deep breathing, as shown in Fig. I-14-2.	
b. Management of pain after surgery	
c. Leg exercises and ambulation	
d. Postoperative equipment and monitoring devices.	

DAY BEFORE SURGERY

| 6. Provide emotional support. Answer questions realistically. Provide spiritual assistance if requested. | Allays client's misconceptions and fears. |

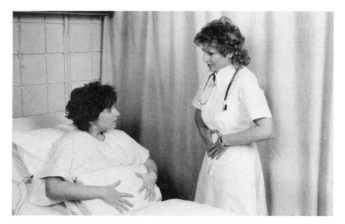

Figure I-14–2   The nurse teaches the client how to splint an incision using a pillow. Supporting the incision reduces pain while deep breathing or coughing.

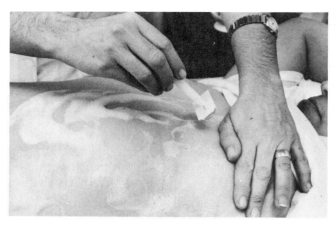

Figure I-14–3   The skin is shaved preoperatively in order to remove hair which harbors microorganisms. Once the integrity of the skin has been compromised during surgery, it is possible for pathogens to enter deeper tissue causing an infection.

7. Follow preoperative dietary restrictions.

Reduces risk of vomiting and aspiration during surgery. Anesthetic agents temporarily depress gastrointestinal function and processes.

8. Prepare for elimination needs during and after surgery.

Anesthetic agents and abdominal surgery interfere with normal elimination function. A urinary catheter inserted preoperatively minimizes risk of inadvertent trauma to bladder during surgery.

9. Shave and prepare the preoperative site, as shown in Fig. I-14-3, if ordered by the physician.

Reduces number of microorganisms present on the skin.

10. Attend to client's special hygiene needs (*i.e.,* use antiseptic cleansing agents).

Decreases potential for infection.

11. Provide for adequate rest.

Minimizes stress prior to surgery.

DAY OF SURGERY

12. Check that proper identification band is on client.

Ensures identity of client.

13. Check that preoperative consent forms are signed and medical record is in order.

Fulfills legal requirement related to informed consent.

14. Check vital signs. Notify physician of any pertinent changes (*e.g.,* rise or drop in blood pressure, elevated temperature, cough, symptoms of infection).

Provides baseline data for comparison.

15. Provide hygiene and oral care. Remind client not to swallow water if NPO for surgery.

Promotes comfort.

16. Continue parenteral nutrition and hydration.

Prepares client for operative procedure.

17. Remove cosmetics and prostheses (*i.e.,* contact lenses, false eyelashes, dentures, and so forth). Assess for loose teeth.

These interfere with assessment and safety during surgery.

18. Have client empty bladder and bowel prior to surgery.

Minimizes risk of injury or complications during and after surgery.

19. Place valuables in appropriate area. Hospital safe is most appropriate place for valuables. They should not be placed in narcotics drawer.

Ensures safety of valuables and personal possessions.

20. Attend to any special preoperative orders.

Prepares client for operative procedure.

21. Complete preoperative checklist, as the nurse in Fig. I-14-4 is doing, and record the client's preoperative preparation.

Ensures accurate documentation.

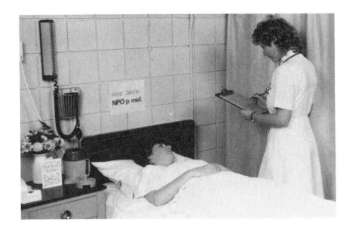

22. Administer preoperative medication as ordered by physician.

Figure I-14-4 The nurse completes a preoperative checklist—a quick and easy way to determine what must still be completed before the client is ready for surgery.

Reduces anxiety, provides sedation, and diminishes respiratory secretions.

SAMPLE DOCUMENTATION

Date	Time	Nurse's note
7/14	0235	15-year-old female admitted through ER accompanied by mother. States, "Having awful pain on R. side." T-103 (0), P-118, R-28, BP 116/70. NPO since last night. 1000 ml of Lactated Ringers infusing at 125 ml/hr in L. arm. Abdomen shaved. Demerol 50 mg. and Phenergan 25 mg. given IM in L. thigh. Preop checklist completed and sent to OR per stretcher. *P. Cleary, RN*

EVALUATION

REASSESSMENT

Before the client leaves the nursing unit, a person from the operating room and the nurse who prepared the client will review the preoperative checklist. Any omitted aspect of the preparation will be clarified before the client is transported. Nurses in the receiving area of the operating room continue to assess, respond, and inform the client as he waits.

EXPECTED OUTCOMES

The client's preparation and routine care are accomplished prior to the scheduled time of surgery.
The client is provided information and explanations that apply to the intraoperative and postoperative period of care.
The client returns the demonstration of effective deep breathing, coughing, and leg exercises.
The client is optimistic about the outcome of the scheduled procedure.

UNEXPECTED OUTCOMES

The client's medical history and physical examination have not been attached to the client's record.
It has not been possible to complete or acquire the results from diagnostic tests.
The objective data reveal a potential health hazard if surgery were to continue as scheduled.

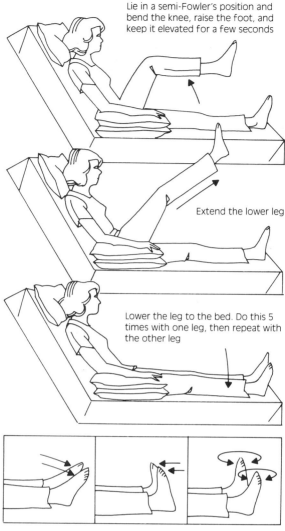

Lie in a semi-Fowler's position and bend the knee, raise the foot, and keep it elevated for a few seconds

Extend the lower leg

Lower the leg to the bed. Do this 5 times with one leg, then repeat with the other leg

A. Point the toes of both feet toward the foot of the bed. Relax both feet

B. Pull toes toward the chin. Relax both feet

C. Make circles with both ankles. First circle to the right, then to the left. Repeat 3 times, Relax feet

Figure I-14–5 This series of drawings explains how to perform leg exercises. The nurse can use a variety of teaching strategies, such as a demonstration and return demonstration or providing the client with a booklet and written instructions.

Legal consent has not been acquired.

The client has recently consumed a quantity of food or liquids.

The client has an unexpected reaction to the preoperative medication.

The client appears extremely frightened or distraught and would benefit from additional teaching or support.

MODIFICATIONS IN SELECTED SITUATIONS

GENERAL VARIATIONS

Many clients are being scheduled for outpatient surgery. Nurses will collect much of the data and provide preoperative teaching a day or more before the surgery.

A plain wedding band can remain on the client's hand. However, it should be secured with tape or gauze so that it cannot fall off.

AGE-RELATED VARIATIONS

A parent or guardian must sign a consent form for a minor.

Children are more likely than adults to have an upper respiratory infection or a communicable disease. Surgery may be postponed if an infection is present.

Use a doll for teaching young children about preoperative, intraoperative, and postoperative care.

Allow a child to take his own stuffed animal, doll, or familiar blanket to the operating room. Communicate with the operating room personnel to promote safe-keeping during surgery and replacement with the child in the recovery room.

Closely observe elderly clients who do not always metabolize or excrete medications as well as others.

HOME-HEALTH VARIATIONS

Clients scheduled for outpatient surgery may perform some preoperative preparation tasks at home, such as self-administering an enema, and bathing or showering with antimicrobial solutions.

RELATED TEACHING

All surgical clients who receive general anesthesia should be taught how to deep breathe, effectively cough, and perform leg exercises, as shown in Fig. I-14-5.

Most hospital clients are fearful of tubes. The nurse should prepare the client for those that are likely to be in place when the client reacts from the anesthesia.

The client should be taught that measures will be used to keep him as comfortable and pain-free as possible. Some forms of analgesics can be instilled through an already established intravenous line and will not require repeated injections.

PERFORMANCE CHECKLIST

When performing preoperative care, the learner:

C	A	U	
[ ]	[ ]	[ ]	Introduces self to the client, his family, and friends.
[ ]	[ ]	[ ]	Checks the client's identification band.
[ ]	[ ]	[ ]	Notes that the water pitcher and glass have been removed from the bedside.
[ ]	[ ]	[ ]	Obtains vital signs and compares them with previous measurements.
[ ]	[ ]	[ ]	Provides privacy when gathering nursing-related information from the client.
[ ]	[ ]	[ ]	Reviews and analyzes the data on the client's record.
[ ]	[ ]	[ ]	Identifies deviations from normal that potentiate surgical risks to the client.
[ ]	[ ]	[ ]	Determines that necessary charts, forms, and laboratory test results are completed.
[ ]	[ ]	[ ]	Notifies appropriate persons when the client's record is incomplete.
[ ]	[ ]	[ ]	Witnesses the consent form.
[ ]	[ ]	[ ]	Teaches the client about: a. Dietary and fluid restrictions b. Deep breathing and coughing c. Leg exercises d. Postoperative equipment and monitoring e. Pain management
[ ]	[ ]	[ ]	Provides the opportunity for personal hygiene, such as bathing and mouth care.
[ ]	[ ]	[ ]	Removes fingernail polish.
[ ]	[ ]	[ ]	Instructs the client to remove any hairpins and artificial items that interfere with assessment.
[ ]	[ ]	[ ]	Assists the client to don a hospital gown and cap.
[ ]	[ ]	[ ]	Prepares the client's skin.

C = competent; A = acceptable; U = unsatisfactory

(Continued)

PERFORMANCE CHECKLIST (Continued)

C	A	U	
[ ]	[ ]	[ ]	Removes or secures rings.
[ ]	[ ]	[ ]	Completes a witnessed inventory and receipt for valuables.
[ ]	[ ]	[ ]	Requests that security personnel deposit valuables within the hospital safe.
[ ]	[ ]	[ ]	Suggests bowel and bladder elimination.
[ ]	[ ]	[ ]	Administers preoperative medications.
[ ]	[ ]	[ ]	Raises the side rails and informs the client to remain on bed rest.
[ ]	[ ]	[ ]	Instructs the client to refrain from smoking.
[ ]	[ ]	[ ]	Provides a cup for the removal of dentures and bridgework before the client is transported to the operating room.

Outcome: [ ] Pass   [ ] Fail

C = competent; A = acceptable; U = unsatisfactory

Comments: _____
_____
_____

_____   _____
Student's Signature   **Date**

_____   _____
Instructor's Signature   **Date**

I-15

Caring for the client postoperatively upon returning to the room

Surgery and anesthesia, though necessary to improve a client's health problem, carry potential risks. The client may also experience unique problems such as pain postoperatively that were not present preoperatively. The nurse implements the nursing process, providing specific skills for caring for the client postoperatively.

PURPOSES OF PROCEDURE

Postoperative care is performed in order to

1. Assess alterations in the client's condition that imply possible complications.
2. Assist the client react and recover from anesthesia safely.
3. Monitor and implement therapeutic measures that promote the restoration of the client's health.
4. Reduce or eliminate the discomfort the client is experiencing.
5. Prevent complications.

ASSESSMENT

OBJECTIVE DATA

- Check the equipment, supplies, and readiness of the room.
- Communicate with the recovery room nurse concerning the stability of the client and the client's progress since leaving the operating room.
- Read the postoperative written medical orders and the summary of the client's condition.
- Identify family members and determine their location.

SUBJECTIVE DATA

- Assess the client's description of discomfort, such as pain, coldness, full bladder, tenderness around the IV site, and so on.
- Analyze the client's and family's response to the outcomes of the surgical procedure based on the information provided by the surgeon.

RELEVANT NURSING DIAGNOSES

Most postoperative clients will have one or several of the following nursing diagnoses:

- *Potential Activity Intolerance*
- *Potential Ineffective Airway Clearance*
- *Altered Comfort*
- *Potential Ineffective Coping*
- *Potential Fluid Volume Deficit*
- *Potential for Infection*
- *Potential for Injury*
- *Impaired Physical Mobility*
- *Potential for Altered Nutrition: Less than Body Requirements*
- *Self-Care Deficit*
- *Sleep Pattern Disturbance*
- *Potential for Altered Tissue Perfusion*
- *Potential for Altered Patterns of Urinary Elimination*

PLANNING

ESTABLISHING PRIORITIES

Because the postoperative client's safety is largely dependent on the nurse, the client's care demands immediate and frequent attention.

SETTING GOALS

- The client's basic needs will be met while recovering from anesthesia.
- The client's safety will be maintained as the level of consciousness improves.
- The client will receive analgesia as prescribed to control discomfort.

PREPARATION OF EQUIPMENT

The following equipment should be available when preparing to care for the postoperative client upon return to the room:

Fresh linen fanfolded to the side of a bed in high position
Emesis basin, tissues, and wastepaper bag at the bedside
Call light attached to the bed in working condition
Fresh water or container of ice
Intake and output recording sheet
Graduated pitcher for measuring urinary output
IV pole, oxygen flow meter, suction machine, if necessary
Sphygmomanometer and stethoscope

Technique for caring for the client postoperatively upon returning to the room

ACTION	RATIONALE
1. Place the client in a safe position on the side with face down and neck slightly extended. Note the client's level of consciousness.	This prevents aspiration of vomitus and airway obstruction.
2. Monitor vital signs and other pertinent information (Fig. I-15-1) frequently. Record information. Assessment order may vary but the usual frequency includes taking vital signs every 15 minutes the first hour, every 30 minutes the next 2 hours, every hour for 4 hours, and finally, every 4 hours.	Comparison with baseline preoperative vital signs may indicate impending shock or hemorrhage.
3. Provide for warmth. Assess skin color and condition.	Depressed level of functioning results in a fall in body temperature.
4. Check dressings for color, odor, and amount of drainage and feel under the client for bleeding, as the nurse in Figure I-15-2 is doing.	Hemorrhage and shock are life-threatening complications of surgery.

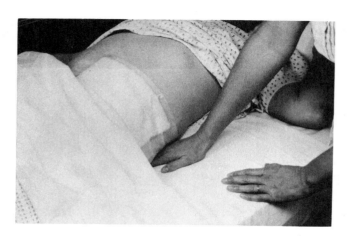

Figure I-15-2 Blood will drain to lower levels under the influence of gravity. Although the dressing may appear dry, by placing the hand under the client, it may be possible for the nurse to assess excessive blood loss from a wound.

Name _____

M.R. # _____

POST-OP
PROGRESS FLOW RECORD

DATE									
TIME									
BP									
PULSE									
RESPIRATIONS									
TEMPERATURE									
I.V.									
WOUND									
DRAIN (S)									
LOC									
PAIN									
NAUSEA									
FOLEY/ OTHER CATH OR VOIDING									
TURN, COUGH DEEP BREATHE									
MOVES ALL EXTREMITIES									
Initials									

Key _____ _____

_____ _____

640-044-830/0800751

Figure I-15-1 This postoperative flow sheet helps the nurse to perform focused assessments following a client's surgery. It helps to have all the data in one place to make quick comparisons and identify trends that are occurring.

5. Verify that all tubes are patent and equipment is operative.

This ensures maintenance of vital functions.

6. Maintain the intravenous infusion at the correct rate.

This provides nutrition and prevents dehydration and electrolyte imbalances.

7. Provide for a safe environment. Keep the bed in the low position with side rails up. Have the call bell within the client's reach. Have a "No Smoking" sign posted if the client is receiving oxygen.

This prevents accidental injury.

8. Relieve pain by administering medications ordered by the physician. Check the record to verify if analgesic medication was administered in the recovery room.

Analgesics are used for relief of postoperative pain.

9. Record assessments and interventions on the chart.

This provides for accurate documentation.

GENERAL

10. Promote optimal respiratory function:

Anesthetic agents may depress respiratory function. Clients who have existing respiratory or cardiovascular disease, abdominal or chest incisions, or are obese, elderly, or in a poor state of nutrition are at greater risk of developing respiratory complications.

    a. Coughing and deep breathing

    b. Use of incentive spirometry

    c. Early ambulation

    d. Frequent position change

    e. Administration of oxygen as ordered.

11. Maintain adequate circulation:

Preventive measures can improve venous return and the circulatory status.

    a. Maintenance of IV therapy

    b. Early ambulation

    c. Application of antiembolic stockings if ordered by the physician

    d. Leg exercises and range-of-motion exercises if not contraindicated

12. Assess urinary elimination status:

Anesthetic agents may temporarily depress bladder tone and response.

    a. Promote voiding by offering the bedpan or urinal at regular intervals.

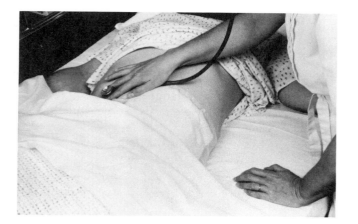

Figure I-15-3 This nurse is auscultating bowel sounds to determine if peristalsis is returning.

b. Monitor catheter drainage if present.

c. Measure intake and output.

13. Promote optimal nutritional status and return of gastrointestinal function:

Anesthetic agents depress peristalsis and normal functioning of the gastrointestinal tract.

a. Assess for return of peristalsis, as shown in Figure I-15-3.

b. Assist with diet progression.

c. Encourage fluid intake.

d. Monitor intake.

e. Medicate for nausea and vomiting as ordered by the physician.

14. Promote wound healing:

Alterations in nutritional, circulatory, and metabolic status may predispose clients to infection and delayed healing.

a. Use surgical asepsis.

b. Assess the condition of the wound.

c. Assess any drainage.

15. Provide for rest and comfort.

This shortens the recovery period and facilitates the return to normal function.

16. Provide emotional and spiritual support.

This facilitates individualized care and the client's return to normal health.

SAMPLE DOCUMENTATION

Date	*Time*	*Nurse's note*
11/09	1340	Returned from recovery room by stretcher. Lethargic but able to assist with transfer to bed. BP 110/72, P-88, R-16. Skin warm and pink. IV infusing well @ 125 ml/hr. Foley catheter to gravity drainage. O$_2$ @ 3 L per nasal cannula. Family at bedside.
		E. Mohr, RN

EVALUATION

REASSESSMENT

The client's condition should be reassessed every 15 minutes for the first hour. If the client's vital signs are unstable, it may be necessary to reassess every 5 minutes. If the vital signs are stable, the client may be reassessed every 30 to 60 minutes according to the agency's policies and procedures.

EXPECTED OUTCOMES

The client's vital signs remain stable and in a range similar to preoperative recordings.
The client is alert, oriented, and responds appropriately to questions or requests.
The client performs deep breathing and leg exercises every 2 hours while awake.
The client's discomfort is maintained within a tolerable range.
The client is able to take fluids and nourishment without nausea, vomiting, or distention.
The client voids within 8 hours of surgery if there is no indwelling catheter.
The client is able to dangle the legs or ambulate within the room on the evening of surgery.

UNEXPECTED OUTCOMES

The client's breathing becomes noisy or labored.
The client's pulse becomes irregular.
The client's vital signs are recorded above or below the ranges for his age.

There is bright red bleeding from the incisional area.

There is less than 50 ml of urine excreted per hour.

Pain, nausea, or vomiting is unrelieved with prescribed measures.

MODIFICATIONS IN SELECTED SITUATIONS

GENERAL VARIATIONS

The bed of a client undergoing orthopedic surgery may be taken to the operating room. The client is then returned to the room in the hospital bed with mechanical devices attached.

Unstable clients or those with complicated procedures may be cared for temporarily in an intensive care unit.

Clients who require emergency surgery or whose surgery may extend beyond the usual staffing time of the recovery room personnel may be observed and cared for in the intensive care unit until stable enough to be sent to the general nursing unit.

Clients undergoing ambulatory surgery will be discharged as soon as they have reacted and are stable.

AGE-RELATED VARIATIONS

Children recover postoperatively in a crib rather than in an adult bed or stretcher.

Parents may be allowed to be with a child in the recovery room.

Expect that elderly or debilitated clients may take longer to react and stabilize after surgery.

HOME-HEALTH VARIATIONS

Remind the client and family that the postoperative individual is not to drive or operate equipment or dangerous appliances for 24 to 36 hours following surgery.

Reinforce the teaching about signs and symptoms of infection and potential complications. Provide the client with a phone number for contacting the nurse or physician if problems should develop.

RELATED TEACHING

Each assessment and its results should be explained at the level and extent to which the client or family is capable of understanding.

Reinforcement of deep breathing, coughing, and leg exercises may be required from time to time if the nurse observes that the client is not performing them correctly.

Explain the principles of measuring intake and output in order to gain the client's cooperation. The client may help record the type and volume of oral liquids on the bedside form. Tell the client that urine should be saved for measuring rather than flushed.

The purpose and schedule of medications may be explained. This is especially important when the client requires relief from pain.

Ambulatory surgical clients should have a thorough understanding of their postoperative care and what symptoms warrant immediate reporting. A written sheet of instructions is recommended as a later reference for the client who may not recall all the necessary verbal information.

Teach the client, family, and friends that smoking is not allowed when oxygen is in use.

PERFORMANCE CHECKLIST

When providing postoperative care, the learner:

C	A	U	
[ ]	[ ]	[ ]	Provides privacy
[ ]	[ ]	[ ]	Calls the client by name and identifies self even if the client seems unresponsive
[ ]	[ ]	[ ]	Washes hands
[ ]	[ ]	[ ]	Positions the client on the side or abdomen if the oral airway is still in place or the client does not seem to be aroused with stimulation
[ ]	[ ]	[ ]	Measures and records blood pressure, pulse, and respiration; takes the temperature if the client is shivering or perspiring or has required hypothermic techniques
[ ]	[ ]	[ ]	Checks the color of the skin and nailbeds
[ ]	[ ]	[ ]	Observes the dressing for bleeding or drainage
[ ]	[ ]	[ ]	Attaches tubes to suction or gravity drainage
[ ]	[ ]	[ ]	Counts intravenous fluid drip rate and confirms that the site is patent and the volume is infusing on schedule
[ ]	[ ]	[ ]	Lowers the bed to low position and raises the side rails
[ ]	[ ]	[ ]	Orients the client to the location of the call bell for assistance
[ ]	[ ]	[ ]	Asks the client to describe level of comfort
[ ]	[ ]	[ ]	Encourages the client to deep breathe and move legs about
[ ]	[ ]	[ ]	Applies antiembolism stockings if ordered
[ ]	[ ]	[ ]	Regulates the administration of humidified oxygen
[ ]	[ ]	[ ]	Washes hands
[ ]	[ ]	[ ]	Records initial assessments
[ ]	[ ]	[ ]	Reassesses the client in increments of time appropriate to the client's condition
[ ]	[ ]	[ ]	Provides mouth swabs or mouth care and oral liquids if allowed
[ ]	[ ]	[ ]	Responds to the client's requests for pain relief, elimination, position change, additional warmth, and so on; notes the response of the client to selected measures
[ ]	[ ]	[ ]	Shares significant information on the client's condition with unit personnel and client's family

Outcome: [ ] Pass   [ ] Fail

C = competent; A = acceptable; U = unsatisfactory

Comments: _____

_____

_____

_____   _____
            Student's Signature   Date

_____   _____
          Instructor's Signature   Date

Administering intravenous fluids and medications

Water is necessary for sustaining life. Many chemicals, such as electrolytes, are distributed within a person's body fluid. When fluid is lost, both the water and the dissolved substances within it require replacement. The nurse is frequently required to plan and implement measures to maintain or restore a client's fluid balance. The intravenous route can also be used to administer dissolved medications for rapid circulation and action.

I-16   *Starting an intravenous infusion*

Fluid replacement as well as medications are prescribed by the physician. It is the nurse's responsibility to access the circulatory system by venipuncture in order to carry out the medical order.

PURPOSES OF PROCEDURE

Starting an intravenous (IV) infusion is performed to

1. Administer fluids and chemical substances when circumstances prevent the client from consuming a normal diet and oral liquids
2. Replace fluids and chemical substances when the client has experienced their loss through vomiting, diarrhea, bleeding, and so on
3. Provide a source of calories for energy when oral consumption is restricted
4. Provide access to the circulatory system if it becomes necessary to administer emergency medications
5. Maintain an access to the circulatory system for the intermittent administration of scheduled medications

ASSESSMENT

OBJECTIVE DATA

- Read the written medical order and identify the volume and type of solution, additives, and the rate of infusion.
- Assess the client's cardiac status, such as blood pressure, pulse rate, and other hemodynamic measurements that are available, such as central venous pressure (CVP) or pulmonary capillary wedge pressure (PCWP), and hematocrit.
- Note the client's renal status, such as the output for the previous day or the trend in hourly output, and the specific gravity of urine.
- Observe the client's level of consciousness and activity to determine the need to use measures for preventing infiltration.
- Weigh the client; examine the skin turgor and the moistness of the mucous membranes.
- Assess the client's respiratory rate. Observe the effort of breathing. Auscultate lung sounds.
- Determine whether it is necessary to use a filter within the infusion tubing.
- Identify the manufacturer's drop factor.
- Identify the client's dominant hand.
- Note any treatment or pathology in an extremity that contraindicates use of the extremity for venipuncture, such as a mastectomy or an arteriovenous fistula used for hemodialysis.
- Determine the client's prior sensitivity to additives in the solution, antimicrobial ointments, or adhesive tape.
- Examine potential infusion sites for the presence of scars, bruises, or swelling. Note the size and condition of the veins.

SUBJECTIVE DATA

- Determine the client's ability to understand an explanation of the procedure.
- Assess the client's perception, anxiety, and fear associated with an IV infusion.
- Ask the client to describe pain or tenderness in a potential infusion site.

RELEVANT NURSING DIAGNOSES

The nurse can consider the following nursing diagnoses as applicable for those clients who require the infusion of IV fluids or medications:

- *Fluid Volume Deficit*
- *Altered Cardiac Output: Decreased*
- *Altered Nutrition: Less than Body Requirements*
- *Altered Oral Mucous Membranes*
- *Self-Care Deficit*
- *Impaired Swallowing*

PLANNING

ESTABLISHING PRIORITIES

Fluid replacement orders should be implemented immediately for those clients who are experiencing severe hypovolemia. The need for priority attention is often related to obvious high volume loss, such as in a burn or hemorrhage, declining vital signs, and a renal output that is <30 ml to 50 ml per hour.

SETTING GOALS

- The solution will infuse safely at the prescribed rate.
- The venipuncture site will remain nontender throughout the infusion.

PREPARATION OF EQUIPMENT

The following equipment should be assembled when preparing to start an IV infusion:

IV solution
IV tubing
IV pole
Needle (angiocatheter, standard needle, butterfly)
Tourniquet
Antiseptic swabs
Tape
Infusion or controller pump, if required
Dressings with povidone–iodine (Betadine) or other antiseptic ointment
Armboard, if needed
Clean, disposable gloves

Technique for starting an intravenous infusion

ACTION	RATIONALE
1. Gather all equipment and bring to the bedside. Check the IV solution and medication additives with the physician's order.	Having equipment available saves time and facilitates accomplishment of the task. Checking ensures that the client receives the correct IV solution and medication as ordered by the physician.
2. Explain the procedure to the client.	Explanation allays the client's anxiety.
3. Wash your hands.	Handwashing deters the spread of microorganisms.
4. Prepare the IV solution and tubing:	
a. Maintain aseptic technique when opening sterile packages and IV solution.	This prevents the spread of microorganisms.
b. Clamp tubing, as shown in Figure I-16-1; uncap the spike and insert it into the entry site on the bag, as shown in Figure I-16-2, or bottle as the manufacturer directs.	This punctures the seal in the IV bag or bottle.
c. Squeeze the drip chamber and allow it to fill at least halfway.	Suction effect causes fluid to move into the drip chamber and also prevents air from moving down the tubing.
d. Remove the cap at the end of the tubing, release the clamp, and allow the fluid to move through the tubing. Allow fluid to flow until all air bubbles have disappeared. Close the clamp and recap the end of the tubing, maintaining sterility of the set-up.	This removes air from the tubing, which can, in larger amounts, act as an air embolus.

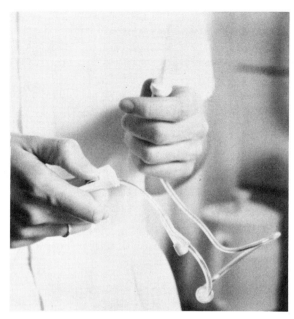

Figure I-16–1 Before the spike is inserted into the solution, the tubing is clamped by tightening the roller clamp.

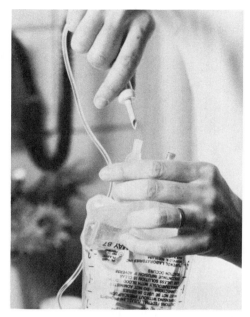

Figure I-16–2 The nurse prepares to insert the spike into a bag of solution.

e. If an infusion or controller pump is to be used, follow the manufacturer's instructions for inserting tubing and setting the infusion rate.

5. Have the client in a supine or low Fowler's position in bed.

6. Select an appropriate site and palpate accessible veins, as illustrated in Figure I-16-3.

7. If the site is hairy and agency policy permits, shave a 2-inch area around the intended site of entry.

8. Apply a tourniquet 2 to 3 inches above the venipuncture site to obstruct venous blood flow and distend the vein. Direct the ends of the tourniquet away from the site of entry. Check to be sure that the radial pulse is still present.

9. Ask the client to open and close his fist. Observe and palpate for a suitable vein. Try the following techniques if a vein cannot be felt:

a. Release the tourniquet and have the client lower his arm below the level of the heart to fill the veins. Reapply the tourniquet and gently tap over the intended vein to help distend it.

b. Remove the tourniquet and place warm compresses over the intended vein for 10 to 15 minutes.

10. Don clean, disposable gloves.

This ensures the correct flow rate and proper use of equipment.

The supine position permits either arm to be used and allows for good body alignment. The low Fowler's position is usually the most comfortable for the client.

The selection of an appropriate site decreases discomfort for the client and possible damage to body tissues.

It is difficult to clean the site of entry in the presence of hair because hair can harbor microorganisms. Adhesive tape will adhere better and may be removed more easily if hair is removed from the site.

Interrupting the blood flow to the heart causes the vein to distend. Interruption of the arterial flow will impede venous filling. Distended veins are easy to see, palpate, and enter. The end of the tourniquet could contaminate the area of injection if directed toward the site of entry.

Contraction of the muscles of the forearm forces blood into the veins, thereby distending them further. Lowering the arm below the level of the heart, tapping the vein, and applying warmth help distend veins by filling them with blood.

Care must be used when handling any blood or body fluids to prevent transmission of HIV and other blood-borne infections.

11. Cleanse the entry site with an antiseptic solution. Use a circular motion to move from the center outward for several inches.

Cleansing that begins at the site of entry and moves outward in a circular motion carries organisms away from the site of entry. Organisms on the skin can be introduced into the tissues or bloodstream with the needle.

12. Use your nondominant hand, placed about 1 or 2 inches below the entry site, to hold the skin taut against the vein.

Pressure on the vein and surrounding tissues helps in preventing movement of the vein as the needle is being inserted.

13. Enter the skin gently with the needle held in your dominant hand, bevel side up, at a 30-degree to 45-degree angle, and when the needle is through the skin, lower the needle until it is nearly parallel to the skin. This step is illustrated in Figure I-16-4. While following the course of the vein, advance the needle or catheter into the vein. A sensation of "give" can be felt when the needle enters the vein.

This allows the needle to enter the vein with minimal trauma and deters passage of the needle through the vein.

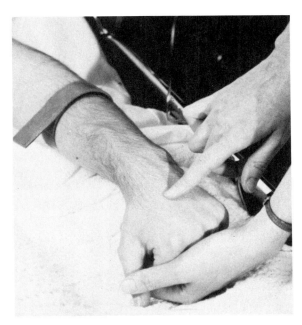

Figure I-16–3 The client's veins are assessed before selecting one for venipuncture.

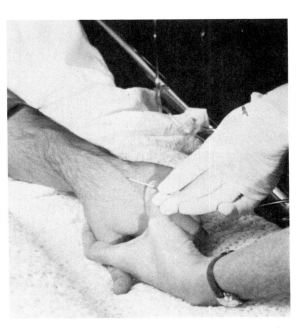

Figure I-16–4 The nurse punctures the vein. The needle is held so that it can be threaded within the blood vessel.

14. When blood returns through the lumen of the needle, advance the needle further into the vein. The exact technique depends on the needle used. With an angiocatheter, the needle is removed leaving the catheter in place.

The tourniquet causes increased venous pressure resulting in automatic backflow. Having the needle placed well into the vein helps prevent dislodgement of the needle.

15. Quickly remove the protective cap from the IV tubing and attach the tubing to the catheter or needle with your nondominant hand and release the tourniquet with your other hand.

Bleeding is minimized and patency of the vein is maintained if the connection is made smoothly between the catheter and tubing.

16. Start the flow of solution promptly by releasing the clamp on the tubing. Examine the tissue around the entry site for signs of infiltration.

Blood will clot readily if IV flow is not maintained. If the needle accidentally slips out of the vein, solution will accumulate and infiltrate into surrounding tissue.

17. Support the needle with a small piece of gauze under the hub, if necessary, to keep the needle properly positioned in the vein.

The pressure of the wall of the vein against the bevel of the needle will interrupt the rate of flow of the solution. The wall of the vein can be easily punctured by the needle.

18. An antiseptic ointment may be applied to the needle's site of entry with a sterile dressing according to agency policy. Remove soiled gloves and discard appropriately.

Dressing and antiseptic ointment reduce skin contamination and protect against infection.

19. Loop the tubing near the site of entry, and anchor it with tape to prevent pull on the needle, as illustrated in Figure I-16-5.

The smooth structure of the vein does not offer resistance to the movement of the needle. The weight of the tubing is sufficient to pull the needle out of the vein if it is not well anchored.

20. Mark the date, time, and type and size of the needle used for the infusion on the tape anchoring the tubing, as shown in Figure I-16-6.

Personnel working with the infusion will know what type of needle is being used and when it was inserted. This protects the client and IV site from infection.

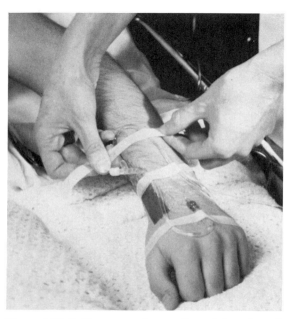

Figure I-16-5 To prevent the needle and the tubing from being caught on objects and pulled from the vein, the nurse secures the tubing by anchoring it to the skin.

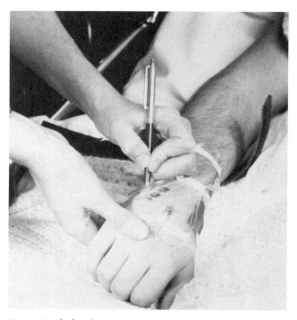

Figure I-16-6 The nurse writes the date, time, type and size of the needle, and initials. This information provides a quick source of information to determine when an IV site should be changed.

21. Anchor the arm to an armboard for support, if necessary.

An armboard protects against change in the position of the vein and acts as a reminder to the client to minimize arm movements.

22. Adjust the rate of solution flow according to the amount prescribed, or follow the manufacturer's directions for adjusting the flow rate on an infusion pump.

The physician prescribes the rate of flow.

23. Remove all equipment and dispose in the proper manner. Wash your hands.

Handwashing deters the spread of microorganisms.

24. Document the procedure and the client's response. Chart the time, site, device used, solution, and rate of flow.

This provides accurate documentation and ensures continuity of care.

25. Return to check flow rate and observe for infiltration $\frac{1}{2}$ hour after starting infusion.

This documents the client's response to the infusion.

SAMPLE DOCUMENTATION

Date	Time	Nurse's note
12/04	1350	#20 angiocath inserted into left dorsal metacarpal vein. 1000 ml of Lactated Ringer's infusing at 125 ml per hour.
		N. English, RN

EVALUATION

REASSESSMENT

The client's condition and the progress of the infusion should be reassessed within 30 minutes after the infusion has been initiated. The frequency of focus assessments, such as vital signs and urine output, depend on the acuity of the client's condition. The infusion may be assessed at hourly intervals to determine that the rate has not slowed or accelerated. The condition of the venipuncture site should be noted and documented by each nurse assigned to the client's care.

EXPECTED OUTCOMES

The fluid infuses according to schedule.

The client's intake approximates the output.

The client's lung sounds remain clear.

The client's blood pressure and pulse return to or are maintained within normal ranges.

The IV site is free of discomfort.

UNEXPECTED OUTCOMES

The venipuncture is not successfully inserted within a vein.

The solution stops infusing.

The rate of the infusion slows or speeds more than 25% of the hourly prescribed rate.

The client's output is <30 ml to 50 ml per hour.

The client's vital signs rise or fall beyond normal ranges.

The client develops difficulty breathing or adventitious lung sounds are heard.

The IV site becomes warm, swollen, or tender, or drainage is noted.

MODIFICATIONS IN SELECTED SITUATIONS

GENERAL VARIATIONS

The client's dominant hand may be used for an IV infusion if extenuating circumstances, such as a prior amputation, interfere with the use of the nondominant side.

The veins of the leg are generally not recommended for use because dependent distal circulation is often impaired or slow. Leg veins are more prone to the formation of thrombi. However, if veins are not accessible in either hand or arm, a leg vein may be the nurse's only choice.

The antecubital vein may be used when other distal sites in the hand or arm are unavailable and the solution is scheduled to infuse in a few hours.

Select a large vein and gauge of needle if the solution is to infuse rapidly or is viscous or likely to irritate the vein due to its concentration.

Use a filter in the IV tubing if the solution contains an additive or component that may form a precipitate.

Hair around the venipuncture site can be trimmed using scissors rather than shaved with a razor.

Transparent dressing material, such as Opsite, may be used to facilitate better assessment of the venipuncture site.

The IV tubing can be labeled with a piece of tape indicating the date, time, and nurse's initials to promote changing the equipment at intervals no longer than 48 hours.

Use 500-ml containers when the rate of infusion is so slow that an entire 1000-ml container will not infuse in 24 hours.

Change any containers of fluid that have hung 24 hours regardless of the volume remaining. This reduces the possibility of pathogen growth within the fluid.

AGE-RELATED
VARIATIONS

Scalp veins may be used in infants to prevent the child from dislocating the needle.

A thick rubberband about the skull, rather than a tourniquet, may be used to distend the scalp veins of an infant.

Use a papoose board or a bath blanket around the arms and chest to temporarily restrain a child before starting an IV infusion.

A hospitalized child should be taken to a treatment room when an IV solution is to be started. This practice helps the child to conclude that his room is a haven from procedures that cause pain or discomfort.

The rate of an infusion is likely to be slower for pediatric and geriatric clients to avoid overloading the circulatory system.

The size and type of venipuncture device may need to be adjusted according to the size and condition of the client's veins. It is not unusual for the veins of elderly clients to be thin walled and fragile.

Protect the venipuncture site, secure the tubing well, and restrain the hand and arm to an armboard to prevent dislodgement when the client is a child or highly active adult.

HOME-HEALTH
VARIATIONS

The nurse in the health-care agency will need to refer the client who requires fluid or IV therapy to a home-health agency prior to discharge.

A heparin lock or port on a long line catheter is often utilized to administer home infusions of IV solutions.

A bottle of isopropyl alcohol and cotton pledgets may be used at home for cleansing the port of a heparin lock.

A peg or hook attached to a wall, door frame, or post may be used to suspend the container of solution.

Make armboard or wristboard splints by covering the IV tubing box with a hand towel or by forming a washcloth into a roll to support the hand.

RELATED TEACHING

Explain the purpose(s) for the infusion and each step before it is performed.

Inform the client of the signs or symptoms that should be reported, such as pain or swelling.

Indicate when a solution or medication can cause irritation or discomfort during its infusion.

PERFORMANCE CHECKLIST

When starting an IV infusion, the learner:

C	*A*	*U*	
[ ]	[ ]	[ ]	Checks the written medical order
[ ]	[ ]	[ ]	Gathers the appropriate solution, tubing, and venipuncture supplies
[ ]	[ ]	[ ]	Explains the procedure to the client
[ ]	[ ]	[ ]	Delivers a portable pole to the room or attaches a stationary IV pole to the client's bed
[ ]	[ ]	[ ]	Provides the client the opportunity to use the bedpan, urinal, or toilet
[ ]	[ ]	[ ]	Applies a gown with sleeves that allows for changing without interfering with the infusion equipment
[ ]	[ ]	[ ]	Washes hands
[ ]	[ ]	[ ]	Tightens the roller clamp on the tubing
[ ]	[ ]	[ ]	Removes the protective coverings from the solution container and tubing without contamination
[ ]	[ ]	[ ]	Connects the tubing to the solution container
[ ]	[ ]	[ ]	Partially fills the drip chamber

C = competent; A = acceptable; U = unsatisfactory

PERFORMANCE CHECKLIST (Continued)

C	A	U	
[ ]	[ ]	[ ]	Opens the clamp and flushes air from the tubing
[ ]	[ ]	[ ]	Hangs the fluid container from the IV pole
[ ]	[ ]	[ ]	Assists the client to a low Fowler's position
[ ]	[ ]	[ ]	Tears pieces of tape for securing the venipuncture device and tubing, and prepares dressing material for covering the site
[ ]	[ ]	[ ]	Raises the bed to a height that promotes proper posture for the nurse
[ ]	[ ]	[ ]	Inspects the client's veins
[ ]	[ ]	[ ]	Selects an appropriate distal site on the hand or arm
[ ]	[ ]	[ ]	Places a clean towel under the hand and arm for absorbing blood
[ ]	[ ]	[ ]	Applies a tourniquet and utilizes other appropriate methods for distending the vein
[ ]	[ ]	[ ]	Dons clean, disposable gloves
[ ]	[ ]	[ ]	Cleanses the site according to proper principles of medical asepsis
[ ]	[ ]	[ ]	Stabilizes the selected vein
[ ]	[ ]	[ ]	Inserts the venipuncture device through the skin and guides its advancement into the vein
[ ]	[ ]	[ ]	Observes for a flashback of blood and threads the needle or catheter within the vein
[ ]	[ ]	[ ]	Compresses the skin over the top of the device to reduce the backflow of blood
[ ]	[ ]	[ ]	Connects the tubing to the venipuncture device without contaminating the tubing or dislodging the needle or catheter
[ ]	[ ]	[ ]	Releases the tourniquet
[ ]	[ ]	[ ]	Opens the roller clamp to allow the slow but gradual infusion of solution
[ ]	[ ]	[ ]	Notes that dripping continues from the container and that the site does not become swollen
[ ]	[ ]	[ ]	Applies a dressing with antiseptic ointment over the venipuncture site
[ ]	[ ]	[ ]	Removes gloves
[ ]	[ ]	[ ]	Secures the dressing and tubing with strips of tape
[ ]	[ ]	[ ]	Adjusts the flow of the infusion to the prescribed rate
[ ]	[ ]	[ ]	Labels the tubing and dressing with required information
[ ]	[ ]	[ ]	Restrains the arm or hand if necessary
[ ]	[ ]	[ ]	Lowers the bed and provides the client with access to the signal device
[ ]	[ ]	[ ]	Returns or disposes of supplies
[ ]	[ ]	[ ]	Records the appropriate information on client's chart

Outcome: [ ] Pass   [ ] Fail

C = competent; A = acceptable; U = unsatisfactory

Comments: _____
_____
_____

_____   _____
Student's Signature   Date

_____   _____
Instructor's Signature   Date

I-17   *Regulating intravenous flow rate*

Before the infusion of the intravenous (IV) solution is begun, the nurse should mathematically convert the rate of infusion prescribed by the physician into comparable drops per minute. It is more accurate and time efficient to regulate a minute-by-minute rate.

PURPOSES OF PROCEDURE

IV flow rates are regulated to

1. Comply with the prescribed rate indicated by the physician in the medical order
2. Maintain an equal and constant rate of fluid administration throughout the duration of the infusion
3. Assist in reassessing the progress of the fluid infusion
4. Prevent circulatory overload or insufficient correction of hypovolemia

ASSESSMENT

OBJECTIVE DATA

In addition to the physical assessments of the client identified in Procedure I-16, the following assessments are pertinent:

• Read the current written medical order for the volume and number of hours for the infusion.
• Determine the tubing manufacturer's drop factor, the ratio of drops per milliliter.
• Check agency policy for how frequently a new order must be written to continue fluid therapy.

RELEVANT NURSING DIAGNOSES

When regulating an IV flow rate, the same nursing diagnoses apply as those associated with Procedure I-16.

PLANNING

ESTABLISHING PRIORITIES

Calculation of the rate of drops per minute is a critical skill associated with the initiation and maintenance of IV fluids. It is synonymous with computing a drug dosage. A miscalculation of a flow rate is as serious (and is considered the same as) a medication error. Each nurse assigned to care for the client continues to be held accountable for maintaining the prescribed rate of flow. Therefore, it is imperative that the nurse's computation is mathematically correct and that the IV drip rate is adjusted and maintained at the correct rate.

SETTING GOALS

• The rate of flow in drops per minute will equal the rate per hour prescribed by the physician.
• The hourly rate of infusion will not deviate by more or less than 25% of the hourly calculated rate.

PREPARATION OF EQUIPMENT

The nurse will need the following:

Paper and pen or pencil
Wristwatch with a second hand
Strip of tape marked in graduated hourly increments
Infusion or controller pump (optional)

Technique for regulating intravenous flow rate

ACTION	RATIONALE
1. Check the physician's order.	This ensures that the correct solution is being given with the correct medications and determines the exact time period for administration of the IV solution.
2. Check the patency of the IV line and needle.	Any interference with the patency of the IV line will influence the IV flow rate.
3. Verify the drop factor (number of drops in 1 ml) of the equipment in use.	The drop factor of the equipment varies according to the manufacturer and will be displayed on the outer package. Equipment labeled microdrop or minidrop is standard and delivers 60 gtt/ml but macrodrip delivery systems vary. Some of the more common types of equipment according to manufacturer are Travenol Macrodrip, 10 gtt/ml; Abbott Macrodrip, 15 gtt/ml; and McGaw Macrodrip, 15 gtt/ml.
4. Calculate the flow rate using the standard formula:	The standard formula for calculating IV flow rate produces the number of gtt/min.

a. *Standard formula*

$$gtt/min = \frac{volume\ (ml) \times drop\ factor\ (gtt/ml)}{time\ in\ minutes}$$

Example—administer 1000 ml 5% D/W over 10 hours (set delivers 60 gtt/1 ml)

b. *Short formula using milliliters/hour*

gtt/min = milliliters (per hour)

$\times$ drop factor (gtt/ml)

Example—administer 1000 ml 5% D/W over 10 hours (set delivers 60 gtt/1 ml)

$$\frac{1000\ ml \times 60\ (gtt/ml)}{600\ min\ (or\ 60\ min \times 10\ hr)} = \frac{60,000}{600} = 100\ gtt/min$$

5. Count the drops per minute in the drip chamber (number of gtt/min). Hold the watch beside the drip chamber.	Holding the watch next to the drip chamber allows the eyes to focus on drops and the second hand on the watch to provide an accurate count.
6. Adjust the IV clamp as needed and recount the drops per minute.	This regulates the flow rate into the drip chamber.
7. Mark the IV container according to the agency policy and manufacturer's recommendations. Use a time tape or label to measure the amount to be infused at timed intervals, as shown in Figure I-17-1.	This allows for comparison of the volume actually infused with the scheduled infusion rate.
8. Monitor the IV flow rate at frequent intervals. Document the client's response to the infusion at the prescribed rate.	This provides for observation of the IV infusion and ensures accurate documentation of the client's response to the IV infusion.

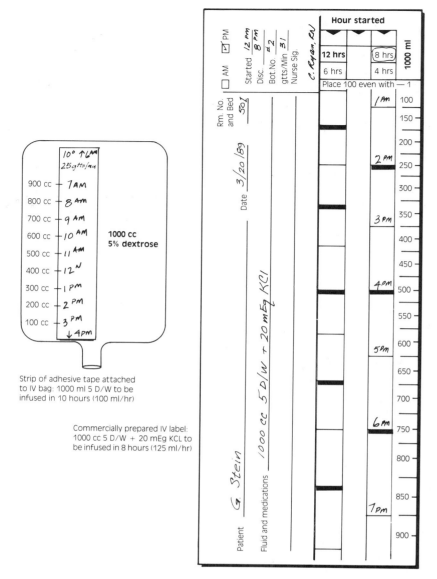

Strip of adhesive tape attached
to IV bag: 1000 ml 5 D/W to be
infused in 10 hours (100 ml/hr)

Commercially prepared IV label:
1000 cc 5 D/W + 20 mEg KCL to
be infused in 8 hours (125 ml/hr)

Figure I-17–1 A time tape enables the nurse to quickly evaluate if
the intravenous solution is infusing according to schedule and to regulate the drip rate if needed.

SAMPLE DOCUMENTATION

Date	Time	Nurse's note
10/02	1500	1000 ml of 5% D/W assessed hourly. Continues to infuse at 42 gtt/min. No tenderness or swelling at site. No dyspnea or shortness of breath. Hourly output between 100–120 ml.
		E. Russo, RN

EVALUATION

REASSESSMENT

It is not uncommon for health agencies to adopt a policy that requires hourly reassessment of an infusion. The volume infused, the rate of flow per minute, the condition of the site, and the client's response should be noted and compared with previous assessments, the medical order, and the agency's protocols concerning IV infusions.

EXPECTED OUTCOMES

The solution infuses according to the calculated schedule.
The tubing and site remain patent.
The client remains comfortable and alert.

UNEXPECTED OUTCOMES

The rate of infusion stops, slows, or speeds.
The client's hemodynamic status changes as indicated by deviations from the normal ranges of blood pressure, pulse rate, central venous pressure (CVP) or pulmonary capillary wedge pressure (PCWP).
The client's respirations become labored.
The client's hourly output becomes low or suppressed.

MODIFICATIONS IN SELECTED SITUATIONS

GENERAL VARIATIONS

The rate during the first hour of infusion should be checked at half-hour or more frequent intervals since the flexibility of the tubing has been shown to alter the initially regulated rate.
The physician may write an order directing the nurse to recalculate the rate of infusion according to the previous hour's urinary output.
The medical order may direct that the rate be adjusted to maintain the client's systolic blood pressure or pulse within a certain range.
An infusion pump, shown in Figure I-17-2, may be used when it is necessary to regulate the administration of small volumes of fluid or drugs that are toxic if the rate of administration is too fast.

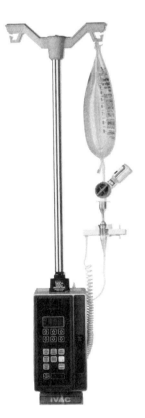

Figure I-17–2 An example of a positive-pressure infusion pump that automatically regulates the flow rate. The alarm on this model is activated by an empty fluid container, an occluded tubing, or an unobtainable drop rate. (Photo courtesy of IVAC Corporation, San Diego, California)

An electronic sensor, shown in Figure I-17-3, monitors the rate continuously.

When a secondary, or piggyback, solution is infused, the primary container is lowered. This change in the height of the primary solution causes the infusion from that container to stop while the higher solution infuses. Temporarily interrupting the rate of flow will alter the total time of the infusion.

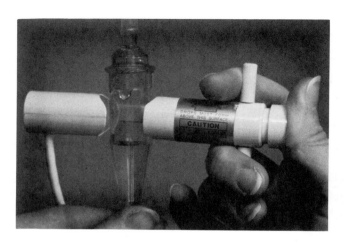

Figure I-17–3 Electronic equipment may be used to regulate and infuse intravenous solution. This sensor is able to count the number of drops as they fall. It compares the actual drops that fall to the number for which the pump is programmed. A discrepancy in the two figures will trigger an automatic alarm.

A portable, battery-operated flow meter can be attached to a drip chamber. This device digitally displays the current per-minute flow rate without requiring that the nurse count the drops.

Consult the respective agency's policy concerning a "keep vein open" (KVO) rate. It is customary to maintain the rate slow enough to keep the vein patent. This may be achieved with a flow rate of as little as 10 ml to 15 ml/hour.

For the nurse's convenience, some agencies provide a conversion chart that correlates the milliliter per hour rate with the drop per minute rate delivered by the equipment used within that agency.

The pharmacy in some agencies provides a computerized label on each container of prescribed solution. Among other information, the drops per minute are listed. The nurse is still held accountable for determining the accuracy of the labeled rate.

AGE-RELATED VARIATIONS

Expect that the rate of flow will be slower for infants, children, and debilitated or geriatric clients to accommodate their cardiovascular and renal capacities.

HOME-HEALTH VARIATIONS

IVs may be intermittent or continuous in the home setting. The nurse may or *may not* remain in the client's home during an infusion. Agency policy should be followed.

If the nurse does not remain in the home, the nurse must assess the ability of a family member to count the drops per minute and regulate the flow rate.

RELATED TEACHING

The client should be instructed to refrain from manipulating the roller clamp that is used to regulate infusion rates. Inform the client to avoid lying on the tubing or the arm in which the solution is infusing. This tends to slow or stop the infusion.

Explain that the distance between the container and the infusion site affects the rate of infusion. The greater the distance, the faster the rate. When the distance becomes smaller, the rate slows.

Instruct the client that if the IV tubing hangs below the infusion site, there may not be enough pressure to infuse the fluid. Venous blood, under greater pressure in that situation, would backfill the tubing. The blood could then clot within the tubing and require that the entire system and site be changed.

PERFORMANCE CHECKLIST

When the rate of infusion is regulated competently, the learner:

C	A	U	
[ ]	[ ]	[ ]	Checks the written medical order
[ ]	[ ]	[ ]	Identifies the drip factor on the intravenous tubing package
[ ]	[ ]	[ ]	Calculates the rate of drops per minute
[ ]	[ ]	[ ]	Counts the number of drops falling into the drip chamber for 1 minute
[ ]	[ ]	[ ]	Tightens or releases the roller clamp until the calculated rate is infusing
[ ]	[ ]	[ ]	Marks the container at hourly increments

Outcome: [ ] Pass   [ ] Fail

C = competent; A = acceptable; U = unsatisfactory

Comments: _____

_____

_____

_____   _____
Student's Signature   Date

_____   _____
Instructor's Signature   Date

I-18

Monitoring an intravenous site and infusion

The nurse is responsible for the continuous, safe administration of the prescribed fluid. Therefore, all the components of the equipment, the intravenous (IV) site, and the client's response require frequent monitoring. Agencies often set policies that determine the regularity and circumstances for changing equipment. The nurse may determine unique factors that justify the modification of the agency's policies. When the policy is not followed, the nurse must validate, in the client's record, those reasons for deviating from the adopted standard for care.

PURPOSES OF PROCEDURE

The IV site and infusion are monitored to

1. Evaluate the client's response to intravenous fluid therapy
2. Ensure safe, adequate, and appropriate standards of care
3. Identify signs of complications that may be reduced through early detection

ASSESSMENT

OBJECTIVE DATA

- Observe the current rate and progress within the overall time schedule for the infusion.
- Inspect the security of all tubing connections.
- Read the dates on the IV solution container, the tubing, and the dressing.
- Examine the condition of the dressing.
- Note the temperature, color, and appearance of the site.
- Review the trends in vital signs.
- Monitor the results of white blood cell (WBC) count.

SUBJECTIVE DATA

- Ask the client to indicate any tenderness, burning, or discomfort at the venipuncture site or the extremity into which it is infusing.

RELEVANT NURSING DIAGNOSES

Typical nursing diagnoses that may be associated with clients who require monitoring of an IV site or infusion include

- *Potential for Altered Comfort*
- *Potential for Infection*
- *Potential Fluid Volume Deficit (or Excess)*
- *Potential for Injury*
- *Potential for Altered Tissue Perfusion*

PLANNING

ESTABLISHING PRIORITIES

An IV site and infusion should be assessed on the first contact with the client. They should be continuously monitored at a minimum of once per hour throughout the day.

SETTING GOALS

- The client will remain free of iatrogenic (treatment-induced) complications.
- All containers of solution, tubing, and the site are within the current safe period of use.

PREPARATION OF
EQUIPMENT

When monitoring the IV site and infusion, the nurse will need

Watch with a second hand or digital timer
Tourniquet or sphygmomanometer to assess for infiltration

Technique for monitoring an intravenous site and infusion

ACTION	RATIONALE
1. Monitor the IV infusion at least once every hour. More frequent checks may be necessary if medication is being infused:	This promotes safe administration of IV fluids and medication. Too rapid administration of medications can result in the development of speed shock.
a. Check the physician's order for IV solution.	This ensures that the correct solution is being given at the correct rate and in the proper sequence with the correct medications.
b. Check the drip chamber and time the drops, as the nurse in Figure I-18-1 is doing, if the IV is not monitored by an infusion-control device.	This ensures that the flow rate is correct.
c. Check the tubing for anything that might interfere with the flow. Be sure that the clamp is in the open position. Observe the dressing for leakage of the IV solution.	Any kink or pressure on the tubing may interfere with the flow. Leakage may occur at the connection of the tubing with the hub of the needle or catheter and allow for loss of IV solution.
d. Observe settings, alarm, and indicator lights on an infusion-control device, shown in Figure I-18-2, if one is being used.	This ensures that the infusion-control device is functioning and that the alarm is in the "On" position.

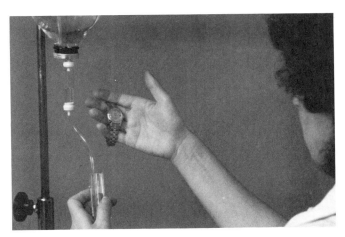

Figure I-18-1   The nurse holds a watch close to the drip chamber and counts the drops that fall.

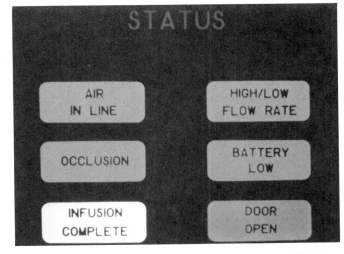

Figure I-18-2   This electronic equipment is able to trouble-shoot information that it monitors. The machine is capable of displaying visual messages for the nurse.

2. Inspect the site for swelling, pain, coolness, or pallor at the site of insertion, which may indicate infiltration of the IV. This necessitates removing the IV and restarting it at another site. Another method of validating whether the IV is infiltrated involves applying a tourniquet above the insertion site. If the IV needle is in the vein, the solution will stop flowing.

The needle may become dislodged from the vein and the IV solution flows into subcutaneous tissue.

3. Inspect the IV site, shown in Figure I-18-3, for redness, swelling, heat, and pain, which may indicate a phlebitis is present. The IV will need to be discontinued and restarted at another site. Notify the physician if you suspect that a phlebitis may have occurred.

Chemical irritation or mechanical trauma cause injury to the vein and can lead to the development of phlebitis.

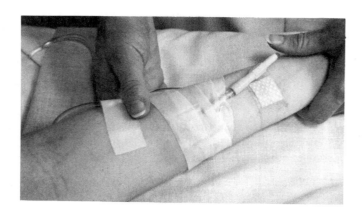

Figure I-18–3 This site shows signs of inflammation. The nurse should discontinue the infusion at this location. The IV can be restarted at another location, preferably in the opposite arm.

4. Check for local or systemic manifestations that indicate an infection is present at the site. The IV will be discontinued and the physician notified. Never disconnect an IV tubing when putting on a client's hospital gown.

Poor aseptic technique may allow bacteria to enter the needle or catheter insertion site or tubing connection.

5. Be alert for additional complications of IV therapy.

a. Circulatory overload can result in signs of cardiac failure and pulmonary edema. Monitor intake and output during IV therapy.

Infusing too much IV solution results in an increased volume of circulating fluid.

b. Bleeding at the site is most likely to occur when the IV is discontinued.

Bleeding may be caused by anticoagulant medication.

6. If possible, instruct the client to call for assistance if any discomfort is noted at the site, solution container is nearly empty, or the flow has changed in any way.

This facilitates cooperation of the client and safe administration of the IV solution.

7. Document the IV infusion, any complications of therapy, and the client's reaction to the therapy.

This provides accurate documentation and ensures continuity of care.

SAMPLE DOCUMENTATION

Date	Time	Nurse's note
9/12	2100	1000 ml normal saline with 40 mEq of KCl infusing at 80 ml per hour. Site remains nontender. No redness or swelling noted. IV dressing removed. Sterile dressing applied to venipuncture site.

B. Gregg, RN

EVALUATION

REASSESSMENT

Besides compliance with the agency's policy for regular reassessment, the nurse should inspect the infusion whenever the client manifests an elevated temperature or describes discomfort at the site. The client's hydration status and ability to supplement fluid intake with oral liquids should be documented and discussed with the physician. The balance between intake and output should be evaluated at the end of each nursing shift and 24-hour period.

The rate and integrity of the system should be inspected whenever the infused volume does not compare with the schedule. Whenever the client is transported and returns from various departments, the nurse should validate that the system is intact and continues to infuse at the predetermined rate. The IV site and infusion warrant frequent reassessment if the client is agitated or hyperactive.

EXPECTED OUTCOMES

The client receives the correct solution at the prescribed rate for the intended period of time.

The client's infusion site remains free of discomfort, redness, pallor, coolness, and swelling.

The container of fluid is changed at least every 24 hours.

The tubing and the IV site remain patent and are changed at least every 24 to 48 hours or as directed by agency policy.

UNEXPECTED OUTCOMES

The client gains or loses more than 5% total body weight (TBW) within 24 hours.

There is a 500-ml difference between total intake and total output.

There is a contradiction between the prescribed solution or additives and what the nurse observes to be infusing.

The connections in the tubing become separated, or the system shows signs of leaking, such as a saturated dressing or moist bed linens.

The safe usage time for the solution, site, or tubing expires and becomes outdated.

The site becomes warm or cool, red or pale, swollen, or tender.

Drainage or bleeding is observed from the infusion site.

MODIFICATIONS IN SELECTED SITUATIONS

GENERAL VARIATIONS

When potential new venipuncture sites are limited, the nurse may elect to leave the needle in its present location longer than 48 hours as long as there is no sign that any complication is occurring. Documentation should include related assessments as well as the rationale for allowing the infusion to continue in the same site.

Any connection with additional sections of tubing should be taped to prevent accidental separation.

If the client develops a fever or there is purulent drainage from an IV site, the wound and a sample of drainage from the removed venipuncture device is cultured to determine its possible connection as a source of infection.

The slowing of some infusions occurs because the bevel of the needle or catheter lodges against the vein wall. Repositioning or rotating the venipuncture device at its insertion site may promote a more accurate infusion rate.

An obstructed needle or catheter may be aspirated in an effort to restore its patency. Irrigation of an obstructed needle is controversial since it can precipitate an embolus.

AGE-RELATED VARIATIONS

Look for a change in behavior, such as crying and restlessness, to indicate that an infant or young child is experiencing discomfort.

HOME-HEALTH VARIATIONS

If the nurse does not remain in the home to monitor the IV, assess the person who will be responsible.

Provide a flow sheet for the family to follow.

Develop written instructions for the procedure to follow if the tubing becomes disconnected, the alarm sounds, the bag empties, or the client experiences problems. Include a telephone number for the family to call if problems or questions occur.

Teach the client and family the signs and symptoms of complications associated with fluid therapy, such as infiltration and fluid overload.

RELATED TEACHING

Inform the client about the schedule for routine monitoring in order to alleviate any unfounded fears that complications are developing.

Explain the necessity for measuring the client's oral intake and urine output. Gain the client's cooperation in recording the type and amount of fluid he consumes and saving his urine for measurement.

Instruct the client that an infusion pump may signal an alarm when there is a change in the pattern of administration. Quick response to an alarm can convey reassurance that the nurse is providing conscientious care.

PERFORMANCE CHECKLIST

When an IV site and infusion are monitored, the learner:

C	A	U	
[ ]	[ ]	[ ]	Checks the medical orders for the most current fluid therapy prescription
[ ]	[ ]	[ ]	Counts the rate of drops per minute
[ ]	[ ]	[ ]	Compares the amount that has infused with the schedule rate
[ ]	[ ]	[ ]	Notes the dates on all infusion equipment
[ ]	[ ]	[ ]	Examines the connections within the components of the intravenous tubing
[ ]	[ ]	[ ]	Inspects the dressing and IV site
[ ]	[ ]	[ ]	Collects objective data relating to the client's response to the fluid administration
[ ]	[ ]	[ ]	Questions the client concerning his perception of discomfort about the IV site
[ ]	[ ]	[ ]	Documents significant objective and subjective information
[ ]	[ ]	[ ]	Responds and trouble-shoots the alarm signals from an infusion pump
[ ]	[ ]	[ ]	Accurately measures and records the volume of infused fluid
[ ]	[ ]	[ ]	Communicates the current status of the fluid infusion, including the amount remaining, to other nurses who assume care for the client

Outcome: [ ] Pass   [ ] Fail

C = competent; A = acceptable; U = unsatisfactory

Comments: _____

_____

_____

_____

_____   _____
Student's Signature   **Date**

_____   _____
Instructor's Signature   **Date**

Changing an intravenous dressing

Whenever the integrity of the skin has been compromised by an invasive procedure, the site becomes a pathway for microorganisms. Care must be taken to prevent an infection at the point of entry made by the needle or catheter. Further, the site must be inspected to detect any signs that may indicate an inflammation of the vein wall due to trauma or clot formation. The venipuncture device is treated as a foreign object by the body. Natural protective mechanisms, such as platelet aggregation, leukocytosis, and so on, occur in the area of the needle or catheter. Cleaning and changing the site with relative frequency tend to prevent complications from occurring.

PURPOSES OF PROCEDURE

The dressing over an intravenous (IV) site is changed to

1. Cleanse the entry site of organisms commonly found on the surface of skin
2. Apply antimicrobial ointment to reduce the growth of microorganisms
3. Provide a barrier from pathogens in the environment to the bloodstream
4. Inspect the condition of the site used for venipuncture

ASSESSMENT

OBJECTIVE DATA

- Review the agency's policy for the recommended schedule routine for changing an IV dressing.
- Examine the current dressing, nurses' notes, or nursing Kardex for the date and time of the most recent dressing change.
- Note the trend in the client's body temperature and pulse rate, being especially concerned about any recent elevations.
- Inspect the dressing for signs of bleeding, drainage, or saturation with fluid.
- Look at the area of the IV site and note if there is redness or swelling.
- Feel the surrounding tissue for areas that feel warm or hard.

SUBJECTIVE DATA

- Encourage the client to describe his level of comfort in relation to the IV site. Tenderness or pain at the infusion area could indicate phlebitis, thrombus, thrombophlebitis, infection, or infiltration.

RELEVANT NURSING DIAGNOSES

The client who needs an IV dressing changed can have any one or more of these nursing diagnoses:

- *Potential for Infection*
- *Potential for Injury*
- *Altered Comfort*
- *Altered Tissue Perfusion*

PLANNING

ESTABLISHING PRIORITIES

An IV dressing should be changed as soon as the nurse detects a cluster of signs and symptoms suggestive of a complication. The nurse should also consider removing the needle or catheter from its site in these cases and restarting the infusion at another site, preferably in the opposite hand or arm.

When the IV dressing is changed in compliance with the agency's policy, it should be changed relatively close to its expiration time. The nurse may select a convenient time within the client's plan for care, preferably after the client's personal hygiene has been completed. If the IV site, tubing, or solution requires changing, the nurse may plan to perform all the procedures at one time.

SETTING GOALS

• The IV site will be inspected, cleansed, and redressed according to the policy of the agency or whenever a need is indicated.

PREPARATION OF EQUIPMENT

When an IV dressing is changed, the nurse will likely need items from the following list:

Sterile gauze (2 × 2 or 4 × 4) or transparent polyurethane dressing
Povidone–iodine (Betadine) solution or swabs
Adhesive remover
Povidone–iodine ointment (or other antiseptic ointment recommended by the agency)
Alcohol swabs
Tape
Clean, disposable gloves

Technique for changing an intravenous dressing

ACTION	RATIONALE
1. Assess the client's need for a dressing change.	Agency policy determines the interval for dressing change (every 24 to 72 hours). The presence of moisture or a nonadhering dressing increases the risk of bacterial contamination at the site.
2. Gather equipment and bring to the bedside.	Having equipment available saves time and facilitates the performance of the task.
3. Explain the procedure to the client.	Explanation allays the client's anxiety.
4. Wash your hands. Don clean, disposable gloves.	Handwashing deters the spread of microorganisms. Gloves prevent transmission of HIV and other blood-borne infections.
5. Carefully remove the old dressing but leave the tape that anchors the IV needle or catheter in place. Discard in the proper manner.	This prevents dislodging of the IV needle or catheter.
6. Assess the IV site for the presence of inflammation or infiltration. Discontinue and relocate the IV if noted.	Inflammation or infiltration causes trauma to tissues and necessitates removal of the IV needle or catheter.
7. Loosen the tape and gently remove it, being careful to steady the catheter or needle hub with one hand.	This stabilizes the needle and prevents its inadvertent dislodging.
8. Use adhesive remover to initiate cleansing procedure at the site.	This removes adhesive residue and facilitates the attachment of a new dressing.

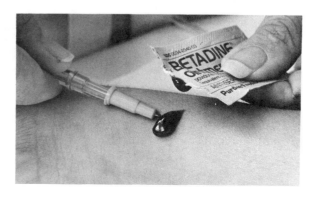

Figure I-19-1 The nurse has placed a drop of povidone–iodine (Betadine) ointment at the needle's entry.

9. Cleanse the entry site with povidone–iodine (Betadine) solution. Use a circular motion to move from the center outward. Follow with alcohol cleansing.

Cleansing in a circular motion while moving outward carries organisms away from the entry site. Use of antiseptic solutions reduces the number of microorganisms on the skin surface.

10. Reapply tape strip to needle or catheter at the entry site.

This anchors the needle or catheter to prevent dislodgement.

11. Apply povidone–iodine (Betadine) ointment to the entry site, as shown in Figure I-19-1.

Antiseptic ointment reduces skin contamination and protects against infection.

12. Apply sterile gauze or a transparent polyurethane dressing, such as the one shown in Figure I-19-2, over the entry site.

This protects the site and deters contamination with microorganisms.

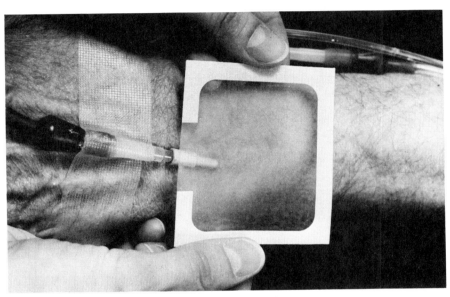

Figure I–19–2 Tegaderm Transparent IV Dressing and Transpore Surgical Tape combine to provide a neat, secure, and visible IV site. (Courtesy of 3M Medical Products Division.)

13. Secure the IV tubing with additional tape if necessary. Label the dressing with the date, time of change, and your initials. Check that the IV flow is accurate and the system is patent.

This documents IV dressing change.

14. Discard equipment properly and wash hands.

Handwashing protects against the spread of microorganisms.

15. Record the client's response to the dressing change and the observation of the site.

This provides accurate documentation and ensures continuity of care.

SAMPLE DOCUMENTATION

Date	Time	Nurse's note
6/15	1035	IV dressing changed according to protocol. Site is free of drainage. No redness, swelling, bleeding or drainage, tenderness noted.

S. L., RN

EVALUATION

REASSESSMENT

When the nurse observes the hourly progress of the infusion, it is also a good opportunity to include a focused assessment of the IV site and dressing. Each assigned nurse should inspect the dressing and change it if it is no longer secure or intact.

EXPECTED OUTCOMES

The client's venipuncture device remains inserted and continues to provide an access for the infusion.

The client's IV site is free of signs associated with infiltration, inflammation, thrombus, or infection.

The client's dressing is sterile, dry, and secure.

UNEXPECTED OUTCOMES

The venipuncture device accidentally becomes displaced from the vein during the removal or replacement of the dressing.

The client's venipuncture site looks red. The area above the insertion site is warm and tender or cool and swollen.

MODIFICATIONS IN SELECTED SITUATIONS

GENERAL VARIATIONS

Change any IV dressing if the date of its application is unknown.

Use the agency's choice of antimicrobial ointment. Other examples of substitutes for povidone–iodine include Mycitracin and Neosporin ointment.

Dressings that may be saturated with a toxic chemotherapeutic agent, such as drugs used to treat oncology clients, should be double wrapped. The wrapped dressing should then be placed in a waterproof bag, labeled with its contents, and returned to the pharmacy for toxic waste disposal. These measures prevent accidental skin absorption of the drug by agency personnel and environmental contamination.

A Band-Aid is sterile and can be substituted for sterile gauze over the venipuncture site.

A transparent adhesive dressing may not adhere well when antimicrobial ointment is used. An antiseptic solution may be used as an alternative aseptic measure. After air drying, the dressing can be applied.

Follow the infection-control policy for obtaining a culture of the needle, catheter, or venipuncture site if purulent drainage or an unexplained fever has occurred.

Apply a warm moist compress to a reddened, swollen, tender site after removing the venipuncture device. Restart the infusion in another location.

AGE-RELATED VARIATIONS

Use a protective device, armboard, or restraint to ensure that an infant or child cannot remove the dressing or needle.

Use a mitt on the hand without the IV to prevent a child from manipulating the IV dressing, roller clamp, and so on. Remove the mitt periodically for exercise when it is possible to observe the child closely.

HOME-HEALTH VARIATIONS

Although the family may be taught to care for certain aspects of IV therapy, it is most common for the nurse to be responsible for changing an IV dressing.

The client should be provided with a list of assessments that indicate potential complications. Include the telephone number where the nurse can be reached in the event that the dressing may need to be changed before a scheduled return visit.

RELATED TEACHING

Explain that changing an IV dressing does not always mean the site will be changed.

Identify the reasons for complying with a pattern for routine dressing changes. Many clients do not understand the concept of prophylactic care.

Instruct the client on the signs or symptoms that indicate a need for changing the site. Encourage the client to communicate any discomfort that occurs.

PERFORMANCE CHECKLIST

When an IV dressing is changed, the learner:

C	A	U	
[ ]	[ ]	[ ]	States the agency's policy concerning the routine for dressing changes
[ ]	[ ]	[ ]	Checks the date indicating the most recent dressing change
[ ]	[ ]	[ ]	Assesses the progress of the IV infusion, the condition of the current dressing, and any untoward signs or symptoms manifested by the client
[ ]	[ ]	[ ]	Explains the procedure to the client and plans the time for the dressing change with the client
[ ]	[ ]	[ ]	Washes hands
[ ]	[ ]	[ ]	Gathers equipment
[ ]	[ ]	[ ]	Tears strips of tape, opens sterile dressing package or Band-Aid and antimicrobial ointment packet
[ ]	[ ]	[ ]	Dons gloves
[ ]	[ ]	[ ]	Removes the current dressing touching only the outside surface
[ ]	[ ]	[ ]	Places the soiled dressing within a lined receptacle
[ ]	[ ]	[ ]	Observes the condition of the IV site
[ ]	[ ]	[ ]	Removes the tape without disturbing the needle or catheter
[ ]	[ ]	[ ]	Swabs the site with povidone–iodine (Betadine), followed by alcohol
[ ]	[ ]	[ ]	Allows the cleansing agents time to evaporate
[ ]	[ ]	[ ]	Secures the needle or catheter with fresh tape
[ ]	[ ]	[ ]	Covers the puncture site with antimicrobial ointment and a dressing or Band-Aid
[ ]	[ ]	[ ]	Covers the gauze dressing and adjacent skin with tape or a transparent adhesive dressing
[ ]	[ ]	[ ]	Loops and secures the distal portion of the IV tubing to avoid any direct pulling and separation at the needle or catheter
[ ]	[ ]	[ ]	Labels the dressing with pertinent information
[ ]	[ ]	[ ]	Discards used supplies; returns unused items to stock
[ ]	[ ]	[ ]	Washes hands
[ ]	[ ]	[ ]	Records the procedure and observations in the client's record

Outcome: [ ] Pass   [ ] Fail

C = competent; A = acceptable; U = unsatisfactory

Comments: _____
_____
_____

_____   _____
Student's Signature   Date

_____   _____
Instructor's Signature   Date

I-20

Changing intravenous solution and tubing

Most agencies follow prophylactic infection-control policies for changing intravenous (IV) solution containers and tubing. It is a common practice to replace a container of solution after it has been hanging 24 hours even if the entire volume has not infused. Tubing is generally changed every 24 to 48 hours. It is customary for a physician to review the IV therapy orders daily. It is possible that changes in the medical orders will require changing the solution containers and tubing.

PURPOSES OF PROCEDURE

IV solution containers and tubing are changed to

1. Prevent the growth of organisms in equipment that is directly connected with the client's circulatory system
2. Infuse newly ordered fluids that are incompatible with previous infusions or types of equipment, such as blood
3. Continue the progress of an infusion that may be slowed or stopped due to the collection of particles within an in-line filter
4. Continue fluid therapy when the solution container has been punctured or connections in the tubing have become separated

ASSESSMENT

OBJECTIVE DATA

- Review the agency policy for the prescribed routine for changing solutions and tubing.
- Determine the expiration dates on the solution and tubing as well as on the venipuncture site and dressing.
- Inspect the solution and the tubing for "floaters," additives that have precipitated, or blood that has backflowed into the distal portion of the tubing.
- Compare the current IV solution prescription with the solution that is infusing.
- Count and validate the rate of infusion.
- Inspect the connections on the tubing to note that they are secure and intact.

SUBJECTIVE DATA

- Ask the client to describe any symptoms of distress or discomfort. Examples of unfavorable reactions may include feeling warm or chilled or burning or pain in the area of the IV site.

RELEVANT NURSING DIAGNOSES

When an IV solution container and tubing require a change, the nurse may be caring for a client with the following nursing diagnoses:

- *Potential for Injury*
- *Potential for Infection*
- *Anxiety*
- *Fear*
- *Knowledge Deficit*
- *Self-Care Deficit*

PLANNING

ESTABLISHING PRIORITIES

The nurse must attend immediately to any life-threatening signs or symptoms that are related to the infusing solution. When noting that the rate of infusion has slowed or stopped, the nurse should simultaneously trouble-shoot the possible reasons. Delay in changing an IV solution or tubing may contribute to inadequate treatment of the client's condition. When there is no particular danger to the client, as when a solution and tubing are due to be changed to comply with the agency's policy, the nurse can exercise flexibility for accomplishing the task.

SETTING GOALS

• The client's new solution or tubing will be changed without contamination or interruption of the infusion.

PREPARATION OF EQUIPMENT

The nurse will need the following:

For solution change
 IV solution as ordered by the physician
For tubing change
 Administration set
 Sterile gauze
 Tape or label
 Sterile dressing and antiseptic solutions/ointments (according to agency recommendations)
 Clean, disposable gloves

Technique for changing intravenous solution and tubing

ACTION	RATIONALE
1. Gather all equipment and bring it to the bedside. Check the IV solution and medication additives with the physician's order.	Having equipment available saves time and facilitates accomplishment of the task. Checking ensures that the client receives the correct IV solution and medication as ordered by the physician.
2. Explain the procedure to the client.	Explanation allays the client's anxiety.
3. Wash your hands.	Handwashing deters the spread of microorganisms.

TO CHANGE IV SOLUTION

4. Carefully remove the protective cover from the new solution container and expose the entry port.	This maintains sterility of the IV solution.
5. Close the clamp on the tubing.	This stops the flow of IV fluid during the change of the solution.
6. Lift the container off the IV pole and invert it. Quickly remove the spike from the old IV container, being careful not to contaminate it.	This maintains sterility of the IV set-up.
7. Steady the new container and insert the spike. Hang the new container on the IV pole.	This allows for uninterrupted flow of the new solution.
8. Reopen the clamp on the tubing and adjust the flow.	This regulates the flow rate into the drip chamber.
9. Label the container according to agency policy. Record on the intake/output record and document on the client's chart according to agency policy. Discard used equipment in the proper manner. Wash your hands.	Labeling ensures accurate continuation and administration of the correct IV solution. Handwashing deters the spread of microorganisms.

TO CHANGE IV TUBING AND SOLUTION

10. Follow Steps 1 to 4.

11. Open the administration set and remove the protective covering from the infusion spike. Using sterile technique, insert the spike into the new container.

This maintains the sterility of the IV set-up.

12. Close the clamp on the new tubing. Hang the IV container on the pole, as the nurse in Figure I-20-1 is preparing to do. Squeeze the drip chamber, shown in Figure I-20-2, to fill it at least halfway.

Gravity and suction cause the fluid to move into the drip chamber. This also prevents air from moving down the tubing.

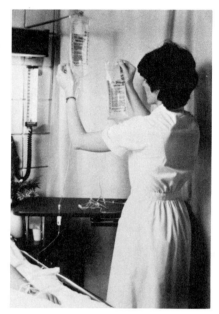

Figure I-20–1 This nurse has brought a new container of solution connected to sterile tubing into the client's room. The previous container of fluid is almost empty.

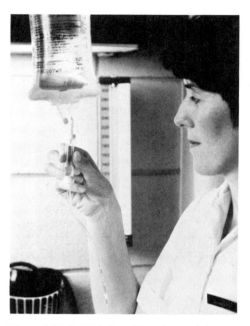

Figure I-20–2 With the tubing clamped, the nurse squeezes the drip chamber so that it is partially filled.

13. Remove the cap at the end of the tubing, release the clamp, and allow the fluid to move through the tubing until all air bubbles have disappeared. Close the clamp and recap the end of the tubing, maintaining sterility of the set-up.

This removes air from the tubing, which can, in larger amounts, act as an air embolus.

14. Carefully remove the tape and dressing from the IV insertion site.

This provides access to the needle hub necessary for the tubing change.

15. Place a sterile gauze square under the needle hub.

The gauze absorbs any leakage when the tubing is disconnected from the needle.

16. Place the new IV tubing close to the client's IV site and slightly loosen the protective cap.

This facilitates the removal of the cap and attachment to the needle hub.

17. Don clean, disposable gloves.

Gloves act as a transmission barrier for blood-borne microorganisms.

18. Clamp the old IV tubing. Steady the needle hub with your nondominant hand until the change is completed. Remove the tubing with your dominant hand, using a twisting motion.

This stabilizes the needle and prevents inadvertently dislodging it.

19. Set the old tubing aside. While maintaining sterility, carefully remove the cap and insert the sterile end of the tubing into the needle hub, as shown in Figure I-20-3. Twist to secure it.

This maintains the sterility of the IV set-up.

20. Open the clamp.

This allows the solution to flow to the client.

21. Remove the gloves, turning them inside out.

This prevents skin contact with blood.

22. Reapply the sterile dressing to the site according to agency protocol. (See Procedure I-19.)

This deters entry of microorganisms at the site.

23. Regulate the IV flow according to the physician's order. (See Procedure I-17.)

This ensures that the client receives the IV solution at the prescribed rate.

24. Attach a tab of tape or label to the IV tubing, stating the date, time, and your initials, as shown in Figure I-20-4. Label the container and record the procedure according to agency policy. Discard the used equipment in the proper manner and wash hands.

This documents the IV tubing change.

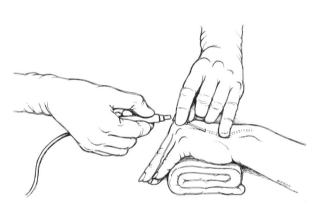

Figure I-20-3 Compressing the vein above the distal end of the venipuncture device will control blood loss during the time that the new tubing is being connected. Note that the tip of the catheter is being stabilized at the same time to avoid its accidental displacement. (Brunner LS, Suddarth DS: The Lippincott Manual of Nursing Practice, 4th ed, p 104. Philadelphia, JB Lippincott, 1986)

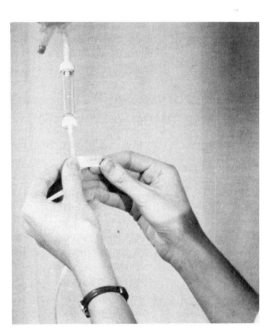

Figure I-20-4 A tab of tape with the date, time, and initials of the nurse lets other caregivers know when the tubing was changed and by whom.

25. Record the client's response to the IV infusion.

This ensures accurate documentation of the client's response.

SAMPLE DOCUMENTATION

Date	Time	Nurse's note
7/01	1204	Results of serum Na, K, Cl levels reported to Dr. Moss. Remaining 200 ml
	1215	of 0.9% normal saline discontinued. 1000 ml of 5% D/.45% saline $\in$ 20 mEq of KCl infusing at 42 gtt/minute according to new fluid orders.
		G. Rappe, RN

EVALUATION

REASSESSMENT

A nurse should check the date on all current IV equipment each shift. When care is given to the client, it is also recommended that the equipment and the infusion be assessed concurrently. Medical orders should be noted frequently, especially those of clients who are acutely ill.

EXPECTED OUTCOMES

The IV system remains sterile.
The client's venipuncture device remains patent.
The client does not experience excessive blood loss during the change from one tubing to another.
The solution continues to infuse without difficulty.

UNEXPECTED OUTCOMES

The sterile areas on the equipment, such as the spike or distal end of the tubing, become contaminated.
The IV needle or catheter is displaced.
The rate-adjustment clamp malfunctions.
The rate slows or stops.

MODIFICATIONS IN SELECTED SITUATIONS

GENERAL VARIATIONS

There may be more than one IV solution infusing at the same time.
Dates on each IV system should be checked for their expiration.
Some pharmacy departments provide personalized labels on IV solution containers noting the current date of the order and the use date. Care should be taken to avoid hanging outdated solutions.
Nurses may obtain IV solutions from a stock supply. In an emergency the nurse may be required to instill additives to the solution, such as potassium chloride (KCl). A special label must be attached indicating the name of the drug, the dose, the date and time, and the name of the person who prepared the solution.
A hemostat may be needed in some situations to separate the old tubing from the hub of the IV needle or catheter. The presence of antibiotic ointment or residue of adhesive sometimes interferes with separating the connection with gloved hands.
Although air within the tubing is not likely to be dangerous, it may be best to relieve a client's anxiety by displacing the air. One method is shown in Figure I-20-5.

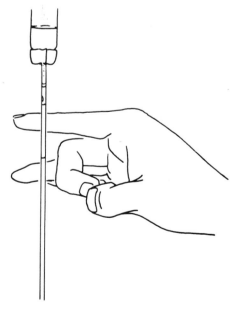

Figure I-20–5 Any air that remains within the IV tubing once a new container of solution has been hung can be removed by thumping the tubing below the lowest level of air and proceeding upward until the air escapes into the drip chamber.

HOME-HEALTH VARIATIONS

If the family is to be taught how to change IV solutions, assess their ability to learn, anxiety level, and potential for compliance. Provide a written schedule that includes the name of the solution, the time it should be hung, and a place for documentation. Emphasize the importance of maintaining the sterility and matching the name on the solution with the written name on the instruction sheet.

In the event that problems occur between regularly scheduled visits, instruct the client on pertinent assessments. Put the instructions in writing. Include the telephone number where the nurse can be reached.

RELATED TEACHING   Explain that air bubbles within the tubing will not be lethal. The minimum quantity of air that would be fatal to humans is not known, but animal experimentation indicates that it is much larger than the quantity that could be present in the entire length of infusion tubing. The average infusion tubing holds about 5 ml of air, an amount not ordinarily considered dangerous.

PERFORMANCE CHECKLIST

When changing an IV solution and tubing, the learner:

C	A	U	
[ ]	[ ]	[ ]	Assesses the progress of the current infusion
[ ]	[ ]	[ ]	Notes the date and time at which the current equipment was first used
[ ]	[ ]	[ ]	Inspects the volume remaining in the current container and determines the projected time for the completion of the infusion
[ ]	[ ]	[ ]	Checks the medical order for the volume and type of the next solution
[ ]	[ ]	[ ]	Explains the need for changing equipment to the client
[ ]	[ ]	[ ]	Washes hands
[ ]	[ ]	[ ]	Selects the replacement solution and tubing
[ ]	[ ]	[ ]	Opens the package of tubing and tightens the rate-adjustment clamp
[ ]	[ ]	[ ]	Inserts the spike on the IV tubing into the container of solution without contaminating either
[ ]	[ ]	[ ]	Elevates the container of solution
[ ]	[ ]	[ ]	Partially fills the drip chamber by compressing it between the thumb and forefinger
[ ]	[ ]	[ ]	Removes the protective cover from the distal end of the tubing
[ ]	[ ]	[ ]	Holds the tip of the tubing securely to avoid touching unsterile areas and releases the clamp
[ ]	[ ]	[ ]	Displaces the air with fluid within the tubing
[ ]	[ ]	[ ]	Tightens the clamp and replaces the protective cap when completed
[ ]	[ ]	[ ]	Hangs the replacement solution and tubing from the IV pole in the client's room
[ ]	[ ]	[ ]	Prepares tape and sterile dressing material
[ ]	[ ]	[ ]	Removes the current dressing to gain access to the hub of the needle or catheter
[ ]	[ ]	[ ]	Positions the tubing for easy access
[ ]	[ ]	[ ]	Dons clean, disposable gloves
[ ]	[ ]	[ ]	Clamps the infusing IV tubing and disconnects it from the hub of the needle or catheter

C = competent; A = acceptable; U = unsatisfactory

(Continued)

PERFORMANCE CHECKLIST (Continued)

C	A	U	
[ ]	[ ]	[ ]	Inserts the new tubing within the needle or catheter without contamination
[ ]	[ ]	[ ]	Opens the clamp to continue the infusion of fluid
[ ]	[ ]	[ ]	Cleans the area of blood and removes gloves
[ ]	[ ]	[ ]	Reapplies a sterile IV dressing
[ ]	[ ]	[ ]	Readjusts the infusion to the prescribed rate of flow
[ ]	[ ]	[ ]	Labels all equipment with recommended information
[ ]	[ ]	[ ]	Removes soiled equipment to receptacles within the utility room
[ ]	[ ]	[ ]	Washes hands
[ ]	[ ]	[ ]	Records new volume, type of fluid, rate of administration, and the condition of the client within the agency's records; records infused volume on the intake and output sheet

Outcome: [ ] Pass   [ ] Fail

C = competent; A = acceptable; U = unsatisfactory

Comments: _____
_____
_____

_____   _____
        Student's Signature   **Date**

_____   _____
        Instructor's Signature   **Date**

I-21

Administering a blood transfusion

Replacing fluids intravenously with crystalloid solutions (solutions in which the solutes completely dissolve in the liquid) may not be adequate in all situations. Some clients may require whole blood, blood products, or other substances found in plasma. The administration of these types of fluids requires specific pretransfusion assessments and specialized nursing techniques throughout the period of infusion.

PURPOSES OF PROCEDURE

Blood transfusions are administered to

1. Replace lost blood volume and cellular components
2. Improve the ability to perfuse the body's cells with oxygen
3. Maintain colloidal osmotic pressure

ASSESSMENT

OBJECTIVE DATA

- Read the medical order prescribing the volume and type of blood product.
- Assess the client's vital signs, including body temperature.
- Observe the client's level of consciousness, appearance and turgor of the skin, and latest trend in urinary output.
- Compare the identification numbers and information on the client's blood type and crossmatch with donated blood held in the blood bank or agency. Confirm information with a second person.
- Review the most recent complete blood cell count or hemoglobin and hematocrit.
- Examine the condition of veins and potential venipuncture sites.
- If the client already has an intravenous (IV) running, check the type of solution that is infusing. Only normal saline is compatible with blood products.

SUBJECTIVE DATA

- Inquire about the client's history of allergies or reactions during previous transfusions.
- Assess the client's knowledge and concerns about receiving blood.

RELEVANT NURSING DIAGNOSES

A client who requires a blood transfusion is likely to have nursing diagnoses such as

- *Activity Intolerance*
- *Altered Cardiac Output: Decreased*
- *Fluid Volume Deficit*
- *Altered Tissue Perfusion*
- *Fear*

PLANNING

ESTABLISHING PRIORITIES

In the presence of active hemorrhage, the administration of blood requires priority attention. It may be necessary to infuse the blood with a pressurized sleeve to ensure that an adequate circulating volume is maintained. For clients with chronic anemia or depression of bone marrow function due to chemotherapy or blood dyscrasias, the replacement of blood may be planned on a routine scheduled basis. Once the blood of the recipient has been crossmatched with that of a donated unit, the donated blood should be infused or released within a few days for someone else's use. A large-gauge needle and blood administration tubing with a filter must be used. Sterile normal saline must be infusing prior to the administration of blood.

SETTING GOALS	• The client's laboratory blood slip and the numbers on the unit of blood will be identical. • The client will remain comfortable, alert, and stable throughout the infusion.
PREPARATION OF EQUIPMENT	The following should be collected prior to administering a blood transfusion: Blood product Blood administration set (tubing with in-line filter and Y-connection for saline administration) 0.9% normal saline IV pole IV line with a #18 or #19 needle or catheter Clean, disposable gloves (if a new IV must be started)

Technique for administering a blood transfusion

ACTION	RATIONALE
1. Explain the procedure to the client. Check for signed consent for transfusion if required by the agency. Advise the client to report any chills, itching, rash, or unusual symptoms.	This provides reassurance and facilitates cooperation. Prompt reporting of any reaction to the transfusion necessitates stopping it immediately.
2. Wash your hands.	Handwashing deters the spread of microorganisms.
3. Hang the container of 0.9% normal saline with blood administration set to initiate the IV infusion and to follow the administration of blood.	Dextrose may lead to clumping of red blood cells and hemolysis. The filter in the blood administration set removes particulate material formed during the storage of the blood.
4. Don gloves and start an IV with a #18 or #19 catheter if not already present. Keep the IV open by starting the flow of normal saline.	A large-bore needle or catheter is necessary for the infusion of blood products. The lumen must be large enough not to cause damage to red blood cells.
5. Secure the blood product from the blood bank according to agency policy.	Blood must be stored in a refrigerated unit at a carefully controlled temperature (4°C).
6. Complete the identification and checks as required by the agency:	Some agencies require two registered nurses to verify information:
a. Identification number	Verifies that unit numbers match
b. Blood group and type	Verifies that ABO group and Rh type are the same
c. Expiration date	Safe storage of blood is limited to 35 days before red blood cells begin to deteriorate.
d. Client's name	Never administer blood to a client without a name band.
e. Inspection of blood for clots	If clots are present, blood should be returned to the blood bank.
7. Take baseline set of vital signs prior to beginning the transfusion.	Any change in vital signs during the transfusion may indicate a reaction.
8. Start the infusion of the blood product:	
a. Prime the in-line filter with blood, as shown in Figure I-21-1.	This is necessary if blood is to flow properly.
b. Start the administration slowly, as shown in Figure I-21-2.	Transfusion reactions typically occur during this period, and a slow rate will minimize the volume of red blood cells infused. If there have been no adverse effects during this time, the infusion rate is increased.

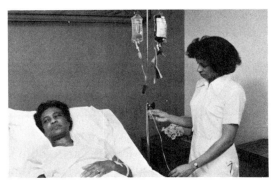

Figure I-21–1 A blood administration set is designed with a **Y**-connection making it possible to alternate between infusing normal saline and blood. A large filter prevents small clots from entering the client's vein.

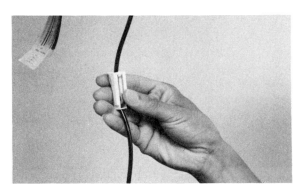

Figure I-21–2 The nurse unclamps the tubing leading to the blood. While letting the blood flow slowly, the nurse can observe the client for a reaction.

c. Check vital signs every 5 minutes for the first 15 minutes, as the nurse in Figure I-21-3 is doing.

If complications occur, they can be observed, and the blood infusion can be stopped immediately.

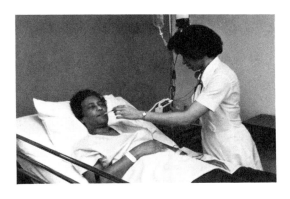

Figure I-21–3 The nurse monitors the client closely for a blood reaction. Vital signs are useful in noting the client's response to the administration of blood.

d. Observe the client for flushing, dyspnea, itching, hives, or rash.

These may be early indications of a transfusion reaction.

9. Maintain the prescribed flow rate as ordered and assess frequently for a transfusion reaction. Stop the blood transfusion and allow the saline to flow if you suspect a reaction. Notify the physician and the blood bank.

Rate must be carefully controlled and the client's reaction monitored on a frequent basis.

10. When the transfusion is complete, infuse 0.9% normal saline.

Saline prevents hemolysis of red blood cells and clears the remainder of the blood in the IV line.

11. Record the administration of blood and the client's reaction as ordered by the agency. Return the blood transfusion bag to the blood bank according to agency policy.

This provides for accurate documentation of the client's response to the blood transfusion.

SAMPLE DOCUMENTATION

Date	Time	Nurse's note
3/18	1830	BP 110/60/56 (right arm), T-98 (oral), P-86, R-24. #18 angiocath inserted into L antecubital vein. Normal saline infusing at 10 gtt/min.

| 1845 | Unit of whole blood obtained from the blood bank. Identification checks verified with D. Cook, RN. Blood infusing at 10 gtt/min. |

B. Swartz, RN

| 1850 | BP 112/64/60, P-88, R-24. Rate of blood administration increased to 20 gtt/min. No signs of dyspnea, urticaria, chills, or discomfort. |

B. Swartz, RN

EVALUATION

REASSESSMENT

The nurse should remain with the client during the first 15 minutes of the blood transfusion assessing vital signs at 5-minute intervals. Vital signs should be rechecked at 15-minute intervals during the next hour if there are no untoward effects. Observations and reassessments should be made with relative frequency during the remaining infusion time.

EXPECTED OUTCOMES

The blood is hung within 30 minutes of its release from the blood bank.
A transfusion reaction does not occur.
The blood infuses within 2 to 4 hours unless a faster rate is specified.
The client's red cell count, hemoglobin, and hematocrit increase within therapeutic ranges 24 hours following the infusion.

UNEXPECTED OUTCOMES

The client suddenly develops dyspnea, chest pain, chills and fever, hypotension, rapid pulse and respiratory rate, hives, or other unusual symptoms related to the concomitant administration of blood.
The infusion is prolonged or stops due to extravasation or obstruction in the passage of the cells through the filter, tubing, or needle.

MODIFICATIONS IN SELECTED SITUATIONS

GENERAL VARIATIONS

The rate of infusion may be slower than usual if the client has cardiopulmonary pathology and the increased volume could overload the client's circulatory status.
Ordinarily a small volume of normal saline is administered after the blood transfusion to flush the maximum amount of blood remaining within the tubing. However, in volume-depleted individuals, the entire remaining normal saline may be infused.
A blood coil may be used to warm blood when a rapid infusion is required.
Take the client's temperature during the infusion if chills develop. The chills may be the result of infusing cold blood. If a fever accompanies the chills, the client is more likely experiencing a pyrogenic reaction.
Individuals who anticipate needing a blood transfusion may have their own blood collected and stored for limited future use. This practice is gaining popularity since information on the blood-borne transmission of human immunodeficiency virus (HIV) has been publicized.
Individuals who object to a blood transfusion on the basis of a religious belief may receive a synthetic blood substitute. An example is Fluosol-DA, which contains substances that carry oxygen, but no red blood cells, and has been used effectively for persons needing the components of whole blood.
Clamp the tubing infusing blood and open the tubing to the saline whenever a transfusion reaction is suspected.
Save all equipment and the client's first voided urine specimen when there has been a transfusion reaction.
It is the policy in some agencies that the empty blood bag be double wrapped when returned after the transfusion.

AGE-RELATED VARIATIONS

Newborns who have developed red blood cell destruction due to maternal antibody production may require blood exchanges involving the total circulating volume.

HOME-HEALTH VARIATIONS

If the nurse does not remain in the home during a transfusion, teach the client and family the signs and symptoms of a blood reaction. It is preferable to write out instructions. Include a telephone number for contacting the nurse.

RELATED TEACHING

Identify the possible signs and symptoms associated with a transfusion reaction.

Explain that donated blood is screened for hepatitis and HIV antibodies.

A vaccine is now available for individuals at risk for acquiring hepatitis B, such as the hemodialysis client.

Blood donors are constantly needed because blood is only stored for 21 to 35 days. The supply becomes critical during periods of high use, such as during holidays when there is a predictably high incidence of trauma-related accidents.

Explain that it is impossible to acquire a blood-borne infection when donating blood. Disposable equipment used to collect blood is sterile and used for only one person.

PERFORMANCE CHECKLIST

When blood is administered, the learner:

C	A	U	
[ ]	[ ]	[ ]	Checks the medical order
[ ]	[ ]	[ ]	Reviews the returned laboratory slips to determine if blood has been typed and crossmatched
[ ]	[ ]	[ ]	Explains the plan for administering blood to the client
[ ]	[ ]	[ ]	Obtains the signature of the client on a consent form, if required by the agency
[ ]	[ ]	[ ]	Gathers equipment for starting an intravenous infusion or that needed to change the solution and tubing, whichever is the case for the client
[ ]	[ ]	[ ]	Washes hands
[ ]	[ ]	[ ]	Connects the blood administration set to normal saline solution
[ ]	[ ]	[ ]	Fills the filter and purges the tubing of air
[ ]	[ ]	[ ]	Hangs the transfusion equipment on an IV pole within the client's room
[ ]	[ ]	[ ]	Takes the client's vital signs
[ ]	[ ]	[ ]	Starts the infusion of normal saline solution
[ ]	[ ]	[ ]	Obtains the blood from the blood bank
[ ]	[ ]	[ ]	Checks identification numbers and labels with a second nurse
[ ]	[ ]	[ ]	Spikes the container of blood
[ ]	[ ]	[ ]	Clamps the tubing from the saline container and opens the tubing from the blood container
[ ]	[ ]	[ ]	Regulates the rate of administration to maintain a slow infusion
[ ]	[ ]	[ ]	Remains with the client
[ ]	[ ]	[ ]	Continues to assess the client at 5-minute intervals
[ ]	[ ]	[ ]	Increases the rate of infusion if no untoward effects are noted
[ ]	[ ]	[ ]	Returns at periodic intervals, specified by the agency's blood administration protocol, to check the client's vital signs and general condition
[ ]	[ ]	[ ]	Clamps the blood tubing and opens the saline tubing when the unit of blood has infused
[ ]	[ ]	[ ]	Flushes the tubing with saline
[ ]	[ ]	[ ]	Checks vital signs before discontinuing the IV

C = competent; A = acceptable; U = unsatisfactory

(Continued)

PERFORMANCE CHECKLIST (Continued)

C	A	U	
[ ]	[ ]	[ ]	Clamps the saline tubing and discontinues the administration
[ ]	[ ]	[ ]	Records the volume infused on the intake and output sheet
[ ]	[ ]	[ ]	Returns the empty blood container to the blood bank
[ ]	[ ]	[ ]	Washes hands
[ ]	[ ]	[ ]	Checks the client's vital signs again after the blood has been discontinued
[ ]	[ ]	[ ]	Documents all pertinent assessments on the client's record

Outcome: [ ] **Pass**   [ ] **Fail**

C = competent; A = acceptable; U = unsatisfactory

Comments: _____
_____
_____

_____   _____
Student's Signature   **Date**

_____   _____
Instructor's Signature   **Date**

Administering parenteral medications

The term *parenteral*, strictly defined, refers to all routes other than the oral route for administering medication. However, the term has come to refer to the administration of medication by injection. Examples of routes for injection are listed in Table I-22-1. This section of procedures focuses on those skills the nurse utilizes in administering parenteral medications by the intradermal, subcutaneous, intramuscular, and intravenous routes.

Table I-22–1
Parenteral medication administration

Method	Location	Term
Parenteral: Given by injection	Corium (under epidermis)	Intradermal
	Subcutaneous tissue	Subcutaneous
	Muscle tissue	Intramuscular
	Vein	Intravenous
	Artery	Intra-arterial
	Heart tissue	Intracardial
	Peritoneal cavity	Intraperitoneal
	Bone	Intraosseous
	Spinal canal	Intraspinal or intrathecal

I-22 _Removing medications from an ampule_

Manufacturers of pharmaceutical products prepare parenteral medications in ampules, vials, or prefilled cartridges. An ampule completely encases medication in a glass container. The medication can be removed only by breaking the thin neck of the ampule. It is impossible to prevent airborne contamination of any unused portion of an opened ampule. Therefore, most ampules contain a single dose of medication. Unused portions of an opened ampule are discarded.

PURPOSES OF PROCEDURE

The technique of removing medication from an ampule is performed to

1. Withdraw injectable medication in a sterile manner
2. Administer a single dose of parenteral medication
3. Provide a route for the quick absorption and distribution of medication

ASSESSMENT

OBJECTIVE DATA

- Review the written medical order. Question any information that may be illegible, unsafe, or ambiguous.
- Review information on the drug from an available reference text or package insert.
- Compare the medical order with the kardex or medication card transcription.
- Read the label on the ampule when removing it from the stock or storage area and at least three times before administering the medication.
- From information on the supplied dose (the dose of the drug per volume of solution) determine if it is necessary to compute a fractional dosage.
- Note the specific injectable route by which the medication within the ampule may be administered.
- Determine that the contents of the ampule are not outdated.
- Observe the ampule for the clarity of the medication.
- Determine that the time of administration will not cause an interaction with other scheduled medication.
- Read the client's chart and note any pathology or laboratory results that would contraindicate the administration of the prescribed medication.
- Scan the nursing history or data-base assessment form for information on the client's recent use of other prescription and over-the-counter drugs to determine a potential for a drug interaction.

SUBJECTIVE DATA

- Interview or examine the client to determine if an "as needed" (prn) administration of a medication is appropriate.
- Refer to the client's medication history or ask the client about any allergies to medication.
- Determine the client's knowledge and prior experience in receiving injectable medication.

RELEVANT NURSING DIAGNOSES

Clients who receive parenteral medications may have nursing diagnoses, such as

- _Anxiety_
- _Potential for Altered Comfort_

- *Fear*
- *Potential for Infection*
- *Potential for Injury*
- *Knowledge Deficit*

PLANNING

ESTABLISHING PRIORITIES

Any stat medication order should be prepared and administered immediately. Medication should be withdrawn from an ampule just prior to its administration. The plan for nursing care must be revised or adapted to allow adequate time for preparing medication.

SETTING GOALS

- The client will receive the correct medication and dosage at the appropriate time and by the appropriate route.
- The client will experience therapeutic effects from the prescribed medication.

PREPARATION OF EQUIPMENT

The nurse will need the following:

Ampule of medication
Medication card or Kardex
Sterile syringe and needle (Size will depend on the medication being administered and the client.)
Alcohol swab or gauze pad

Technique for removing medication from an ampule

ACTION	RATIONALE
1. Gather equipment. Check the medication card against the original physician's order.	This comparison helps to identify errors that may have occurred when orders were transcribed.
2. Wash your hands.	Handwashing deters the spread of microorganisms.
3. Tap the stem of the ampule, shown in Figure I-22-1, or twist your wrist quickly while holding the ampule vertically.	This facilitates movement of medication in the stem to the body of the ampule.
4. Wrap a small gauze pad or dry alcohol swab around the neck of the ampule, as shown in Figure I-22-2.	This protects the nurse's fingers from the glass as the ampule is broken.

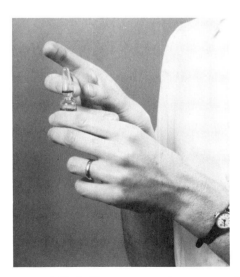

Figure I-22–1 The nurse taps the upper portion of the ampule to remove air bubbles and move all of the medication below the neck of the glass container. A twisting motion can be used as an alternative.

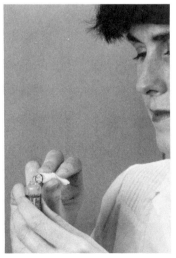

Figure I-22–2 The ampule is wrapped with a gauze pad to protect the nurse as the ampule is opened.

5. Use a snapping motion to break off the top of the ampule along the prescored line at its neck. Always break away from your body.

This protects the nurse's face and fingers from any shattered glass fragments.

6. Remove the cap from the needle by pulling it straight off. Insert the needle into the ampule being careful not to touch the rim.

The rim of the ampule is considered contaminated.

7. Withdraw the medication in the amount ordered. Do not inject any air into the solution. Use either of the following methods:

The nurse carries out the written medical order. Injecting air would cause a loss of volume or frothing within the solution.

a. Insert the tip of the needle into the ampule, which is *upright* on a flat surface, and withdraw fluid into the syringe, as shown in Figure I-22-3.

The contents of the ampule are not under pressure; therefore, air is unnecessary and will cause the contents to overflow.

b. Insert the tip of the needle into the ampule and *invert* the ampule, as shown in Figure I-22-4. Keep the needle centered and not touching the sides of the ampule. Remove the prescribed amount of medication.

Surface tension holds fluid in the ampule when inverted. If the needle touches the side or is removed and then reinserted into the ampule, surface tension will be broken and fluid will run out.

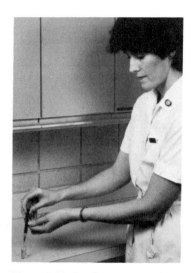

Figure I-22-3 The contents of a glass ampule can be removed easily by inserting a needle into the center of the opened container.

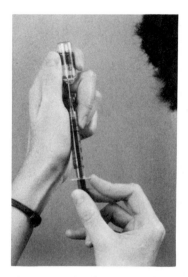

Figure I-22-4 The nurse withdraws medication from an ampule by using this alternative method. Note that the ampule is held vertically and the needle does not touch the rim.

8. Do not expel any air bubbles that may form in the syringe. Wait until the needle has been withdrawn to tap the syringe and expel the air carefully. Check the amount of medication in the syringe and discard any surplus.

Ejecting air from the syringe into the solution will increase pressure in the ampule and can force the medication to spill out over the ampule.

9. Discard the ampule in a suitable container after comparing it with the medication card or Kardex.

If all of the medication has not been removed from the ampule, it must be discarded because there is no way to maintain the sterility of the contents in an opened ampule.

10. Cap the needle on the syringe.

This prevents contamination of the needle.

11. Wash your hands.

Handwashing deters the spread of microorganisms.

SAMPLE DOCUMENTATION

Date	Time	Nurse's note
12/26	1220	R-32, lung sounds are wheezy throughout. Brethine 0.25 mg administered subcutaneously into the left lateral deltoid as per stat order.

F. Littlefield, RN

EVALUATION

REASSESSMENT

The information on the label of the ampule should be reread before withdrawing the contents and before discarding the glass ampule. Reanalyze the appropriateness of the calculated dosage before discarding any remaining portion within the ampule. The client should be reassessed following any administration of medication. Since parenterally administered medications are quickly absorbed, the nurse should observe the client's response. Any adverse reactions should be reported to the physician immediately.

EXPECTED OUTCOMES

The neck of the ampule snaps without loss of its contents.
No injuries occur when opening the ampule.
The client does not experience an adverse reaction.

UNEXPECTED OUTCOMES

The delivered medication contains precipitate or is discolored, or it is past its expiration date.
Shards of glass fall into the reservoir of medication when the neck of the ampule is broken.
The nurse sustains cut fingers when opening the ampule.
The client experiences an allergic reaction or undesirable side-effects to the prescribed medication.

MODIFICATIONS IN SELECTED SITUATIONS

GENERAL VARIATIONS

A file may be used to score the neck of the ampule before snapping it open. This serves to fracture the glass partially thereby facilitating a clean break.
Some agencies require that a needle and syringe with a filter be used when withdrawing the medication from an ampule. The filter traps small glass particles, which prevents the administration of foreign material that is too small to be seen. The needle and filter used to withdraw the medication are discarded and replaced with another sterile needle before administering the drug.

AGE-RELATED VARIATIONS

Expect that dosages for children and geriatric clients will be smaller than the usual range of adult doses.
The appropriateness of a child's dosage can be determined by computing the dose according to the child's age, weight, or body surface area. The latter two are considered more accurate.
Double check the computation of a child's fractional dosage with another nurse or a pharmacist.

HOME-HEALTH VARIATIONS

If not all of the medication in the ampule is required for the client's dose, discard the extra medication into the lavatory or waste receptacle rather than leaving the medication in the ampule.

RELATED TEACHING

Explain the desired effects of the drug, common unusual effects, and the schedule for the administration of newly prescribed medication.
Identify the various sites that may be used for the administration of the medication. Allow the client to select the site from appropriate alternatives.

PERFORMANCE CHECKLIST

When medication is withdrawn from an ampule, the learner:

C	A	U	
[ ]	[ ]	[ ]	Compares the medical order with its transcription on the medication kardex or medication card.
[ ]	[ ]	[ ]	Reviews the literature on the drug, if unfamiliar with its action, usual dosage, method of administration, side-effects, and nursing implications.
[ ]	[ ]	[ ]	Reads the information on the ampule label.
[ ]	[ ]	[ ]	Assembles the type of syringe and size of needle appropriate for the administration of the medication.
[ ]	[ ]	[ ]	Washes hands.
[ ]	[ ]	[ ]	Locates the medication to the base of the ampule.
[ ]	[ ]	[ ]	Protects the finger with alcohol swabs or pads.
[ ]	[ ]	[ ]	Snaps the neck of the ampule away from the hands.
[ ]	[ ]	[ ]	Re-reads the label for the name and dosage of medication contained within the ampule.
[ ]	[ ]	[ ]	Inserts the uncapped needle and syringe.
[ ]	[ ]	[ ]	Avoids touching the shaft of the needle to the rim of the ampule.
[ ]	[ ]	[ ]	Withdraws the appropriate volume from the ampule.
[ ]	[ ]	[ ]	Expels the air and excess volume from the syringe.
[ ]	[ ]	[ ]	Re-reads the information on the ampule one more time.
[ ]	[ ]	[ ]	Changes the needle used for withdrawing the medication, if necessary.
[ ]	[ ]	[ ]	Discards the glass fragments and needle in a puncture-resistant container.
[ ]	[ ]	[ ]	Replaces a protective cap on the needle.
[ ]	[ ]	[ ]	Washes hands.

Outcome: [ ] Pass   [ ] Fail

C = competent; A = acceptable; U = unsatisfactory

Comments: _____

_____

_____

_____   _____
Student's Signature   Date

_____   _____
Instructor's Signature   Date

I-23 — *Removing medication from a vial*

A vial is a glass container of medication designed for parenteral administration. A vial has a self-sealing rubber stopper through which medication is withdrawn. Vials may contain single or multiple doses of medication. The rubber stopper acts as a transmission barrier against the entry of pathogens. The contents of multiple-dose vials remain sterile and can be used for a period of time.

PURPOSES OF PROCEDURE

Medication is removed from a vial to

1. Administer a parenteral dose of medication
2. Safely protect any remaining medication needed for the client in the near future

ASSESSMENT

OBJECTIVE DATA

- Review the written medical order. Question any information that may be illegible, unsafe, or ambiguous.
- Review information on the drug from an available reference text or package insert.
- Compare the medical order with the Kardex or medication card transcription.
- Read the label on the vial when removing it from the stock or stored area.
- From information on the supplied dose (the dose of the drug per volume of solution) determine if it is necessary to compute a fractional dosage.
- Note the specific injectable route by which the medication within the vial may be administered.
- Determine that the contents of the vial are not outdated.
- Observe that the contents of the vial are uniformly mixed. Some medications intended for intramuscular use will not be transparent; however, the solute should be evenly distributed throughout the solution. There should not be any solid particles.
- Determine that the time of administration will not cause an interaction with other scheduled medication.
- Scan the nursing history or data-base assessment form for information on the client's recent use of other prescription and over-the-counter drugs to determine a potential for a drug interaction.

SUBJECTIVE DATA

- Interview and examine the client to determine if an "as needed" (prn) administration of a medication is appropriate.
- Refer to the client's medication history or ask the client about any allergies to medication.
- Determine the client's knowledge and prior experience in receiving injectable medication.

RELEVANT NURSING DIAGNOSES

Clients who receive parenteral medications may have nursing diagnoses, such as

- *Anxiety*
- *Potential for Altered Comfort*
- *Fear*
- *Potential for Infection*
- *Potential for Injury*
- *Knowledge Deficit*

PLANNING **ESTABLISHING PRIORITIES**	A stat medication must be administered as soon as possible. The nurse can adapt the plan for client care to allow sufficient time for the preparation of routinely scheduled medications.
SETTING GOALS	• The client will receive the correct medication and dosage at the appropriate time and by the appropriate route. • The contents of the vial as well as the needle and syringe will remain sterile.
PREPARATION OF EQUIPMENT	The nurse will need the following: Vial of medication Medication card or kardex Sterile syringe and needle (Size will depend on the medication being administered and the client.) Alcohol swab

Technique for removing medication from a vial

ACTION	RATIONALE
1. Gather equipment. Check the medication card against the original physician's order.	This comparison helps identify errors that may have occurred when orders were transcribed.
2. Wash your hands.	Handwashing deters the spread of microorganisms.
3. Remove the metal cap on the vial that protects the rubber stopper.	The metal cap prevents contamination of the rubber top.
4. Swab the rubber top with an alcohol swab.	Alcohol removes surface bacterial contamination. This step is not necessary the first time the rubber stopper is entered but subsequent reentries into the vial require use of alcohol cleansing.
5. Remove the cap from the needle by pulling it straight off.	Before fluid is removed, the injection of an equal amount of air is required to prevent the formation of a partial vacuum, because a vial is a sealed container. If not enough air is injected, the negative pressure makes it difficult to withdraw the medication.

6. Pierce the rubber stopper in the center with the needle tip and inject measured air into the space above the solution, as shown in Figure I-23-1. (Do not inject air into the solution.) The vial may be positioned
 	
   a. Upright on a flat surface
   b. Inverted
	Air bubbled through the solution could result in withdrawal of an inaccurate amount of medication.

7. Invert the vial and withdraw the needle tip slightly so that it is below the fluid level.	This prevents air from being aspirated into the syringe.
8. Draw up the prescribed amount of medication while holding the syringe vertically at eye level, as illustrated in Figure I-23-2.	Holding the syringe at eye level facilitates accurate reading, and the vertical position makes removal of air bubbles from the syringe easy.
9. If any air bubbles accumulate in the syringe, tap the barrel of the syringe sharply and move the needle past the fluid into the air space to reinject the air bubble into the vial. Return the needle tip to the solution and continue withdrawal of the medication.	Removal of air bubbles is necessary to ensure an accurate dose of medication.
10. Once the correct dose is withdrawn, remove the needle from the vial and cap it. If a multiple-dose vial	Since the vial is sealed, the medication inside remains sterile and can be used for future injections.

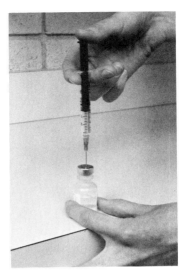

Figure I-23–1 The nurse injects a volume of air equal to the amount of drug that will be withdrawn from the vial.

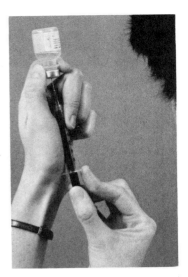

Figure I-23–2 The nurse has inverted the vial and is holding the syringe vertically at eye level to ensure accuracy in removing medication from a vial.

is used, store the vial containing the remaining medication according to the manufacturer's recommendations.

11. Wash your hands.　　　　　　　　　　Handwashing deters the spread of microorganisms.

SAMPLE DOCUMENTATION

Date	*Time*	*Nurse's note*
2/25	0315	Vial of normal saline obtained and used to demonstrate the technique for self-administration of insulin. Practiced cleansing stopper, instilling air, withdrawing prescribed volume. Needs to review rotating solution before instilling air.
		G. Smythe, RN

EVALUATION

REASSESSMENT

The information on the label of a vial should be reread before withdrawing any contents and once again before returning or discarding the vial. The client should be reassessed within the expected period of time for the drug to act.

EXPECTED OUTCOMES

The medication mixes homogenously throughout the solution.
The quantity of medication withdrawn from the vial equals the desired dose.
Medication in an open vial that is not immediately used is labeled with the date and the nurse's initials and returned to a medication drawer for future administration to the same client.
The volume of drug within a vial is comparable to the supply dose indicated on the label.
The client experiences a therapeutic effect from the prescribed medication.

UNEXPECTED OUTCOMES

The vial contains undissolved particles.
The vial contains less volume than indicated on the label.
The vial has not been stored according to the manufacturer's directions.
The client experiences an allergic reaction or undesirable effects in response to the administration of medication.

MODIFICATIONS IN SELECTED SITUATIONS

GENERAL VARIATIONS

Vials occasionally are delivered to the nursing unit containing powdered medication that must be reconstituted according to the directions on the label. The nurse who mixes the solute and solvent must write the supply dosage (weight of the drug per volume of solution), the date, and initials on the label.

To prevent deterioration, the unused contents of some vials should be stored in the refrigerator or protected from exposure to light. Follow the manufacturer's directions or the agency's policy.

Change the needle used for withdrawing the medication when it may be irritating to the layers of tissue through which it must pass during the injection.

HOME-HEALTH VARIATIONS

Ensure the availability of supplies and medication for subsequent visits.

Teach the client and family about the intended and untoward effects of the medication.

RELATED TEACHING

Explain the desired effects of the drug, common unusual effects, and the schedule for the administration of newly prescribed medication.

Identify the various sites that may be used for the administration of the medication. Allow the client to select the site from appropriate alternatives.

PERFORMANCE CHECKLIST

When medication is withdrawn from a vial, the learner:

C   *A*   *U*

[ ]   [ ]   [ ]   Compares the medical order with its transcription on the medication Kardex or medication card

[ ]   [ ]   [ ]   Reviews the literature on the drug if unfamiliar with its action, usual dosage, routes of administration, side-effects, and nursing implications.

[ ]   [ ]   [ ]   Reads the information on the label of the vial

[ ]   [ ]   [ ]   Assembles the type of syringe and size of needle appropriate for the administration of the medication

[ ]   [ ]   [ ]   Washes hands

[ ]   [ ]   [ ]   Removes the protective cap if using a new vial

[ ]   [ ]   [ ]   Cleanses the rubber stopper if using an already opened vial

[ ]   [ ]   [ ]   Fills the syringe with the volume of air equal to the amount of medication that will be withdrawn

[ ]   [ ]   [ ]   Inserts the needle through the rubber stopper

[ ]   [ ]   [ ]   Inverts the vial so that the tip of the needle is above the liquid contents

[ ]   [ ]   [ ]   Instills air within the vial

[ ]   [ ]   [ ]   Positions the needle within the medication

[ ]   [ ]   [ ]   Controls the plunger of the syringe so that the barrel fills with the desired volume of medication

[ ]   [ ]   [ ]   Removes the needle and syringe from the vial

[ ]   [ ]   [ ]   Caps or changes the needle without contamination

[ ]   [ ]   [ ]   Stores or discards the vial

[ ]   [ ]   [ ]   Washes hands

Outcome: [ ] Pass   [ ] Fail

C = competent; A = acceptable; U = unsatisfactory

Comments: _____

_____

_____

_____   _____
Student's Signature   Date

_____   _____
Instructor's Signature   Date

I-24   *Mixing insulins in one syringe*

Some individuals with diabetes mellitus must receive insulin daily to control the level of blood sugar. Several types of insulin are available. Insulin comes in short-acting, intermediate-acting, and long-acting forms. It is prepared in multiple-dose vials for parenteral administration. It is possible that some diabetics require a mixture of two types of insulin.

PURPOSES OF PROCEDURE

Insulins are mixed in one syringe to

1. Avoid dual injections of daily medication
2. Reduce the discomfort associated with multiple injection sites
3. Slow the process of tissue trauma, such as lipoatrophy or lipohypertrophy, associated with a lifetime of daily injections

ASSESSMENT

OBJECTIVE DATA

- Read the medical order for the type, dosage, and time for the administration of insulin.
- Read the label on the insulin vials to confirm that the correct type of insulin has been supplied.
- Note the expiration date on the vial.
- Note the client's fasting blood sugar, glucometer reading, or the level of glucose and acetone in the urine prior to preparing the insulin.
- Identify the last site where insulin was administered.
- Inspect the previous injection site for signs of a local allergic reaction. Redness, warmth, and induration can be observed as long as 24 hours after the previous injection.
- Observe the client for signs associated with hypoglycemia or hyperglycemia; the latter is more likely when insulin has not been administered since the previous day. Common signs of hyperglycemia include warm, flushed, dry skin; rapid breathing; and drowsiness. Common signs of hypoglycemia include excessive perspiration, trembling, tachycardia, slurred speech, and confusion.

SUBJECTIVE DATA

- Ask the client to indicate if he is experiencing common symptoms associated with hyperglycemia, such as thirst, hunger, and drowsiness; ask about common symptoms of hypoglycemia, such as headache, faintness, anxiety, and emotional irritability.
- Question the client concerning discomfort or stinging at a previous injection site, which is also associated with a local allergic reaction to insulin.

RELEVANT NURSING DIAGNOSES

The client who receives insulin may have any of the following nursing diagnoses:

- *Anxiety*
- *Altered Comfort*
- *Fear*
- *Knowledge Deficit*
- *Disturbance in Self-Concept*
- *Potential for Impaired Skin Integrity*
- *Potential for Infection*
- *Potential for Altered Tissue Perfusion*

The nurse must also consider the following collaborative problems:

- *Potential for Hypoglycemia*
- *Potential for Hyperglycemia*

PLANNING

ESTABLISHING PRIORITIES

The onset of hyperglycemia is usually insidious. However, the nurse working in the emergency department may encounter a client in the late stages of ketoacidosis. The administration of fast-acting insulin and other medications is a life-saving measure in this instance. Once diabetes is controlled, the nurse should plan to administer insulin at approximately the same time daily. A morning administration is generally injected approximately $\frac{1}{2}$ hour before the client will eat breakfast.

SETTING GOALS

- The exact prescribed amounts of insulin will be removed from each vial.
- The contents of one vial will not become mixed with the contents of the other vial.
- The client will receive the combined total of both insulins in one syringe within 15 minutes of mixing.
- The client will eat food within $\frac{1}{2}$ hour following the administration of insulin.

PREPARATION OF EQUIPMENT

The nurse will need the following:

Two vials of insulin
Medication card or Kardex
Sterile insulin syringe with a $\frac{1}{2}$-inch or $\frac{5}{8}$-inch, 25-gauge to 27-gauge needle
Alcohol swabs

Technique for mixing insulins in one syringe

ACTION	RATIONALE
1. Gather equipment. Check the medication order against the original physician's order.	This comparison helps to identify errors that may have occurred when orders were transcribed.
2. Wash your hands.	Handwashing deters the spread of microorganisms.
3. If necessary, remove the metal cap that protects the rubber stopper on each vial.	The metal cap prevents contamination of the rubber top.
4. Rotate each vial (other than regular insulin) between the palms of the hands prior to withdrawing insulin.	Shaking vials creates froth that may interfere with withdrawal of an accurate dose. Regular insulin is clear because it does not contain any modifying agent to slow its absorption.
5. Cleanse the rubber tops of previously opened vials with an alcohol swab.	Alcohol removes surface bacterial contamination. This is not necessary the first time the metal cap is removed, but subsequent reentries into the vial require use of alcohol cleansing.
6. Remove the cap from the needle. Inject air into the modified insulin vial equal to the amount of medication to be withdrawn, as shown in Figure I-24-1. Do not allow the needle to touch the medication in the vial. Remove the needle.	Regular insulin should never be adulterated with modified insulin containing added protein. Placing air in the vial of modified insulin first without allowing the needle to contact the insulin ensures that the regular insulin will not be adulterated.
7. Inject air into the regular insulin vial equal to the amount of the medication to be withdrawn, as shown in Figure I-24-2. Do not bubble through the medication.	An equal amount of air must be injected into the vacuum to allow easy withdrawal of medication.
8. Invert the vial of regular insulin and aspirate the amount prescribed, as shown in Figure I-24-3. Remove the needle from the vial.	Regular insulin that contains no additional protein is not contaminated by insulin containing globulin or protamine.

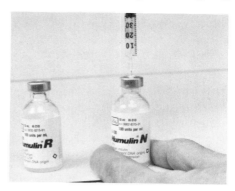

Figure I-24–1 Air is instilled into the vial containing the modified insulin. The needle is prevented from touching the insulin.

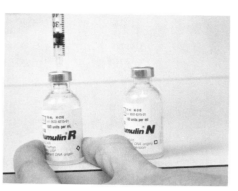

Figure I-24–2 The same needle and syringe are used to inject air into the vial containing the unmodified insulin.

9. Cleanse the rubber top of the modified insulin vial. Insert the needle and withdraw the medication, as shown in Figure I-24-4. Cap the needle.

The previous addition of air eliminates the need to create positive pressure.

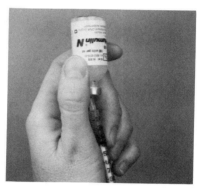

Figure I-24–3 Without withdrawing the needle from the unmodified insulin, the vial is inverted and the insulin is withdrawn.

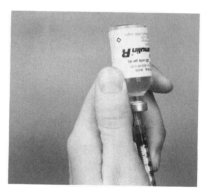

Figure I-24–4 The partially filled syringe is inserted back into the modified insulin and the remaining volume is withdrawn into the syringe.

10. Store vials according to the manufacturer's recommendations.

Insulin need not be refrigerated, but needs to be protected from temperature extremes.

11. Wash your hands.

Handwashing deters the spread of microorganisms.

SAMPLE DOCUMENTATION

Date	Time	Nurse's note
5/26	0730	5 U Humulin R mixed with 20 U Humulin N. Insulin administered subcutaneously 2″ lateral and left of the umbilicus.
		V. Ruggles, RN

EVALUATION

REASSESSMENT

Any container of medication should be reexamined before withdrawing the drug and before putting the container away. Checking the type and volume of insulin with a second nurse is a special reassessment when administering medication, such as insulin, that may cause adverse effects in even small excess amounts.

The client should be assessed for signs of hypoglycemia at the time when the onset of the insulin's action is likely to occur. Reassessment should also take place at the time when the peak effect of the insulin is expected. A local allergic reaction may be noted within an hour to 24 hours postinjection.

EXPECTED OUTCOMES

The regular insulin will remain clear and free of any modified insulin.
The withdrawn volumes and types of insulin are checked and confirmed by a second nurse.
The prescribed volume of insulin is contained within one syringe.

UNEXPECTED OUTCOMES

Modified insulin becomes mixed within the vial of unmodified insulin.

MODIFICATIONS IN SELECTED SITUATIONS

GENERAL VARIATIONS

Mixed insulins must be discarded if not administered within 15 minutes because the two insulins will bond.
The schedule, type, and amounts of insulin may be adjusted daily by the physician when a client is newly diagnosed or is difficult to control.
A carbohydrate snack may be scheduled in the afternoon or at bedtime to compensate for the drop in blood sugar expected at the time of the insulin's peak action.
A longer needle, $\frac{5}{8}$ to 1 inch, or a 90-degree angle may be used when administering insulin to an individual weighing over 190 lb to make sure that the insulin is injected subcutaneously.

AGE-RELATED VARIATIONS

Children who develop diabetes mellitus are insulin dependent. The nurse must assess the juvenile client's response to the administration of insulin frequently because exercise, erratic mealtimes, and dietary noncompliance increase the risk for hypoglycemic or hyperglycemic reactions.
Expect that older diabetics are likely to experience an acceleration of the complications associated with diabetes, such as diabetic retinopathy and cataract formation. The ability to self-administer insulin accurately may be affected by changes in vision.

HOME-HEALTH VARIATIONS

Periodically verify the ability of the client and caregivers to identify the signs and symptoms of hyperglycemia and hypoglycemia.
Before contacting a physician regarding the possibility of adjusting an insulin dosage, check the client's blood sugar using a glucometer.
A loading gauge may be helpful for the visually impaired client who self-administers his own insulin.
An individual who self-administers insulin should have another vial available in case he is unable to obtain a refill of his prescription in adequate time. The unused insulin vial may be stored in the refrigerator until the one being used is empty.
Insulin may be wrapped in a soft cloth and placed in a thermos with a supply of sterile syringes and alcohol pledgets when traveling. This protects the insulin from deterioration due to exposure to heat. It also helps keep all the diabetic's equipment organized in one location.

RELATED TEACHING

Insulin injection sites should be rotated daily. The diagram in Figure I-24-5 shows examples of alternative sites.
Teach the diabetic client to develop a regular schedule for testing blood sugar, administering insulin, eating meals, and performing exercise.
Instruct the diabetic to carry a quickly metabolized form of glucose, such as chocolate candy or sugar cubes, in case he experiences an insulin reaction.
The client should be referred to the Medic-Alert Foundation International, 2323 Colorado, Turlock, California 95380, for a bracelet identifying him as a diabetic.
Advise the client to monitor blood glucose levels frequently when experiencing an infection or stress. Low or high levels should be reported immediately.
Explain that the client should notify the physician if unable to eat.

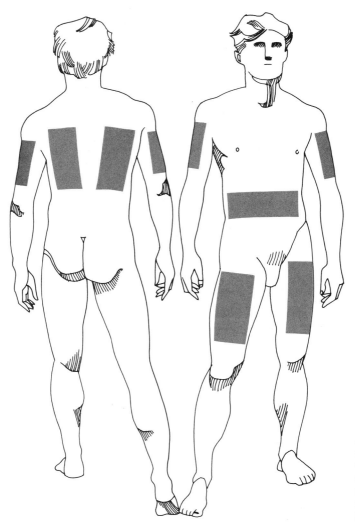

Figure I-24–5 The shaded areas on this diagram indicate sites where subcutaneous injections can be given. Diabetics should rotate from one area of the body to another with each subsequent injection.

The client should be referred to the dietitian for an explanation of his calorie-controlled diet and exchange lists. The client may be allowed to adjust food intake upwardly prior to an activity that involves a great deal of exercise.

Any diabetic should be encouraged to have regular examinations by an ophthalmologist and family practitioner to detect the onset of systemic complications associated with diabetes, such as arteriosclerosis, peripheral vascular disease, coronary artery disease, nephropathy, and neuropathy.

PERFORMANCE CHECKLIST

When insulins are mixed, the learner:

C	A	U	
[ ]	[ ]	[ ]	Compares the medical order with its transcription on the medication Kardex or medication card
[ ]	[ ]	[ ]	Reviews the literature for the time of onset and peak action of the prescribed insulin, if unfamiliar with the drug
[ ]	[ ]	[ ]	Notes the blood glucose level obtained prior to the scheduled administration of insulin
[ ]	[ ]	[ ]	Reviews the client's record for the location of the last administration of insulin
[ ]	[ ]	[ ]	Obtains the two vials of insulin, an insulin syringe, and alcohol swabs
[ ]	[ ]	[ ]	Reads the labels to ensure that the prescribed types of insulin have been supplied
[ ]	[ ]	[ ]	Washes hands
[ ]	[ ]	[ ]	Rotates any vial containing modified insulin
[ ]	[ ]	[ ]	Rereads the label
[ ]	[ ]	[ ]	Instills air into the modified insulin equal to the volume that will be withdrawn
[ ]	[ ]	[ ]	Withdraws the needle and repeats the above step with the vial containing the unmodified (regular) insulin
[ ]	[ ]	[ ]	Inverts the vial of unmodified insulin, withdrawing the prescribed amount
[ ]	[ ]	[ ]	Requests that a second nurse check the volume and type of insulin and compares it with the written order
[ ]	[ ]	[ ]	Inserts the needle into the vial of modified insulin and withdraws the prescribed amount
[ ]	[ ]	[ ]	Double checks the total dose and type of insulin in the vial of modified insulin with the second nurse
[ ]	[ ]	[ ]	Checks the labels on the vials one last time
[ ]	[ ]	[ ]	Recaps the needle
[ ]	[ ]	[ ]	Washes hands

Outcome: [ ] Pass   [ ] Fail

C = competent; A = acceptable; U = unsatisfactory

Comments: _____

_____

_____

_____   _____
Student's Signature   Date

_____   _____
Instructor's Signature   Date

I-25

Administering an intradermal injection

The longest absorption rate by any parenteral route occurs with an intradermal injection. Medication injected below the epidermis is slowly absorbed through the capillaries in the area. Intradermal sites, such as the inner surface of the forearm, upper chest, and upper back, facilitate the assessment of a local reaction since they are easily observed.

PURPOSES OF PROCEDURE

Intradermal injections are performed to

1. Identify allergens to which the client may be hypersensitive
2. Diagnose individuals who have developed antibodies against specific pathogens, such as the tubercle bacillus
3. Infiltrate superficial layers of the skin with a local anesthetic, such as 1% Xylocaine, prior to performing a venipuncture

ASSESSMENT

OBJECTIVE DATA

- Review the written medical order.
- Read the label on the pharmaceutical product; note the name, strength, supply dose, and expiration date.
- Verify that the five rights of medication administration, identified in Table I-25-1, are followed.

Table 25–1
The five rights of medication administration

1. *Right* drug
2. *Right* dose
3. *Right* route
4. *Right* time
5. *Right* client

- Examine the skin of potential injection sites for areas that are irritated, bruised, open, draining, unusually pigmented, or excessively hairy.
- Review the literature to determine the expected and unexpected effects associated with the injection if unfamiliar with the drug.
- Determine that a physician is available for assistance if a potential allergic reaction is possible.
- Identify the location of emergency medication, oxygen, and an artificial airway.

SUBJECTIVE DATA

- Interview the client concerning his history of allergies and his unique types of reactions.
- Determine the client's knowledge and response to explanations about the technique for administering an intradermal injection.

RELEVANT NURSING DIAGNOSES

An individual receiving an intradermal injection may have nursing diagnoses, such as

- *Anxiety*
- *Fear*
- *Potential for Altered Cardiac Output*
- *Potential for Injury*
- *Knowledge Deficit*
- *Potential for Ineffective Airway Clearance*

PLANNING

ESTABLISHING PRIORITIES

Intradermal injections are generally not given during emergency situations. Therefore, the nurse may plan to perform this procedure with some flexibility.

SETTING GOALS

- The client will receive the specified strength and dosage of the ordered preparation within the dermis of the skin.

PREPARATION OF EQUIPMENT

The following should be gathered when preparing to administer an intradermal injection:

Medication
Medication card or kardex
Sterile syringe and needle (Size will depend on the medication being administered and the client; it is common to use a $\frac{1}{2}$-inch to $\frac{3}{8}$-inch, 26-gauge or 27-gauge needle with a tuberculin syringe.
Alcohol swab
Acetone and 2 × 2 gauze square (optional)

Technique for administering an intradermal injection

ACTION	RATIONALE
1. Assemble equipment and check the physician's order.	This ensures that the client receives the right medication at the right time by the proper route. Many intradermal drugs are potent allergens and may cause a significant reaction if given in an incorrect dosage.
2. Explain the procedure to the client.	An explanation encourages cooperation and reduces apprehension.
3. Wash your hands.	Handwashing deters the spread of microorganisms.
4. If necessary, withdraw medication from an ampule or vial as described in Procedures I-22 and I-23.	Pharmaceutical products for parenteral administration are supplied in various containers.
5. Select an area on the inner aspect of the forearm. The upper chest and upper back beneath the scapulae are also sites for intradermal injections.	The forearm is a convenient and easy location for introducing an agent intradermally.
6. Cleanse the area with an alcohol swab while wiping with a firm, circular motion and moving outward from the injection site. Allow the skin to dry. If the skin is oily, cleanse the area with a pledget moistened with acetone.	Pathogens on the skin can be forced into the tissues by the needle. Introducing alcohol into tissues irritates the tissues and is uncomfortable for the client. Acetone is effective for removing oily substances from the skin.
7. Use your nondominant hand to spread the skin taut.	Taut skin provides an easy entrance into intradermal tissue.
8. Remove the needle cap with your nondominant hand by pulling it straight off.	This protects the needle from contact with microorganisms.

9. Place the needle almost flat against the client's skin, bevel side up, and insert the needle beneath the skin so that the point of the needle can be seen through the skin, as shown in Figure I-25-1. Insert the needle only about ⅛ inch.

Intradermal tissue will be entered when the needle is held as near parallel to the skin as possible and is inserted about ⅛ inch.

10. Slowly inject the agent while watching for a small wheal or blister to appear, as shown in Figure I-25-2. If none appears, withdraw the needle slightly.

If a small wheal or blister appears, the agent is in intradermal tissue.

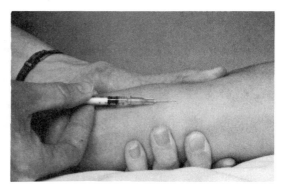

Figure I-25–1   The nurse is giving an intradermal injection. Note that the needle is almost parallel to the client's forearm.

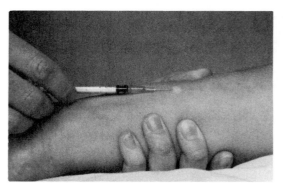

Figure I-25–2   When the needle is placed correctly within the intradermal layers, a wheal appears when the solution is injected.

11. Withdraw the needle quickly at the same angle that it was inserted.

Withdrawing the needle quickly and at the angle at which it entered the skin minimizes tissue damage and discomfort for the client.

12. Do not massage the area after removing the needle.

Massaging the area where an intradermal injection is given may interfere with test results by spreading medication to underlying subcutaneous tissue.

13. Do not recap the used needle. Discard the needle and syringe in an appropriate receptacle.

Most accidental puncture wounds occur when recapping the needles. Leaving the needle uncapped protects the nurse from accidental injury with the needle.

14. Assist the client to a position of comfort.

The nurse considers the well-being of the client.

15. Wash your hands.

Handwashing deters the spread of microorganisms.

16. Chart the administration of the medication.

Accurate documentation is necessary to prevent a medication error.

17. Observe the area for signs of a reaction at ordered intervals, usually at 24-hour to 72-hour periods. Inform the client of this inspection. In some agencies, a circle may be drawn on the skin around the injection site.

A circle easily identifies the site of intradermal injections and allows for careful observation of the exact area.

SAMPLE DOCUMENTATION

Date	Time	Nurse's note
8/24	1640	Intradermal Mantoux test administered by injecting 0.1 ml PPD-tuberculin under the skin of L forearm.
		J. Fabres, RN

EVALUATION

REASSESSMENT

The product label should be reexamined before withdrawing the medication and again before replacing or discarding the container.

Stay with the client for at least 15 minutes following an intradermal injection of a substance that is a known allergen or if the individual has a history of allergic reactions. Insist that the client remain in an outpatient clinic, physician's office, or health clinic for 30 minutes after an intradermal injection to detect delayed reactions.

Reexamine the site of a tuberculin test in 24 hours and again in 48 hours. Measure the area of redness and swelling. Report any areas more than 10 mm in diameter.

EXPECTED OUTCOMES

A small wheal, approximately the size of a mosquito bite, is evident in the area of the injection.

The client remains free of allergic symptoms following the injection.

UNEXPECTED OUTCOMES

The bevel of the needle is not placed deeply enough; a wheal does not form, or the volume escapes from the injection site.

The site bleeds or becomes bruised.

The client experiences an allergic reaction, such as itching, rash, hives, dyspnea, wheezing, hypotension, or loss of consciousness.

MODIFICATIONS IN SELECTED SITUATIONS

GENERAL VARIATIONS

Some diagnostic preparations are supplied in multiple-dose vials, the contents of which are used for many different clients.

Avoid aspiration prior to the injection. There are no veins or arteries located in the dermis. The needle is larger than the diameter of the capillaries so direct injection into the vascular system is unlikely.

Write the date on a newly opened multiple-dose vial to avoid the repeated use of a biologic product after an extended period of time.

HOME-HEALTH VARIATIONS

In accordance with agency policy and the physician's orders, ensure that appropriate medication is available in the event that the client experiences an allergic reaction.

RELATED TEACHING

Explain the purpose of the injection and expected and unexpected after-effects.

Inform the client that a reaction to a tuberculin test less than 10 mm is not significant. Even larger reactions do not indicate that the client has an active case of tuberculosis but require additional testing, such as a chest x-ray or sputum examination.

Explain that once a client has a positive reaction to a tuberculin test, it will remain positive throughout his lifetime.

(Performance checklist next page)

PERFORMANCE CHECKLIST

When an injection is given intradermally, the learner:

C   A   U

[ ]   [ ]   [ ]   Reads the medical order written by the physician

[ ]   [ ]   [ ]   Compares the transcribed information on the medication card or Kardex with the medical order

[ ]   [ ]   [ ]   Reviews the usual strength and dosage of the prescribed medication, if unknown, in reference literature

[ ]   [ ]   [ ]   Checks the client's identification band

[ ]   [ ]   [ ]   Explains the purpose and technique for administering an intradermal injection to the client

[ ]   [ ]   [ ]   Inspects potential injection sites

[ ]   [ ]   [ ]   Washes hands

[ ]   [ ]   [ ]   Gathers the needed equipment

[ ]   [ ]   [ ]   Reads the label on the material for injection and notes the name, strength, supply dose, expiration date, and clarity of the solution

[ ]   [ ]   [ ]   Re-reads the label before withdrawing the medication

[ ]   [ ]   [ ]   Withdraws the solution in the appropriate manner for those supplied within an ampule or vial

[ ]   [ ]   [ ]   Reads the label one last time before replacing or discarding the medication container

[ ]   [ ]   [ ]   Pulls the privacy curtain and shuts the door to the client's room

[ ]   [ ]   [ ]   Washes hands

[ ]   [ ]   [ ]   Cleanses the client's skin with alcohol or acetone

[ ]   [ ]   [ ]   Inserts the bevel of the needle at a 5-degree to 15-degree angle approximately $\frac{1}{8}$ inch below the surface of the skin

[ ]   [ ]   [ ]   Instills the medication, forming a well-defined wheal

[ ]   [ ]   [ ]   Removes the needle from the site

[ ]   [ ]   [ ]   Notes the time of the injection

[ ]   [ ]   [ ]   Washes hands

[ ]   [ ]   [ ]   Remains with the client for the purpose of observing the site and any untoward reactions

[ ]   [ ]   [ ]   Provides the client with a signal device to inform the nurse of adverse symptoms

[ ]   [ ]   [ ]   Records the administration of the intradermal injection

[ ]   [ ]   [ ]   Returns to observe the client for signs of a local or systemic reaction

Outcome: [ ] Pass   [ ] Fail

C = competent; A = acceptable; U = unsatisfactory

Comments: _____

_____

_____

_____   _____

Student's Signature   Date

_____   _____

Instructor's Signature   Date

I-26

Administering a subcutaneous injection

Subcutaneous tissue lies between the skin and the muscle. The same sites as shown earlier in Figure I-24-5 can be used for injecting any medication intended for subcutaneous tissue. Heparin and insulin are examples of drugs commonly injected by this parenteral route. Most subcutaneous injections contain no more than 1 ml of medication. Larger amounts contribute to greater discomfort during the injection and slower absorption.

PURPOSES OF PROCEDURE

A subcutaneous injection is administered to

1. Provide the client with medication that cannot be absorbed by the oral route
2. Allow for the proper rate of absorption of certain medications

ASSESSMENT

OBJECTIVE DATA

- Read the medical order.
- Compare the transcribed information on the medication card or kardex with the physician's written order.
- Review the action of the drug, side-effects, contraindications, usual dosage, route(s) of administration, and other pertinent information in an appropriate pharmacology reference if unfamiliar with the medication.
- Note the results of all pertinent laboratory tests and the effect that the prescribed medication is likely to produce. Note any pathology or laboratory tests that would contraindicate the administration of the prescribed medication.
- Identify the client by checking his admission armband.
- Inspect the client's potential sites for injection, such as the upper arm, anterior aspects of the thigh, the lower abdominal wall, and upper back.
- Read the medication label to verify that the right medication and the right dosage will be administered by the right route to the right client, at the right time.

SUBJECTIVE DATA

- Interview the client to determine his prior experience in receiving injections and any history of allergies to medications.
- Explore the client's site preference, if appropriate.

RELEVANT NURSING DIAGNOSES

A client who requires a subcutaneous injection may have nursing diagnoses such as

- *Anxiety*
- *Altered Comfort*
- *Fear*
- *Potential for Injury*
- *Knowledge Deficit*

PLANNING

ESTABLISHING PRIORITIES

Medications administered by subcutaneous injection are generally scheduled on a routine timetable. Therefore, the nurse should administer the injection as closely as possible to the agency's established schedule. Any medication ordered for stat administration, such as epinephrine, takes precedence over other usual nursing actions. When a client requests a drug ordered on a prn (as needed) basis, the nurse should investigate and comply with the request as soon as possible, if that is appropriate.

SETTING GOALS

- The client will receive the prescribed dose of medication within $\frac{1}{2}$ hour of the scheduled time.
- The medication will be injected into the subcutaneous layer of tissue.

PREPARATION OF EQUIPMENT

The nurse will need the following:

Medication
Medication card or Kardex
A sterile syringe and needle (Size will depend on the medication being administered and the client; it is common to use a $\frac{1}{2}$-inch to 1-inch, 25-gauge needle, with an insulin, tuberculin, or 1-ml to 3-ml syringe.)
Alcohol swabs

Technique for administering a subcutaneous injection

ACTION	RATIONALE
1. Assemble equipment and check the physician's order.	This ensures that the client receives the right medication at the right time by the proper route.
2. Explain the procedure to the client.	An explanation encourages client cooperation and reduces apprehension.
3. Wash your hands.	Handwashing deters the spread of microorganisms.
4. If necessary, withdraw the medication from an ampule or vial as described in Procedures I-22 and I-23.	Parenteral medications are generally supplied in ampules, vials, or prefilled cartridges.
5. Add 0.1 to 0.2 ml of air to the filled syringe according to agency policy.	The air bubble will force the total volume of medication from the syringe; none will be trapped in the needle.
6. Identify the client carefully. Close the curtain to provide privacy.	This nursing responsibility guards against error.
7. Have the client assume a position appropriate for the site selected:	Injection into a tense muscle causes discomfort.
a. Outer aspect of upper arm—the client's arm should be relaxed at this side.	
b. Anterior thigh—the client may sit or lie with the leg relaxed.	
c. Abdomen—the client may lie in a semirecumbent position.	
d. Scapular area—the client may be prone, on the side, or assume a sitting position.	
8. Locate the site of choice and ensure that the area is not tender and is free of lumps or nodules.	Good visualization is necessary to establish the correct location of the site and avoid damage to tissues. Nodules or lumps may indicate a previous injection site where absorption was inadequate.
9. Clean the area of the skin around the injection site with an alcohol swab, as illustrated in Figure I-26-1. Use a firm, circular motion while moving outward from the injection site. Allow the antiseptic to dry. Leave the alcohol swab in a clean area for reuse when withdrawing the needle.	Friction helps clean the skin. A clean area is contaminated when a soiled object is rubbed over its surface.
10. Remove the needle cap with the nondominant hand, pulling it straight off.	This protects the needle from contact with microorganisms.

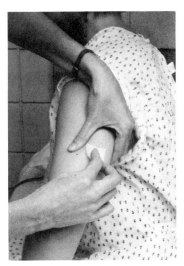

Figure I-26–1 An alcohol swab is used to cleanse the upper arm before administering a subcutaneous injection.

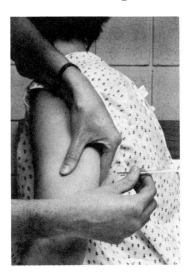

Figure I-26–2 The nurse is injecting a medication subcutaneously. Note how the tissue is bunched. The nurse holds the syringe like a dart to pierce the skin and tissue quickly.

11. Grasp and bunch the area surrounding the injection site, as the nurse in Figure I-26-2 is doing, or spread the skin at the site.

12. Hold the syringe in the dominant hand between the thumb and the forefinger. Insert the needle quickly at an angle of 45 degrees to 90 degrees, depending on the amount and turgor of the tissue and the length of the needle, as illustrated in Figure I-26-3.

This provides for easy, less painful entry into the subcutaneous tissue. The decision to pinch or spread the tissue at the injection site will depend on the size of the client. If obese, the skin needs to be bunched to allow the needle to penetrate below the fatty layer in subcutaneous tissue.

Subcutaneous tissue is abundant in well-nourished, well-hydrated persons and sparse in emaciated, dehydrated, or very thin persons.

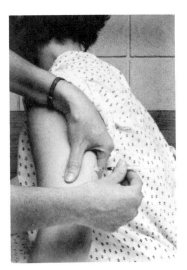

Figure I-26–3 This syringe is being held at a 90-degree angle to locate the needle within the subcutaneous tissue of this client.

13. After the needle is in place, release the grasp on the tissue and immediately move your nondominant hand to steady the lower end of the syringe. Slide your dominant hand to the tip of the barrel.

Injecting the solution into compressed tissues results in pressure against the nerve fibers and creates discomfort. Your nondominant hand secures the syringe and allows for smooth aspiration.

14. Aspirate by pulling back gently on the plunger of the syringe to determine whether the needle is in a blood vessel. If blood appears, the needle should be withdrawn and discarded, and a new syringe should be prepared with new medication.

Discomfort and possibly a serious reaction may occur if a drug intended for subcutaneous use is injected into a vein.

15. If no blood appears, inject the solution slowly.

Rapid injection of the solution creates pressure in the tissues, resulting in discomfort.

16. Withdraw the needle quickly at the same angle it was inserted.

Slow withdrawal of the needle pulls the tissues and causes discomfort. Applying countertraction around the injection site helps prevent pulling on the tissue as the needle is withdrawn. Removing the needle at the same angle it was inserted minimizes tissue damage and discomfort for the client.

17. Massage the area gently with the alcohol swab.

Massaging helps distribute the solution and hastens its absorption.

18. Do not recap the used needle. Discard the needle and syringe in an appropriate receptacle.

Most accidental puncture wounds occur when recapping needles. Leaving the needle uncapped protects the nurse from an accidental needle-stick.

19. Assist the client to a position of comfort.

This provides for the well-being of the client.

20. Chart the administration of medication.

Accurate documentation is necessary to prevent a medication error.

21. Evaluate the response of the client to the medication within an appropriate time frame.

A reaction to the medication given subcutaneously may occur within 15 to 30 minutes after injection.

SAMPLE DOCUMENTATION

Date	Time	Nurse's note
1/09	1152	Dilaudid 2 mg administered subcutaneously into L upper arm for "sharp pain" in abdominal incisional area.
		G. Murphy, RN

EVALUATION

REASSESSMENT

The information on the medication label should always be checked before withdrawing the drug and again before replacing or discarding the container.

The condition of the site used for the injection should be inspected and any alteration, such as redness, warmth, swelling, or induration, should be documented in the client's record.

The client's response to the intended action of the medication should be observed within an appropriate time, usually 15 to 30 minutes, following the injection. A description of the reassessment data should be documented in the client's record.

EXPECTED OUTCOMES

The client experiences the intended effects of the drug and no ill effects.

UNEXPECTED OUTCOMES

Blood enters the syringe at the time of aspiration.

Discomfort at the injection site intensifies or becomes prolonged. Signs and symptoms, such as pain, redness, itching, swelling, numbness and tingling, or bruising, become evident.

The client experiences undesirable effects in response to the injected medication.

MODIFICATIONS IN SELECTED SITUATIONS

The nurse can exercise judgment and administer a subcutaneous injection at a 90-degree angle with a ½-inch needle when a client weighs more than 190 lb, rather

GENERAL VARIATIONS

than the more usual 45-degree angle with a $\frac{5}{8}$-inch needle for clients of average weight. Either technique will locate the needle in subcutaneous tissue.

The administration of heparin is accompanied by certain modifications in the usual technique for administering a subcutaneous injection:

Change the needle after removing heparin from a vial or ampule.

Ice may be placed in a clean rubber glove and applied to the site for 10 minutes prior to injecting heparin to reduce local bleeding.

Avoid aspirating a syringe when injecting heparin, which could lead to local bleeding.

Refrain from massaging the injection site when removing a syringe containing heparin.

HOME-HEALTH
VARIATIONS

Construct a hand-drawn chart of injection sites with dates indicating when each site should be used.

Prefill and date a supply of syringes with medication when the client has difficulty withdrawing accurate dosages.

RELATED TEACHING

Explain the purpose of the injection and expected and unexpected after-effects to the client.

Teach the client receiving heparin to observe for signs of bleeding, such as bruising, bleeding gums, blood in the stool, and so on.

Inform the client as to the schedule for administering any new medication. Instruct the client to identify when he feels the need for a medication prescribed on a prn basis.

Indicate the subsequent assessments that will be useful in determining the client's response to the medication.

PERFORMANCE CHECKLIST

When a medication is injected subcutaneously, the learner:

C	A	U	
[ ]	[ ]	[ ]	Reads the medical order written by the physician.
[ ]	[ ]	[ ]	Compares the medical order with the information transcribed to the medication card or Kardex.
[ ]	[ ]	[ ]	Reviews pertinent drug information in an appropriate text if unfamiliar with the medication.
[ ]	[ ]	[ ]	Explains to the client the action of the medication, expected effects, method of administration, and schedule for receiving the drug.
[ ]	[ ]	[ ]	Inspects potential sites and notes the amount of tissue pad at the selected site when the skin is bunched.
[ ]	[ ]	[ ]	Washes hands.
[ ]	[ ]	[ ]	Selects an appropriate size and gauge needle and syringe according to the type of medication, the size of the client, and the volume of the medication.
[ ]	[ ]	[ ]	Reads the label on the container of medication when removing it from its stocked location.
[ ]	[ ]	[ ]	Re-reads the label before withdrawing medication.
[ ]	[ ]	[ ]	Withdraws the medication into the syringe according to the manner in which the drug has been supplied.

C = competent; A = acceptable; U = unsatisfactory

(Continued)

PERFORMANCE CHECKLIST (Continued)

C	A	U	
[ ]	[ ]	[ ]	Reads the label on the drug container one last time before replacing or discarding it.
[ ]	[ ]	[ ]	Identifies the client by checking the identification band.
[ ]	[ ]	[ ]	Pulls the privacy curtain and shuts the door.
[ ]	[ ]	[ ]	Washes hands.
[ ]	[ ]	[ ]	Cleanses the skin with alcohol in a circular motion.
[ ]	[ ]	[ ]	Bunches or stretches the skin.
[ ]	[ ]	[ ]	Inserts the needle quickly at either a 45-degree or 90-degree angle.
[ ]	[ ]	[ ]	Releases the pad of tissue.
[ ]	[ ]	[ ]	Steadies the lower end of the syringe.
[ ]	[ ]	[ ]	Aspirates to check for blood (unless injecting heparin).
[ ]	[ ]	[ ]	Injects the medication.
[ ]	[ ]	[ ]	Removes the needle.
[ ]	[ ]	[ ]	Massages the site with an alcohol pledget (unless the drug is heparin).
[ ]	[ ]	[ ]	Assists the client to a comfortable position and provides him with the signal device.
[ ]	[ ]	[ ]	Disposes of the needle, its cover, and the syringe in a puncture-resistant container.
[ ]	[ ]	[ ]	Washes hands.
[ ]	[ ]	[ ]	Records the administration of the medication on appropriate forms.
[ ]	[ ]	[ ]	Checks the client within 15 to 30 minutes to evaluate his response to the medication.

Outcome: [ ] Pass   [ ] Fail

C = competent; A = acceptable; U = unsatisfactory

Comments: _____
_____
_____

_____	_____
Student's Signature	**Date**
_____	_____
Instructor's Signature	**Date**

I-27
Administering an intramuscular injection

The intramuscular route is often used for drugs that are irritating, since there are few nerve endings in deep tissue. Absorption occurs more rapidly than with a subcutaneous injection because muscle tissue is more vascular. A volume of 3 ml is considered the maximum amount that is given in one injection.

The sites for intramuscular injections are limited to those well-developed muscles that anatomically are located away from large nerves, bones, and major blood vessels. Repeated injections should be rotated to promote absorption and lessen discomfort.

PURPOSES OF PROCEDURE

Intramuscular injections are administered to

1. Promote faster absorption of medication as compared with the subcutaneous route
2. Facilitate the instillation of a larger volume of medication than in the subcutaneous layer of tissue
3. Reduce the discomfort associated with the injection of irritating medications

ASSESSMENT

OBJECTIVE DATA

- Read the medical order.
- Compare the transcribed information on the medication card or Kardex with the physician's written order.
- Review the action of the drug, side-effects, contraindications, usual dosage, route(s) of administration, and other pertinent information in an appropriate pharmacology reference if unfamiliar with the medication.
- Read the client's record and review diagnostic test results to determine the therapeutic reason for the administration of the medication.
- Note any pathology or laboratory results that would contraindicate the administration of the prescribed medication.
- Examine the chart to discover the locations of previous injections.
- Inspect the potential sites for injection, such as the dorsogluteal and ventrogluteal areas, the vastus lateralis and deltoid muscles, or, as a last resort, the rectus femoris muscle in an adult. Exclude the deltoid and the dorsogluteal sites in infants and children since the muscles are not adequately developed for the instillation of a large volume of medication.
- Palpate the potential site. Eliminate a tender site or one that feels contracted, firm, or tense.
- Read the medication label to verify that the correct medication in an appropriate supply dose prepared for intramuscular injection has been delivered for the intended client.

SUBJECTIVE DATA

- Interview the client to determine his prior experience in receiving injections and any history of allergies to medications.
- Explore the client's site preference, if a choice is appropriate.

RELEVANT NURSING DIAGNOSES

A client who receives an intramuscular injection may have nursing diagnoses, such as

- *Anxiety*
- *Potential Altered Comfort*
- *Fear*
- *Potential for Injury*
- *Knowledge Deficit*

PLANNING

ESTABLISHING PRIORITIES

Most intramuscular injections are scheduled for repeated times throughout the day. The nurse should allow adequate time for the preparation and administration of medication within a half hour of the scheduled routine. Stat medications should be given immediately.

SETTING GOALS

- The client will receive the right medication, the right dosage, by the right route, at the right time.
- The selected site will be well visualized, relaxed, and free of any irritation or inflammation.
- The site will not develop any indication of abscess, necrosis, skin slough, nerve injury, lingering pain, or periostitis.

PREPARATION OF EQUIPMENT

The following will be needed when administering an intramuscular injection:

Medication
Medication card or Kardex
Sterile syringe and needle (Size will depend on medication being administered and the anatomical characteristics of the client; commonly the nurse will need a 1-ml to 3-ml syringe with a 1-inch to 1½-inch, 20-gauge to 22-gauge needle.)
Alcohol swab

Technique for administering an intramuscular injection

ACTION	RATIONALE
1. Assemble the equipment and check the physician's order.	This ensures that the client receives the right medication at the right time via the proper route.
2. Explain the procedure to the client.	An explanation encourages cooperation and alleviates apprehension.
3. Wash your hands.	Handwashing deters the spread of microorganisms.
4. If necessary, withdraw the medication from an ampule or vial as described in Procedures I-22 and I-23.	Medications for parenteral administration are generally supplied in ampules, vials, or prefilled cartridges.
5. Add 0.1 to 0.2 ml of air to the syringe.	The air bubble will force the medication out of the needle shaft and helps to trap it in the muscle tissue. Some experts question this practice and feel that it interferes with the administration of an accurate dose.
6. Provide for privacy. Have the client assume a position appropriate for the site selected:	Injection into a tense muscle causes discomfort.

a. Dorsogluteal, shown in Figure I-27-1—The client may lie prone with toes pointing inward or on the side with the upper leg flexed and placed in front of the lower leg.

b. Ventrogluteal—The client may lie on his back or side with the hip and knee flexed.

c. Vastus lateralis or rectus femoris—The client may lie on his back or assume a sitting position.

d. Deltoid—The client may sit or lie with the arm relaxed.

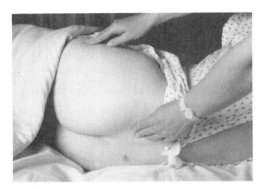

Figure I-27–1 The dorsogluteal site and surrounding anatomical structures are identified. The site of the injection is lateral and slightly superior to the midpoint of the line drawn from the trochanter to the posterior superior iliac spine. It is important to avoid injury to the sciatic nerve, which is also located near the dorsogluteal site.

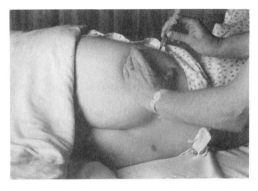

Figure I-27–2 The nurse spreads the skin, making it taut. The needle will enter the tissue under less resistance, reducing the client's discomfort.

7. Locate the site of choice and ensure that the area is not tender and is free of lumps or nodules.

Good visualization is necessary to establish the correct location of the site and avoid damage to tissues. Nodules or lumps may indicate a previous injection site where absorption was inadequate.

8. Clean the area thoroughly with an alcohol swab, using friction.

Pathogens present on the skin can be forced into the tissues by the needle.

9. Remove the needle cap by pulling it straight off.

This protects the needle from contact with microorganisms.

10. Spread the skin at the site using your nondominant hand, as shown in Figure I-27-2.

Spreading makes the tissue taut and minimizes discomfort.

11. Hold the syringe in your dominant hand between the thumb and forefinger. Quickly dart the needle into the tissue at a 90-degree angle.

A quick injection is less painful. Inserting the needle at a 90-degree angle facilitates entry into muscle tissue.

12. As soon as the needle is in place, move your nondominant hand to hold the lower end of the syringe, as the nurse in Figure I-27-3 is doing. Slide the dominant hand to the top of the barrel.

Steadying the syringe allows for ease of aspiration.

13. Aspirate by slowly pulling back on the plunger, as shown in Figure I-27-3, to determine whether the needle is in a blood vessel. If blood is aspirated, discard the needle, syringe, and medication; prepare a new sterile set-up; and inject another site.

Discomfort and possibly a serious reaction may occur if a drug intended for intramuscular use is injected into a vein.

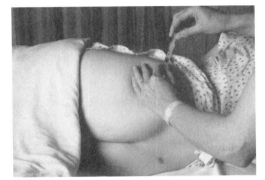

Figure I-27–3 The nurse pulls back on the plunger to assess if the needle has entered a blood vessel.

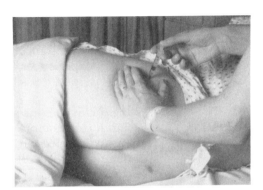

Figure I-27-4 If no blood is aspirated, the nurse injects the solution slowly, followed by the air bubble.

14. If no blood is aspirated, inject the solution slowly, as shown in Figure I-27-4 on page 173.

Injecting slowly helps reduce discomfort by allowing time for the solution to disperse in the tissues.

15. Remove the needle quickly.

Slow removal of the needle pulls the tissues and may cause discomfort.

16. Massage the injection site with the alcohol swab using gentle pressure.

Massaging helps distribute the solution and hastens its absorption by increasing blood flow to the area.

17. Do not recap the used needle. Discard the needle and syringe in an appropriate receptacle.

Leaving the needle uncapped protects the nurse from an accidental needle-stick. Most accidental puncture wounds occur when recapping needles.

18. Assist the client to a position of comfort.

The client's well-being is maintained.

19. Wash your hands.

Handwashing deters the spread of microorganisms.

20. Chart the administration of the medication.

Accurate documentation is necessary to prevent a medication error.

21. Evaluate the client's response to the medication within an appropriate time frame.

Reaction to medication given via the intramuscular route is likely to be evident within 15 to 30 minutes after injection.

SAMPLE DOCUMENTATION

Date	Time	Nurse's note
6/19	1040	Penicillin G 600,000 U injected intramuscularly into the dorsogluteal site in the R buttock.
		S. O'Malley, LPN

EVALUATION

REASSESSMENT

The information on the supplied medication should be re-read before withdrawing the medication and again before replacing or discarding the container.
The client's response to the intended action of the medication should be observed and documented within the first 30 minutes after the injection.
The condition of the integument and more specifically the site of previous injections should be observed as part of the daily head-to-toe assessment.

EXPECTED OUTCOMES

The medication is injected easily within the selected site, when no blood has been aspirated.
The client experiences a therapeutic response to the medication.

UNEXPECTED OUTCOMES

A blood vessel is entered when the needle is inserted. Blood mixes with the medication during aspiration and must be discarded.
The needle meets with resistance, possibly due to contact with bone, when inserted.
The site becomes inflamed, indurated, or painful after the injection.
The client experiences numbness, tingling, or altered muscle function in the area of the injection, possibly due to nerve irritation.

MODIFICATIONS IN SELECTED SITUATIONS

GENERAL VARIATIONS

Use the rectus femoris site only when others are contraindicated since many clients find it causes more postinjection discomfort.
Intramuscular injections into the deltoid muscle should be limited to 1 ml of solution due to the relatively smaller size of the muscle.
Use the **Z**-track method, described in Procedure I-28, for trapping medications that are particularly irritating to tissue.
The characteristics of the client's anatomy should dictate the length of the needle. The principle guiding needle length is that the tip should be able to reach the targeted muscle.

Avoid injecting any medication into a part of the body that is paralyzed. Also select an alternative site when the client has had surgery, such as a mastectomy, or other treatment, such as radiation. Any condition that may compromise the absorption of the medication at the site or jeopardize the potential integrity of the remaining tissue can be a basis for excluding an ordinarily acceptable site for an injection.

AGE-RELATED VARIATIONS

The upper arm and the dorsogluteal sites should be avoided in infants and children because muscles in these areas are not developed enough to absorb medication adequately.

HOME-HEALTH VARIATIONS

Ensure proper storage of medication according to the manufacturer's instructions.
Clients who must self-administer intramuscular injections at home may have no other choice but using the rectus femoris site because of its accessibility over the others. Locating other sites is impossible when the injection must be performed without assistance.

RELATED TEACHING

Explain the purpose of the injection and expected and unexpected after-effects.
Explain why one injection site may be more preferable among alternative sites.
Inform the client as to the schedule for administering any new medication. Instruct the client to inform the nurse when feeling the need for a medication prescribed on a prn (as needed) basis.
Indicate the subsequent assessments that will be useful in determining the client's response to the medication.

PERFORMANCE CHECKLIST

When an intramuscular injection is performed, the learner:

C	A	U	
[ ]	[ ]	[ ]	Reads the medical order written by the physician.
[ ]	[ ]	[ ]	Compares the medical order with the information transcribed to the medication card or Kardex.
[ ]	[ ]	[ ]	Reviews pertinent drug information in an appropriate reference text if unfamiliar with the medication.
[ ]	[ ]	[ ]	Explains to the client the action of the medication, expected effects, method of administration, and schedule for receiving the drug.
[ ]	[ ]	[ ]	Inspects potential injection sites and notes the size and condition of the tissue.
[ ]	[ ]	[ ]	Washes hands.
[ ]	[ ]	[ ]	Assembles an appropriate size needle and syringe according to the type of medication, the size of the client, and the volume of medication.
[ ]	[ ]	[ ]	Reads the label on the container of medication at least three times.
[ ]	[ ]	[ ]	Withdraws the supplied medication into a syringe.
[ ]	[ ]	[ ]	Identifies the client by checking the identification band.
[ ]	[ ]	[ ]	Pulls the privacy curtain and shuts the door.
[ ]	[ ]	[ ]	Washes hands.
[ ]	[ ]	[ ]	Cleanses the skin with alcohol in a circular motion.
[ ]	[ ]	[ ]	Spreads the skin over the site.

C = competent; A = acceptable; U = unsatisfactory

(Continued)

PERFORMANCE CHECKLIST (Continued)

C	A	U	
[ ]	[ ]	[ ]	Holds the syringe similarly to the manner in which a dart is held.
[ ]	[ ]	[ ]	Inserts the needle quickly at a 90-degree angle.
[ ]	[ ]	[ ]	Steadies the lower end of the syringe.
[ ]	[ ]	[ ]	Aspirates to check for blood.
[ ]	[ ]	[ ]	Injects the medication if no blood is seen on aspiration.
[ ]	[ ]	[ ]	Removes the needle.
[ ]	[ ]	[ ]	Massages the site with an alcohol swab.
[ ]	[ ]	[ ]	Assists the client to a comfortable position and provides him with the signal device.
[ ]	[ ]	[ ]	Disposes of the needle, its cover, and the syringe in a puncture-resistant container.
[ ]	[ ]	[ ]	Washes hands.
[ ]	[ ]	[ ]	Records the administration of the medication on the client's record.
[ ]	[ ]	[ ]	Checks the client within 30 minutes to evaluate his response to the medication.

Outcome: [ ] Pass   [ ] Fail

C = competent; A = acceptable; U = unsatisfactory

Comments: _____
_____
_____

_____   _____
Student's Signature   Date

_____   _____
Instructor's Signature   Date

I-28

Performing a Z-track injection

The **Z**-track or zig-zag technique is a modification of the method for performing an intramuscular injection. It acquired its name because the technique results in manipulating the tissue somewhat like the letter **Z**. Any intramuscular injection can be administered using this method. However, there are specific medications that should always be administered using this technique.

PURPOSES OF PROCEDURE

An intramuscular injection is given by **Z**-track to

1. Administer medications that are irritating to subcutaneous tissue, such as iron–dextran injection (Imferon) or chlorpromazine hydrochloride (Thorazine)
2. Avoid depositing irritating medication through superficial layers of tissue during the insertion of the needle
3. Seal medication within the muscle so that it cannot leak back through the upper layers of tissue following the path of the withdrawn needle
4. Prevent bruising or staining superficial layers of tissue

ASSESSMENT

Refer to Procedure I-27, Administering an Intramuscular Injection, with the following exception:

• Inspect and palpate only a large muscle as a potential site, such as the dorsogluteal area or vastus lateralis muscle.

RELEVANT NURSING DIAGNOSES

A client who receives an intramuscular injection by **Z**-track may have nursing diagnoses, such as

• *Anxiety*
• *Potential Altered Comfort*
• *Fear*
• *Potential for Injury*
• *Knowledge Deficit*

PLANNING

ESTABLISHING PRIORITIES

Medications administered by intramuscular injection are generally ordered to be administered stat (immediately), one time, several times during a day on a schedule of evenly spaced intervals, or prn (as needed). Any stat order requires priority attention and necessitates that the nurse modify or delegate other responsibilities in order to administer the medication. Scheduled medications should be administered as closely as possible to the routine established by the clinical agency.

SETTING GOALS

• The client will receive the right medication, the right dosage, by the right route, at the right time.
• The medication will be deposited within a large, well-developed muscle.
• The tissue will be manipulated successfully to trap the deposition of medication well within the muscle.
• The client will not manifest any irritation, bruising, or staining of superficial tissue.

PREPARATION OF EQUIPMENT

The nurse will need the following equipment when performing the **Z**-track technique for administering an intramuscular injection:

Medication
Medication card or Kardex
Two needles (1½-inch to 3-inch, 20-gauge to 22-gauge)
3-ml syringe
Alcohol swab

Technique for performing a Z-track injection

ACTION	RATIONALE
1. Assemble the equipment and check the physician's order.	This is one step for ensuring that the client receives the right medication at the right time by the proper route.
2. Explain the procedure to the client.	An explanation encourages cooperation and alleviates apprehension.
3. Wash your hands.	Handwashing deters the spread of microorganisms.
4. If necessary, withdraw the medication from an ampule or vial as described in Procedures I-22 and I-23.	Medications for parenteral administration are generally supplied in ampules, vials, or prefilled cartridges.
5. Replace the needle used for filling the syringe with another long sterile needle.	The outer surface of the needle must be free of irritating medication and long enough to be inserted deeply within the intended muscle.
6. Create an air bubble, shown in Figure I-28-1, by adding 0.2 ml of air to the quantity of medication in the syringe.	The air bubble ensures that the irritating medication will be sealed into the muscle and not leak back through the path of the needle.

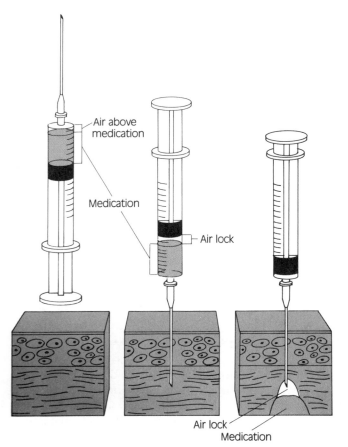

Figure I-28–1 An air bubble added to the syringe after the medication has been accurately measured helps expel solution that is trapped in the shaft of the needle when the injection is given. It also helps trap irritating medication within the tissue.

7. Cleanse the skin over a wide area, approximately 3 to 4 inches, of the selected injection site.

A wider area of the skin must be manipulated, so the area that is cleansed should be of a comparable amount.

8. Grasp the muscle and pull it laterally about 1 inch, until it is taut, as shown in Figure I-28-2. Hold the tissue in that position.

This provides a straight path during the time of the injection.

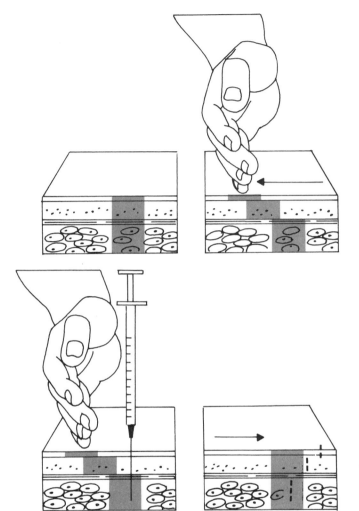

Figure I-28–2 The **Z**-track method of giving an intramuscular injection involves pulling the skin to one side rather than spreading it taut. When the needle is withdrawn and the displaced tissue returns to its original position, the injection site settles away from the deposited medication, preventing the solution from escaping through the injection site and irritating other layers of tissue.

9. Insert the needle at a 90-degree angle using a dart-like motion.

This directs the tip of the needle deeply within the muscular layer of tissue.

10. Use the last three fingers of the hand holding the syringe to steady the barrel. Use the thumb and index finger on the same hand to aspirate.

The nondominant hand must not be released from its hold on the tissue.

11. Inject the medication with slow even pressure if no blood appears in the barrel of the syringe.

Slow instillation allows time for the medication to become evenly distributed within the muscle.

12. Wait about 10 seconds with the needle still in place.

Pausing allows the medication to be distributed widely from the needle tip.

13. Withdraw the needle and immediately release the skin.

The injection track now becomes a diagonal path sealing the original route of entry with layers of released tissue.

14. Apply pressure to the site unless the manufacturer of the medication indicates that the site may be massaged.

Massaging the site may cause some of the trapped medication to leak from the pocket where it has been deposited and irritate surrounding tissue.

SAMPLE DOCUMENTATION

Date	Time	Nurse's note
4/06	0900	Imferon 250 mg administered by **Z**-track into the vastus lateralis of the R leg.
		P. Moore, RN

EVALUATION

REASSESSMENT

The information on the supplied medication should be re-read before withdrawing the medication and again before replacing or discarding the container.

The client's response to the intended action of the medication should be observed and documented within the first 30 minutes after the injection. Iron injected by **Z**-track is absorbed slowly over as long as 6 months. However, if the injected iron produces a therapeutic effect, the client's hemoglobin should increase by 2 g in 3 weeks.

The condition of the integument and more specifically the site of any previous injections should be observed as part of the daily head-to-toe assessment.

EXPECTED OUTCOMES

The medication is injected easily within the selected site when no blood has been aspirated.

The site of the needle insertion does not bleed or leak medication.

The client experiences minimal discomfort at the time of the injection and for only a brief period afterwards.

The client experiences a therapeutic response to the medication.

UNEXPECTED OUTCOMES

The muscle is not held laterally during the injection.

Blood is aspirated within the syringe.

Medication leaks from the puncture site.

The client experiences prolonged discomfort, bruising, and staining of the tissue at the injection site.

The client experiences undesirable side-effects to the medication.

MODIFICATIONS IN SELECTED SITUATIONS

GENERAL VARIATIONS

When selecting the dorsogluteal site for an injection, discomfort can be reduced by positioning the client on the abdomen with the feet pointing inward.

Some nurses prefer to steady the base of the syringe with the thumb and forefinger of the hand being used to manipulate the position of the tissue. The ulnar side of that hand is used to control the placement of the tissue.

HOME-HEALTH VARIATIONS

Ensure that needed supplies and medications are available for subsequent injections.

Store medication in accordance with the manufacturer's instructions.

Periodically verify that the client or members of the client's family can recall the intended and untoward effects of the medications being administered.

RELATED TEACHING

Explain the purpose of the injection and expected and unexpected after-effects.

Explain why one injection site may be more preferable among other alternative sites.

Inform the client as to the schedule for administering any new medication.

Indicate the subsequent assessments that will be useful in determining the client's response to the medication.

PERFORMANCE CHECKLIST

When an intramuscular injection is administered using the Z-track technique, the learner:

C	A	U	
[ ]	[ ]	[ ]	Reads the medical order written by the physician
[ ]	[ ]	[ ]	Compares the medical order with the information transcribed to the medication card or Kardex
[ ]	[ ]	[ ]	Reviews pertinent drug information in an appropriate reference text if unfamiliar with the medication
[ ]	[ ]	[ ]	Explains to the client the action of the medication, expected effects, method of administration, and schedule for receiving the drug
[ ]	[ ]	[ ]	Inspects and palpates the dorsogluteal area and vastus lateralis muscle on both sides of the body to select a potential injection site
[ ]	[ ]	[ ]	Washes hands
[ ]	[ ]	[ ]	Assembles the equipment, including a second needle of adequate length to reach the muscle at the intended injection site
[ ]	[ ]	[ ]	Reads the label on the container of medication when removing it from its stocked location
[ ]	[ ]	[ ]	Withdraws the medication in the syringe after reading the label a second time
[ ]	[ ]	[ ]	Re-reads the label once more before discarding or replacing the container
[ ]	[ ]	[ ]	Adds 0.2 ml of air to the medication within the syringe
[ ]	[ ]	[ ]	Replaces the needle used for withdrawing the medication
[ ]	[ ]	[ ]	Disposes of the used needle within a puncture-resistant receptacle
[ ]	[ ]	[ ]	Identifies the client by checking the identification band
[ ]	[ ]	[ ]	Pulls the privacy curtain and shuts the door
[ ]	[ ]	[ ]	Washes hands
[ ]	[ ]	[ ]	Cleanses the skin in a circular motion with alcohol over a wide area of the injection site
[ ]	[ ]	[ ]	Pulls the skin laterally with the nondominant hand
[ ]	[ ]	[ ]	Inserts the needle with the dominant hand
[ ]	[ ]	[ ]	Steadies the syringe with the last three fingers of the hand used to insert the needle
[ ]	[ ]	[ ]	Aspirates the syringe with the thumb and forefinger of the dominant hand
[ ]	[ ]	[ ]	Injects the medication if no blood is aspirated
[ ]	[ ]	[ ]	Waits 10 seconds
[ ]	[ ]	[ ]	Withdraws the needle and immediately releases the tissue being held with the nondominant hand
[ ]	[ ]	[ ]	Applies pressure to the injection site with an alcohol swab
[ ]	[ ]	[ ]	Assists the client to a comfortable position and provides the client with a signal device
[ ]	[ ]	[ ]	Disposes of the needle, its cover, and the syringe in an appropriate container
[ ]	[ ]	[ ]	Washes hands
[ ]	[ ]	[ ]	Records the administration of the medication on the client's record
[ ]	[ ]	[ ]	Checks the client within 30 minutes to evaluate response to the medication

C = competent; A = acceptable; U = unsatisfactory

(Continued)

PERFORMANCE CHECKLIST (Continued)

Outcome: [ ] Pass   [ ] Fail

Comments: _____
_____
_____

_____   _____
Student's Signature   Date

_____   _____
Instructor's Signature   Date

I-29

Adding medications to an intravenous solution container

The intravenous (IV) route is potentially the most dangerous parenteral route because the drug is placed directly in the bloodstream. IV medication can be added to a large volume of fluid and infused over a period of time. Dilution of the medication can temper an adverse reaction that the client may experience.

PURPOSES OF PROCEDURE

Medications are added to an IV solution to

1. Administer a drug for immediate distribution by the vascular system
2. Provide a uniform, sustained level of medication within the bloodstream
3. Rapidly treat the client's medical problem
4. Reduce the client's discomfort by avoiding repeated injections of medication into subcutaneous or muscular tissue

ASSESSMENT

OBJECTIVE DATA

- Read the physician's order.
- Compare the transcribed information on the medication card or Kardex with the written medical order.
- Review the action of the drug, side-effects, contraindications, usual dosage by the IV route, and other pertinent information in an appropriate pharmacology reference if unfamiliar with the medication.
- Note the types of solutions that are compatible when mixed with the medication.
- Determine if the medication can cause irritation to the vein while being infused.
- Note any actions that should be taken if the medication infiltrates into the surrounding subcutaneous tissue.
- Know the location of any drug or equipment that may be needed to counteract an adverse reaction to the prescribed medication.
- Read the client's chart and note any pathology or laboratory results that would contraindicate the administration of the prescribed medication.
- Examine the site of an already infusing IV solution and verify that the needle or catheter is definitely within the vein.
- Obtain vital signs for a baseline comparison.
- Confirm that the client's output is adequate and that no other factors will interfere with the circulation, metabolism, or excretion of the drug.
- Weigh the client if it is necessary to calculate the dosage based on kilograms of body weight; measure and weigh the client if the dosage of medication is based on body surface area (BSA).

SUBJECTIVE DATA

- Interview the client to determine his prior experience with receiving IV medication.
- Ask the client about any history of drug allergies and a description of the types of symptoms experienced during prior allergic reactions.

RELEVANT NURSING DIAGNOSES

A client who receives IV medication may have nursing diagnoses such as

- *Anxiety*
- *Fear*

- *Potential for Injury*
- *Knowledge Deficit*
- *Potential Fluid Volume Excess*

PLANNING

ESTABLISHING PRIORITIES

Medications added to a large volume of IV fluid, such as 500 ml or 1000 ml of solution, are generally intended to infuse over several hours. The nurse must calculate the rate of infusion in order to regulate the administration of the medication in equal amounts over the total period of time. Refer to Procedure I-17, Regulating Intravenous Flow Rate. If the infusion should slow or stop, the nurse has an obligation to determine the cause and resume the administration as soon as possible.

SETTING GOALS

- The client will receive the correct dosage of medication mixed within a safe volume of a compatible solution.
- The medicated solution will infuse on time over the period specified by the physician.

PREPARATION OF EQUIPMENT

The following will be needed when adding medication to a container of IV solution:

Medication prepared in a syringe with a 19-gauge to 21-gauge needle
Alcohol swab
IV fluid container (bag or bottle)
Label to be attached to the IV container

Technique for adding medications to an intravenous solution container

ACTION	RATIONALE
1. Check the medication card or Kardex with the physician's order.	Checking ensures that the client receives the correct medication at the correct time in the right manner.
2. Gather all equipment and bring to the bedside.	Having equipment available saves time and facilitates performance of the task.
3. Explain the procedure to the client.	An explanation allays the client's anxiety.
4. Wash your hands.	Handwashing deters the spread of microorganisms.
5. Identify the client by checking the client's wristband and asking the client his name.	Checking identification ensures that the medication is given to the right client.
6. Add the medication to the IV solution that is infusing:	Mixing dilutes the drug within the solution.
a. Check that the volume in the bag or bottle is adequate.	The volume should be sufficient to dilute the drug.
b. Close the IV clamp, shown in Figure I-29-1.	Clamping prevents the administration of improperly diluted medication directly to the client.
c. Cleanse the medication port with an alcohol swab, as shown in Figure I-29-2.	Cleansing deters the entry of microorganisms when the needle punctures the port.
d. Steady the container, uncap the needle, and insert it into the port. Inject the medication, as the nurse is doing in Figure I-29-3.	Stabilizing the container ensures that the needle enters the port and the medication is dispersed within the solution.
e. Remove the container from the IV pole and gently rotate the solution, as shown in Figure I-29-4.	Rotation mixes the medication throughout the solution.
f. Rehang the solution, open the clamp, and readjust the flow rate.	Readjustment ensures that the solution with medication infuses at the prescribed rate.

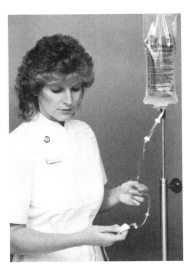

Figure I-29–1 The nurse closes the IV clamp to ensure that the medication that is added will be diluted within the solution that is hanging rather than travel directly into the vein in a concentrated amount.

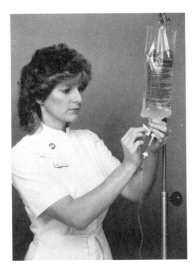

Figure I-29–2 The nurse wipes the injection port with an alcohol swab preparatory to adding medication to the container of IV solution. The system and all equipment must be kept sterile so that pathogens are not introduced into the vascular system.

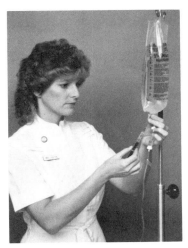

Figure I-29–3 The needle is placed through a self-sealing port. The nurse must be careful when plastic bags are used. Accidental puncture with the needle could cause a slow leak to occur.

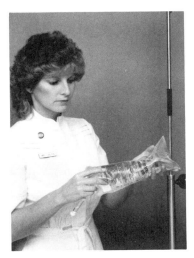

Figure I-29–4 The nurse promotes the dilution and homogenous distribution of the medication by rotating the solution.

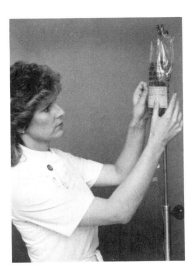

Figure I-29–5 The nurse attaches a drug label to the container of solution. IV medications can have a rapid effect because they are absorbed instantly into the bloodstream. Being able to refer to the information on the label helps in identifying the medication as a potential cause if an adverse reaction occurs.

g. Attach a label to the container, as shown in Figure I-29-5, so that the dosage of the medication that has been added is apparent.

Labeling confirms that the prescribed dose of medication has been added to the IV solution.

Add medication to an IV solution prior to its infusion:

a. Carefully remove any protective cover and locate the injection port.

Careful removal deters the entry of microorganisms when the needle punctures the port.

b. Uncap the needle and insert it into the injection port. Inject the medication.

This facilitates the entry of the needle into the container so the medication can be dispersed into the solution.

c. Withdraw the needle and insert the spike into the proper entry site on the bag or bottle.

The spike punctures the seal in the IV bag or bottle.

d. With the tubing clamped, gently rotate the IV solution in the bag or bottle.

Rotation mixes the medication with the solution.

e. Attach a label to the container so that the dosage of medication that has been added is apparent.

Labeling confirms the prescribed dose of medication has been added to the IV solution.

7. Dispose of the equipment according to agency policy.

Proper disposal prevents inadvertent injury from the equipment.

8. Wash your hands.

Handwashing deters the spread of microorganisms.

9. Chart the addition of medication to the IV solution.

Accurate documentation is necessary to prevent medication errors.

10. Evaluate the client's response to the medication within the appropriate time frame.

Clients require careful observation because medication given by the IV route may have a rapid effect.

SAMPLE DOCUMENTATION

Date	Time	Nurse's note
10/30	0245	2 ml of Berocca added to remaining 450 ml of lactated Ringer's. Infusing well at 22 gtt/min.
		M. Brown, RN

EVALUATION

REASSESSMENT

The label of any medication container should be read at least three times before actually administering the drug to the client. Once the drug is infusing, observe the client receiving an IV medication for the first time or who has had a history of allergic reactions to similar medications throughout the first 15 minutes of the infusion. IV infusions and the response of the client should be assessed at least hourly throughout the administration.

EXPECTED OUTCOMES

The medication mixes uniformly throughout the IV solution.
The solution infuses at the regulated rate over the prescribed period of time.
The client remains free of any drug-related reactions.
The client experiences the therapeutic effects from the infused medication.

UNEXPECTED OUTCOMES

A precipitate forms when the medication and the solution are mixed.
The medicated solution infiltrates into subcutaneous tissue.
The client experiences an allergic reaction or undesirable side-effects to the medication.
The client feels uncomfortable sensations in the vein used for the infusion.

MODIFICATIONS IN SELECTED SITUATIONS

GENERAL VARIATIONS

When the client has no preexisting IV site, the nurse can refer to Procedure I-16, Starting an Intravenous Infusion.

Pharmacists in many clinical agencies mix IV medications and solutions. The mixing is often performed under special ultraviolet lights and air-flow control units to ensure the sterility of the fluid.

Pharmaceutical manufacturers are now supplying premixed medication in IV solution.

Solutions of very toxic drugs or medications that must be administered in small amounts may be regulated by using an infusion pump.

The nurse may need to collaborate with the laboratory when the physician requests the blood level of a medication that has been infusing in a solution. Report the results of the blood level to the physician as soon as it is available.

AGE-RELATED VARIATIONS

Restrain a client, immobilize the arm or hand, or protect the infusion device if the client is very young, restless, or uncooperative.

Expect that the medication dosage will be lower for children and individuals with low body weight.

The volume will be smaller and rate of infusion may be slower for pediatric and geriatric clients.

Very young, elderly, or debilitated clients should be assessed frequently because variations in drug absorption, metabolism, and distribution may alter the expected responses to IV medication.

HOME-HEALTH VARIATIONS

Follow the agency policy regarding additions of medications to an IV solution. Usually drugs are added to the solution by a pharmacist. However, the nurse or a family member may be responsible for adding the medication to the solution at the client's residence.

RELATED TEACHING

Explain the purpose of the infusion and expected and undesirable effects.

Inform the client about the signs of infiltration and the need to notify personnel if any discomfort is experienced around the IV site.

Instruct the client that hourly or more frequent checks will be made during the infusion.

PERFORMANCE CHECKLIST

When medication is added to an IV solution container, the learner:

C	A	U	
[ ]	[ ]	[ ]	Reads the medical order written by the physician.
[ ]	[ ]	[ ]	Compares the medical order with the information transcribed to the medication card or Kardex.
[ ]	[ ]	[ ]	Reviews pertinent drug information in an appropriate reference text if unfamiliar with the medication.
[ ]	[ ]	[ ]	Explains the action of the medication, expected effects, method of administration, and schedule for receiving the drug to the client.
[ ]	[ ]	[ ]	Washes hands.
[ ]	[ ]	[ ]	Examines the IV site, the patency of the venipuncture device, the dates on the solution, tubing, and dressing.
[ ]	[ ]	[ ]	Performs related physical assessments, such as vital signs, weight, urine output, and so on.
[ ]	[ ]	[ ]	Washes hands.

C = competent; A = acceptable; U = unsatisfactory

(Continued)

PERFORMANCE CHECKLIST (Continued)

C	A	U	
[ ]	[ ]	[ ]	Gathers equipment.
[ ]	[ ]	[ ]	Reads the label of the drug container at least three times.
[ ]	[ ]	[ ]	Withdraws the supplied medication into a syringe.
[ ]	[ ]	[ ]	Checks the identification of the client.
[ ]	[ ]	[ ]	Clamps the tubing of an already infusing solution.
[ ]	[ ]	[ ]	Removes the bag or bottle of an existing infusion from the IV pole.
[ ]	[ ]	[ ]	Cleanses the injection port of the bag or bottle of IV solution.
[ ]	[ ]	[ ]	Inserts the needle through the port designed for adding medication and instills the drug.
[ ]	[ ]	[ ]	Rotates the solution to distribute the medication uniformly, and spikes a new container of solution with the IV tubing.
[ ]	[ ]	[ ]	Hangs the solution and opens the clamp.
[ ]	[ ]	[ ]	Adjusts the flow at the calculated rate.
[ ]	[ ]	[ ]	Attaches a label to the container identifying the date, time, name of the medication, dosage of medication added, and the nurse's initials.
[ ]	[ ]	[ ]	Observes the client's immediate response.
[ ]	[ ]	[ ]	Provides the client with a signal device.
[ ]	[ ]	[ ]	Disposes of equipment appropriately.
[ ]	[ ]	[ ]	Washes hands.
[ ]	[ ]	[ ]	Documents the medication administration.
[ ]	[ ]	[ ]	Returns to reassess the infusion and the client's response.

Outcome: [ ] Pass   [ ] Fail

C = competent; A = acceptable; U = unsatisfactory

Comments: _____

_____

_____

_____   _____
Student's Signature   Date

_____   _____
Instructor's Signature   Date

I-30

Adding a bolus IV medication to an existing IV

Only a physician can administer a medication directly into a vein. The closest nursing approximations to this technique are the administration of a bolus of medication to an existing IV line and instilling medication through a heparin lock. The latter is described in Procedure I-33. Having a preexisting infusion of solution is a safeguard in case emergency measures are needed.

PURPOSES OF PROCEDURE

Adding a bolus IV medication is done to:

1. Administer a drug for immediate distribution by way of the vascular system.
2. Rapidly treat a client's medical problem.
3. Achieve high blood levels of a medication in a short period of time.

ASSESSMENT

Refer to Procedure I-29, Adding Medications to an IV Solution Container.

RELEVANT NURSING DIAGNOSES

A client who receives a bolus IV medication may have nursing diagnoses such as:

- *Anxiety*
- *Fear*
- *Potential for Injury*
- *Knowledge Deficit*

PLANNING

ESTABLISHING PRIORITIES

The nurse should plan to carry out a STAT medication order immediately. Scheduled medications may be given within a half hour of the agency's routine.

SETTING GOALS

- The client will receive the correct dosage of medication at the correct time by the intravenous route.
- The drug will be injected no more rapidly than 1 ml per minute.
- The drug will mix compatibly with the solution within the IV tubing.

PREPARATION OF EQUIPMENT

The following equipment will be needed for this procedure:

Medication prepared in a syringe with a #23–25 gauge, 1-inch needle
Alcohol swab
Watch with a second hand

Technique for adding a bolus IV medication to an existing IV

ACTION	RATIONALE
1. Check the medication order with the physician's order.	Checking ensures that the client receives the correct medication at the correct time in the right manner.
2. Gather the equipment and bring to the client's bedside.	Having equipment available saves time and facilitates performance of the task.
3. Explain the procedure to the client.	An explanation allays a client's anxiety.

4. Wash your hands.

Handwashing deters the spread of microorganisms.

5. Identify the client by checking his wristband and asking the client his name.

Checking identification ensures the medication is given to the right person.

6. Assess the IV site for the presence of inflammation or infiltration.

IV medication must be given into a vein for safe administration.

7. Select the injection port on the tubing that is closest to the venipuncture site. Cleanse the port with an alcohol swab, as shown in Fig. I-30-1.

Using the port closest to the needle insertion site minimizes dilution of the medication. Cleansing with alcohol deters entry of microorganisms when the needle punctures the port.

8. Uncap the syringe. Steady the port with the nondominant hand while inserting the needle into the center of the port.

Supporting the injection port lessens the risk of accidentally dislodging the IV or entering the port incorrectly.

9. Move the nondominant hand to the section of the IV tubing just below the injection port. Fold the tubing between the fingers to temporarily stop the flow of IV solution, as shown in Fig. I-30-2.

Occluding the tubing minimizes the dilution of IV medication with the IV solution.

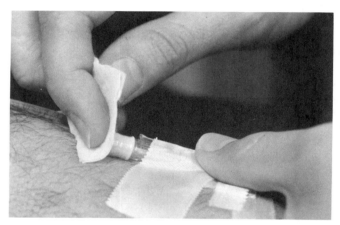

Figure I-30–1 Pathogens are removed from the injection port by using an alcohol swab and friction.

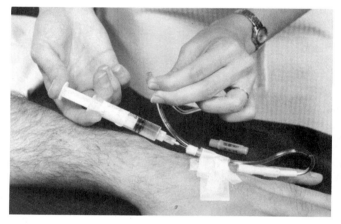

Figure I-30–2 The nurse steadies the injection port while pinching the IV tubing. The nurse then slowly administers the bolus of medication while watching the second hand on the watch.

10. Pull back slightly on the plunger just until blood appears in the tubing.

Aspirating assures that the venipuncture device is within a vein.

11. Inject the medication at the prescribed rate.

Slow administration delivers the correct amount of medication over a safe period of time.

12. Remove the needle. Do not cap it. Release the tubing and allow the IV to flow at the proper rate.

Leaving the needle uncapped prevents an accidental needle stick.

13. Dispose of needle and syringe in a proper receptacle.

Proper disposal prevents accidental injury and spread of microorganisms.

14. Wash your hands.

Handwashing deters the spread of microorganisms.

15. Chart the administration of medication.

Accurate documentation is necessary to prevent medication errors.

16. Evaluate the client's response to medication within the appropriate time frame.

The client requires careful observation because medications given by an IV bolus injection may have a rapid effect.

SAMPLE DOCUMENTATION

Date	Time	Nurse's note
12/13	0900	40 mg. Lasix administered IV push. IV continues to infuse at 32 gtts./min. following the infusion. IV site does not appear swollen, pale, or tender.

L. Lionel, R.N

EVALUATION

REASSESSMENT

Reading the label on any medication container at least three times before its administration is a good reassessment practice to ensure that the client receives the correct medication.

Because a bolus administration of a medication is likely to produce an immediate effect, the client should be observed closely. A desired or undesired response to the action of a drug may be evident even during its administration.

Return to check on the client soon after an uneventful administration to gather data indicating his response.

EXPECTED OUTCOMES

The IV line is patent.
A blood return is observed in the tubing when the syringe is aspirated.
The medication infuses freely through the port.
The client experiences no discomfort or untoward reactions during medication administration.

UNEXPECTED OUTCOMES

The IV site is swollen and tender.
There is no sign of a blood return in the tubing when the syringe is aspirated.
The medication forms a precipitate when instilled through the port.
Resistance is felt when pushing the plunger of the syringe.

MODIFICATIONS IN SELECTED SITUATIONS

GENERAL VARIATIONS

Some drugs should be injected at a rate slower than 1 ml/min. Consult a reliable pharmacology reference or a registered pharmacist if the safe rate of administration is unclear or unknown.

The tubing and needle or catheter may be flushed with 10 ml of sterile normal saline if the medication is incompatible with the infusion solution. This step should be repeated after the injection of the medication as well. Care must be taken that the tubing to the container of the solution remains clamped during the process of injecting an incompatible medication.

If a drug must be instilled over several minutes, release the pinched tubing to allow some fluid to periodically infuse. This will help to keep the needle or catheter from becoming obstructed with blood. This same action may help relieve the burning that some client's experience when a concentrated drug is administered.

AGE-RELATED VARIATIONS

Expect the medication dosage to be lower for children and persons with low body weight. Check any mathematical computation of a divided dosage with another nurse in order to maintain accuracy when administering intravenous medication.

HOME-HEALTH VARIATIONS

Ensure that equipment and supplies are available for subsequent doses of intravenous medication.

RELATED TEACHING

Explain the purpose of the infusion, and expected and undesirable effects.
Inform the client to notify personnel if any unusual symptoms are experienced closely following the injection of the medication.
Instruct the client about the kinds of assessments that will be noted to evaluate his response to the medication.

PERFORMANCE CHECKLIST

When administering an IV bolus of medication, the learner:

C	A	U	
[ ]	[ ]	[ ]	Reads the medical order written by the physician.
[ ]	[ ]	[ ]	Compares the medical order with the information transcribed to the medication card or Kardex.
[ ]	[ ]	[ ]	Reviews pertinent drug information in an appropriate reference text, if unfamiliar with the medication.
[ ]	[ ]	[ ]	Explains the action of the medication, expected effects, method of administration, and schedule for administering the drug to the client.
[ ]	[ ]	[ ]	Washes hands.
[ ]	[ ]	[ ]	Examines the IV site, the patency of the venipuncture device, the dates on the solution, tubing, and dressing.
[ ]	[ ]	[ ]	Performs related physical assessments, such as vital signs, weight, urine output, and so on.
[ ]	[ ]	[ ]	Washes hands.
[ ]	[ ]	[ ]	Gathers equipment.
[ ]	[ ]	[ ]	Reads the label of the drug container at least three times.
[ ]	[ ]	[ ]	Withdraws the supplied medication into a syringe.
[ ]	[ ]	[ ]	Checks the identification of the client.
[ ]	[ ]	[ ]	Locates the port closest to the needle or catheter.
[ ]	[ ]	[ ]	Cleanses the injection port.
[ ]	[ ]	[ ]	Inserts the needle.
[ ]	[ ]	[ ]	Pinches the tubing above the port.
[ ]	[ ]	[ ]	Aspirates to assess for a blood return.
[ ]	[ ]	[ ]	Notes the position of the second hand on a clock or watch.
[ ]	[ ]	[ ]	Depresses the plunger of the syringe instilling the medication slowly over the recommended period of time.
[ ]	[ ]	[ ]	Releases the tubing and permits the IV solution to infuse.
[ ]	[ ]	[ ]	Removes the needle from the port.
[ ]	[ ]	[ ]	Validates that the IV continues to infuse at the prescribed rate.
[ ]	[ ]	[ ]	Disposes of the equipment in a puncture-resistant receptacle.
[ ]	[ ]	[ ]	Washes hands.
[ ]	[ ]	[ ]	Records the medication administration.
[ ]	[ ]	[ ]	Reassesses the client's response to the medication.

Outcome: [ ] Pass   [ ] Fail

C = competent; A = acceptable; U = unsatisfactory

Comments: _____

_____

_____

_____   _____
Student's Signature   Date

_____   _____
Instructor's Signature   Date

Administering medications by IV piggyback

Medications can be administered by intermittent infusion. The drug is mixed with a small volume of solution, such as 50 ml to 100 ml, and administered over 30 minutes to 60 minutes. These types of medications are generally scheduled for repeated administrations throughout the day. The small volume of medication is joined in tandem to the main IV tubing. The main IV is lowered while the secondary solution infuses, hence the term "piggyback."

PURPOSES OF PROCEDURE

Medications are given by piggyback to:

1. Administer a drug for immediate distribution by way of the vascular system.
2. Maintain therapeutic blood levels of medications that are metabolized and excreted within several hours of administration.
3. Reduce the client's discomfort by avoiding repeated injections into muscular tissue or unwanted gastrointestinal effects by the oral route.
4. Retain the potency of drugs that may deteriorate if mixed and infused over a long period of time.

ASSESSMENT

Refer to Procedure I-29, Adding Medications to an IV Solution Container.

RELEVANT NURSING DIAGNOSES

A client who receives intravenous medication may have nursing diagnoses such as:

- *Anxiety*
- *Fear*
- *Potential for Injury*
- *Knowledge Deficit*

PLANNING

ESTABLISHING PRIORITIES

Medication must be conscientiously administered according to the physician's orders and the agency's schedule. It is the nurse's responsibility to requisition the medication so it is available before the scheduled time. The nurse may delegate another nursing team member to pick up the drug or prepared solution from the pharmacy so as to not deviate more than one half hour from the time it should be administered.

SETTING GOALS

- The client will receive the correct medication at the scheduled time by the intravenous route.
- The medicated solution will infuse within 30 minutes to 60 minutes.

PREPARATION OF EQUIPMENT

The following will be needed when administering a piggyback solution of medication:

Medication preparation in a labeled piggyback solution (50 ml to 100 ml)
Secondary infusion tubing
Hanger to lower the primary solution
Sterile needle (#21 to #23 gauge)
Alcohol swab
Tape

Technique for administering medications by IV piggyback

ACTION	RATIONALE
1. Check the medication order with the physician's order.	Checking ensures that the client receives the correct medication at the correct time in the correct manner.
2. Gather all equipment and bring to the client's bedside.	Having equipment available saves time and facilitates the performance of the task.
3. Explain the procedure to the client.	An explanation allays the client's anxiety.
4. Wash your hands.	Handwashing deters the spread of microorganisms.
5. Assess the IV site for the presence of inflammation or infiltration.	IV medication must be given into a vein for safe administration.
6. Attach the secondary infusion tubing to the piggyback set containing diluted medication, as shown in Fig. I-31-1. Fill the drip chamber. Open the clamp and prime the tubing.	Purging with fluid removes the air from the tubing.
7. Hang the piggyback container from the IV pole. Position it higher than the primary IV, as shown in Fig. I-31-2.	The position of the container influences the flow of IV fluid.

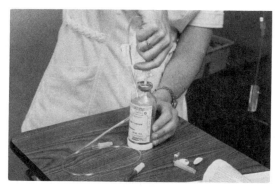

Figure I-31-1 The nurse inserts secondary tubing into a small container of IV fluid mixed with medication. The piggyback will be administered intermittently over a relatively short period of time.

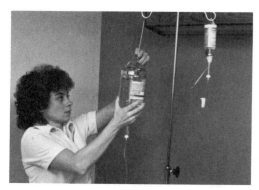

Figure I-31-2 The medication in the small container on the left side will infuse before the solution in the lower container.

8. Identify the client by checking his identification band and asking the client his name.	Identification ensures that the medication is given to the right person.
9. Use an alcohol swab to cleanse the port for the secondary IV.	Cleansing deters the entry of microorganisms when the needle punctures the port.
10. Remove the cap and insert the needle into the port, as shown in Fig. I-31-3. Use a strip of tape to secure the secondary tubing within the primary infusion tubing.	Tape stabilizes the needle in the infusion port and prevents it from slipping out.

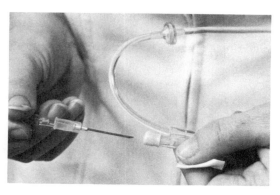

Figure I-31-3 A needle is used to connect the secondary tubing with the primary tubing. Because the needle could be pulled from the port fairly easily, most nurses tape the connection for greater stability.

11. Open the clamp on the secondary tubing and regulate the prescribed rate of flow. Monitor the medication infusion at periodic intervals.

Delivery over a 30-minute to 60-minute interval is a safe method of administering the medication within a small volume of solution.

12. Clamp the tubing on the piggyback set when the solution has infused. Follow the agency policy regarding disposal of equipment.

Leaving the tubing in place reduces the risk of contaminating the primary IV and the secondary tubing in case it is needed for subsequent use.

13. Readjust the flow rate of the primary IV.

Piggyback medication administration interrupts the normal flow rate of the primary IV. Readjustment of the rate may be necessary.

14. Wash your hands.

Handwashing deters the spread of microorganisms.

15. Chart the administration of medication.

Accurate documentation is necessary to prevent medication errors.

16. Evaluate the client's response to the medication within an appropriate time frame.

Clients require careful observation because medication given by the IV route may have a rapid effect.

SAMPLE DOCUMENTATION

Date	Time	Nurse's note
2/26	1500	1 Gm. Kefzol added to 100 mL of 5%D/Lactated Ringer's. Infusing at 100 mL/hr (25 gtts/min) through secondary port. *D. Merritt, RN*

EVALUATION

REASSESSMENT

Drug labels should be read several times before administering medication. Once an infusion has begun, the nurse should observe the client's immediate response. If the initiation of the infusion is uneventful, the client can be checked in 15-minute to 30-minute intervals until the total volume in the piggyback container infuses. Any alteration in the schedule of infusing fluids needs to be resolved immediately. An IV that slows or stops prevents the client from receiving an adequate or full amount of medication.

EXPECTED OUTCOMES

The IV is patent and located within the vein.
The piggyback solution infuses at the proper rate over the prescribed period of time.
The client remains free of undesirable effects related to the medication.

UNEXPECTED OUTCOMES

The IV slows or stops infusing.
The IV shows signs of infiltration.
The client experiences an allergic reaction or side-effects to the infusing medication.

MODIFICATIONS IN SELECTED SITUATIONS

GENERAL VARIATIONS

When the same drug is scheduled for repeated administrations during the day, the solution container and tubing may be left in place after the infusion. The new solution container is then spiked with the previously used tubing. Care must be taken that the tubing is not reused for a piggyback solution of different medication. Tubing should not be reused longer than 24 hours. The nurse should apply a tab of tape with the date, time, and initials so that asepsis is maintained.

Piggyback solutions may be prepared in advance and stocked in the nursing unit's refrigerator. Remove the solution $\frac{1}{2}$ hour before its scheduled infusion to allow it to return to room temperature.

A secondary solution may be administered with an infusion pump. In that situation, the primary fluid container need not be lowered. Both fluids will infuse simultaneously. The rate of the smaller volume solution is under the control of the pump. Hydrostatic pressure, influenced by the height of the primary fluid container, controls the infusion rate of the main solution.

Extension tubing is needed if the secondary fluid container will be administered with an infusion pump.

The physician may order a peak and trough level measurement to determine the client's lowest and highest blood levels of medication. The blood sample for the trough is drawn immediately before hanging the piggyback solution; the peak is drawn immediately after the solution infuses. The nurse should coordinate the medication administration with the laboratory personnel so that the test results are not invalid.

Y-connected tubing can be used instead of the combination of primary and secondary infusion tubing.

AGE-RELATED VARIATIONS

Expect the medication dosage to be lower for children and persons with low body weight.

The volume and rate of infusion will probably be less for a pediatric and geriatric client.

Small volumes of medication may be administered using an infusion pump.

Very young, elderly, and debilitated clients should be assessed frequently because variations in drug absorption, metabolism, and distribution may alter the expected responses to IV medication.

HOME-HEALTH VARIATIONS

Piggyback solutions that have been commercially prepared may be used in order to avoid adding medication to a solution.

RELATED TEACHING

Explain the purpose of the infusion, and expected and common undesirable effects.

Inform the client about the signs of infiltration and the need to notify personnel if any discomfort is experienced around the IV site.

Explain that once the secondary container of fluid is finished infusing, the primary fluid will automatically resume.

Instruct the client that frequent checks will be made during the infusion.

PERFORMANCE CHECKLIST

When administering medication by IV piggyback, the learner:

C	A	U	
[ ]	[ ]	[ ]	Reads the medical order written by the physician.
[ ]	[ ]	[ ]	Compares the medical order with the information transcribed to the medication card or Kardex.
[ ]	[ ]	[ ]	Reviews pertinent drug information in an appropriate reference text, if unfamiliar with the medication.
[ ]	[ ]	[ ]	Explains the action of the medication, common undesirable effects, method of administration, and the schedule for administering the drug to the client.
[ ]	[ ]	[ ]	Washes hands.
[ ]	[ ]	[ ]	Examines the IV site, the patency of the venipuncture device, the dates on the solution, tubing, and dressing.
[ ]	[ ]	[ ]	Performs physical assessments pertinent to the medication about to be administered.
[ ]	[ ]	[ ]	Washes hands.
[ ]	[ ]	[ ]	Gathers equipment.
[ ]	[ ]	[ ]	Reads the label on the solution container at least three times.
[ ]	[ ]	[ ]	Spikes the piggyback solution with secondary tubing.
[ ]	[ ]	[ ]	Fills the drip chamber.
[ ]	[ ]	[ ]	Attaches a needle to the end of the secondary tubing.
[ ]	[ ]	[ ]	Flushes the air from the tubing.
[ ]	[ ]	[ ]	Clamps the secondary tubing.
[ ]	[ ]	[ ]	Hangs the piggyback solution from the IV pole.
[ ]	[ ]	[ ]	Cleanses the injection port on the upper portion of the main IV tubing.
[ ]	[ ]	[ ]	Pierces the injection port with the needle.
[ ]	[ ]	[ ]	Tapes the needle within the port.
[ ]	[ ]	[ ]	Lowers the primary bag or bottle of IV solution.
[ ]	[ ]	[ ]	Opens the clamp on the secondary tubing and adjusts the rate of flow.
[ ]	[ ]	[ ]	Observes the condition of the client.
[ ]	[ ]	[ ]	Disposes of the used alcohol gauze pad; returns the tape.
[ ]	[ ]	[ ]	Washes hands.
[ ]	[ ]	[ ]	Documents the administration of the medication.
[ ]	[ ]	[ ]	Returns to reassess the client.
[ ]	[ ]	[ ]	Restores the primary solution to its original height after the piggyback infuses.

Outcome: [ ] Pass   [ ] Fail

C = competent; A = acceptable; U = unsatisfactory

Comments: _____

_____

_____

_____   _____
Student's Signature   Date

_____   _____
Instructor's Signature   Date

I-32

Administering IV medications by a volume-control set

A volume-control set is a cylindrical chamber located below the IV solution container. It can be filled with a small proportion of fluid from time to time. IV medication can be added to the fluid within the volume-control set. The section of tubing above the volume-control set is clamped allowing only the contents in the small volume chamber to infuse. This process is comparable to infusing intermittent medication without the added volume of a second piggyback container.

PURPOSES OF PROCEDURE

Intravenous medication is administered by a volume-control set to:

1. Provide immediate distribution of the drug by way of the vascular system.
2. Avoid administering a separate secondary container of fluid.
3. Repeat the administration of medications that are metabolized and excreted within several hours.
4. Retain the potency of a drug that may deteriorate if mixed and infused over several hours.
5. Reduce the client's discomfort by avoiding repeated injections into muscular tissue or unwanted gastrointestinal effects of administration by the oral route.

ASSESSMENT

Refer to the discussion in Procedure I-29, Adding Medications to an IV Solution Container.

RELEVANT NURSING DIAGNOSES

A client who receives IV medication by a volume-control set may have nursing diagnoses, such as:

- *Anxiety*
- *Fear*
- *Potential for Injury*
- *Knowledge Deficit*
- *Potential Fluid Volume Excess*

PLANNING

ESTABLISHING PRIORITIES

Medication must be administered as closely to the scheduled time as possible. To accommodate the medication schedule, the nurse may delay performing less important responsibilities, seek the assistance of another member of the nursing team, or delegate nursing tasks to another comparably qualified nurse. Any STAT administration of medication should receive immediate attention.

SETTING GOALS

- The client will receive the correct dosage of medication mixed within a safe volume of compatible solution.
- The medicated solution will infuse over the time period specified by the physician.

PREPARATION OF EQUIPMENT

The nurse will need the following:

Volume-control administration set
Medication

Syringe with #20 to #21 gauge needle attached
Alcohol swab
Medication label

Technique for administering IV medication by volume-control set

ACTION	RATIONALE
1. Check the medication card or Kardex with the physician's order.	Checking ensures that the client receives the correct medication at the correct time and in the correct manner.
2. Gather all equipment and bring it to the client's bedside.	Having the equipment available saves time and facilitates the performance of the task.
3. Explain the procedure to the client.	An explanation allays the client's anxiety.
4. Wash your hands.	Handwashing deters the spread of microorganisms.
5. Assess the IV site for the absence of inflammation or infiltration.	IV medication must be given into the vein for safe administration.
6. Withdraw the medication from the vial or ampule into a syringe. Refer to Procedure I-22 or I-23.	The correct dose must be prepared for dilution in the IV solution.
7. Identify the client by checking the identification wristband and asking the client his name.	Checking the wristband ensures that the medication is given to the right person.
8. Open the clamp between the solution and the volume-control set, as shown in Fig. I-32-1. Fill with the desired amount of IV solution.	Solution from the IV fluid dilutes the medication.
9. Close the clamp between the volume-control chamber and the IV solution container.	Clamping prevents the continued addition of fluid to the volume needed to mix with the medication.
10. Use an alcohol swab to cleanse the injection port on the volume-control set.	Cleansing deters the entry of microorganisms when the needle punctures the port.
11. Remove the cap and insert the needle into the port while holding the syringe steady. Inject the medication, as shown in Fig. I-32-2. Gently mix the solution in the small volume container.	Mixing ensures that the medication is evenly distributed within the solution.

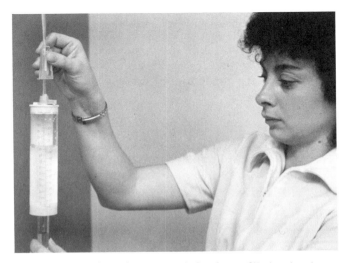

Figure I-32–1 The volume control chamber is filled with solution from the primary container. Once the desired amount enters the volume control chamber, the flow from the primary container is clamped.

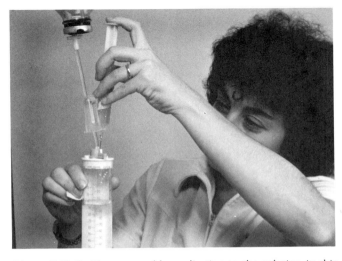

Figure I-32–2 The nurse adds medication to the solution in this volume-control set. The client receives the medication more quickly in this manner than if the drug has been mixed with the entire amount of solution in the bottle.

12. Open the clamp below the volume-control set and regulate the flow at the prescribed delivery rate. Monitor the medication infusion at periodic intervals.

Delivery over a 30-minute to 60-minute interval is a safe method of administering IV medication.

13. Attach a label to the volume-control device.

Labeling indicates that medication has been added and is infusing.

14. Place the syringe with the needle uncapped in a designated container.

Leaving the needle uncapped prevents an inadvertent needle stick.

15. Wash your hands.

Handwashing deters the spread of microorganisms.

16. Chart the administration of medication.

Accurate documentation is necessary to prevent medication errors.

17. Evaluate the client's response to the medication within an appropriate time frame.

Clients require careful observation because medications given by the IV route may have a rapid effect.

18. Return to refill the volume-control chamber or permit the fluid in the large container to infuse.

It is necessary to release the clamp above the volume-control chamber to resume the continued infusion of fluid.

SAMPLE DOCUMENTATION

Date	Time	Nurse's note
6/03	1300	Solu-Medrol 500 mg. added to 50 mL of 5%D/W in Volutrol. Infusing at 1 mL/min.

C. Shelski, RN

EVALUATION

REASSESSMENT

The information on the medication label should be read and reread at least three times. This reassessment practice helps to ensure that the correct medication has been supplied.

The infusion of fluid in a volume-control set must be reassessed frequently. Once the small volume infuses, there is no way for the remainder of the fluid to begin infusing again until the clamp above the volume-control set is released.

Stay with the client as the infusion begins and observe for signs of an allergic reaction or adverse effects to the medication. The client should be reassessed frequently during the short period while the medication is infusing.

EXPECTED OUTCOMES

The medication mixes compatibly with the solution in the volume-control set.

The client receives the correct medication and dosage in the recommended time.

The client experiences no side-effects, allergic reaction, or untoward effects to the medication.

UNEXPECTED OUTCOMES

The medication forms a precipitate when mixed with the fluid in the volume-control set.

The fluid in the volume-control set infuses more rapidly than desired.

The administration of the solution infuses slower than the recommended time.

The client receives only part of the medication due to an infusion that stops or infiltrates.

The client experiences undesirable effects from the medication.

MODIFICATIONS IN SELECTED SITUATIONS

GENERAL VARIATIONS

The clamp above the volume-control set can be opened and adjusted to infuse fluid continuously when no special intermittent medications are being administered.

AGE-RELATED
VARIATIONS

When very slow rates of infusion are ordered (*e.g.*, 10 ml/hour), the nurse must adjust the time when the medication is added to the volume-control set. To be extremely accurate, the nurse must account for the time it will take the volume in the tubing to infuse before the medication will be infusing. Intravenous tubing holds approximately 5 ml of solution.

Restrain a client, or immobilize the arm or hand, or protect the infusion site if the client is very young, restless, or uncooperative.

HOME-HEALTH
VARIATIONS

Should agency policy and the client's condition permit the nurse to leave the residence before the completion of the infusion of the medication in a volume-control set, provide written instructions for the family. Identify how to monitor and regulate the flow of the primary IV solution. Include a telephone number where the nurse can be reached.

RELATED TEACHING

Explain the purpose of the infusion and expected and undesirable effects of the medication.

Inform the client about the signs of infiltration and the need to notify personnel if any discomfort is experienced around the IV site.

Instruct the client that when the volume-control set is nearly empty, he should turn on his call signal.

PERFORMANCE CHECKLIST

When IV medication is administered by a volume-control set, the learner:

C	A	U	
[ ]	[ ]	[ ]	Reads the medical order written by the physician.
[ ]	[ ]	[ ]	Compares the medical order with the information transcribed to the medication card or Kardex.
[ ]	[ ]	[ ]	Reviews pertinent drug information in an appropriate reference text, if unfamiliar with the medication.
[ ]	[ ]	[ ]	Explains the action of the medication, expected effects, method of administration, and schedule for administering the drug to the client.
[ ]	[ ]	[ ]	Washes hands.
[ ]	[ ]	[ ]	Examines the IV site, the patency of the venipuncture device, the dates on the solution, tubing, and dressing.
[ ]	[ ]	[ ]	Performs physical assessments related to the medication about to be administered.
[ ]	[ ]	[ ]	Washes hands.
[ ]	[ ]	[ ]	Gathers equipment.
[ ]	[ ]	[ ]	Reads the drug label at least three times.
[ ]	[ ]	[ ]	Withdraws the supplied medication into a syringe.
[ ]	[ ]	[ ]	Checks the identification of the client.
[ ]	[ ]	[ ]	Fills the volume-control chamber with the appropriate amount of solution from the larger volume container.
[ ]	[ ]	[ ]	Clamps the tubing above the volume-control set.
[ ]	[ ]	[ ]	Cleanses the injection port on the volume-control set.
[ ]	[ ]	[ ]	Inserts the needle through the port of the volume-control set and instills the medication.

C = competent; A = acceptable; U = unsatisfactory

(Continued)

PERFORMANCE CHECKLIST (Continued)

C	A	U	
[ ]	[ ]	[ ]	Rotates the chamber to uniformly mix the medication throughout the solution.
[ ]	[ ]	[ ]	Adjusts the clamp regulating the calculated rate of flow from the volume-control set.
[ ]	[ ]	[ ]	Attaches a label to the container, identifying the date, time, name of the medication, dosage of medication added, and nurse's initials.
[ ]	[ ]	[ ]	Observes the client's immediate response.
[ ]	[ ]	[ ]	Provides the client with a signal device.
[ ]	[ ]	[ ]	Disposes of equipment appropriately.
[ ]	[ ]	[ ]	Washes hands.
[ ]	[ ]	[ ]	Documents the medication administration.
[ ]	[ ]	[ ]	Returns to reassess the client, release the clamp, and continue the infusion of the IV solution.

Outcome: [ ] Pass   [ ] Fail

C = competent; A = acceptable; U = unsatisfactory

Comments: _____

_____

_____

_____   _____
Student's Signature   Date

_____   _____
Instructor's Signature   Date

Introducing drugs through a heparin lock and performing a heparin flush

A heparin lock is a device that provides constant access to venous circulation without the continuous infusion of solution. Bolus medications and intermittent small volume containers of medication, ordinarily given by piggyback administration, can be given through a heparin lock. Care must be taken to prevent clotting around the needle or catheter that is within the vein.

PURPOSES OF PROCEDURE

A heparin lock is used to:

1. Administer IV medications at intermittent periods.
2. Provide continuous access to the venous circulation in case the administration of emergency medications becomes necessary.
3. Avoid the infusion of unneeded fluid.
4. Promote the comfort and freedom of movement not possible with IV tubing, solution container, and pole.

ASSESSMENT

Refer to Procedure I-29, Adding Medications to an IV Solution Container, with the following exception:
• The patency and placement of the needle or catheter is assessed with a syringe containing saline during the implementation stage of the procedure.

RELEVANT NURSING DIAGNOSES

The client who receives IV medication through a heparin lock may have nursing diagnoses, such as:

• *Anxiety*
• *Fear*
• *Potential for Injury*
• *Potential for Altered Tissue Perfusion*
• *Knowledge Deficit*

PLANNING

ESTABLISHING PRIORITIES

A heparin lock must be flushed once each 8 hours if it has not been used for the intermittent administration of IV medication. This is best scheduled at specific times to ensure a similar number of hours between each flush.

Medications should always be administered as near to the scheduled time as possible. Implementation of other nursing responsibilities should be planned in order to accommodate time for the safe preparation and administration of scheduled medications. Client care may be revised, modified, or delegated when a STAT medication requires immediate administration.

SETTING GOALS

• The heparin lock will be patent before and after the procedure is performed.
• The client will receive the correct dosage of medication at the scheduled time.
• The medication and flush solutions will infuse easily through the heparin lock.

PREPARATION OF EQUIPMENT

The following will be necessary when using a heparin lock:

Medication (optional if just flushing the heparin lock)
Medication card or Kardex
Sterile syringe and needle (#25 gauge) with 1 ml of diluted heparin solution (usually 1:1000 dilution or 10 U/ml)
Sterile syringe and needle (#25 gauge) with 2 ml of sterile saline and an extra #25 gauge needle.
Watch with second hand or digital readout if giving a bolus of medication
Alcohol swabs

Technique for introducing drugs through a heparin lock and performing a heparin flush

ACTION	RATIONALE
1. Assemble equipment and check the physician's order.	Checking the written order ensures that the client receives the right medication at the right time by the proper route.
2. Explain the procedure to the client.	An explanation alleviates the client's apprehension.
3. Wash your hands.	Handwashing deters the spread of microorganisms.
4. Withdraw the heparin solution and sterile saline from appropriate vials into syringes.	Using proper technique maintains the sterility of the syringes and solutions.
5. Cleanse the injection port of the heparin lock with an alcohol swab, as shown in Fig. I-33-1.	Cleansing removes surface bacteria at the entry site.

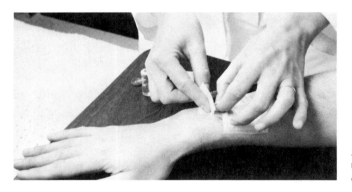

Figure I-33–1 The heparin lock has already been inserted within the venipuncture device. Before instilling saline, heparin, or medication, the port on the heparin lock is cleansed to remove pathogens.

6. Remove the needle cap by pulling it straight off.	Avoiding contact with microorganisms protects the sterility of the needle.
7. Stabilize the injection port with the nondominant hand, and insert the needle of the syringe containing 2 ml of sterile normal saline into the injection port.	Stabilization allows for the careful insertion of the needle into the center circle of the port without pulling the needle or catheter out of the vein.
8. Aspirate gently and inject 1 ml of saline if a blood return is observed in the syringe. If the lock is obstructed, it will have to be changed. Do not force saline through a lock that is not patent.	A blood return indicates that the heparin lock is still patent and in the vein. Forcing the instillation of saline may dislodge a clot that has formed.
9. Remove the needle, and replace it with a second sterile #25 gauge needle.	Each time the injection port is pierced a sterile needle should be used.
10. If medication is to be given via the heparin lock, cleanse the port with an alcohol swab, insert the needle, and inject the medication (Fig. I-33-2) using a watch to verify the correct injection rate.	After patency has been established and the site has been cleansed, the medication can be administered. A slow rate of infusion allows the nurse to assess for adverse reactions to the drug.

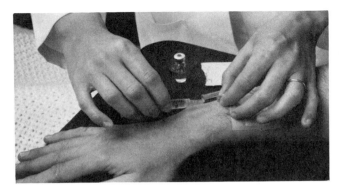

Figure I-33-2 The nurse steadies the heparin lock and the venipuncture device while preparing to flush the lumen with heparin.

11. Withdraw the empty medication syringe, cleanse the port, and reinsert the syringe containing the saline.

The use of sterile equipment and surgical asepsis reduces the potential for introducing pathogens within the bloodstream.

12. Inject 1 ml of saline.

Instilling saline flushes the entire dose of medication into the vein and prevents any incompatibility reaction to the forthcoming instillation of heparin.

13. Remove the empty syringe and needle, cleanse the port, and insert the needle with the syringe containing 1 ml of heparin. Inject the heparin.

Injecting heparin ensures the patency of the lock between injections by preventing the formation of blood clots in the needle or catheter. One milliliter usually fills the chamber within the heparin lock.

14. Dispose of the needles and syringes in an appropriate puncture-resistant container.

Proper disposal prevents accidental needle-stick and transmission of blood-borne diseases.

15. Wash your hands.

Handwashing deters the spread of microorganisms.

16. The injection site and heparin lock should be checked and flushed at least every 8 hours with saline and heparin if medication is not given at least that often.

Periodic flushing ensures the patency of the system for continuing injections.

17. The heparin lock, should be changed at least every 48 hours. An obstructed lock should be changed immediately.

Changing a heparin lock regularly and having it free of clotted blood reduces the dangers of infection and emboli in the circulating blood.

18. Chart the administration of the heparin flush or medication.

Accurate documentation is necessary to prevent medication error.

SAMPLE DOCUMENTATION

Date	Time	Nurse's note
6/21	0947	Heparin lock patent and flushes well. Apical pulse rate 120. Lanoxin 1 mg. administered IV push through heparin lock as first digitalizing dose.
		S. Lane, RN

EVALUATION

REASSESSMENT

The patency and placement of a heparin lock is reassessed before each use and at least every 8 hours when medications are not regularly administered.

The information on the IV drug label should be read at least three times to ensure that the client receives the right drug, the right dosage, by the right route.

When any drug is administered intravenously, the client should be observed closely during and immediately after the injection. The drug effects following a bolus administration may be detected within 5 minutes to 30 minutes. Therefore, the nurse should reassess the client's response soon after disposing of the used equipment and charting the administration of the drug.

Blood levels may be drawn by laboratory personnel to measure the serum concentration of some drugs. The physician may modify the dosage or the schedule for drug administration based on the nurse's clinical observations and laboratory results.

The distal location of a central venous catheter, sealed with a heparin lock, may be confirmed by x-ray.

EXPECTED OUTCOMES

The insertion date of the needle or catheter is within the safe period for use.

A blood return is observed indicating the needle or catheter is patent and located within the vein.

Sterile normal saline used for flushing infuses easily through the heparin lock.

The medication is administered over the recommended period of time without adverse consequences.

Diluted heparin instills easily through the resealable injection port.

UNEXPECTED OUTCOMES

The date indicating the insertion of the needle or catheter, and heparin lock is beyond the agency's policy for safe use.

The area around the heparin lock is tender.

No blood is evident during aspiration.

An attempt to flush with normal saline is met with resistance.

The client experiences an allergic reaction or undesirable effects to the medication.

MODIFICATIONS IN SELECTED SITUATIONS

GENERAL VARIATIONS

Any venipuncture device can be converted to a heparin lock by aseptically removing the IV tubing, inserting the lock, and instilling heparin.

A heparin lock can be inserted into the end of a long catheter placed in the subclavian or other central vein. A central line is kept patent by intermittently instilling a more concentrated solution of heparin, such as 100 U/ml.

If a drug is compatible with heparin, the lock need not be flushed with saline before and after the drug's administration. However, for reasons of safety, some agencies require that a saline flush be used regardless of the drug's compatibility.

Some nurses withdraw 1 ml of saline into two separate syringes. A piece of tape, different colored protective needle cap, or other identifying mark is applied to distinguish the syringes containing heparin and medication.

HOME-HEALTH VARIATIONS

Ensure the availability of supplies and heparin for subsequent use of a heparin lock.

Prefilled syringe cartridges of heparin may be given to clients for maintaining the patency of intravenous devices or central catheters when home administration of medication is required.

RELATED TEACHING

Explain that the heparin lock allows intermittent administration of IV medication or access to the vein in the case of an emergency.

Inform the client that the dilute volume of heparin is designed to keep the needle or catheter open, and is so small an amount that it will not inhibit his own ability to control bleeding.

Identify the name of the drug, the effects of the medication, possible adverse effects, and the frequency of their administration.

Instruct the client to notify the nurse if his hand or arm becomes tender, painful, or swollen.

PERFORMANCE CHECKLIST

When administering medications through a heparin lock or performing a heparin flush, the learner:

C	A	U	
[ ]	[ ]	[ ]	Reads the medical order written by the physician.
[ ]	[ ]	[ ]	Compares the medical order with the information transcribed to the medication card or Kardex.
[ ]	[ ]	[ ]	Reviews the pertinent drug information in an appropriate reference text, if unfamiliar with the medication.
[ ]	[ ]	[ ]	Explains the action of the medication, expected effects, method of administration, and schedule for administering the drug to the client.
[ ]	[ ]	[ ]	Gathers appropriate number and sizes of syringes and needles.
[ ]	[ ]	[ ]	Washes hands.
[ ]	[ ]	[ ]	Prepares syringes with saline, medication (omitted if only flushing the lock), and heparin.
[ ]	[ ]	[ ]	Checks the identification of the client.
[ ]	[ ]	[ ]	Obtains the physical assessments pertinent to the type of medication that will be injected.
[ ]	[ ]	[ ]	Examines and palpates the area of the venipuncture device.
[ ]	[ ]	[ ]	Cleanses the injection port, inserts the syringe with saline, aspirates, and instills 1 ml of saline following a blood return.
[ ]	[ ]	[ ]	Changes the needle if a second syringe of saline has not been prepared.
[ ]	[ ]	[ ]	Repeats the cleansing prior to the insertion and instillation of medication. (This step and the two which follow are omitted if the heparin lock is only being flushed to maintain its patency.)
[ ]	[ ]	[ ]	Observes the client's immediate response to the administration of the medication.
[ ]	[ ]	[ ]	Cleanses the port, inserts and instills the remaining saline.
[ ]	[ ]	[ ]	Repeats the above sequence of steps with the syringe containing heparin.
[ ]	[ ]	[ ]	Makes the client comfortable, raises the side rails, and provides the client with a signal device.
[ ]	[ ]	[ ]	Disposes of needles and syringes in an appropriate receptacle.
[ ]	[ ]	[ ]	Washes hands.
[ ]	[ ]	[ ]	Documents the medication administration or the heparin flush.
[ ]	[ ]	[ ]	Returns to reassess the client's response to the medication.

Outcome: [ ] Pass   [ ] Fail

C = competent; A = acceptable; U = unsatisfactory

Comments: _____

_____

_____

_____   _____
       Student's Signature   Date

_____   _____
       Instructor's Signature   Date

I-34 *Transferring a client*

When a client's condition changes, for better or worse, he may be transferred. Transfers usually occur when the client has a reduced need for specialized care. However, the opposite may be true. Clients may also be moved from one area on a unit to another to facilitate better observation or to accommodate a personal request. Room transfers are not subject to the details involved in an interagency transfer or the transfer of a client from one unit to another.

PURPOSES OF PROCEDURE

A transfer is conducted to:

1. Locate the client in a health-care agency or unit that is best suited to provide for his specialized nursing care.
2. Place the client where there is the most appropriate utilization of available personnel and services.
3. Match the intensity of nursing care with the client's level of need.

ASSESSMENT

OBJECTIVE DATA

- Note the physician's written order to transfer the client.
- Analyze the client's need for skilled or basic care.
- Observe the client's ability to participate in self-care.
- Identify the specialized equipment and services that are being used for the client's care and determine which facilities can provide similar care.
- Determine that the potential agency (or agencies) has the ability to accept a new client.

SUBJECTIVE DATA

- Discuss the client's feelings concerning extended care.
- Consult the client's preference for alternative agencies for care.

NURSING DIAGNOSES

The client who is being transferred may have nursing diagnoses, such as:

- *Anxiety*
- *Impaired Adjustment*
- *Ineffective Family Coping*
- *Altered Family Processes*
- *Impaired Home Maintenance Management*
- *Impaired Physical Mobility*
- *Self-Care Deficit*

PLANNING

ESTABLISHING PRIORITIES

When a client's acuity level intensifies, it is imperative that the transfer occurs as quickly and efficiently as possible. Rapid transfers are now being facilitated not only by ambulance but by helicopters as well. The details of the transfer must be coordinated in order to accommodate the vehicle's expected time of arrival (ETA). When the condition of the client warrants less critical time-management, the transfer can be arranged when it is most convenient for the client and the staff.

SETTING GOALS

- The client and family will be consulted and collaborate on the potential transfer site.

208

- The transfer form, shown in Fig. I-34-1, will be completed $\frac{1}{2}$ hour before the scheduled transfer.

- The client will be transferred safely, comfortably, and expeditiously to the new location.

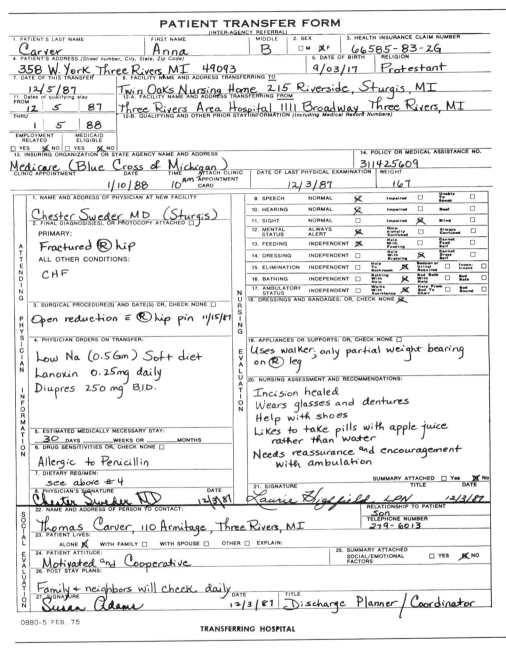

Figure I-34-1 The patient transfer form is used when clients are referred from one health agency to another. It illustrates the type of information the receiving agency needs to make continuity of care possible. (Lewis LW, Timby BK: Fundamental Skills and Concepts in Patient Care, 4th ed, p 157. Philadelphia, JB Lippincott, 1988)

PREPARATION OF EQUIPMENT

When the nurse prepares the client for transfer, the following are needed:

Interagency transfer form
Client's personal items, such as clothing, valuables, hygiene products, plants, flower arrangements, and get-well cards

Prescriptions or limited supply of prescribed medications
Hospital equipment that may be kept for personal use, such as a urinal and thermometer

Technique for transferring a client

ACTION	RATIONALE
1. Verify that a transfer order has been written by the physician.	The physician determines when it is in the best interest of the client to transfer him to another facility.
2. Determine that the client and his family have received information about the transfer.	Communication promotes cooperation when there is a change in the client's condition.
3. Gather the client's personal belongings.	Carelessness can lead to loss of the client's property.
4. Notify the referral personnel that arrangements are being made for the client's transfer.	Other personnel should be provided time to plan and adjust their schedules so the transferred client will feel welcome and unhurried.
5. Summarize the significant information about the client to the new personnel, such as the medical diagnosis and treatment, nursing diagnoses, current care plan, diet, and medications.	New personnel may not have time to read the chart thoroughly before assuming responsibility for the client's care.
6. Complete the charting on the client's record.	Legally the client's permanent record must contain accurate documentation of his care in the agency.
7. Fill in all areas of information on the transfer form.	The transfer form provides a written summary of the current status of the client.
8. Assist in transferring the client to a wheelchair or stretcher.	The safety of the client is ensured by assisting his mobility.
9. Notify other departments within the hospital, such as the dietary department and switchboard, of the client's transfer.	Services, such as phone calls, will need to be redirected.
10. Record the circumstances and condition of the client when transferred.	The chart should reflect the client's care and responses.

SAMPLE DOCUMENTATION

Date	Time	Nurse's note
4/07	1330	Transferred by ambulance with personal belongings to Pine View Home. Alert and comfortable. Remaining digoxin and Lasix sent with client. *K. Frye, RN*

EVALUATION

REASSESSMENT

A conscientious nurse may call the receiving agency and inquire about the condition of the client and ask that they convey personal regards for his welfare. Communication also provides an opportunity to clarify written information on the transfer form. When the client is transferred to another unit within the facility, the nurse can visit the transferred client from time to time.

EXPECTED OUTCOMES

The client and his family are pleased with the prospect of the transfer.
The client is comfortable while being transported from one facility or unit to another.

UNEXPECTED OUTCOMES	The client or his family react negatively to the potential plans for transfer. There is no vacancy to accommodate the client's transfer. The client experiences discomfort, delay, or inconvenience during the transfer.
MODIFICATIONS IN SELECTED SITUATIONS GENERAL VARIATIONS	Critically ill clients may be accompanied by the primary care nurse during a transfer. Family members may wish to accompany a client during a transfer. They may follow in a personal car, or in some instances, ride in the ambulance. The nurse may write a summary of the client's condition and provide an updated nursing care plan and current medication schedule for the new nursing unit or agency when a transfer form is not used. The client's head should be covered, and the client's body should be covered with several blankets if the weather is windy or cold. The source for oxygen may be temporarily switched to a tank during a transfer in an ambulance.
AGE-RELATED VARIATIONS	Infants may be transported in an isolette which can be returned later.
HOME-HEALTH VARIATIONS	Follow agency policy and requirements of third-party payors as to whether a physician's order is needed to transfer a client. Agency policies usually prohibit the nurse from transporting a client in a private vehicle. Transfer from the home setting may be for a few hours to attend a clinic or workshop or for an extended period of time if readmission to a hospital or nursing home is necessary. Sometimes home care clients are transferred to a nursing home while the family takes a vacation. The client will need to be readmitted to a home health agency following his stay in a hospital or nursing home.

(Performance checklist next page)

PERFORMANCE CHECKLIST

When participating in the transfer of a client, the learner:

C	A	U	
[ ]	[ ]	[ ]	Verifies the written medical order.
[ ]	[ ]	[ ]	Contacts the discharge coordinator.
[ ]	[ ]	[ ]	Assesses the client's physical condition and his response to the plan for transfer.
[ ]	[ ]	[ ]	Consults with the client and family concerning preferences for relocation, if appropriate.
[ ]	[ ]	[ ]	Contacts the agency or unit where the client will be transferred.
[ ]	[ ]	[ ]	Informs the client and his family of the projected time for the transfer.
[ ]	[ ]	[ ]	Completes the plan of care scheduled up to the time of transfer.
[ ]	[ ]	[ ]	Contacts an ambulance or helicopter service if the client's family cannot or should not assume the risks involved in transferring the client.
[ ]	[ ]	[ ]	Completes the transfer form or summary information.
[ ]	[ ]	[ ]	Gathers all the client's personal items and equipment using the clothing and valuable list to avoid omissions.
[ ]	[ ]	[ ]	Provides the transport personnel or the family with prescriptions, medications, or medical supplies the client will need in the near future.
[ ]	[ ]	[ ]	Dresses the client appropriately.
[ ]	[ ]	[ ]	Assists in transferring the client to a wheelchair or stretcher.
[ ]	[ ]	[ ]	Directs a responsible family member or accompanies the client, if his condition permits, to the business office if being transferred to another agency.
[ ]	[ ]	[ ]	Escorts the client from the agency or unit.
[ ]	[ ]	[ ]	Charts the specifics of the transfer.
[ ]	[ ]	[ ]	Notifies related agency departments of the transfer.
[ ]	[ ]	[ ]	Strips the client's room so that it can be cleaned and prepared for another admission.

Outcome: [ ] Pass   [ ] Fail

C = competent; A = acceptable; U = unsatisfactory

Comments: _____
_____
_____

_____   _____
Student's Signature   Date

_____   _____
Instructor's Signature   Date

I-35   *Discharging a client from a health-care agency*

The procedure for discharging a client is only one small aspect of the discharge process. Clients generally are admitted with high acuity levels yet receive fewer days of treatment than before implementation of the prospective Diagnostic Related Group (DRG) payment system. Therefore it is crucial that the discharge be planned early. It is not uncommon for nurses to project potential discharge needs at the time of admission.

PURPOSES OF PROCEDURE

A client is discharged in order to:

1. Return the person to a state of independent living.
2. Provide continued care by home-health nurses, or family assistance.

ASSESSMENTS

OBJECTIVE DATA

- Review the discharge planning form, if one is available.
- Discuss the possible options after discharge, such as returning home for independent living, an adult day-care facility, a small residential adult foster care home, a skilled or basic nursing home, or intermittent home care.
- Determine if the client or his family have the knowledge and skills necessary to maintain or improve the current level of health. Explore dietary changes, medication administration, use and care of technical equipment.
- Identify if assistive devices, such as a walker or commode, have been obtained.
- Check to see if the home environment has been modified to avoid structural barriers, such as stairs.
- Assess if the client can obtain transportation for subsequent health care.
- Check if the client has had contact with a social worker for assistance with finances, insurance, or Medicare.
- Determine if the client has been referred to appropriate community services.

SUBJECTIVE DATA

- Interview the client to determine his perceptions concerning discharge and recovery.
- Explore the client's and family's attitudes and beliefs that affect health and illness.

RELEVANT NURSING DIAGNOSES

Examples of nursing diagnoses when a client is being discharged from the hospital are:

- *Self-Care Deficit*
- *Knowledge Deficit*
- *Ineffective Family Coping*
- *Potential for Noncompliance*
- *Impaired Home Maintenance Management*

PLANNING

ESTABLISHING PRIORITIES

It is important to begin preparing the client for discharge as soon as possible. Clients tend to be overwhelmed when lengthy instructions are provided immediately before leaving the facility. Optimum learning occurs by providing graduated amounts of information, building from simple to complex, repetition and practice. The nurse should develop a teaching plan which can be implemented gradually each day. Any teaching and the client's learning should be documented.

SETTING GOALS
- Before the day of discharge the client and his family will be prepared for obtaining the highest potential for wellness.
- Before the day of discharge the client will be referred to services that will maintain continuity of care for any lingering health problems.

PREPARATION OF EQUIPMENT

When discharging the client, the nurse will need:

Written discharge instructions
Prescriptions for medications (optional)
Diet instruction booklet (optional)
Written cards identifying the place, date, and time of future appointments for medical care or referral services
Medical supplies or list of suppliers in the immediate area
Clothing and valuables list
Wheelchair (optional)
Cart for personal belongings

Technique for discharging a client from a health-care agency

ACTION	RATIONALE
1. Check to see that the client has a discharge order.	It is the physician's responsibility to discharge a client.
2. Make sure the client or support person has had discharge instructions (*i.e.,* regarding diet, medications).	The client or a support person should be able to continue with necessary care after discharge when properly instructed.
3. Have all necessary equipment and supplies ready for the client.	Having equipment and supplies ready saves time and the annoyance of having to wait for them when the client is ready to leave.
4. Check to see that proper financial arrangements have been made by the client or support person. Obtain valuables. Observe agency policies.	These actions help to avoid legal problems.
5. Assist the client to dress and pack belongings. Make sure the client has all personal belongings.	Assisting the client conserves client strength. Time and trouble are saved when the client leaves with all belongings.
6. If the client needs reimbursement for future home visits, be sure the physician has given a written order for all services.	There must be a physician's order for reimbursement by Medicare and other third-party payers.
7. Transport the client and belongings to a car and assist the client into the car as necessary.	Assisting the client conserves the client's strength. Such assistance is courteous and helps the client feel that personnel are interested in his welfare.
8. Make necessary recordings on the client's records and complete the discharge summary, shown in Fig. I-35-1.	It is important legally that the client's permanent hospital record is complete.

Doe, Jane   Age 73
1200 West Elm
Jackson, Mo.
00011000

ST. FRANCIS MEDICAL CENTER
211 ST. FRANCIS DRIVE
CAPE GIRARDEAU, MO. 63701

**PATIENT
DISCHARGE SUMMARY**

		MORNING						AFTERNOON					EVENING / NIGHT						
I MEDICATION (NAME/DOSAGE)	6 AM	7 AM	8 AM	9 AM	10 AM	11 AM	12 NOON	1 PM	2 PM	3 PM	4 PM	5 PM	6 PM	7 PM	8 PM	9 PM	10 PM	11 PM	12 PM	1 AM
ASA gr XV			X				X						X							
Lanoxin 0.125 mg			X																	
Diuril 500 mg			X										X							
Cefaclor 500 mg			X								X								X	

WEEKLY SCHEDULE (For alternating dosage)

NAME / DOSAGE	SUNDAY	MONDAY	TUESDAY	WEDNESDAY	THURSDAY	FRIDAY	SATURDAY

[X] PRESCRIPTION GIVEN TO PATIENT   [X] HOME MEDICATIONS RETURNED   [X] HANDOUT GIVEN IF APPLICABLE

MEDICATIONS SHOULD BE TAKEN IN ACCORDANCE WITH YOUR PHYSICIAN'S PRESCRIPTION. THIS FORM IS PROVIDED AS A SERVICE BY ST. FRANCIS MEDICAL CENTER. ANY CHANGE IN AMOUNT OR DOSAGE OF MEDICATION MUST BE APPROVED BY YOUR PHYSICIAN.

II   SPECIAL DISCHARGE INSTRUCTIONS (Side Affects to Medications, Activities, Diabetes, Cardiac Rehab., P.T., R.T., Wound or Dressing Care, Irrigation, etc.)

1) Take antibiotic (Cefaclor) with food; report rash or GI upset to MD
2) Use good handwashing to prevent spread of infection and dispose of sputum and tissues in paper bag
3) Rest for one hour each afternoon
4) Drink extra fluids for this week

INSTRUCTED BY *P. LeMone   R.N.*   PATIENT UNDERSTANDS [X] YES [ ] NO   CARBON COPY GIVEN TO PATIENT [X]

III   M.D. OFFICE VISIT   [ ] NO   [X] YES   1 week — appointment made

IV   METHOD OF DISCHARGE

[X] RELEASE SIGNED
[ ] AMA WITH RELEASE SIGNED BY PATIENT [ ] YES [ ] NO

DR. NOTIFIED   Date _____   Time _____

D/C BY DR. *James*
D/C DATE *12-2-89*   Time *1000*
HOW D/C [X] VOLUNTEER, OTHER *and husband*
TRANSPORTED BY [ ] STRETCHER [X] W/C [ ] AMBULATORY

V   DISCHARGED TO:
[X] HOME WITH WHOM *husband*
[ ] NURSING HOME _____
[ ] TRANSFER TO OTHER FACILITY _____

VI   GENERAL CONDITION ON DISCHARGE

[X] ALERT	[ ] LETHARGIC	[X] PAIN CONTROLLED	[ ] DECUBITUS [X] SELF
[X] ORIENTED	[ ] COMATOSE	[X] AFEBRILE	[ ] INCISION HEALING [ ] WITH HELP
[ ] CONFUSED	[ ] PAIN FREE	[ ] RASH	[ ] DRAINING WOUND [ ] ROOM ONLY
			[X] AMBULATORY [ ] HALL

Signature *P. LeMone R.N.*   Date *12-2-89*

640-260-812/0800048   **CHART**

Figure I-35–1 On the patient discharge summary information is provided that will help the client to maintain his restored level of health.

SAMPLE DOCUMENTATION

Date	Time	Nurse's note
2/09	1345	Teaching completed. Able to state the name, dosage, frequency, purpose, expected and undesired effects of Parnate. Discharged per wheelchair to home. Prescription for Parnate and MAO inhibitor diet instructions sent with client. Given written card indicating the date and time of office appointment c̄ Dr. Silvers. Provided with Mental Health Association hotline number.
		N. Gleason, RN

EVALUATION

REASSESSMENT

In some institutions, the primary care nurse or the discharge coordinator may make a follow-up phone call, send a questionnaire, or arrange a home visit to the discharged client. The client should always be encouraged to call the nursing unit to discuss the progress or problems after discharge. Some community agencies return a form to the referring facility describing the status of the discharged client.

EXPECTED OUTCOMES

The client looks forward to returning home.
The client or his family understand and demonstrate competence in carrying out the care necessary to maintain health.
The client's home has been prepared for his unique limitations.
The client and his family have a plan for obtaining assistance if difficulties develop following discharge.

UNEXPECTED OUTCOMES

The client cannot return to home living.
The client has no family or significant friends who can provide assistance.
Neither the client nor his family can perform the required care.
Placement is not available in an extended care or adult foster care facility.
The client develops new complications.

MODIFICATIONS IN SELECTED SITUATIONS

GENERAL VARIATIONS

If the client is leaving without a physician's consent, check to see that the proper form has been completed. Because a competent person cannot be held legally in an institution against his wishes, a properly signed form releases the agency and physician from responsibility should problems arise because the client refused further care. If the client refuses to sign the form, document the explanation given to the client and his refusal to sign the release form. Notify the physician.

HOME-HEALTH VARIATIONS

In order for a home care referral to be made and subsequent home visits to be reimbursed, there must be a written order by the physician for all services.
Clients must meet certain criteria to have home care services reimbursed by Medicare and other third-party payors. Examples include: The client must be homebound; the care must be intermittent.
All persons in a family become the focus of the home health nurse. Of particular concern is the primary caregiver who often needs respite care. The nurse can assist by involving other family members, neighbors, or a home health aide to help. The home health nurse must use skill and creativity in finding less expensive but equally effective methods of carrying out treatments.

RELATED TEACHING

The client should be instructed on the disease, safety, emergency measures, basic nursing care, preventive measures, instructions on all treatments, medications, and diet.

PERFORMANCE CHECKLIST

When a client is discharged, the learner:

C	A	U	
[ ]	[ ]	[ ]	Notes the discharge order written by the physician.
[ ]	[ ]	[ ]	Contacts the discharge coordinator.
[ ]	[ ]	[ ]	Reviews the discharge planning form and teaching plan for any uncompleted aspects.
[ ]	[ ]	[ ]	Consults with the client and family concerning the time and place for discharge.
[ ]	[ ]	[ ]	Completes unfinished teaching.
[ ]	[ ]	[ ]	Validates the client's understanding of information by having the client verbally list, describe, write the main points, or return a demonstration.
[ ]	[ ]	[ ]	Contacts the provider for transportation.
[ ]	[ ]	[ ]	Gathers the client's personal belongings.
[ ]	[ ]	[ ]	Provides the client or his family with prescriptions, appointment cards, medical supplies or sources for them.
[ ]	[ ]	[ ]	Assists the client to dress appropriately for the seasonal weather.
[ ]	[ ]	[ ]	Assists the client to walk or provides a wheelchair.
[ ]	[ ]	[ ]	Helps the client locate the business office to complete financial arrangements, if necessary.
[ ]	[ ]	[ ]	Aids in safely transferring the client from the health-care facility into a private car or ambulance.
[ ]	[ ]	[ ]	Charts the specifics of the discharge on the client's record.

Outcome: [ ] Pass   [ ] Fail

C = competent; A = acceptable; U = unsatisfactory

Comments: _____
_____
_____

_____   _____
Student's Signature   Date

_____   _____
Instructor's Signature   Date

Performing postmortem care

After a client dies, the nurse is responsible for postmortem care. This literally means care after death. The extent of postmortem care is related to variable factors, such as the circumstances of the death, personal or religious customs of the family, and the time span between death and care of the body by the mortician.

PURPOSES OF PROCEDURE

Postmortem care is performed to:

1. Prepare the body in a manner that will reduce the family's distress when viewing the body.
2. Prevent distortions in the body's appearance during later viewing at the funeral home.

ASSESSMENTS

OBJECTIVE DATA

- No response to stimulation
- Absence of pulse, respirations, and blood pressure
- Dilated, fixed pupils
- Flat electroencephalogram (EEG) in the presence of artificial ventilation

RELEVANT NURSING DIAGNOSES

Nurses consider the other persons who are significant to the client as potential recipients for nursing care. Therefore, any one in the family or a friend of the deceased client may have nursing diagnoses, such as:

- *Anticipatory Grieving*
- *Dysfunctional Grieving*
- *Hopelessness*
- *Ineffective Individual Coping*

PLANNING

ESTABLISHING PRIORITIES

The nurse should always respond immediately to the sudden clinical death of a client. An exception would be when the physician has written a "Do not resuscitate" (DNR) order on the record after consulting with the client and his family.

The nurse should be attending the dying client quite closely. One of the greatest fears of terminally ill clients is that they will die alone. The nurse should contact the family or assign one of the nursing team personnel to remain with the client when death is imminent. Once death has occurred, the nurse should note the time and be prepared to comfort the client's family and friends. Meeting their emotional needs takes precedence over care of the body.

SETTING GOALS

- The client's body will be clean and free of all equipment used for treatment within $\frac{1}{2}$ to 1 hour following the pronouncement of death.
- The body will be transported with respect to the morgue or mortuary.

PREPARATION OF EQUIPMENT

The nurse will need the following:

Towels, washcloth, basin
Soap and water
Clean, disposable gloves
Waterproof bag for soiled equipment

Disposable absorbent pads
Identification tags
Paper shroud or clean cotton sheet

Technique for performing postmortem care

ACTION	RATIONALE
1. Notify the doctor of the signs of death.	The physician should notify the family if they have not been with the client.
2. Transfer any client who shared a room with the deceased temporarily to another location, if possible.	The client may be upset by his roommate's death. The family will appreciate privacy with the body.
3. Contact any persons involved in organ procurement.	Organs must be removed and preserved as quickly as possible to ensure their usefulness.
4. Inform the designated mortician.	The mortician may indicate that the body will be removed from the nursing unit or picked up at the morgue.
5. Determine that the family and clergy have spent all the time they want with the body.	Some persons request that certain religious services be performed at the time of death.
6. Assemble the equipment for cleaning, wrapping, and identifying the body.	The body is prepared in a clean condition before it is transferred to the mortuary.
7. Place the body supine with the arms extended at the side or folded over the abdomen.	A normal anatomical position prevents discoloration of the skin from pooling blood in the areas visible in a casket.
8. Remove hairpins or clips.	Sharp objects about the face can scratch and detract from its appearance.
9. Close the eyelids by applying gentle pressure.	The eyes may not be easily closed if the time between death and preparation of the body is prolonged.
10. Replace or retain dentures within the mouth or label and send them with the body.	Dentures maintain the natural contour of the face. They may be difficult to insert several hours after death.
11. Use a small towel under the chin to close an open mouth.	If the mouth is allowed to remain open, it may resist closing later.
12. Apply gloves and remove soiled dressings or other potential sources of pathogens.	Live pathogens continue to be present even though the client is dead.
13. Remove venipuncture devices, indwelling catheter, monitor leads, and so on.	Only the body should be delivered to the mortician.
14. Remove gloves and discard them with the removed articles.	Soiled gloves are a source of infection transmission if disposed improperly.
15. Dispose of all contaminated and soiled items in appropriate containers.	A container acts as a transmission barrier to control the spread of organisms.
16. Wash your hands thoroughly.	Handwashing deters the spread of microorganisms.
17. Cleanse any obviously soiled areas of the body.	Because the body is washed by the mortician a complete bath is not required.
18. Apply disposable pads in the perineal area.	Stool or urine may be released after death when the sphincter muscles relax.
19. Remove or make an inventory of the valuables still attached to the body.	All personal valuables must be accounted for.
20. Wrap the body in a shroud or cover it with a clean, cotton sheet.	Covering the body promotes respect by preventing its observation by curious onlookers.

21. Attach an identification tag according to agency policy.

Tagging facilitates determining the identity of one body from another.

22. Transport the body to the morgue or await the arrival of the mortician's assistants.

The body may be held temporarily in the morgue or transported directly from the unit.

23. Lock removed valuables in a safe, and note their location on the client's record.

Valuables must be safeguarded until they can be returned to the family.

24. Complete charting indicating the disposition of the body.

The permanent record should note where and to whom the body was transferred.

25. Prepare the room for terminal disinfection.

The unit must be cleaned and disinfected for subsequent use.

SAMPLE DOCUMENTATION

Date	Time	Nurse's note
5/01	0753	Wife and son ⊆ client. Last rites administered by clergy. No BP or pulse obtainable. Pupils are fixed and dilated. Dr. Roche informed of death. Zeiler Funeral Home notified. Wedding ring and wristwatch given to wife along with clothing. Postmortem care performed. Body wrapped and identified. Taken to morgue.

G. Porter, RN

EVALUATION

REASSESSMENT

At the time of death it is common for family members or close friends to experience shock and disbelief. Much of the information concerning the circumstances of the death are likely to seem unreal and unclear. It is becoming a practice to invite the recently bereaved to return to the hospital 6 weeks after the death of a loved one. Gathering again with agency personnel provides the opportunity to ask questions and verbally express stifled emotions. To resolve grief, it is necessary to experience the "pain." Nurses and other personnel can use this time to assess the progress of persons in resolving their grief. It may be helpful to refer persons who may be experiencing dysfunctional grieving to mental health counselors.

EXPECTED OUTCOMES

The body appears clean and peaceful.
The client's family or friends are provided the opportunity to express their grief by whatever manner they deem appropriate.
The family views, touches, holds, or speaks to the body of the deceased.
The nurse shares a description of the client's care, treatment, and responses before death.

UNEXPECTED OUTCOMES

The family cannot be notified before the body is delivered to the morgue or mortuary.

MODIFICATIONS IN SELECTED SITUATIONS

GENERAL VARIATIONS

The client may have indicated a desire to donate organs for transplant. The next of kin must give consent. An organ procurement team must be notified as soon as possible following death.
The physician may request permission for an autopsy. A coroner has the right to order that an autopsy be performed if the death involved a crime, was of a suspicious nature, or occurred without any prior medical attention.
It is the practice in some facilities to leave the body in the same condition as when the death occurred until the family has arrived. The presence of treatment equipment provides evidence that the care of the client was not neglected.
Some morticians allow family members to bathe, dress, and coif the hair of the deceased.

AGE-RELATED
VARIATIONS

Photograph a stillborn infant or one who dies soon after birth. The photograph may be attached to the medical record. Copies can be offered to the parents.

Wrap an infant in a cotton receiving blanket, and give the parents the opportunity to hold and examine the child.

HOME-HEALTH
VARIATIONS

Family members who are involved in the care of a terminally ill client have a headstart on resolving their grief. Anticipating and dealing with the potential loss before it occurs aids in earlier emotional healing. Many families are assisted by hospice nurses and volunteers.

Follow the agency's policy and state laws regarding who may legally pronounce the client dead and release the body from the home setting.

RELATED TEACHING

Explain that it is healthy to talk with children and other family members about death. Open communication prepares persons to deal with death as a realistic part of life.

Encourage young children to draw a picture of their dead relative. This helps others to know the child's impression of death and provides a basis for communication.

Inform persons that it is healthy to consider the circumstances of their own death. Those who feel philosophically inclined may be referred to organ donation societies or associations that provide living will documents.

(Performance checklist next page)

PERFORMANCE CHECKLIST

When performing postmortem care, the learner:

C   A   U

[ ]   [ ]   [ ]   Assesses signs that confirm death.

[ ]   [ ]   [ ]   Notifies the physician and funeral home.

[ ]   [ ]   [ ]   Gathers equipment.

[ ]   [ ]   [ ]   Dons clean gloves.

[ ]   [ ]   [ ]   Removes equipment and soiled articles from the body.

[ ]   [ ]   [ ]   Removes valuables from the body or records an inventory of what has been left in place.

[ ]   [ ]   [ ]   Cleanses the body.

[ ]   [ ]   [ ]   Places the body in supine position.

[ ]   [ ]   [ ]   Closes the eyelids.

[ ]   [ ]   [ ]   Inserts clean dentures.

[ ]   [ ]   [ ]   Straightens the bed linen.

[ ]   [ ]   [ ]   Disposes of soiled equipment.

[ ]   [ ]   [ ]   Washes hands.

[ ]   [ ]   [ ]   Meets the family and accompanies them to the location of the body.

[ ]   [ ]   [ ]   Returns personal belongings and valuables to a responsible family member.

[ ]   [ ]   [ ]   Covers the body in a shroud or with a clean sheet.

[ ]   [ ]   [ ]   Attaches an identification tag.

[ ]   [ ]   [ ]   Transfers the body to a stretcher.

[ ]   [ ]   [ ]   Requests that an assistant hold an empty elevator.

[ ]   [ ]   [ ]   Closes the doors to other rooms while wheeling the body down the hall.

[ ]   [ ]   [ ]   Uses the "express" mode to transport the body in the elevator preventing it from opening for passengers.

[ ]   [ ]   [ ]   Delivers the body to the appropriate area in the morgue.

[ ]   [ ]   [ ]   Completes charting.

[ ]   [ ]   [ ]   Strips the room and informs the housekeeping department concerning terminal cleaning.

Outcome: [ ] Pass   [ ] Fail

C = competent; A = acceptable; U = unsatisfactory

Comments: _____
_____
_____

_____   _____
       Student's Signature   **Date**

_____   _____
     Instructor's Signature   **Date**

RELATED LITERATURE

**PROCEDURE I-1
ADMITTING A CLIENT
TO A HEALTH-CARE
FACILITY**

Anderson R, Zimbra C: Same day surgery; coordinating the admission process. Nursing Management 17(12):23–25, December 1987

Dombrowski B: Knock, knock. American Journal of Nursing 87(2):205–206, February 1987

Galton R: Documentation: the key to reimbursement. Caring 6(2):68–70, February 1987

Gato L, Braun K: Nursing home without walls . . . long-term care services in homes. Journal of Gerontological Nursing 13(1):6–9, January 1987

Gull HJ: The chronically ill patient's adaptation to hospitalization. Nursing Clinics of North America 22(3):593–601, September 1987

Omdahl DJ: Preventing home care denials. American Journal of Nursing 87(8):1031–1033, August 1987

Robinson PD, Roe H, Boys LJ: The focus of hospitals on family care. Health Values 11(2): 19–24, March–April 1987

Worley B: Pre-admission testing and teaching: more satisfaction at less cost . . . surgical admissions. Nursing Management 17(12):32–33, December 1986

**PROCEDURE I-2
ASSESSING BODY
TEMPERATURE**

Boylan A, Brown P: Student observations: temperature. Nursing Times 81:36–40, April 17–23, 1985

Closs J: Oral temperature measurement. Nursing Times 83(1):36–39, January 7–13, 1987

Criss E, Lee S, Joyce SM: Prehospital temperature monitoring. Emergency Medical Services 16(4):38–39, 56, May 1987

Haddock B: Vincent P, Merrow D: Axillary and rectal temperatures of full term neonates: are they different? Neonatal Network 5(4):43, February 1987

Lipsy JG: It's vital! Journal of Practical Nursing 36:26–29, June 1986

Samples JF, VanCott ML, Long C: Circadian rhythms: basis for screening for fever . . . routine temperature assessments in hospitals. Nursing Research 34:377–379, November–December 1985

Siebenaler ME: Taking a baby's temperature: is it common knowledge? American Journal of Maternal Child Nursing 10:71, January–February 1985

Stone S: A new concept in routine vital signs measurement. Nursing Management 17:28–29, February 1986

The pitfalls of armpit temperatures. Emergency Medicine 16:76, December 15, 1984

**PROCEDURE I-3
ASSESSING RADIAL
PULSE**

Birdsall C: How do you interpret pulses? American Journal of Nursing 85(7):785–786, July 1985

Davis-Rollans C, Cunningham SG: Physiologic responses of coronary care patients to selected music. Heart & Lung: Journal of Critical Care 16(4):370–378, July 1987

Schneider JR: Effects of caffeine on heart rate, blood pressure, myocardial oxygen consumption, and cardiac rhythm in acute myocardial infarction patients. Heart & Lung: Journal of Critical Care 16(2):167–174, March 1987

Toney J: Monitoring cardiac rhythms *part 1.* AD Nurse 2(2):8–16, March–April 1987

Toney J: Monitoring cardiac rhythms *part 2.* AD Nurse 2(3):20–30, May–June 1987

Valle BK, Lemberg L: Cardiac manifestations of AIDS *part 2*. Heart & Lung: Journal of Critical Care 16(5):584–589, September 1987

Van Parys E: Assessing the failing state of the heart. Nursing 87 17(2):42–50, February 1987

Yacone LA: Cardiac assessment: what to do, how to do it. RN Magazine 50(5):42–48, May 1987

**PROCEDURE I-4
ASSESSING THE
APICAL PULSE RATE**

Joffe M: Pediatric digoxin administration. Dimensions of Critical Care Nursing 6(3):136–146, May–June 1987

Lewis VC: Monitoring the patient with acute myocardial infarction. Nursing Clinics of North America 22(1):15–32, March 1987

**PROCEDURE I-5
ASSESSING THE
RESPIRATORY RATE**

Bloch H: Phenomena of respiration: historical overview to the twentieth century. Heart & Lung: Journal of Critical Care 16(4):419–423, July 1987

Boylan A, Brown P: Student observations: respiration. Nursing Times 81:35–38, March 13–19, 1985

Hahn K: Slow-teaching the C.O.P.D. patient. Nursing 87 17(4):34–42, April 1987

Hopp LJ, Williams M: Ineffective breathing pattern related to decreased lung expansion. Nursing Clinics of North America 22(1):193–206, March 1987

Lareau S, Larson JL: Ineffective breathing pattern related to airflow limitation. Nursing Clinics of North America 22(1):179–191, March 1987

Larson JL, Kim MJ: Ineffective breathing pattern related to respiratory muscle fatigue. Nursing Clinics of North America 22(1):207–223, March 1987

Mlynczak BA: Ventilation disorders: a guide you can use with an air of confidence. Nursing 85 15(4):12–13, April 1985

Richman E: Dyspnea: sorting out the diagnosis. Patient Care 21(9):22–25, 28–29, 32–36, May 15, 1987

Riley HD, Selbst SM, Wingert WA: Pediatric respiratory distress. Patient Care 21(3):84–89, 93–94, 96–99+, August 15, 1987

Spearing C, Cornell DJ: Incentive spirometry: inspiring your patient to breathe deeply. Nursing 87 17(9):50–51, September 1987

**PROCEDURE I-6
ASSESSING BLOOD
PRESSURE**

Blood-pressure monitors . . . suitable for home use. Consumers Report 52(5):314, 316–319, May 1987

Boylan A, Brown P: Student observations: more than "doing the obs" . . . the significance of pulse and blood pressure measurement. Nursing Times 81:24–25, February 13–19, 1985

Boylan A, Brown P: Student observations: the pulse and blood pressure. Nursing Times 81: 26–29, February 13–19, 1985

Bruya MA, Demand JK: Nursing decision making in critical care: traditional versus invasive blood pressure monitoring. Nursing Administration Quarterly 9:19–31, Summer 1985

Clochesy JM: Systemic blood pressure in various lateral recumbent positions: a pilot study. Heart & Lung: Journal of Critical Care 15(6):593–594, November 1986

Downey KK, Davis BK: Measuring blood pressure via sensory detection. Journal of Gerontological Nursing 12(11):8–11, November 1986

Draper P: Not a job for juniors. Nursing Times 83(10):58–59, 62, March 11–17, 1987

Mancia G: Parati G, Pomidossi G: Alerting reaction and rise in blood pressure during measurement by physician and nurse. Hypertension 9(2):209–215, February 1987

Rottenberg RF: Sphygmomanometers: which to choose? Patient Care 21(8):67–70, 75–76, April 30, 1987

The 1984 Report of the Joint National Committee on Detection, Evaluation, and Treatment of High Blood Pressure. Nursing Practice 10:9–10, 13–14, 19–20, July 1985

Weber EM, Dipette DJ: Clinical use of 24-hour ambulatory blood pressure monitoring. Nurse Practitioner: American Journal of Primary Health Care 12(2):30, 34, 36–37, February 1987

**PROCEDURE I-7
HANDWASHING**

Bartzokas CA, Corkhill JE, Makin T: Evaluation of the skin disinfecting activity and cumulative effect of chlorhexidine and triclosan handwash preparations on hands artificially contaminated with *Serratia marcescens*. Infection Control 8(4):163–167, April 1987

Burnie JP: *Candida* and hands. Journal of Hospital Infection 8(1):1–4, July 1986

Donowitz LG: Handwashing technique in a pediatric intensive care unit. American Journal of Diseases of Children 14(6):683–686, June 1987

Gidley C: Now, wash your hands! Nursing Times 83(29):40–42, July 22–28, 1987

Larson E: Change and infection control. American Journal of Infection Control 8(1):1–4, July 1986

Recommended practices: Basic aseptic technique. Journal of American Operating Room Nurses 45(3):784, 786, 788–789, March 1987

Reybrouck G: Handwashing and hand disinfection. Journal of Hospital Infection 8(1):5–23, July 1986

PROCEDURE I-8 CLEANING AND DISINFECTING A GLASS THERMOMETER

Greene VW: Reuse of disposable medical devices: historical and current aspects. Infection Control 7(10):508–513, October 1986

Guidelines for the reuse of disposable medical devices. Infection Control 7(11):562, November 1986

Mayhall CG: Commentary: types of disposable medical devices reused in hospitals. Infection Control 7(10):491–494, October 1986

Radany MH, Perry S, McCallum: Is it safe to reuse disposables? American Journal of Nursing 87(1):35–38, January 1987

PROCEDURE I-9 CARING FOR A CLIENT ON ISOLATION PRECAUTIONS

DeCrosta T: Nosocomial infections: every patient is a target. Fighting the problem *part 2*. Nursing Life 7(1):48–53, January–February 1987

Fuchs PC: Will the real infection rate please stand? Infection Control 8(6):235–236, June 1987

Jackson MM, Lynch P, McPherson DC: Why not treat all body substances as infectious? American Journal of Nursing 87(9):1137–1139, September 1987

Maki DG, Alvarado C, Hassemer C: Double-bagging of items from isolation rooms is unnecessary as an infection control measure: a comparative study of surface contamination with single and double bagging. Infection Control 7(11):535–537, November 1986

McCreight LM: Stepping up to new challenges in public health nursing. Nursing & Health Care 204(2):69–72, February 1987

Webster M: Are A.I.D.S. patients getting good nursing care? Nursing Life 7(1):48–53, January–February 1987

PROCEDURE I-10 MAKING AN UNOCCUPIED BED

Pottle B: When the sheets were changed . . . absorbent sheets designed for incontinent patients. Nursing Times 82(48):64, 66, November 26–December 2, 1986

Webster O, Cowan M, Allen J: Dirty linen . . . microbiological contamination of duvets and associated linen. Nursing Times 82(44):36–37, October 29–November 4, 1986

PROCEDURE I-11 MAKING AN OCCUPIED BED

Bolyard EA, Townsend TR, Horan T: Airborne contamination associated with in-use air-fluidized beds: a descriptive study. American Journal of Infection Control 15(2):75–78, April 1987

Cuzzell JZ, Willey T: Pressure relief perennials . . . mattress choices. American Journal of Nursing 87(9):1157–1160, September 1987

Howie D: Trial of a mattress for the chronically disabled . . . the Aqua Dome water-filled mattress. Nursing Times 83(16):51–52, April 22–28, 1987

Wirtz BJ: Effects of air and water mattresses on thermoregulation. Journal of Gerontological Nursing 13(5):13–17, May 1987

PROCEDURE I-12 DONNING AND REMOVING STERILE GLOVES

Guenther SH, Hendley JO, Wenzel RP: Gram-negative bacilli as nontransient flora on the hands of hospital personnel. Journal of Clinical Microbiology 25(3):488–490, March 1987

Mooney BR, Armington LC: Infection control: how to prevent nosocomial infections. RN magazine 50(9):20–23, September 1987

**PROCEDURE I-13
DONNING A
STERILE GOWN**

Campbell VG: Covergowns for newborn infection control? American Journal of Maternal Child Nursing 12(1):54, January–February 1987

Haberstich N: Preventing of infection during major construction and renovation of a large hospital. American Journal of Infection Control 15(2):36A–38A, April 1987

Mailhot CB, Slezak LG, Copp G: Cover gowns: researching their effectiveness. Journal of American Operating Room Nurses 46(3):482–483, 1987

Nurses, surgeons, anesthesiologists meet to discuss operating room problems. Journal of American Operating Room Nurses 46(1):19, 22–24, 26+, July 1987

Recommended practices: basic aseptic technique. Journal of American Operating Room Nurses 45(3):784, 786, 788–789, March 1987

**PROCEDURE I-14
CARING FOR
THE CLIENT
PREOPERATIVELY**

Bonner M: Can my friend go with me . . . to help prepare young children for their treatment. Nursing Times 82(40):75–76, October 1–7, 1986

Dean AF: The aging surgical patient: historical overview, implications, and nursing care . . . in the ambulatory setting. Perioperative Nursing Quarterly 3(1):1–7, March 1987

Harvey CK: Future trends in perioperative nursing and technology. Nursing Administration Quarterly 11(2):38–41, Winter 1987

Hathaway D, Powell S: An evaluation of a perioperative assessment program. Perioperative Nursing Quarterly 3(2):56–64, June 1987

Ivey DF: Local anesthesia: implications for the perioperative nurse . . . home study program. Journal of American Operating Room Nurses 45(3):682–689, 692–695, March 1987

Kuhn PL: Standing ovation . . . patient needing emergency surgery. Today's OR Nurse 9(2):43–44, February 1987

Recommended practices: documentation of perioperative nursing care. Journal of American Operating Room Nurses 45(3):777, 779, 781, March 1987

Tupa DF: Alleviating the fears of pediatric patients. Today's OR Nurse 9(7):33–36, July 1987

**PROCEDURE I-15
CARING FOR
THE CLIENT
POSTOPERATIVELY
UPON RETURNING
TO THE ROOM**

Aimino PA: Perioperative nursing documentation: developing the record and using nursing care plans. American Journal of Operating Room Nurses 46(1):73, 76–81, 84–86, July 1987

Gray-Vickrey M: Color them special: a sensible guide to caring for elderly patients. Nursing 87 17(5):59–62, May 1987

Hernandez CMG: Surgery and diabetes: minimizing the risks. American Journal of Nursing 87(6):788–792, June 1987

Hylka SC: Discharge instructions for ambulatory patients. Perioperative Nursing Quarterly 2(3):61–64, September 1986

Latz PA, Wyble SJ: Elderly patients: perioperative nursing implications. Journal of American Operating Room Nurses 46(2):238, 240, 242+, August 1987

Mortensen M, McCullin C: Discharge score for surgical outpatients. American Journal of Nursing 86(12):1347–1349, December 1986

Wachenstein J: Care of the elderly surgical patient. Geriatric Nursing: American Journal of Care for the Aging 7(4):12–14, April 1987

**PROCEDURE I-16
STARTING AN
INTRAVENOUS
INFUSION**

Ballenger MJ: IV insight. Emergency 18(11):51, 54, November 1986

Coggin S: Evaluating and selecting IV equipment. Journal of the National Intravenous Therapy Association 10(1):49–51, January–February 1987

Knox LS: Implantable venous access devices. Critical Care Nurse 7(1):70–73, January–February 1987

Krakowska G: Practice versus procedure . . . setting up intravenous infusions. Nursing Times 82(49):64, 66, 69, December 3–9, 1986

Lampinen J: Once you hit the streets . . . starting an IV line in the field. Emergency 18(11):51, 54, November 1986

Larkin M: Home I.V. therapy. Journal of the National Intravenous Therapy Association 10(3):171, May–June 1987

Schulmeister L: A comparison of skin preparation procedures for accessing implanted ports. Journal of the National Intravenous Therapy Association 10(1):45–47, January–February 1987

Taylor JP, Taylor JE: Vascular access devices . . . uses and aftercare. Journal of Emergency Nursing 13(3):160–167, May–June 1987

Wildblood RA, Strezo PL: The how-to's of home IV therapy. Pediatric Nursing 13(1):42–46, 68, January–February 1987

PROCEDURE I-17 REGULATING IV FLOW RATE

Byers RH, Burke EH, Overstake SK: Reading the amount of fluid in polyvinyl chloride IV bags. Journal of the National Intravenous Therapy Association 9(6):484–487, November–December 1986

Cheung P: Learning your tables . . . dosage rates for intravenous infusion. Nursing Times 82(42):40–41, October 15–21, 1986

Green LM: Calculation of dosage and infusion rate in continuous intravenous medications. Journal of Post Anesthesia Nursing 2(3):210–215, August 1987

Nortridge JA: Calculating I.V. medications with confidence. Nursing 87 17(9):55–57, September 1987

Rimar JM: Guidelines for the intravenous administration of medications used in pediatrics. American Journal of Maternal Child Nursing 12(5):322–340, September–October 1987

PROCEDURE I-18 MONITORING AN IV SITE AND INFUSION

Millam DA, Warren J: Irrigating peripheral IVs: sensible or foolhardy? Nursing Life 6(6): 24–25, November–December 1986

Mylotte JM, McDermott C: *Staphlococcus aureus* bacteremia caused by infected intravenous catheters. American Journal of Infection Control 15(1):1–6, February 1987

Persons CB: Preventing infection from intravascular devices. Nursing 87 17(4):75, 77–78, April 1987

Vlahov D, Cervino KN, Standiford HC: Accuracy of patient recall for date of peripheral intravenous catheter insertion. American Journal of Infection Control 15(1):26–28, February 1987

PROCEDURE I-19 CHANGING AN IV DRESSING

Crow S: Infection risks in IV therapy. Journal of the National Intravenous Therapy Association 10(2):101–105, March–April 1987

Messner RL, Gorse GJ: Nursing management of peripheral intravenous sites. Focus on Critical Care 14(2):25–33, April 1987

PROCEDURE I-20 CHANGING IV SOLUTION AND TUBING

Beckwith N: Fundamentals of fluid resuscitation. Nursing Life 7(3):49–56, May–June 1987

Bryan CS: CDC says . . . the case of IV tubing replacement. Infection Control 8(6):255–256, June 1987

Infusion: do you have the correct solution? The Nurse, The Patient & The Law pp 10–11, June 1987

Snydman DR, Donnelly-Reidy M, Perry LK: Intravenous tubing containing burettes can be safely changed at 72 hour intervals. Infection Control 8(3):113–116, March 1987

Weinstein S: Intravenous filters. Infection Control 8(5):220–221, May 1987

PROCEDURE I-21 ADMINISTERING A BLOOD TRANSFUSION

Bello K: Managing an autologous blood program. Medical Laboratory Observer 19(2):63–66, February 1987

Landier WC, Barrell ML, Styffe EJ: How to administer blood components to children. American Journal of Maternal Child Nursing 12(3):178–184, May–June 1987

Mahoney DH Jr: Blood component therapy: redefined guidelines for pediatric patients. Consultant 27(1):130–132, 135–136, 138+ January 1987

McVan BW: How we give blood transfusions at home. RN Magazine 50(8):79–80, 82, August 1987

Peck NL: Action STAT! Blood transfusion reaction. Nursing 87 17(1):33, January 1987

Phillips A: Are blood transfusions really safe? Nursing 87 17(6):63–64, June 1987

Taylor BN, Wagner PL, Kraus CL: Development of a standard for time-effective patient assessment during blood transfusion. Journal of Nursing Quality Assurance 1(2):66–71, February 1987

Webster A: Banking your own blood. Nursing Times 83(31):36–37, August 5–11, 1987

PROCEDURE I-22
REMOVING
MEDICATION FROM
AN AMPULE

McGovern K: 10 steps for preventing medication errors. Nursing 86 16(12):36–39, December 1986

Rousseau P: Pharmacologic alterations in the elderly: special considerations. Hospital Formulary 22(6):543–545, June 1987

Scherer P: New drugs: hands-on experience *part 2*. American Journal of Nursing 87(5):644–649, May 1987

Wong DL: The significance of dead space in syringes. American Journal of Nursing 82(8): 1237, August 1982

PROCEDURE I-23
REMOVING
MEDICATION FROM
A VIAL

Henrietta G: Lab tests you can't overlook *part 2*. Nursing 87 17(3):48–51, March 1987

Wieland D, Cohen M, Wieman R: Medication errors: what happens afterward? Nursing Life 7(2):41–42, March–April 1987

Young FE: Experimental drugs for the desperately ill. FDA Consumer 21(5):2–3, June 1987

PROCEDURE I-24
MIXING INSULINS
IN ONE SYRINGE

Hernandez CMG: Surgery and diabetes: minimizing the risks. American Journal of Nursing 87(6):788–792, June 1987

Insulin edema. Nurses' Drug Alert 11(3):19, March 1987

Kronsick A: Diabetes treatment update: switching to biosynthetic human insulin. Consultant 27(7):78–80, 83, 86–87, July 1987

Skelly AH, VanSon AR: Insulin allergy in clinical practice. Nurse Practitioner: American Journal of Primary Health Care 12(4):14, 16–18, 23, April 1987

Thatcher G: Insulin injections: the case against random rotation. American Journal of Nursing 85(8):690–692, August 1985

PROCEDURE I-25
ADMINISTERING AN
INTRADERMAL
INJECTION

Huber K, Sumner W II: Recapping the accidental needlestick problem. American Journal of Infection Control 15(3):127–130, June 1987

Krasinski K, LaCouture R, Holzman RS: Effects of changing needle disposal systems on needle puncture injuries. Infection Control 8(2):59–62, February 1987

Ribner BS, Landry MN, Gholson GL: Impact of a rigid, puncture resistant container system on needlestick injuries. Infection Control 8(2):63–66, February 1987

PROCEDURE I-26
ADMINISTERING A
SUBCUTANEOUS
INJECTION

Rogers AG: The use of continuous subcutaneous infusion of narcotics in chronic cancer pain. Journal of Pain Symptom Management 2(3):167–168, Summer 1987

Wisinger MM: Hypodermoclysis in the elderly: a means of hydration. Nursing Homes 33(3): 32–33, May–June 1987

PROCEDURE I-27
ADMINISTERING AN
INTRAMUSCULAR
INJECTION

Creagh T: Just a little job. Nursing Times 82(49):50, December 3–9, 1986

deCarteret JC: Needle-stick injuries: an occupational health hazard for nurses. Journal of American Association of Occupational Health Nurses 35(3):119–123, March 1987

Farley HF, Joyce N, Long B: Will that IM needle reach the muscle? American Journal of Nursing 86(12):1327, 1331, December 1986

Feldman HR: Practice may make perfect but research makes a difference . . . IM injection in the ventrogluteal site. Nursing 87 17(3):46–47, March 1987

Megel ME, Wilken MK, Volcek MK: Nursing students' performance: administering injections in laboratory and clinical area. Journal of Nursing Education 26(7):288–293, September 1987

PROCEDURE I-28
PERFORMING A Z-
TRACK INJECTION

Chaplin G, Shull H, Welk P: How safe is the air-bubble technique for IM injections? Nursing 85 15(9):559, September 1985

Shepherd MJ, Swearingen PL: Z-track injections. American Journal of Nursing 84(6):746–747, June 1984

PROCEDURE I-29
ADDING MEDICATIONS
TO AN IV SOLUTION
CONTAINER

Cohen MR: Improperly mixed IV additives. Nursing 87 17(5):16, May 1987

Darbyshire P: Handle with care . . . cytotoxic drugs. Nursing Times 82(40):37–38, October 1–7, 1987

Kasmer RJ, Hoisington LM, Jukniewicz S: Home parenteral antibiotic therapy: drug preparation and administration considerations. Home Healthcare Nurse 5(1):19–23, 26–29, January–February 1987

**PROCEDURE I-30
ADDING A BOLUS IV
MEDICATION TO AN
EXISTING IV**

Ballenger MJ: IV insight. Emergency 19(8):19–22, August 1987

Cohen MR: Improperly mixed IV additives. Nursing 87 17(5):16, May 1987

Kosloski G, Nelson LA: Guideline for monitoring parameters for commonly used intravenous drugs in the ED setting. Journal of Emergency Nursing 12(6):382–386, November–December 1986

Lunn JK, Wilson A: Retrograde medication administration: a predictable and simple system for pediatric drug delivery. Focus on Critical Care 13(6):59–63, December 1986

Nahata MC: Drug delivery by retrograde intravenous infusions: implications for therapy. Journal of the National Intravenous Therapy Association 10(3):198–201, May–June 1987

Weinstein SM: Biohazards of working with antineoplastics. Home Healthcare Nurse 5(1): 30–34, January–February 1987

**PROCEDURE I-31
ADMINISTERING
MEDICATIONS BY
IV PIGGYBACK**

Cohen MR: Improperly mixed IV additives. Nursing 87 17(5):16, May 1987

Kasmer RJ, Hisington LM, Yukniewicz S: Home parenteral antibiotic therapy: drug preparation and administration considerations. Home Healthcare Nurse 5(1):19–23, 26–29, January–February 1987

Wachs T, Watkins S, Hickman RO: No more pokes: a review of parenteral access devices. Nutritional Support Services 7(6):12–13, 18, June 1987

Zenk KE: Special delivery: administering IV antibiotics to children. Nursing 86 16(12): 50–52, December 1986

**PROCEDURE I-32
ADMINISTERING
MEDICATIONS BY A
VOLUME-CONTROL SET**

Axton SE, Fugate T: A protocol for pediatric IV meds. American Journal of Nursing 87(7): 943A–944B, 946D, July 1987

Beckwith N: Fundamentals of fluid resuscitation. Nursing Life 7(3):49–56, May–June 1987

Demling RH: The principles of fluid resuscitation after thermal injury. Emergency Care Quarterly 1(3):12–21, November 1985

Fulks KD, Kenady DE: Techniques of chemotherapy delivery for cancer patients. Hospital Formulary 22(3):248–254, March 1987

Gaysek SJ: I.V. team management of patient-controlled analgesia. Journal of National Intravenous Therapy Association 10(2):142–144, March–April 1987

**PROCEDURE I-33
INTRODUCING DRUGS
THROUGH A HEPARIN
LOCK AND
PERFORMING A
HEPARIN FLUSH**

Cyganski JM, Donahue JM, Heaton JS: The case for the heparin flush. American Journal of Nursing 87(6):796–797, June 1987

Dunn DL, Lenihan SF: The case for the saline flush. American Journal of Nursing 87(6):798–799, June 1987

**PROCEDURE I-34
TRANSFERRING A
CLIENT**

Champion HI: Helicopter triage. Emergency Care Quarterly 2(3):13–21, November 1986

Craney JM, Greck DL: Easing the transfer from CCU. American Journal of Nursing 87(5): 618–619, May 1987

Deckshot P, Feige KE: Centralizing patient transfer promotes efficiency and control. Health Progress 68(1):104, 106, 108, January–February 1987

Desmond M: Preparing patients for travel. Patient Care 21(11):217–219, 223–224, 227+, June 15, 1987

Hart MA, Haynes D, Schwaitzberg SD: Air transport of the pediatric patient. Emergency Care Quarterly 3(1):21–26, May 1987

Schactman M: Transfer stress in patients after myocardial infarction. Focus on Critical Care 14(2):34–37, April 1987

**PROCEDURE I-35
DISCHARGING A
CLIENT FROM A
HEALTH-CARE AGENCY**

Barnett D: Opening the communication line . . . from hospital to community nursing staff. Nursing Times 82(45):56, 58, November 5–11, 1986

Jupp M, Sims S: Discharge planning: going home. Nursing Times 82(40):40–42, October 1–7, 1986

McCarthy S: Discharge planning for medically fragile children. Caring 5(11):38–39, 41, November 1986

Mortensen M, McMullin C: Discharge score for surgical outpatients. American Journal of Nursing 86(12):1347–1349, December 1986

Pellegrino RM, Buckley TF: Hospital to home: a partnership in discharge planning. Caring 6(5):10–13, May 1987

**PROCEDURE I-36
PERFORMING
POSTMORTEM CARE**

Bosse LA: A disaster with few survivors . . . no one was "ready" for morgue duty. American Journal of Nursing 87(7):918–919, July 1987

Bourne ED: What a dying patient needs from you. RN Magazine 50(6):65–66, June 1987

Burson N: Sharing death. Nursing 87 17(4):58–59, April 1987

Coolican MB: Katie's legacy . . . organ donation helped this family begin to resolve the tragedy. American Journal of Nursing 87(4):483–485, April 1987

Neuberger J: Never say die? . . . nurse's clinical judgement can be used to report a death. Nursing Times 83(29):22, July 22–28, 1987

Ward CL: Issues on death and dying. Imprint 34(6):93, 96, April–May 1987

II   *Procedures pertaining to the senses*

II-1 *Administering an eye irrigation*

The receptors for the sense of sight are located in the eye. The cornea is the transparent portion that lies on the surface of the eye over the iris, or colored part of the eye. The conjunctiva lines the inner lids and covers the sclera to the margin of the cornea. The cornea can be extremely painful if injured. Therefore, instillations to the eye are generally applied to the conjunctiva.

PURPOSES OF PROCEDURE

An eye irrigation may be done to:

1. Instill medicated solutions to treat conditions affecting the conjunctiva or cornea.
2. Cleanse dried secretions from the lid margins.
3. Remove chemicals or solid substances that may irritate or traumatize the surface of the eye.
4. Reduce swelling or discomfort by the application of a warm or cool solution.

ASSESSMENTS

OBJECTIVE DATA

- Observe the client for excessive tearing or rubbing the eyes.
- Examine the lids for the outward or inward growth of eyelashes, any redness or swelling of the hair follicles, or flakiness around the eyelid margin.
- Determine the client's ability or resistance to opening the eyelids. Note if the client can close the margins of his eyelids together.
- Inspect the conjunctiva for color, moistness and characteristics of secretions, and swelling.
- Look at the tissue beneath the orbit for puffiness which may be associated with contactant allergies.
- Ask if the client has recently changed the use or type of eye makeup or facial soap.
- Ask any client who wears contact lenses to describe the hygiene practices used to cleanse them.

SUBJECTIVE DATA

- Ask the client to indicate if he has or is experiencing blurred vision, itching, burning, or sensitivity to light.
- Inquire concerning any prior history of allergies; recent upper respiratory infections; exposure to smoke, dust, or wind.

RELEVANT NURSING DIAGNOSES

The client who receives an eye irrigation may have nursing diagnoses, such as:

- *Altered Comfort*
- *Potential for Infection*
- *Potential for Injury*
- *Sensory Perceptual Alteration: Visual*
- *Self-Care Deficit*

PLANNING

ESTABLISHING PRIORITIES

When the eyes are splashed with a chemical, the nurse must immediately flush the surface of the eye with tap water for at least 30 minutes. Other eye problems are less of an emergency and can be treated with periodic irrigations throughout the day. The client is more apt to experience an increase of thick secretions and particulate matter in the morning. During sleep, the closed eyelids tend to trap and accumulate exudate.

SETTING GOALS

• The eye(s) will be flushed safely and comfortably with solution.

PREPARATION OF
EQUIPMENT

The following equipment will be needed:

Sterile irrigating solution (warmed to 37°C or 98.6°F)
Sterile irrigation set (sterile container and irrigating or bulb syringe
Cotton balls
Emesis basin or irrigation basin
Disposable gloves (optional)
Waterproof pad
Towel

Technique for administering an eye irrigation

ACTION	RATIONALE
1. Explain the procedure to the client.	An explanation facilitates cooperation and provides reassurance for the client.
2. Assemble equipment.	Gathering equipment provides for an organized approach to the task.
3. Wash your hands.	Handwashing deters the spread of microorganisms.
4. Have the client sit or lie with his head tilted toward the side of the affected eye.	Gravity will aid the flow of solution away from the unaffected eye and from the inner canthus of the affected eye toward the outer canthus.
5. Don disposable gloves if an infection is present. Clean the lids and the lashes with a cotton ball moistened with normal saline or the solution ordered for the irrigation. Wipe from the inner canthus, as shown in Fig. II-1-1, to the outer canthus. Discard each cotton ball after one wipe.	Materials lodged on the lids or in the lashes may be washed into the eye. This cleansing motion protects the nasolacrimal duct and the other eye from the transmission of substances containing pathogens.

Figure II-1-1 When an eye irrigation has been ordered, the client may either sit up, as this client is doing, or lie in bed. The nurse is cleaning the lids and lashes from the inner to the outer canthus. A disposable, absorbent pad has been draped over the client's chest and shoulder area to protect the linen and clothing from dampness.

6. Place the curved basin at the cheek on the side of the affected eye to receive the irrigating solution. If the client is sitting up, ask him to support the basin.	Gravity will aid the flow of solution. A properly positioned basin will collect the solution and limit the saturation of the linen and the client's clothing.
7. Expose the lower conjunctival sac and hold the upper lid open with your nondominant hand.	The solution is directed onto the lower conjunctival sac because the cornea is very sensitive and easily injured. This also prevents reflex blinking.
8. Hold the irrigator about 2.5 cm (1 inch) from the eye. Direct the flow of the solution from the inner canthus to the outer canthus along the conjunctival sac, as shown in Fig. II-1-2.	This distance minimizes the risk of injury to the cornea. By directing the solution toward the outer canthus, the nurse helps prevent the spread of contamination to the lacrimal sac, the lacrimal duct, and the nose.

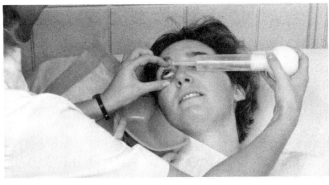

Figure II-1-2 The client tilts her head to the side and holds an emesis basin under her cheek to collect the draining irrigation solution. This position helps carry debris and organisms away from the lacrimal duct.

9. Irrigate until the solution is clear or all has been used. Use only sufficient gentle force to remove secretions from the conjunctiva. Avoid touching any part of the eye with the irrigating tip.

Directing the solution with force may cause discomfort. Touching the eye may cause pain or injury.

10. Have the client close his eye periodically during the procedure.

Movement of the eye when the lids are closed helps to move the solution over the surface of the eye. It also aids removal of secretions from areas other than where the irrigation is being instilled.

11. Dry the area after the irrigation with cotton balls or a gauze sponge. Offer a towel to the client if his face and neck have become wet.

Leaving the skin moist after an irrigation is uncomfortable for the client.

12. Wash your hands.

Handwashing deters the spread of microorganisms.

13. Chart the irrigation, the appearance of the eye, characteristics of the drainage, and the client's response.

Charting provides accurate documentation on the implementation of treatment and the client's progress.

SAMPLE DOCUMENTATION

Date	Time	Nurse's note
1/09	1730	Conjunctiva is red. Dried granular secretions noted on both lid margins. Accumulation of yellow drainage in the inner canthus of OD. OD irrigated with 200 mL of sterile, warmed normal saline. Secretions and drainage removed. States, "Oh, that feels so much better." *C. Morris, RN*

EVALUATION

REASSESSMENT

Note the appearance, sensation, and characteristics of the eyes, eyelids, and periorbital areas after the irrigation. Reassessment should also be conducted before each subsequent irrigation.

EXPECTED OUTCOMES

The eyes are irrigated without injury.
The client will indicate that his eyes feel soothed during and after the irrigation.

UNEXPECTED OUTCOMES

The client describes an increase in pain or burning within the eyes.
The client's eyelids are so swollen that they cannot be separated.

MODIFICATIONS IN SELECTED SITUATIONS

GENERAL VARIATIONS

Protect an unaffected eye during an irrigation with transparent plastic wrap secured with tape if there is a possibility that contaminated droplets may splash into the healthy eye.
A large volume of irrigating solution can be administered by directing sterile intravenous solution through IV tubing.

AGE-RELATED
VARIATIONS

Secure a child's arms to his chest with a towel or bath blanket before beginning an irrigation. This will help keep the child from quick movements which may result in injury from the irrigating syringe.

HOME-HEALTH
VARIATIONS

Ensure the availability of supplies and equipment for an irrigation.

Check that expiration dates on the solution and sterile equipment have not become outdated and that the wrappers are intact.

If eye irrigations are ordered to treat an infectious process, observe the eyes of family members and caregivers. Cross contamination may occur.

RELATED TEACHING

Tell the client to avoid home remedies. If eye symptoms are such that a person considers self-treatment, it is serious enough to be evaluated by medical professionals.

Use a topical anesthetic for ocular pain only as directed. Excessive use can delay healing and may result in a rebound of more intense pain.

Do not share a common face cloth or towel in order to avoid transmitting pathogens among infected and noninfected persons.

Most eye infections are transmitted from contaminated hands. Use paper towels or warm air dryers in lieu of rolled cloth towels in public restrooms.

PERFORMANCE CHECKLIST

When performing an eye irrigation, the learner:

C   *A*   *U*

[ ]   [ ]   [ ]   Reads the written medical order.

[ ]   [ ]   [ ]   Assesses the client.

[ ]   [ ]   [ ]   Gathers the equipment.

[ ]   [ ]   [ ]   Washes hands.

[ ]   [ ]   [ ]   Warms the solution.

[ ]   [ ]   [ ]   Explains the procedure to the client.

[ ]   [ ]   [ ]   Provides for privacy during the procedure.

[ ]   [ ]   [ ]   Positions the client either sitting or lying.

[ ]   [ ]   [ ]   Turns the head toward the affected eye.

[ ]   [ ]   [ ]   Protects the client's clothing and bed linen.

[ ]   [ ]   [ ]   Dons gloves, if appropriate.

[ ]   [ ]   [ ]   Cleans the eye from the inner to outer canthus using one cotton ball for each wipe.

[ ]   [ ]   [ ]   Places an emesis basin below and to the outer side of the eye.

[ ]   [ ]   [ ]   Separates the eyelids.

[ ]   [ ]   [ ]   Fills the syringe with irrigating solution.

[ ]   [ ]   [ ]   Without touching the eye, directs the solution so it flows from the nasal side to the temporal side of the eye.

[ ]   [ ]   [ ]   Intermittently stops the irrigation and instructs the client to close his eyes and move them about beneath the lids.

[ ]   [ ]   [ ]   Removes gloves, if used.

[ ]   [ ]   [ ]   Dries the client's face and assists him to a position of comfort.

[ ]   [ ]   [ ]   Changes wet linen.

[ ]   [ ]   [ ]   Empties the drained solution into the client's toilet or a hopper in the soiled utility room.

[ ]   [ ]   [ ]   Disposes of used equipment and wet linen in appropriate areas.

[ ]   [ ]   [ ]   Washes hands.

[ ]   [ ]   [ ]   Records pertinent assessments, the specifics of the procedure, and the response of the client.

Outcome: [ ] Pass   [ ] Fail

C = competent; A = acceptable; U = unsatisfactory

Comments: _____

_____

_____

_____   _____
Student's Signature   Date

_____   _____
Instructor's Signature   Date

II-2 *Instilling ophthalmic medications*

Eye medications can be applied topically either in the form of an ointment or as eye drops. To avoid injuring the cornea, direct application of a solution or ointment is not recommended. Instead, medications are instilled into the lower conjunctival sac. Although the eye is never free of microorganisms, the tip of the applicator is never touched and is capped after each use to ensure its sterility.

PURPOSES OF PROCEDURE

Ophthalmic medications are administered to:

1. Dilate or constrict the pupil.
2. Treat or prevent inflammation or infection of the surface structures of the eye.
3. Anesthetize the cornea.
4. Apply a fluorescent stain to assist in detecting embedded foreign objects, corneal lacerations, or ulcers.

ASSESSMENTS

OBJECTIVE DATA

- Read the physician's written order to determine the name of the medication, the amount of medication, the percent of concentration, the schedule for administration, and the eye(s) in which the medication is to be administered.
- Consult a pharmacology reference for pertinent information about the drug if it is not known.
- Compare the information on the drug label with the written medical order and its transcription on the medication card or Kardex.
- Examine the periorbital area, the eyelids, and the eyelashes. Note color, presence of swelling, and drainage characteristics.
- Use a penlight and note the response of the pupils to light.
- Inspect the eye for contact lenses which may be on the cornea or displaced in other areas of the eye.
- Observe the client for tearing, rubbing of the eyes, or an effort to keep his eyes closed.

SUBJECTIVE DATA

- Ask the client to indicate if he is experiencing blurred vision, itching, burning, or sensitivity to light.
- Obtain the client's history of prior eye diseases or conditions; hygiene about the face; recent exposure to allergens, irritants, or others with similar eye symptoms.
- Inquire as to the use, type, and care of contact lenses.

RELEVANT NURSING DIAGNOSES

The client who receives eye medication is likely to have nursing diagnoses, such as:

- *Altered Comfort*
- *Potential for Infection*
- *Potential for Injury*
- *Sensory Perceptual Alteration: Visual*
- *Self-Care Deficit*

PLANNING

ESTABLISHING
PRIORITIES

Whenever it is suspected that a foreign body remains in the eye, examination by a physician should be initiated immediately. The client is likely experiencing so much pain and discomfort that inspection will be limited until a topical anesthetic has been instilled. Patch both eyes to limit ocular movement until the client is examined.

Preoperative eye medications are administered as often as 5 minutes apart. Their application must be closely coordinated with the time of surgery to achieve the optimum action of the drug at the time of the operative procedure. Scheduled medications can be administered within a half-hour range of the routine established by the clinical facility.

SETTING GOALS

- The client will receive the correct medication, the prescribed concentration and amount, by the correct route and time.
- Medication will be instilled without injury or systemic absorption.

PREPARATION OF
EQUIPMENT

The nurse will need the following:

Medication card or Kardex
Paper tissues
Sterile cotton balls or 2 × 2 gauze squares
Medication
Eyedropper (omit if the applicator is attached to the medication container)

Technique for administering eye medications

ACTION	RATIONALE
1. Check and compare the written medical order with the medication card or Kardex.	Checking ensures that the nurse implements the physician's order as it has been written.
2. Compare the information on the medication label with what has been delivered from the pharmacy.	Checking a drug label at least three times ensures that the correct medication is administered.
3. Warm the medication by rolling the container between the hands for a minute or two if the medication storage area is unusually cool.	Instilling cold medication into the eye is startling and uncomfortable.
4. Wash your hands.	Handwashing deters the spread of microorganisms.
5. Identify the client by checking the wristband.	Proper identification ensures that the correct client receives the medication.
6. Darken the room if the light causes discomfort.	Clients may experience photosensitivity when the eyes are exposed to bright light.
7. Position the client in a supine or sitting position. Have the client tilt his head back and slightly to the side into which the medication will be instilled.	Positioning prevents the loss of medication down the cheek or into the nasolacrimal duct.
8. Clean the lids and lashes prior to instilling medication. Use one cotton ball for each wipe.	Cleansing avoids introducing organisms or debris into the eye.
9. Move the cotton ball from the inner canthus to the outer canthus.	Wiping removes secretions, residual medications from previous instillations, and organisms away from the nasolacrimal duct.
10. Instruct the client to look toward the ceiling.	Looking upward tends to prevent stimulating the blink reflex and loss of medication.
11. Place the thumb or two fingers of the nondominant hand below the margin of the eyelashes under the lower lid and exert pressure downward over the bony prominence of the cheek, as the nurse in Fig. II-2-1 is doing.	Lowering the lid creates a pouch in the conjunctiva. This small area is a convenient pocket into which the medication may be placed.

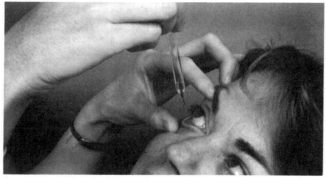

Figure II-2-1 The client tilts her head back and looks upward while receiving eyedrops.

12. Move the medication container from below the line of vision or from the side of the eye.

Keeping the moving object out of the client's direct vision prevents the client from becoming startled and moving away.

13. Hold the tip of the container steady above the conjunctival sac without actually touching the eye itself.

The tip of the container may injure the cornea if it touches the eye. Touching the eye also contaminates the applicator.

14. Deposit the prescribed number of drops into the center of the conjunctival sac or squeeze a ribbon of ointment from the inner to the outer canthus.

Placing the drug in this manner facilitates its distribution throughout the eye when the traction is released from the client's face.

15. Instruct the client to close his eyelids gently and move the eye after the medication has been instilled.

Gentle closing prevents blinking the medication onto the cheek. Moving the eye within the orbit delivers the drug over the surface of the eye.

16. Apply gentle pressure over the opening to the nasolacrimal duct.

Nasal occlusion prevents systemic absorption of the medication through the mucous membrane of the nose.

17. Provide the client with a clean tissue to catch any medication or tears that may escape from the eye and roll down the face.

A clean tissue absorbs liquids that may be irritating or uncomfortable.

18. Instruct the client to avoid rubbing the eyes after the medication has been instilled.

Pressure may cause additional irritation of the eye.

SAMPLE DOCUMENTATION

Date	Time	Nurse's note
6/10	1035	States, "I feel like there's glass in my R eye." Eyes tearing. Resists opening lid for exam. Ophthaine 0.5% gtt. i instilled into OD. Fluoroscein strip wet with sterile normal saline and applied to lower conjunctival lid of OD.

P. Zook, RN

EVALUATION

REASSESSMENT

When medications are administered to alter the size and response of the pupils, the nurse can use a penlight generally 20 minutes later to detect the effect. Fluorescein dye may be seen to fluoresce a green color almost immediately in the presence of cobalt blue light.

Cultures may be taken to determine the response of the client with an eye infection to topical antibiotic medications. The nurse could use clinical signs such as reduced redness and swelling, diminished drainage, and relief of subjective symptoms like burning as evidence of a therapeutic response. Observations should be documented before each subsequent administration of any medication.

EXPECTED OUTCOMES	The prescribed number of drops are instilled within the lower conjunctival sac without injury or discomfort.
	The client responds therapeutically to the medication.

UNEXPECTED OUTCOMES

The tip of the applicator touches the cornea.

The client blinks or squeezes his eye shut forcing the medication onto the surface of the cheek.

Medication drains into the nasolacrimal duct and is systemically absorbed.

The client experiences an untoward reaction to the medication.

MODIFICATIONS IN SELECTED SITUATIONS

GENERAL VARIATIONS

Rather than squeeze a ribbon of ointment along the lower lid margin, the lower lid can be everted and the ointment applied within the conjunctival sac.

Eye medications may be administered with an eyedropper. However, for aseptic reasons, any excess medication within the eyedropper should be discarded and not returned to the original solution.

Hold an eyedropper with the tip lateral to the eye so that if contact is made, it will be less damaging than if the point of the tip directly touches the cornea.

Eye medications are now supplied in small volume, generally from 2 ml to 15 ml. This avoids extended use of liquid drugs that may deteriorate or grow pathogens over time.

HOME-HEALTH VARIATIONS

It is the nurse's responsibility to determine that the client's physician is aware that the client is using a prescribed medication from another physician or is self-medicating.

Tactfully decline from assisting the client with the instillation of ophthalmic medications without a physician's order.

For persons who have difficulty in self-administration of eye drops, devices that rest the container of medication on the bridge of the nose or the bony orbit above the eye help to position the applicator tip without corneal injury.

RELATED TEACHING

The client should be instructed to bring sunglasses if the eyes will be dilated during a routine eye examination. Most mydriatic drugs, which interfere with the eye's ability to constrict in the presence of bright light, do not wear off for several hours.

Emphasize that safety goggles or glasses should always be worn around machinery where there is the potential for injury from projectiles.

Children should be taught to never point toys that shoot objects near the face.

Teach clients to place removed tips from eye medication upside down on a clean surface. Remind them to replace the caps as soon as possible after each use of the medication.

Instruct clients to use a clean tissue to catch medication or tears that may roll down the cheek. However, clients should be told not to use the same tissue for other purposes.

(Performance checklist next page)

PERFORMANCE CHECKLIST

When administering eye medications, the learner:

C	A	U	
[ ]	[ ]	[ ]	Checks the written medical order.
[ ]	[ ]	[ ]	Compares the written prescription with the drug transcription on the medication card or Kardex.
[ ]	[ ]	[ ]	Researches information on an unfamiliar drug.
[ ]	[ ]	[ ]	Reads the drug label at least three times.
[ ]	[ ]	[ ]	Washes hands.
[ ]	[ ]	[ ]	Checks the identification of the client.
[ ]	[ ]	[ ]	Explains the procedure to the client.
[ ]	[ ]	[ ]	Assesses the status of the eye(s).
[ ]	[ ]	[ ]	Positions the client appropriately.
[ ]	[ ]	[ ]	Cleanses the lids if necessary from the inner to the outer canthus.
[ ]	[ ]	[ ]	Gently pulls the lower lid down.
[ ]	[ ]	[ ]	Instructs the client to look upward.
[ ]	[ ]	[ ]	Brings the applicator upward from below the line of vision.
[ ]	[ ]	[ ]	Instills the prescribed amount of medication within the conjuctival sac without touching any structures of the eye OR Squeezes a ribbon of ointment across the lower lid margin.
[ ]	[ ]	[ ]	Allows the lid to gently close.
[ ]	[ ]	[ ]	Applies light pressure to the inner canthus.
[ ]	[ ]	[ ]	Wipes away any excess medication.
[ ]	[ ]	[ ]	Returns the medication container to its stocked location.
[ ]	[ ]	[ ]	Washes hands.
[ ]	[ ]	[ ]	Records the medication administration.
[ ]	[ ]	[ ]	Returns to reassess the client in a reasonable period of time.

Outcome: [ ] Pass   [ ] Fail

C = competent; A = acceptable; U = unsatisfactory

Comments: _____

_____

_____

_____   _____

Student's Signature   Date

_____   _____

Instructor's Signature   Date

II-3 *Inserting a hearing aid*

Some clients may require the use of a hearing aid. This device does not replace the complete quality of hearing but can be an adequate substitute. Hearing aids are designed to be worn in many different ways. Most people choose one that is constructed within the frames of eyeglasses, worn behind the ear as shown in Fig. II-3-1, or placed completely within the ear. The nurse should understand the basics for inserting and caring for a hearing aid when the client is unable to function independently.

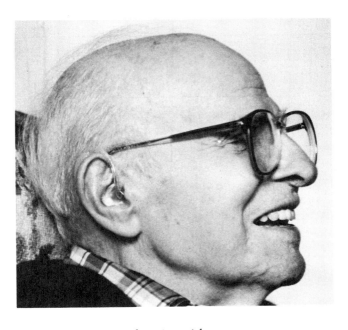

Figure II-3-1 A postauricular hearing aid is one of the most popular types in use because it is so compact and less noticeable than others.

PURPOSES OF PROCEDURE

The nurse inserts a hearing aid to:

1. Improve the client's ability to understand verbal communication.
2. Ensure proper and comfortable fit within the ear.
3. Avoid loud or shrill sounds coming from the hearing aid.

ASSESSMENT

OBJECTIVE DATA

- Inspect the auditory canal for the accumulation of cerumen.
- Determine the manufacturer's design for insertion.
- Locate the on and off control mechanism.
- Determine the length of time that the current battery has been in use.
- Examine the outer surface of the hearing aid for body oil, dust, and cerumen.

SUBJECTIVE DATA

- Ask the client to describe the quality of the sound he hears as compared to prior periods when using his hearing aid.
- Question the client about his level of comfort in relation to the position of the hearing aid.

RELEVANT NURSING DIAGNOSES

The client who is wearing a hearing aid with a low battery or whose hearing is not adequately improved with its use, may have nursing diagnoses, such as:

- *Impaired Communication*
- *Sensory Perceptual Alteration: Auditory*
- *Impaired Social Interaction*

PLANNING

ESTABLISHING PRIORITIES

Most persons remove a hearing aid when retiring for the night. The nurse should assist the client with its insertion as soon as possible in the morning so that the quality of verbal communication and interaction can be maintained. The ability to hear sound is also a factor in preventing injury.

SETTING GOALS

- The client's ability to hear and communicate will be improved by wearing the hearing aid.
- The client will experience comfort wearing the hearing aid.

PREPARATION OF EQUIPMENT

The nurse will need:

Hearing aid
Soap, water, and clean face cloth (optional)

Technique for inserting a hearing aid

ACTION	RATIONALE
1. Inspect the external ear, and clean it if cerumen has accumulated.	Accumulation of cerumen can interfere with sound conduction.
2. Test the ability of the hearing aid to function by turning it on.	A functioning hearing aid produces a continuous whistle when not being worn.
3. Make sure the hearing aid is turned off and the volume is turned down before insertion.	A sudden loud sound can be annoying and uncomfortable for a client who uses a hearing aid.
4. Insert the hearing aid in the external ear. The earlobe should be pulled downward while pressing the hearing aid inward.	The hearing aid is custom molded to fit snugly so that sound does not escape. Feedback, a loud, shrill noise, occurs when a hearing aid is not positioned correctly.
5. Turn the hearing aid on and gradually increase the volume.	The client can best judge the volume that is most comfortable.
6. Turn the hearing aid off when it is removed from the ear.	The life of the hearing aid battery can be prolonged by turning the device off during periods of nonuse.

SAMPLE DOCUMENTATION

Date	Time	Nurse's note
2/02	0630	Hearing aid inserted into R ear and turned on. States, "The sounds aren't as loud or clear as they were last week." Battery changed. No improvement noted. Maintenance representative from hearing and speech clinic notified.
		D. Potts, RN

EVALUATION

REASSESSMENT

The hearing aid should be inspected closely when a battery is replaced. A cracked case can cause variations in the sound level. Hearing tests may be scheduled periodically with an audiologist when the hearing aid seems to function mechanically but the client does not seem to hear as well as in the past.

EXPECTED OUTCOMES

The client understands words spoken in conversational tone and responds appropriately.

The hearing aid does not produce feedback or whistling noises.

UNEXPECTED OUTCOMES

The hearing aid is dropped or damaged.

The hearing aid does not produce a shrill sound when being turned on and tested.

The hearing aid does not improve the client's ability to hear.

The hearing aid emits annoying noises.

Areas of the client's ear become sore or red from pressure or movement of the hearing aid within the ear.

MODIFICATIONS IN SELECTED SITUATIONS

GENERAL VARIATIONS

Hearing aids molded to fit entirely within the ear come with a special tool for removing cerumen that may accumulate.

Persons with unilateral hearing loss may hear better with the hearing aid placed in the ear with normal hearing. When a hearing aid is placed in the ear with diminished hearing, there is a tendency to turn up the volume. The unequal perception of sound tends to distort the ability to hear and discriminate sounds.

AGE-RELATED VARIATIONS

Some children with profound deafness wear hearing aids in both ears to intensify the amplification of sound.

HOME-HEALTH VARIATIONS

Telephones can be specially adapted for the hearing impaired. Clients can be referred to their local telephone company or electronics specialists. A flashing light is one method for calling the deaf person's attention to an incoming call. Dogs are also being trained to attract the response of a deaf person to a door bell or ring of the telephone.

Computers are now available that can convert a phone message into words on a monitor when special phone devices are not adequate for improving hearing.

RELATED TEACHING

Persons should be told that the ability to hear decreases with age.

Hygiene for healthy ears includes washing, rinsing, and drying. No objects should be placed into the ear canal. Cerumen is pushed to the outer areas of the auditory canal as it continues to be manufactured.

Tell a person with a hearing aid to avoid exposing the hearing aid to extreme heat, water, cleaning chemicals, or hair spray.

Explain that shrill noises can be caused by a hearing aid that fits loosely within the ear, volume that is not adequately adjusted, or defective electronic components.

Remind clients to replace batteries on a routine basis.

(Performance checklist next page)

PERFORMANCE CHECKLIST

When inserting a hearing aid, the learner:

C	A	U	
[ ]	[ ]	[ ]	Assesses the cleanliness of the ear.
[ ]	[ ]	[ ]	Cleans the ear with a corner of a washcloth, soap, and water.
[ ]	[ ]	[ ]	Inspects the hearing aid.
[ ]	[ ]	[ ]	Checks that the hearing aid is turned off and the volume is turned down.
[ ]	[ ]	[ ]	Cleans the hearing aid with a soft, dry cloth or paper tissue.
[ ]	[ ]	[ ]	Pulls the earlobe down while inserting the hearing aid.
[ ]	[ ]	[ ]	Adjusts the volume within the client's range of comfort.

Outcome: [ ] Pass   [ ] Fail

C = competent; A = acceptable; U = unsatisfactory

Comments: _____

_____

_____

_____   _____
Student's Signature   Date

_____   _____
Instructor's Signature   Date

II-4 *Administering an ear irrigation*

The external auditory canal of the ear is a channel that normally accumulates cerumen. Ordinary hygiene practices, such as bathing, tend to keep this area clean.

An irrigation may be required in certain circumstances. Occasionally some persons produce excessive amounts of cerumen or that which is produced lacks sufficient water content to retain its moist, fluid characteristics. Foreign objects may be accidentally lodged in the auditory canal. Respiratory infections or allergies can cause swelling and drainage within the middle ear. If the volume of drainage creates enough pressure, the tympanic membrane can rupture, depositing the accumulated drainage within the ear canal.

PURPOSES OF PROCEDURE

An ear irrigation is performed to:

1. Remove material that blocks the external ear canal.
2. Cleanse the ear canal of drainage.
3. Reduce local discomfort.

ASSESSMENT

OBJECTIVE DATA

- Note any elevation in body temperature indicating an infection may be present.
- Inspect the external auditory canal of both ears with a penlight. Note the color, presence, and characteristics of drainage or foreign body. Observe the client's response to manipulation of the ears.
- Examine the tympanic membrane using an otoscope, as shown in Fig. II-4-1.

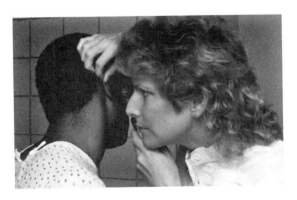

Figure II-4-1 The nurse uses an otoscope to examine the deeper areas of the auditory canal and the tympanic membrane.

- Palpate the neck area below the ear for the presence of enlarged lymph nodes.
- Note the client's general ability to hear while sitting approximately 3 feet to the side of the client.
- Perform the Weber test by striking a tuning fork and placing it in the middle of the upper forehead. Request that the client indicate the location of the sound. Hearing the sound louder in one or the other ear indicates diminished hearing.

SUBJECTIVE DATA

- Inquire as to the presence of pain, vertigo, nausea associated with position changes, or other abnormalities with hearing, such as tinnitus, or itching.
- Palpate the bony mastoid area behind each pinna for signs of tenderness, and note if the client experiences pain or tenderness.

- Ask the client to describe his history of ear, sinus, or respiratory infections; ear, tonsil adenoid surgery; recent head trauma; and airplane travel.
- Determine if the client has ever been told that either ear drum was perforated.
- Question a parent as to whether an irritable child has repeatedly tugged at one or both ears recently.

RELEVANT NURSING DIAGNOSES

The client who requires an ear irrigation is likely to have one or several of the following nursing diagnoses:

- *Potential for Injury*
- *Altered Comfort*
- *Impaired Communication*
- *Altered Health Maintenance: Ear Hygiene*
- *Sensory Perceptual Alteration: Auditory*
- *Impaired Social Interaction*

PLANNING

ESTABLISHING PRIORITIES

The presence of a live insect within the auditory canal requires immediate attention because the noise and possible stinging affect physical comfort and safety. A live insect may be killed by instilling room temperature mineral oil into the external ear prior to the irrigation. The oil will smother the insect.

When the client has a chronic problem, such as impacted cerumen or drainage, the ear irrigation can be scheduled after other nursing interventions that meet the client's needs for nutrition, hydration, elimination, and so on. If the ear drum is perforated, delay irrigation and inform the physician.

SETTING GOALS

- The client's external ear will be clean and free of irritating substances.
- The client will experience comfort from the instillation of warm solution.
- The client will describe a reduction or elimination of disturbing symptoms, such as itching or tinnitus.
- The client's hearing will improve.

PREPARATION OF EQUIPMENT

Locate and obtain the following:

Prescribed warmed (37°C or 98.6°F) irrigating solution
Irrigation set consisting of a container and syringe
Emesis basin
Cotton-tipped applicators
Cotton balls
Waterproof pad

Technique for administering an ear irrigation

ACTION	RATIONALE
1. Explain the procedure to the client.	An explanation facilitates cooperation and provides reassurance for the client.
2. Assemble equipment. Protect the client and bed linens with a waterproof pad.	Gathering necessary supplies provides for an organized approach to the task.
3. Wash your hands.	Handwashing deters the spread of microorganisms.
4. Have the client lie down or sit up with his head tilted toward the side of the affected ear.	Gravity causes the irrigating solution to flow from the ear to the basin.
5. Clean the pinna and the meatus of the auditory canal as necessary with an applicator or soft cloth dipped in normal saline or the irrigating solution.	Materials lodged on the pinna and at the meatus can be moved into the ear if not removed.
6. Have the client support a basin under his ear to receive the draining solution.	Assistance from the client frees the nurse to position the ear and use the irrigation equipment.

7. Fill the syringe with solution. If an irrigating container is used, allow air to escape from the tubing.

Air forced into the ear canal is noisy and therefore unpleasant for the client.

8. Straighten the auditory canal, as shown in Fig. II-4-2, by pulling the pinna up and back for an adult, or down and back for a child under 3 years of age.

Straightening the ear canal allows the solution to reach all areas of the canal easily.

9. Direct a steady, slow stream of solution against the roof of the auditory canal, as illustrated in Fig. II-4-3, using only sufficient force to remove secretions. Do not occlude the auditory canal with the irrigating nozzle. Allow the solution to flow out unimpeded.

Solution directed at the roof of the canal aids in preventing injury to the tympanic membrane. Continuous in-and-out flow of the irrigating solution helps to prevent pressure in the canal.

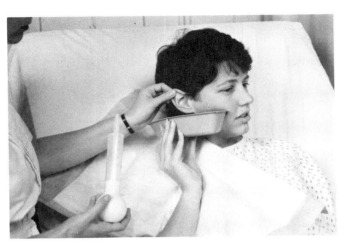

Figure II-4-2 The irrigation will be more effective if the adult client's ear canal is straightened by pulling the pinna up and back.

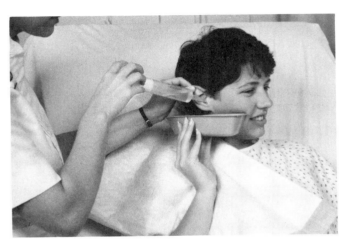

Figure II-4-3 The nurse instills a steady stream of warm irrigating solution at the roof of the auditory canal. Excess force or pressure can cause discomfort or injury to the client.

10. When the irrigation is completed, place a cotton ball loosely in the auditory meatus and have the client lie on the side of the affected ear on a towel or an absorbent pad.

A cotton ball absorbs fluid, and gravity allows the remaining solution in the canal to escape from the ear.

11. Chart the irrigation, appearance of the drainage, and the client's response.

Charting provides accurate documentation of the client's care.

12. Return in 10 minutes to 15 minutes to remove the cotton ball and assess the drainage.

Drainage or pain may indicate injury to the tympanic membrane.

SAMPLE DOCUMENTATION

Date	Time	Nurse's note
1/06	1130	250 ml of warm normal saline instilled into L ear. Solution returned clear with sm. flecks of cerumen. Cotton inserted loosely into L ear. Instructed to lie on L side for 15 minutes.
	1145	Cotton removed. Hardened cerumen approx. size of pea evident. Stated, "Gosh, everything sounds so much louder now."

S. York, RN

EVALUATION

REASSESSMENT

The nurse should repeat the objective inspection of the external auditory canal and assessment of hearing after performing the procedures. Observe the characteristics of the drained solution. Inspect the drainage present on the removed cotton. Determine the client's perception of pain relief or other subjective symptoms.

EXPECTED OUTCOMES

The solution instills and drains freely.
The client remains comfortable throughout the procedure.
Dried blood, secretions such as hardened cerumen, or foreign substances such as an insect or small object, accompany the draining fluid.
The ear canal is patent and intact.
Pain, itching, and discomfort are relieved.
Hearing improves.

UNEXPECTED OUTCOMES

The client experiences an increased level of discomfort upon instillation of the solution.
Foreign or irritating substances remain within the ear.

MODIFICATIONS IN SELECTED SITUATIONS

GENERAL VARIATIONS

Observe the client for nausea and dizziness when the fluid is instilled. The warmth of the solution should be carefully maintained to near body temperature. Avoid unnecessary motion or activity. Assist with ambulation. Reschedule the irrigation for early or late in the day when the client has an empty stomach.
When drainage appears clear and head trauma is suspected, test the fluid with a chemstrip for the presence of glucose. If glucose is present, the drainage may be cerebrospinal fluid. This is an indication for postponing the irrigation until the client can be examined by a physician.

AGE-RELATED VARIATIONS

Use alternate methods for straightening the ear canal when the client is a child, as described within the procedure.

HOME-HEALTH VARIATIONS

Occasionally clients request that the nurse carry out certain treatments, like an ear irrigation. Explain that this type of procedure requires a physician's order.

RELATED TEACHING

Emphasize that objects, such as hairpins, should not be used for removing material from the ear.
Explain that regular use of the tip of a face cloth moistened with soap and water may be used to cleanse the external ear canal of accumulating cerumen.
Inform the client that over-the-counter (OTC) liquid drugs are available to restore and maintain cerumen in a softened state.
Caution a client with ear problems that sneezing should never be stifled by holding the nose. The pressure created can rupture the tympanic membrane.

PERFORMANCE CHECKLIST

When the ear is irrigated, the learner:

C	A	U	
[ ]	[ ]	[ ]	Assesses the appearance of the external canal and eardrum.
[ ]	[ ]	[ ]	Confirms the medical order for an ear irrigation.
[ ]	[ ]	[ ]	Washes hands and assembles the equipment.
[ ]	[ ]	[ ]	Reads and double checks the label of the prescribed solution at least three times.
[ ]	[ ]	[ ]	Warms the solution to the desired temperature.
[ ]	[ ]	[ ]	Identifies the client by checking the identification bracelet and asking the client his name.
[ ]	[ ]	[ ]	Explains the procedure to the client.
[ ]	[ ]	[ ]	Provides privacy.
[ ]	[ ]	[ ]	Positions the client with the affected ear up.
[ ]	[ ]	[ ]	Swabs excess secretions from the ear.
[ ]	[ ]	[ ]	Drapes the client and protects the bed and clothing from becoming wet.
[ ]	[ ]	[ ]	Expels air from the tubing or nozzle of the syringe.
[ ]	[ ]	[ ]	Straightens the ear canal appropriately.
[ ]	[ ]	[ ]	Allows a small volume of solution to flow against the roof of the auditory canal, while observing the client's response.
[ ]	[ ]	[ ]	Instills a slow but steady stream of solution.
[ ]	[ ]	[ ]	Applies cotton loosely within the ear.
[ ]	[ ]	[ ]	Repositions the client on his affected ear.
[ ]	[ ]	[ ]	Changes any wet linen or bed clothing.
[ ]	[ ]	[ ]	Removes soiled equipment.
[ ]	[ ]	[ ]	Washes hands.
[ ]	[ ]	[ ]	Returns and reassesses the condition of the client after 15 minutes to 30 minutes.
[ ]	[ ]	[ ]	Documents the procedure and the client's response.
[ ]	[ ]	[ ]	Provides health teaching to promote an increased level of future wellness.

Outcome: [ ] **Pass**   [ ] **Fail**

C = competent; A = acceptable; U = unsatisfactory

Comments: _____
_____
_____

_____   _____
Student's Signature   Date

_____   _____
Instructor's Signature   Date

II-5 *Instilling ear medication*

When identifying the structures of the ear, it is common to refer to three divisional compartments: the external ear, the middle ear, and the internal ear. Drugs are instilled into the auditory canal of the external ear. The external ear extends to the tympanic membrane, or eardrum, which is intact in most persons.

PURPOSES OF PROCEDURE

Medications are instilled within the ear to:

1. Soften dried cerumen.
2. Reduce inflammation.
3. Treat an infection.
4. Relieve discomfort.

ASSESSMENT

OBJECTIVE DATA

- Read the written medical order.
- Compare the information transcribed to the medication card or Kardex with the order written by the physician.
- Review pertinent drug information in a pharmacology reference, if unfamiliar with the drug.
- Read the drug label at least three times; note especially the drug name, strength of the medication, and that it is intended for otic use.
- Inspect the external ear for color, swelling, characteristics of secretions, appearance of objects, and integrity of the eardrum if it can be seen.
- Palpate the structures in the areas adjacent to the ears.
- Test the client's ability to hear as described in Procedure II-4, Administering an Ear Irrigation.

SUBJECTIVE DATA

- Ask the client to indicate if he is experiencing local itching, pain, dizziness, nausea, diminished hearing, or annoying noises.
- Inquire if the client has had a prior or recent history of upper respiratory infection, allergies, ear infections, or airplane travel.
- Note the response of an infant or child when the ear is manipulated during the physical assessment.

RELEVANT NURSING DIAGNOSES

The client receiving ear medication may have nursing diagnoses, such as:

- *Altered Comfort*
- *Potential for Injury*
- *Impaired Communication*
- *Impaired Social Interaction*
- *Sensory Perceptual Alteration: Auditory*

PLANNING

ESTABLISHING PRIORITIES

Medications may be administered within $\frac{1}{2}$ hour of their scheduled time. The nurse may want to plan the client's care to permit the medication to dwell in the ear at least 5 minutes to 15 minutes. Changing the head or body position immediately after instillation may reduce the contact of the medication within the deeper areas of the ear canal.

SETTING GOALS
- The client will receive the correct type and amount of medication within the indicated ear(s) at the prescribed time.
- The client will experience a therapeutic response to the prescribed medication.

PREPARATION OF EQUIPMENT

The following will be needed when instilling ear medication:

Medication card or Kardex
Medication container
Dispensing dropper
Paper tissue
Cotton ball (optional)

Technique for instilling ear medication

ACTION	RATIONALE
1. Check the written medical order.	Checking ensures accuracy in administering medication according to the physician's directions.
2. Compare the transcribed information on the medication card or Kardex.	Comparing information prevents errors in administration due to misinterpretation.
3. Review drug information.	The nurse should know the action, purpose, usual dose, side-effects, contraindications, and nursing implications of all medications the client receives.
4. Wash your hands.	Handwashing deters the spread of microorganisms.
5. Gather equipment.	Organization is a component of time management.
6. Read the label on the medication container at least three times.	Repetitive reading ensures that the delivered medication matches the physician's prescription.
7. Identify the client by reading the wristband.	Proper identification prevents administering the drug to the wrong client.
8. Provide privacy.	The client should be protected from being seen by others during his care and treatment.
9. Assess the client.	Gathering data assists in identifying problems and provides a baseline for comparing future observations.
10. Warm the medication to room temperature.	Cold medication instilled within the ear can cause discomfort, dizziness, and nausea in some clients.
11. Clean the outer ear with a cotton ball or paper tissue.	The ear may contain dried secretions or drainage that may interfere with the absorption of the drug.
12. Fill the dispenser with sufficient medication.	Most ear medications are instilled using a medication dropper.
13. Position the client on his side with the ear into which the instillation is to be made uppermost.	This prevents loss of any medication from the effect of gravity.
14. Straighten the ear canal. Gently pull the ear upward and backward for an adult or downward and backward for a child under 3 years of age.	Straightening helps the medication reach the lowest area of the ear canal and become distributed over all the surfaces.
15. Hold the dropper with the tip above the ear canal, as shown in Fig. II-5-1.	Touching the ear would contaminate the dispenser and may cause the client to move and become injured.
16. Instill the prescribed number of drops to fall on the side of the ear canal.	When drops fall directly on the eardrum they may cause an unpleasant sensation.
17. Encourage the client to remain in this position for 5 minutes.	Maintaining the position allows time for medication to flow to the lowest area of the ear canal, avoiding the possibility of excessive loss from the ear.

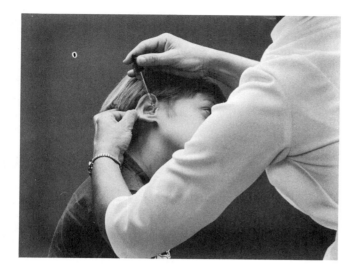

Figure II-5–1 To instill eardrops in a child, the nurse pulls the ear downward and backward and drops the solution along the side of the ear canal.

18. Massage the cartilage below the opening to the ear canal.

Massage promotes the movement and distribution of the drug.

19. Insert cotton loosely within the ear if it is likely the medication will drain out after the client assumes an upright position.

The cotton wick will trap the medication within the ear canal and prevent its loss after instillation.

20. Wait 5 minutes before instilling medication into the opposite ear.

Sufficient time must be allowed to prevent immediate loss of medication from its site of instillation.

SAMPLE DOCUMENTATION

Date	Time	Nurse's note
3/19	0900	Dark brown cerumen at the base of R ear canal. Unable to visualize the eardrum. Mineral oil gtts. vi administered into R ear. Cotton loosely packed within external ear following instillation.

G. Peabody, RN

EVALUATION

REASSESSMENT

The nurse should remove and inspect the cotton 30 minutes after the instillation. Reinspect the ear daily. Determine the client's perception of his comfort and hearing ability after the medication has been administered. Note changes in the type and amount of drainage.

EXPECTED OUTCOMES

The client's ear canal is free of drainage.
The client's ear is not tender or painful.
The client's hearing in his affected ear is comparable to that in the unaffected ear.

UNEXPECTED OUTCOMES

The client's ear canal shows evidence of retained or reaccumulated secretions.
The client continues to experience pain or pressure in the area of the ear.
The client's hearing is diminished in the affected ear.

MODIFICATIONS IN SELECTED SITUATIONS

GENERAL VARIATIONS

Write explanations for the client who has a severe hearing loss. Speak clearly while facing the client who has a moderate hearing deficit.
Ear medication should be administered cautiously to a person whose tympanic membrane is not intact.
Any excess medication drawn into the dispenser should be discarded rather than returned to the original container.

AGE-RELATED VARIATIONS

Straighten the auditory canal of a child under 3 years of age by pulling the cartilaginous portion of the pinna up and back. For children over 3 years of age, pull the ear downward and backward.

For an infant or an irrational or restless client, protect the dropper with a piece of soft tubing to help prevent injury to the ear.

When a child is uncooperative, restrain the arms and head from moving during the time when the medication is administered.

HOME-HEALTH VARIATIONS

It is not uncommon for clients in the home setting to self-medicate. If a client is using over-the-counter ear medication, determine the reason for the practice. Notify the physician of the condition and the medication the client is using.

Tactfully decline from assisting the client with the administration of a treatment or medication without a physician's order.

RELATED TEACHING

Emphasize that objects, such as hairpins, should not be used for removing material from the ear.

Explain that the tip of a face cloth moistened with soap and water may be used to cleanse the external ear canal of accumulating cerumen.

Inform the client that over-the-counter (OTC) liquid drugs are available to restore and maintain cerumen in a softened state.

Caution a client with ear problems that sneezing should never be stifled by holding the nose. The pressure created can rupture the tympanic membrane.

Explain that chewing gum or swallowing during an airplane's take-off and landing can equalize the pressure in the middle ear and promote comfort and hearing. An infant can be offered a bottle or pacifier as a substitute.

Diving and underwater swimming should be avoided by persons with a perforated eardrum unless an ear plug has been inserted in the affected ear(s).

(Performance checklist next page)

PERFORMANCE CHECKLIST

When instilling ear medications, the learner:

C	A	U	
[ ]	[ ]	[ ]	Checks and compares the written order with the transcribed information and drug label.
[ ]	[ ]	[ ]	Washes hands and assembles equipment.
[ ]	[ ]	[ ]	Checks the client's identification.
[ ]	[ ]	[ ]	Provides privacy.
[ ]	[ ]	[ ]	Assesses appropriate objective signs and subjective symptoms.
[ ]	[ ]	[ ]	Cleans the client's external ear, if necessary.
[ ]	[ ]	[ ]	Positions the client in order to have access to the affected ear.
[ ]	[ ]	[ ]	Straightens the ear canal using the appropriate technique for the client's age.
[ ]	[ ]	[ ]	Instills the prescribed number of drops.
[ ]	[ ]	[ ]	Presses on the tragus a few times after instilling the medication.
[ ]	[ ]	[ ]	Packs cotton loosely within the ear.
[ ]	[ ]	[ ]	Instructs the client to maintain his position for at least 5 minutes.
[ ]	[ ]	[ ]	Removes equipment and disposes or returns it to the appropriate location after carrying out the medication order.
[ ]	[ ]	[ ]	Washes hands.
[ ]	[ ]	[ ]	Charts the drug administration.
[ ]	[ ]	[ ]	Returns in 30 minutes to remove the cotton wick and reassess the client.

Outcome: [ ] Pass   [ ] Fail

C = competent; A = acceptable; U = unsatisfactory

Comments: _____

_____

_____

_____   _____
Student's Signature   Date

_____   _____
Instructor's Signature   Date

RELATED LITERATURE

**PROCEDURE II-1
ADMINISTERING AN
EYE IRRIGATION**

Garcia GE: Ophthalmology for the nonophthalmologist: minor office emergencies *part 1.* Emergency Medicine 19(7):62–66, 68–69, 73–76, April 1987

Teutsch E, Hill M: Sjogren's syndrome: adding moisture to your life. American Journal of Nursing 87(3):326–329, March 1987

**PROCEDURE II-2
INSTILLING
OPHTHALMIC
MEDICATIONS**

Can I use homemade saline on my contacts? Patient Care 21(10):81 May 30, 1987

Donelly D: Instilling eyedrops: difficulties experienced by patients following cataract surgery. Journal of Advanced Nursing 12(2):235–243, March 1987

Misuse of steroid eye medications. Nurses' Drug Alert 11(1):7, January 1987

Osis M: Drugs and vision: unexplained symptoms—are they due to eye meds? Gerontion 2(1):14–16, Spring 1987

Smith S: How drugs act: drugs and the eye. Nursing Times 83(25):48–50, June 24–30, 1987

**PROCEDURE II-3
INSERTING A
HEARING AID**

Fountain D: Hearing aids and their care. Geriatric Nursing Home Care 7(2):12–14, February 1987

Gough KH, McKim HR: Staff observations help assess residents' hearing handicap. Dimensions in Health Service 63(8):42–44, November 1986

Mahoney DF: One simple solution to hearing impairment. Geriatric Nursing: American Journal of Care for the Aging 8(5):242–245 September–October 1987

Murphy K: Problems of impaired hearing. Geriatric Nursing Home Care 7(2):9–11, February 1987

Rubin W: Noise-induced deafness . . . major environmental problem. Hospital Medicine 23(7):19–21, 25–27, 30–32+, July 1987

**PROCEDURE II-4
ADMINISTERING AN
EAR IRRIGATION**

Richman E: Swimmer's ear: timely management tips. Patient Care 21(10):28–31, 34, 36+, May 30, 1987

Vernick DM, Warfield CA: Diagnosis and treatment of otalgia. Hospital Practice 22(3):170–172, 175, 178, March 15, 1987

**PROCEDURE II-5
INSTILLING EAR
MEDICATION**

Harrison CJ: Tympanoplasty tubes—to use or not to use. Consultant 27(3):143–144, March 1987

Neff J: Laceration, pharyngitis, and otalgia . . . standardized care plans. Journal of Emergency Nursing 12(6):400–404, November–December 1986

III

Procedures pertaining to the integument

III-1 *Assisting the client with oral care*

Traditional hygiene practices include routinely performed mouth care. The conscientious nurse assists a client with oral hygiene at whatever level is required. Most clients only need the nurse to gather the materials they use for oral hygiene. There are times when care of the mouth must be modified to meet the specific needs of the client.

PURPOSES OF PROCEDURE

The client is assisted with oral care to:

1. Cleanse the teeth of food residue and microorganisms.
2. Prevent dental caries.
3. Refresh the mouth.
4. Improve the pleasure of eating.
5. Maintain or improve self-concept.

ASSESSMENT

OBJECTIVE DATA

- Examine the lips, gums, and buccal mucosa for moisture, color, swelling, lesions, exudate, or bleeding.
- Note the presence and characteristics of unusual mouth odor.
- Observe for loose or missing teeth and the state of dental care.
- Identify the presence of dentures or other orthodontic devices.
- Observe the adequacy of mastication and swallowing.
- Examine the tongue for color, symmetry, movement, texture, and evidence of any lesions.
- Inspect the hard and soft palates for intactness, color, patches, lesions, and petechia.
- Examine the oropharynx. Note the movement of the uvula and the condition of the tonsils if present.
- Note any sensory, cognitive, endurance, mobility, or motivation deficit that interferes with the client's ability to perform hygiene practices.

SUBJECTIVE DATA

- Ask the client to describe his past experiences with oral problems or treatment.
- Determine the client's usual oral hygiene practices, such as brushing, flossing, use of rinses, care of orthodontic devices, frequency of dental examinations, and so on.
- Question the client concerning pain or stinging in mouth structures that occurs with biting, chewing, or swallowing.

RELEVANT NURSING DIAGNOSES

The client who requires assistance with oral care may have nursing diagnoses, such as:

- *Impaired Health Maintenance Management*
- *Altered Comfort*
- *Potential for Infection*
- *Altered Oral Mucous Membrane*
- *Disturbance in Self-Concept*

PLANNING

ESTABLISHING PRIORITIES

Mouth care should be provided immediately after a client vomits. Expectoration of copious amounts of sputum is also an indication for frequent mouth care. Ideally routine oral hygiene should be performed when arising, after each meal, and before bedtime. Some clients may never have learned acceptable oral hygiene practices or may have become lax in its performance.

SETTING GOALS

• The client will maintain oral hygiene practices which promote oral health and general well-being.
• The client will perform effective daily oral hygiene.

PREPARATION OF EQUIPMENT

When assisting with oral care, the nurse will need various items from the following list:

Toothbrush
Toothpaste
Emesis basin
Glass with cool water
Towel
Mouthwash (optional)
Dental floss (optional)
Denture cleansing equipment (if necessary):
    Denture cup
    Denture cleaner
    4 × 4 gauze
    Washcloth or paper towel
Petroleum jelly (optional)

Technique for assisting a client with oral care

ACTION	RATIONALE
1. Explain the procedure to the client.	An explanation facilitates cooperation.
2. Assemble equipment on the overbed table within the client's reach.	Organization facilitates the performance of the task.
3. Wash your hands.	Handwashing deters the spread of microorganisms.
4. Provide privacy for the client.	The client may be embarrassed if cleansing involves removal of dentures.
5. Lower the side rail, and assist the client to a sitting position if permitted, or help him turn on his side. Place a bath towel across the chest. Raise the bed to a comfortable working position.	A sitting or a side-lying position prevents aspiration of fluids into the lungs. The towel protects the client from dampness. Raising the bed promotes efficient body mechanics.
6. Encourage the client to brush his own teeth, or assist if necessary.	The nurse should encourage the client to exercise as much independence as possible.
a. Moisten the toothbrush, and apply toothpaste to the bristles.	Water softens the bristles.
b. Place the brush at a 45-degree angle to the gum line, and brush from the gum line to the crown of each tooth, as shown in Fig. III-1-1. Brush the outer and inner surfaces of the teeth. Brush back and forth across the biting surface of each tooth, as shown in Fig. III-1-2.	Brushing facilitates the removal of plaque and tartar. Angling the brush permits cleansing of all surfaces of the teeth.
c. Brush the tongue gently with the toothbrush.	This removes any coating that may be on the tongue. Gentle motion does not stimulate the gag reflex.

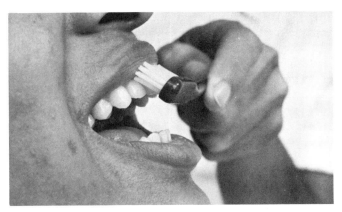

Figure III-1–1 Holding the toothbrush at a 45-degree angle to the gum line helps to remove plaque and tartar.

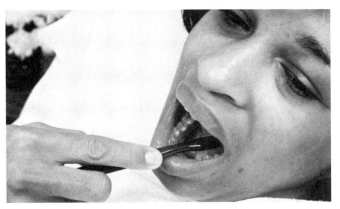

Figure III-1–2 Brushing back and forth cleans food trapped in crevices on the chewing surfaces of the teeth.

d. Have the client rinse vigorously with water and spit into the emesis basin. Repeat until clear.

Vigorous swishing helps remove loosened debris.

e. Assist the client to floss the teeth if necessary, as shown in Fig. III-1-3.

Flossing aids in the removal of plaque and promotes healthy gum tissue.

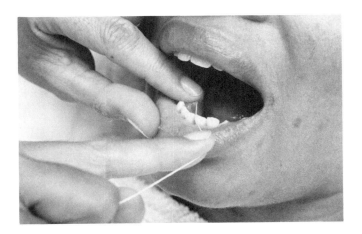

Figure III-1–3 Using dental floss is an important part of daily prophylactic dental hygiene. The floss is wrapped around the middle fingers and inserted with a see-saw motion between adjacent teeth throughout the mouth.

f. Offer mouthwash if the client prefers.

Flavored mouthwash leaves a pleasant aftertaste.

7. Assist the client with the removal and cleansing of dentures if necessary.

Artificial dental devices can be more thoroughly cleaned when removed from the mouth.

a. Apply gentle pressure with a 4 × 4 gauze to grasp and remove the upper denture plate. Place it immediately in a denture cup. Lift the lower denture using a slight rocking motion and place in the denture cup.

A rocking motion breaks the suction between the denture and gum. Using a 4 × 4 gauze prevents slippage and discourages the spread of microorganisms.

b. If the client prefers, add denture cleanser to the cup with water and follow the package directions for cleaning, or brush all areas thoroughly with a toothbrush and toothpaste. Place paper towels or a washcloth in the sink while brushing.

Dentures collect food and microorganisms and require daily cleansing. A paper towel or washcloth in the sink protects against breakage.

c. Rinse dentures thoroughly with water and return them to the client.

Water aids in the removal of debris and the cleansing agent.

d. Offer mouthwash if the client prefers.

Flavored mouthwash leaves a pleasant aftertaste.

e. Apply petroleum jelly to the lips, if needed.

Petroleum jelly prevents cracking and drying of the lips.

8. Remove the equipment, and assist the client to a comfortable position. Record any unusual bleeding or signs of inflammation. Raise the side rail and lower the bed.

Removing soiled material maintains medical asepsis. Reassessment is a method of evaluating the effectiveness of the procedure. Elevated side rails and a lowered bed position maintain the safety of the client.

9. Wash your hands.

Handwashing deters the spread of microorganisms.

SAMPLE DOCUMENTATION

Date	Time	Nurse's note
12/29	0730	Mouth inspected. Mucous membranes appear moist, pink, and intact. All permanent teeth have erupted. Teeth are in good repair. No abnormalities noted on tongue or palate. Tonsils have been removed. Uvula in midline and freely moveable. Provided with materials for oral hygiene. Technique for cleaning teeth is adequate.
		S. Soult, RN

EVALUATION

REASSESSMENT

While carrying out the daily plan for care, the nurse has the opportunity for ongoing assessment of the client's oral cavity and the effectiveness of its care. Observe the client's performance of oral hygiene. Determine whether the mouth and teeth appear clean. Note the improvement of any inflamed or open lesion. Ask the client if he feels the schedule that has been developed for performing oral care is adequate to meet his needs.

EXPECTED OUTCOMES

All surfaces of the teeth are brushed and look clean, shiny, and smooth.
The mouth is thoroughly rinsed of toothpaste residue and cleansing debris.
The client is able to expectorate the toothpaste and rinse without choking or aspiration.
The client's breath smells pleasant.

UNEXPECTED OUTCOMES

The client refuses oral care.
The mouth is not completely cleaned.
The client experiences difficulty in manipulating the toothbrush.
The client has difficulty coordinating the collection of fluid within the mouth or expectorating oral hygiene products.
The gums or mucosa bleed during the process of mouth care.

MODIFICATIONS IN SELECTED SITUATIONS

GENERAL VARIATIONS

A pulsating water device may be helpful in removing particles of food that adhere to braces and mouth appliances.
Enlarge the handle or devise a method to enable the client to grip or hold a toothbrush. The nurse may experiment with wrapping a washcloth about the toothbrush handle. Efforts to secure the toothbrush to the hand may be achieved by inserting the brush within tube stockinette or elastic bandage material that encircles the hand.
Persons with braces can prevent oral lacerations by applying dental wax to sharp areas of their appliances.
When cleansing dentures, avoid the use of hot water which can alter the shape of the synthetic materials used in their construction.
Dentures should be stored in water to prevent drying and warping of plastic materials. A deodorant solution of water and a few drops of ammonia or white vinegar can be used. A few drops of peppermint extract may be added also.
Avoid mechanical injury with a stiff-bristled brush or dental floss when the client is receiving anticoagulant therapy, has a blood dyscrasia, or painful lesions within the mouth.

Motor-driven toothbrushes, electric or battery-operated, have been found to be simple to use and as good as hand brushes in removing debris and plaque.

Clients who receive anticholinergic drugs are likely to experience dry oral mucous membranes. They may require mouth care as frequently as every 2 hours. Chewing gum or sucking on tart hard candy or ice chips may help restore salivation and moisture within the mouth.

AGE-RELATED VARIATIONS

The nurse can apply a finger cot, cover it with a 4 × 4 gauze, moisten the gauze in normal saline or mouthwash, and swab the mouth of a child under 2 years of age.

HOME-HEALTH VARIATIONS

Each person's toothbrush should be replaced at least every 6 months. Locating the toothbrush of a sick person separate from others is a sound medical aseptic practice.

RELATED TEACHING

Recommend regular dental examinations and prophylactic cleaning as important health-care practices to ensure the integrity and longevity of natural teeth.

Instruct adults and children under 9 years of age to consume at least two milk products daily; children 9 to 12 years of age should have three or more servings; teenagers and pregnant or lactating women require four daily servings of dairy products. Dairy products supply calcium for strong dentition.

Explain that foods, such as eggs, meat, milk, and whole grains are good sources of riboflavin and other B complex vitamins which prevent cheilosis. Cheilosis is a vitamin deficiency disease characterized by ulceration of the lips with reddened fissures at the angles of the mouth.

In areas where natural fluoride is deficient in the water or soil, the teeth of young children can benefit from topical applications of fluoride, fluoride added to vitamins, and fluoride toothpaste or rinses.

Teach clients if they notice white or red patches, persistent sores, bleeding, numbness, or pain in the mouth to see their dentist right away. Oral malignancies should be distinguished from benign mouth problems early.

Parents should begin teaching children to brush their own teeth at the age of 2 years.

Explain that concentrated sweets that remain in contact with the surfaces and crevices of teeth increase the risk of dental caries. It is best to limit their consumption, to clean the mouth after eating sweets, or, at the very least, to rinse the mouth thoroughly with plain water.

Advise parents to avoid putting an infant to bed with a bottle of juice or milk. If a bottle is comforting to the child, it should be filled with water to avoid tooth decay.

Inform clients to avoid chewing ice cubes or other hard materials, like partially popped kernels of corn, to avoid fracturing teeth.

If a tooth is broken free, tell the person to rinse the tooth in tap water, place it back in its original area of the gum, and retain it there by biting on a clean handkerchief while contacting the dentist. The tooth should not be allowed to dry. If the tooth is held within the cheek, it may be able to be reattached and saved.

Explain to persons that there is no significant difference between the ability of waxed and unwaxed dental floss to remove plaque. Waxed floss is thicker than unwaxed making it harder to insert into narrow spaces. Unwaxed floss frays somewhat more quickly. The choice is a personal preference.

(Performance checklist next page)

PERRFORMANCE CHECKLIST

When assisting a client with oral care, the learner:

C	A	U	
[ ]	[ ]	[ ]	Introduces self to the client.
[ ]	[ ]	[ ]	Explains the purpose for the interaction.
[ ]	[ ]	[ ]	Provides privacy.
[ ]	[ ]	[ ]	Washes hands.
[ ]	[ ]	[ ]	Inspects the mouth.
[ ]	[ ]	[ ]	Obtains the client's dental history and a description of his pattern for oral hygiene.
[ ]	[ ]	[ ]	Determines the client's preferences concerning the frequency for oral care and the materials he generally uses.
[ ]	[ ]	[ ]	Assembles equipment.
[ ]	[ ]	[ ]	Positions the client to facilitate oral care.
[ ]	[ ]	[ ]	Encourages the client to participate in self-care at whatever level is possible.
[ ]	[ ]	[ ]	Brushes and rinses the teeth, if the client cannot perform this independently.
[ ]	[ ]	[ ]	Offers mouthwash and dental floss, if the client prefers its use.
[ ]	[ ]	[ ]	Applies lubricant to the lips, if needed.
[ ]	[ ]	[ ]	Provides for the safety of the client by lowering the bed, raising the side rails, and securing the signal device within reach.
[ ]	[ ]	[ ]	Removes and cleans oral hygiene materials.
[ ]	[ ]	[ ]	Replaces the client's personal items used for oral care.
[ ]	[ ]	[ ]	Washes hands.
[ ]	[ ]	[ ]	Charts pertinent information.

Outcome: [ ] Pass   [ ] Fail

C = competent; A = acceptable; U = unsatisfactory

Comments: _____

_____

_____

_____   _____
Student's Signature   Date

_____   _____
Instructor's Signature   Date

III-2

Providing oral care for the dependent client

Some clients must rely on the nurse to meet their basic or specialized needs for oral care. Clients at high risk for oral problems include those who are seriously ill, comatose, confused, depressed, or paralyzed. If the client is helpless, the nurse will need to make certain that close attention is given to the condition of the client's mouth as often as is necessary to keep it clean and moist. For some, this may be as frequently as every hour or two.

PURPOSES OF PROCEDURE

The dependent client is assisted with mouth care to:

1. Cleanse the teeth and mouth.
2. Maintain oral moisture and integrity of the tissue.
3. Prevent oral infection.
4. Relieve discomfort from inflamed lesions.

ASSESSMENT

Refer to Procedure III-1, Assisting the Client with Oral Care, plus the following:

OBJECTIVE DATA

• Note the potential for oral side-effects which may occur with drugs, such as dry mouth from anticholinergic drugs, stomatitis from toxic cancer chemotherapy agents, and secondary fungal infections from anti-inflammatory or antibiotic medication.
• Identify treatment interventions that increase the potential for oral problems, such as the use of oxygen, a nasogastric tube, oral airway or endotracheal tube, oral surgery, or mechanical fixation of the jaw due to trauma.

RELEVANT NURSING DIAGNOSES

Dependent clients needing oral care may have nursing diagnoses, such as:

• *Self-Care Deficit*
• *Altered Oral Mucous Membrane*
• *Potential for Infection*
• *Impaired Swallowing*
• *Unilateral Neglect*
• *Impaired Physical Mobility*

PLANNING

ESTABLISHING PRIORITIES

Oral hygiene is a major aspect of caring for a dependent client. Actual or potential oral problems necessitate more frequent and thorough mouth care than the client's usual pattern for oral hygiene. The nurse may need to improvise the procedure in order to maintain the relative safety of the client who has the potential for complications such as choking and aspiration.

SETTING GOALS

• The client's teeth will be free of accumulated secretions and debris.
• The oral mucous membranes will be moist and intact.
• The lips will be smooth and lubricated.

PREPARATION OF EQUIPMENT

The nurse may select those materials from the following list that are relevant to the unique care of a specific client:

> Toothbrush
> Toothpaste
> Emesis basin
> Disposable gloves (optional)
> Cup with cool water
> Towel
> Mouthwash
> Denture cleansing equipment (if necessary)
>> Denture cup
>> Denture cleaner
>> 4 × 4 gauze
>> Washcloth or paper towel
> Sponge toothette or tongue blades padded with 4 × 4 gauze
> Irrigating syringe with rubber tip (optional)
> Cleansing agent (hydrogen peroxide at half strength)
> Lubricating jelly
> Suction catheter with suction apparatus (optional)

Technique for providing oral care for the dependent client

ACTION	RATIONALE
1. Explain the procedure to the client.	An explanation facilitates cooperation.
2. Assemble the equipment on the overbed table within easy reach.	Organization facilitates performance of the task.
3. Wash your hands and, if preferred, don disposable gloves.	Handwashing and disposable gloves deter the spread of microorganisms.
4. Provide privacy for the client. Adjust the height of the bed to a comfortable position for the nurse. Lower one side rail and position the client on his side with his head turned toward the nurse and tilted toward the mattress. Place a bath towel across the chest and an emesis basin in position under the client's chin.	A side-lying position with the head turned downward prevents aspiration of fluid into the lungs. A towel and emesis basin protect the client from dampness.
5. Open the mouth and gently insert a padded tongue blade between the back molars, if necessary, as the nurse in Fig. III-2-1 is doing.	A padded tongue blade keeps the mouth open for easier cleaning and prevents the client from biting the nurse's fingers.

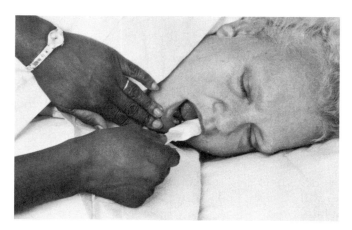

Figure III-2-1 The nurse has taken appropriate safety precautions while administering oral care to the dependent client. The client has been placed in a side-lying position, and the mouth is held open with a padded tongue blade.

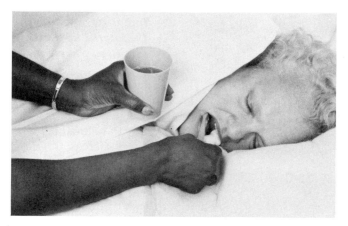

Figure III-2-2 The nurse uses a moistened padded tongue blade to clean the client's teeth.

6. If the client has his natural teeth, clean them carefully with a moistened padded tongue blade as the nurse is doing in Fig. III-2-2. Remove dentures, if present, and clean (Fig. III-2-3). Use a toothette or gauze-padded tongue blade moistened with hydrogen peroxide to gently cleanse the gums, mucous membranes, and tongue.

A toothbrush and padded tongue blade provide friction necessary to clean areas where plaque and tartar accumulate. Hydrogen peroxide solution effectively cleans and removes encrustations from the oral cavity.

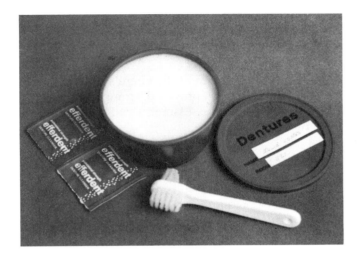

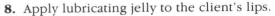

Figure III-2-3 Dentures should be stored in water to prevent warping. Many health-care agencies provide denture cups for storage and cleaning. Soaking dentures in special cleaning preparations helps remove stains and hardened particles.

7. Use a gauze-padded tongue blade dipped in mouthwash solution to rinse the oral cavity, as shown in Fig. III-2-4. If desired, insert the rubber tip of an irrigating syringe into the mouth, as shown in Fig. III-2-5, and gently rinse with a small amount of water. Position the head to the side to allow return drainage of the water or use a suction catheter.

Rinsing helps to cleanse debris from the mouth. A solution that is forcefully irrigated may cause aspiration.

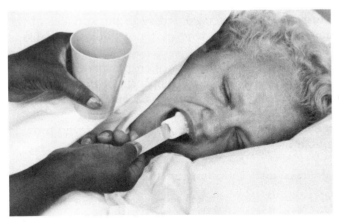

Figure III-2-4 A padded tongue blade can absorb and remove the secretions and moisture that collects during brushing. Using a flavored, aromatic mouthwash creates a refreshing effect.

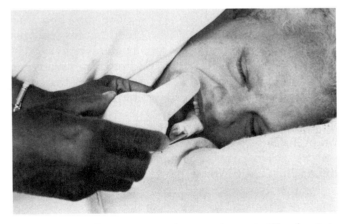

Figure III-2-5 The nurse uses an Asepto syringe to instill and aspirate rinse water from the mouth.

8. Apply lubricating jelly to the client's lips.

Lubrication prevents drying and cracking of the lips.

9. Remove the equipment and return the client to a comfortable position. Raise the side rail and lower the bed. Record any unusual bleeding or inflammation.

Caring for soiled equipment maintains medical asepsis. Raising the side rail and lowering the bed maintain safety.

10. Wash your hands.

Handwashing deters the spread of microorganisms.

SAMPLE DOCUMENTATION

Date	Time	Nurse's note
4/01	2130	Multiple ulcerations on buccal mucosa. Swelling and pain interfere with speaking and eating. Only able to only drink liquids with a straw. Mouth cleansed with swabs moistened in dilute hydrogen peroxide followed with viscous xylocaine rinse. Petroleum jelly applied to lips.
		G. H. olloway, RN

EVALUATION

REASSESSMENT

The nurse has the opportunity for ongoing assessment of the client's oral cavity and the effectiveness of its care each time mouth care is provided. Comparing changes in the characteristics of the objective and subjective assessments will provide a basis for revising the plan and provision of oral hygiene.

EXPECTED OUTCOMES

The client's mouth is clean.
The client's mouth smells fresh.

UNEXPECTED OUTCOMES

Oral secretions and debris remain within the mouth.
The client chokes or aspirates saliva or rinsing solution.

MODIFICATIONS IN SELECTED SITUATIONS

GENERAL VARIATIONS

Commercially prepared oral hygiene swabs may be used, but sparingly. Most contain glycerin which is a mild astringent. This substance can eventually cause the mucous membrane to lose its moisture and defeats one of the purposes for its use.

Aspirating toothbrushes may be useful. These contain a suction tip within the bristle area.

Milk of magnesia or an antacid, such as Maalox, may be used topically to protect the lips and oral mucous membrane.

Once daily, use dental floss on the client's teeth.

AGE-RELATED VARIATIONS

The nurse can apply a finger cot with a gauze square and swab the surfaces of the teeth, gums, and buccal mucosa of children who may not tolerate usual oral hygiene practices.

Children may prefer ginger ale as a substitute for hydrogen peroxide to liberate substances that accumulate in the mouth. Using a diet form of the carbonated beverage avoids instilling a solution with a high sugar content.

HOME-HEALTH VARIATIONS

Offer frequent positive reinforcement to family members or caregivers who provide oral care for the dependent client.

RELATED TEACHING

Refer to the suggestions listed in Procedure III-1, Assisting the Client with Oral Care.

PERFORMANCE CHECKLIST

When assisting the dependent client with oral care, the learner:

C	A	U	
[ ]	[ ]	[ ]	Greets the client and explains the proposed activities pertaining to oral care.
[ ]	[ ]	[ ]	Provides privacy.
[ ]	[ ]	[ ]	Washes hands.
[ ]	[ ]	[ ]	Assembles the necessary equipment.
[ ]	[ ]	[ ]	Checks the function of the suction equipment.
[ ]	[ ]	[ ]	Attaches a suction catheter.
[ ]	[ ]	[ ]	Positions the client to promote drainage of oral secretions and prevent aspiration.
[ ]	[ ]	[ ]	Protects the linen and the client from wetness with a towel or absorbent pad.
[ ]	[ ]	[ ]	Dons clean gloves (optional).
[ ]	[ ]	[ ]	Inserts a padded tongue blade to open and separate the upper and lower teeth.
[ ]	[ ]	[ ]	Brushes the teeth.
[ ]	[ ]	[ ]	Instills rinsing solution with a bulb or Asepto syringe.
[ ]	[ ]	[ ]	Suctions the rinsing solution from the oral cavity.
[ ]	[ ]	[ ]	Swabs the lips and mucous membrane with lubricating or protective substances, if appropriate.
[ ]	[ ]	[ ]	Returns the client to a safe and comfortable position.
[ ]	[ ]	[ ]	Removes and cleans oral hygiene materials.
[ ]	[ ]	[ ]	Replaces cleaned, reusable items in their proper location.
[ ]	[ ]	[ ]	Empties the oral suction container as necessary.
[ ]	[ ]	[ ]	Washes hands.
[ ]	[ ]	[ ]	Charts pertinent information.

Outcome: [ ] Pass   [ ] Fail

C = competent; A = acceptable; U = unsatisfactory

Comments: _____
_____
_____

_____   _____
Student's Signature   Date

_____   _____
Instructor's Signature   Date

III-3   *Giving the bed bath*

Illness and hospitalization may demand that some clients remain in bed during treatment periods. In these situations, the nurse needs to plan modifications that meet the client's needs for personal hygiene. The nurse who assists a client respects individual client preferences and administers only that amount of care that the client cannot or should not provide for himself.

PURPOSES OF PROCEDURE

A bed bath is given to

1. Cleanse the body
2. Refresh the client
3. Stimulate circulation
4. Exercise muscles and joints
5. Provide tactile stimulation
6. Promote comfort and relaxation
7. Improve self-concept
8. Facilitate head-to-toe assessment

ASSESSMENT

OBJECTIVE DATA

- Examine the skin; note its integrity, color, cleanliness, distribution of body hair, presence of bruises or lesions, scars, evidence of moisture, and thickness of subcutaneous tissue.
- Feel the skin to determine variations in temperature, texture, elasticity, and turgor.
- Note evidence of body odor caused by perspiration, bowel or bladder incontinence, or skin excretion of substances, such as urea.
- Identify the client's personal hygiene practices, such as the frequency and time during the day for bathing, preference for a tub bath or shower, and use of soap, deodorant, or other hygiene products.
- Determine any sensory, cognitive, endurance, mobility, or motivational deficit that interferes with the client's ability to perform personal hygiene.

SUBJECTIVE DATA

- Ask the client about any prior history of skin problems involving rashes, lumps, itching, dryness, lesions, ecchymoses, masses, or specific changes in hair or nails.
- Identify the client's history of verified allergic skin reactions to substances like soap or cosmetics.
- Ask the client to identify and describe any areas covered by skin that are painful, itch, burn, or are overly or less sensitive to touch.
- Determine the client's response to sun exposure.

RELEVANT NURSING DIAGNOSES

A client who must be assisted with a bed bath may have nursing diagnoses, such as

- *Activity Intolerance*
- *Self-Care Deficit*
- *Actual or Potential Impaired Skin Integrity*
- *Impaired Physical Mobility*
- *Unilateral Neglect*
- *Disturbance in Self-Concept*
- *Impaired Health Maintenance Management*
- *Sensory Perceptual Alteration: Tactile*

PLANNING

ESTABLISHING
PRIORITIES

The need for bathing is not a life-threatening emergency. Therefore, the client's other needs may demand priority attention. The nurse should attend to bathing the client as soon as possible when there has been excessive soiling or when the client manifests diaphoresis and excessive perspiration.

Most acute health-care agencies provide for daily bathing. However, different individuals possess different ideas regarding personal cleanliness. The nurse should avoid imposing personal values concerning hygiene on the client. The nurse should strive for congruence between the client's prior hygiene practices and the current situation. Exceptions would be made if the illness places the client at high risk for potential impairment of the integument.

SETTING GOALS

- The client's skin will be free of dirt, secretions, and excretions.
- The client's skin will remain intact and well lubricated.
- The client will feel relaxed and refreshed.

PREPARATION OF
EQUIPMENT

The nurse should gather the following items:

Wash basin
Soap and soap dish
Washcloths
Bath blanket
Gown or pajamas
Bed linen
Towels (2)
Personal hygiene supplies (deodorant, lotion, and so on)
Bedpan or urinal
Laundry bag or cart

Technique for giving the bed bath

ACTION	RATIONALE
1. Discuss the procedure with the client and assess the client's ability to assist in bathing as well as with personal hygiene preferences.	This discussion promotes reassurance and provides knowledge about the procedure. Dialogue also encourages client participation and allows for individualized nursing care.
2. Bring the necessary equipment to the bedside stand or overbed table.	Bringing everything to the bedside conserves time and energy. Arranging items nearby is convenient, saves time, and helps prevent stretching and twisting the nurse's muscles.
3. Close the curtains around the bed and close the door if possible.	This ensures the client's privacy and lessens the possibility of loss of body heat during the bath.
4. Offer the bedpan or urinal.	Voiding or defecating before a bath lessens the likelihood that the bath will be interrupted, since the warm bath water may stimulate the urge to void.
5. Wash your hands.	Handwashing deters the spread of microorganisms.
6. Raise the bed to the high position.	Having the bed in a high position prevents strain on the nurse's back.
7. Lower the side rail nearer to you and assist the client to the side of the bed where you will work. Have the client lie on his back.	Having the client positioned near the nurse and lowering the side rail help prevent unnecessary stretching and twisting of muscles on the part of the nurse.
8. Loosen top covers and remove all the linen except the top sheet. Place the bath blanket over the client and then remove the top sheet while the client holds the	The client is not exposed unnecessarily and warmth is maintained. If a bath blanket is not available, the top sheet may be used in place of the bath blanket.

bath blanket in place. If linen is to be reused, fold it over a chair. Place the soiled linen in a laundry bag.

9. Assist the client with oral hygiene as necessary, as described in Procedures III-1 and III-2.

This helps maintain the teeth and gums in good condition, alleviates unpleasant odor and taste, and may improve the appetite. Some clients may prefer oral care after the bath is completed.

10. Remove the client's gown, keeping the bath blanket in place. If the client has an intravenous (IV) line, remove the gown from the other arm first. Lower the IV container and pass the gown over the tubing and container. Rehang the IV and check the drip rate.

Removing clothing provides access during the bath. Covering with a bath blanket maintains the warmth of the client. IV fluids must be maintained at the prescribed rate.

11. Raise the side rail. Fill the basin with sufficient comfortably warm water (between 43°C and 46°C [110°F to 115°F]). Change the water as necessary throughout the bath. Lower the side rail closer to you when you return to the bedside to begin the bath.

Warm water is comfortable and relaxing for the client. It also stimulates circulation and provides for more effective cleansing. Side rails maintain client safety.

12. Fold the washcloth like a mitt, as shown in Figure III-3-1.

Having loose ends of a washcloth drag across the client's skin is uncomfortable. Loose ends cool quickly and will feel cold to the client.

13. Lay a towel across the client's chest and on top of the bath blanket.

A towel prevents chilling and keeps the bath blanket dry.

14. With no soap on the washcloth, wipe one eye from the inner part of the eye, near the nose, to the outer part, as shown in Figure III-3-2. Rinse or turn the cloth before washing the other eye.

Rinsing or turning the cloth prevents spreading organisms from one eye to the other. Soap is irritating to the eyes. Moving from the inner to the outer aspect of the eye prevents carrying debris toward the nasolacrimal duct.

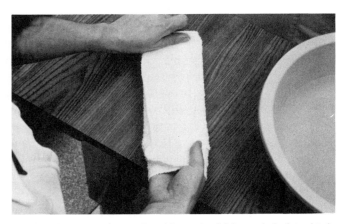

Figure III-3-1 To form a thumbless mitt, fold a washcloth in thirds, slip the hand into the pocket, flip the remainder of the washcloth over the fingers and palm, and place the extra length of washcloth between the palm and the folded washcloth, as this nurse demonstrates.

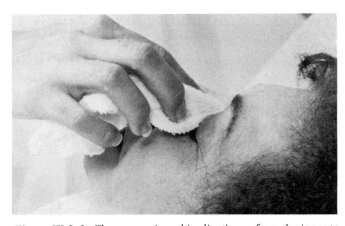

Figure III-3-2 The nurse wipes this client's eye from the inner to the outer corner using a dampened corner of the washcloth without any soap. Another area of the cloth is used for the other eye.

15. Bathe the client's face, neck, and ears. Avoid soap on the face if the client prefers.

Soap can be drying and may be avoided as a matter of personal preference.

16. Expose the client's far arm and place the towel lengthwise under it. Using firm strokes, wash, rinse, and dry the arm and axilla.

The towel helps to keep the bed dry. Washing the far side first eliminates contaminating a clean area once it is washed. Gentle friction stimulates circulation and muscles and helps remove dirt, oil, and organisms. Long, firm strokes are relaxing and more comfortable than short, uneven strokes.

17. Place a folded towel on the bed next to the client's hand and put the hand in the basin as shown in Figure III-3-3. Wash, rinse, and dry the hand.

18. Repeat Steps 16 and 17 for the arm nearer to you.

19. Spread the towel across the client's chest. Lower the bath blanket to the umbilical area. Wash, rinse, and dry the chest. Keep the chest covered with a towel between the washing and rinsing. Pay special attention to the skin folds under a female client's breasts.

20. Lower the bath blanket to cover the perineal area. Place the towel over the client's chest.

21. Wash, rinse, and dry the client's abdomen. Carefully inspect and cleanse the umbilical area and any abdominal folds or creases.

22. Return the bath blanket to the original position and expose the client's far leg. Place the towel under the far leg. Using firm strokes, wash, rinse, and dry the leg from the ankle to the knee and the knee to the groin.

23. Fold the towel near the foot area and place the basin on the towel. Place the foot in the basin while supporting the ankle and heel in your hand and the leg on your arm. Wash, rinse, and dry the foot, paying particular attention to the areas between the toes.

24. Repeat Steps 22 and 23 for the other leg and foot.

25. Make sure the client is covered with a bath blanket. Change the water at this point or earlier if necessary. Assist the client onto his side.

26. Assist the client to a prone or side-lying position. Position the bath blanket and towel so as to expose only the client's back and buttocks.

27. Wash, rinse, and dry the client's back, as shown in Figure III-3-4, and the buttocks area. Pay particular attention to cleansing between the gluteal folds and observe for any indication of redness or skin breakdown in the sacral area.

Placing the hand in the basin of water is comfortable and relaxing for the client and allows for a thorough washing of the hand and between the fingers, as well as facilitating removal of debris from under the nails.

Exposing, washing, rinsing, and drying one part of the body at a time avoids unnecessary exposure and chilling. Skin-fold areas may be sources of odor and skin breakdown if not cleansed and dried properly.

Keeping the bath blanket and towel in place avoids exposure and chilling.

Skin-fold areas may be sources of odor and skin breakdown if not cleansed and dried properly.

The towel protects the linens and prevents the client from feeling uncomfortable from a damp or wet bed. Washing from ankle to groin with firm strokes promotes venous return.

Supporting the foot and leg helps reduce strain and discomfort for the client. Placing the feet in a basin of water is comfortable and relaxing and allows for a thorough cleaning of the feet, the areas between the toes, and under the nails.

The bath blanket maintains warmth and privacy. Clean, warm water prevents chilling and maintains the client's comfort.

Positioning of the towel and bath blanket protects the client's privacy and provides warmth.

Fecal material near the anus may be a source of microorganisms. Prolonged pressure on the sacral area or other bony prominences may compromise circulation and lead to the development of a decubitus ulcer.

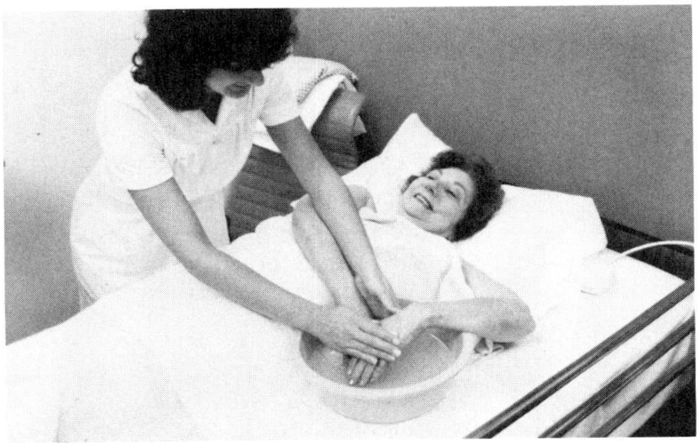

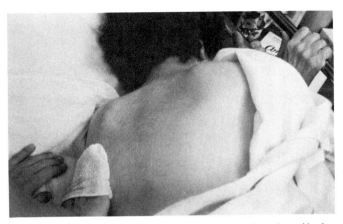

Figure III-3-3 Although the client is not able to bathe in a tub or shower, the client's hands and feet can be soaked in a basin of warm water.

Figure III-3-4 The nurse has turned the client on the side and bathes the back. This provides an excellent opportunity for assessing the condition of the skin on the posterior of the body.

28. If not contraindicated, give the client a back rub, as described in Procedure III-7. A back massage may be given also after perineal care.

A back rub improves circulation to the tissues and is an aid to relaxation. A back rub may be contraindicated in clients with cardiovascular disease or musculoskeletal injuries.

29. Refill the basin with clean water. Discard the washcloth and towel.

The washcloth, towel, and water are contaminated after washing the gluteal area. Changing to clean supplies decreases the spread of organisms from the anal area to the genitals.

30. Clean the perineal area as described in Procedure III-8, or position the client so he can complete the perineal care.

Providing perineal self-care may decrease the embarrassment for the client. Effective perineal care reduces odor and decreases the chance of infection through contamination.

31. Help the client put on a clean gown and attend to the personal hygiene needs.

A clean gown promotes the warmth and comfort of the client.

32. Protect the pillow with a towel, and groom the client's hair.

Hair is lost during the process of combing. The towel collects loose hair.

33. Change bed linens, as described in Procedure I-11.

Providing clean linen promotes medical asepsis and the comfort of the client.

34. Record any significant observations and communication on the client's chart.

A careful record is important for planning and individualizing the client's care.

SAMPLE DOCUMENTATION

Date	Time	Nurse's note
3/13	1800	Experiencing periods of dizziness. BP 120/68/60 when lying down and 90/40/40 upon rising. Assisted with bed bath. Skin is pink, warm, dry, and elastic. No petechiae, lesions, or excoriations noted. *E. Knudsen, RN*

EVALUATION

REASSESSMENT

The nurse should use incidental contacts with the client to determine if bathing is being provided often enough to promote personal hygiene. Factors that may indicate a need to revise the nursing orders for bathing include a change in the client's level of care, newly identified skin problems, or inability to achieve the client-centered goals.

EXPECTED OUTCOMES

The client is completely bathed.
The client's skin is clean and intact.
The client feels more comfortable.

UNEXPECTED OUTCOMES

The client feels cold or exhausted and indicates a desire to discontinue bathing.
Body odor remains after cleansing.
Skin areas over bony prominences appear red and do not return to normal color when pressure is relieved.
The client's skin is dry and flakey, and itches.
The skin manifests areas of rash or open lesions.

MODIFICATIONS IN SELECTED SITUATIONS

GENERAL VARIATIONS

Tepid baths or soaks may relieve skin inflammation and itching.
Substitute using a detergent for soap on persons who are sensitive to the ingredients in soap.
Cold creams liquefy on the skin and loosen and suspend dirt, oily secretions, perspiration, bacteria, cosmetics, dead cells, and other foreign material. These sub-

stances can be applied to areas such as the face and then removed with a tissue or soft cloth rather than bathing with soap and water.

Certain clients may not be able to tolerate lying flat in bed during the bed bath. The position may be modified to accommodate the needs of the client.

If a client receiving an IV is not wearing a gown that snaps at the sleeve, the tubing and the container of solution must be threaded through the sleeve as the gown is removed. Perform the procedure in reverse to replace the gown. Place the clean gown on the unaffected arm first and thread the IV tubing and bag or bottle from inside the arm of the gown on the involved side. *Never* disconnect the IV tubing to change a gown because this causes a break in the sterile system and potentiates the risk for infection.

AGE-RELATED VARIATIONS

When bathing an infant or young child, have all supplies within easy reach and support or hold the child securely at all times to ensure safety. Never leave a child alone during bathing.

Check the temperature of bath water carefully when bathing clients with sensory deficits or altered tissue perfusion. Clients with these problems experience an insensitivity to perception of heat and can easily be burned.

Bath oil may be added to the water for the elderly person with dry skin. Use an emollient, such as lanolin, to soften, soothe, and protect dry skin after cleansing. Emollients leave a film on the skin that retards normal moisture evaporation and scaling of skin.

The adolescent with acne should wash the skin and shampoo hair frequently with soap or detergent and hot water to remove oil and debris.

HOME-HEALTH VARIATIONS

A number of over-the-counter products are available for individuals with sensitive skin or skin problems. The client should be advised to read the labels well and follow the directions carefully. Professional attention should always be sought if the skin problems fail to improve or worsen with self-treatment.

Pad the bed with waterproof material or absorbent towels to prevent the linen and mattress from becoming wet with bath water.

Use proper body mechanics when bathing a client on a low, nonadjustable bed.

RELATED TEACHING

Instruct individuals with dry and easily injured skin to avoid applying defatting agents, such as alcohol.

Explain that wearing garments made of woolen fabrics tends to irritate dry skin.

Inform individuals with dry skin that increasing oral fluid intake and adding moisture to the air with a humidifier may relieve the problem.

Tell adolescents with skin eruptions to use cosmetics sparingly to avoid further blocking of sebaceous gland ducts.

Advise clients who experience intermittent rashes, which may be described as flat or raised, pruritic or nonpruritic, local or systemic, wet or dry areas, that the skin condition may be a response to an allergen. To identify a cause-and-effect relationship, a referral to an allergist may prove helpful.

Tell clients that expensive cleansing agents have not been found to be superior to less expensive ones like soap or detergents.

Vitamin A promotes healthy hair and skin and maintains the integrity of the epithelium. Inform clients to eat a well-balanced diet and include a vegetable high in beta-carotene, a precursor of Vitamin A, every other day. Examples of these include carrots, yellow squash, broccoli, and brussel sprouts.

Explain that the prime requisite for preventing body odors involves keeping the body and clothing clean. Deodorants and antiperspirants may be used after the skin is clean. Recommend that individuals discard cosmetics after they are approximately four months old, especially those applied near the eyes. It has been found that cosmetics often become contaminated with bacteria and fungi.

PERFORMANCE CHECKLIST

When assisting with a bed bath, the learner:

C	A	U	
[ ]	[ ]	[ ]	Greets and introduces self to the client
[ ]	[ ]	[ ]	Explains the purpose of the interaction
[ ]	[ ]	[ ]	Washes hands
[ ]	[ ]	[ ]	Provides privacy
[ ]	[ ]	[ ]	Obtains objective and subjective data
[ ]	[ ]	[ ]	Confers with the client on the frequency, time, and materials preferred for bathing while in the facility, if appropriate
[ ]	[ ]	[ ]	Assembles equipment according to the client's preferences
[ ]	[ ]	[ ]	Positions the client in a supine position
[ ]	[ ]	[ ]	Prevents drafts
[ ]	[ ]	[ ]	Raises the bed and lowers the nearer side rail
[ ]	[ ]	[ ]	Covers the client with a bath blanket
[ ]	[ ]	[ ]	Removes bed clothing and top linen
[ ]	[ ]	[ ]	Assists the client to bathe the face, followed by the arms and hands, chest, abdomen, legs, and feet
[ ]	[ ]	[ ]	Rinses the soap from the washed areas
[ ]	[ ]	[ ]	Dries the washed areas thoroughly
[ ]	[ ]	[ ]	Changes the wash water whenever it becomes cool or soiled
[ ]	[ ]	[ ]	Turns the client to a lateral or prone position
[ ]	[ ]	[ ]	Bathes the back and buttocks
[ ]	[ ]	[ ]	Provides a back massage
[ ]	[ ]	[ ]	Repositions the client on his back
[ ]	[ ]	[ ]	Replaces the water
[ ]	[ ]	[ ]	Offers the client the opportunity to bathe the genitals and perineum (or performs this for the dependent client)
[ ]	[ ]	[ ]	Raises the side rails and leaves while the client washes the genitalia
[ ]	[ ]	[ ]	Removes and cleans the wash basin
[ ]	[ ]	[ ]	Replaces the cleaned, reusable supplies in their proper location within the client's bedside unit
[ ]	[ ]	[ ]	Assists the client with donning clean bed clothing
[ ]	[ ]	[ ]	Provides the client with other materials for grooming and hygiene, such as razor, toothbrush, hairbrush, and cosmetics
[ ]	[ ]	[ ]	Changes bed linen
[ ]	[ ]	[ ]	Lowers the bed, elevates the side rails, and provides the client with a signal device
[ ]	[ ]	[ ]	Deposits soiled bed linen in an appropriate receptacle
[ ]	[ ]	[ ]	Washes hands
[ ]	[ ]	[ ]	Documents the assessment data, care given, the extent of the client's participation, and the client's response

Outcome: [ ] Pass [ ] Fail

C = competent; A = acceptable; U = unsatisfactory

(Continued)

PERFORMANCE CHECKLIST (Continued)

Comments: _____

_____

_____

_____   _____
Student's Signature   Date

_____   _____
Instructor's Signature   Date

III-4 *Shampooing hair*

Hair accumulates the same dirt and oil as the skin. It should be washed as often as necessary to keep it clean. A weekly shampoo may be sufficient for some persons whereas others may prefer to perform this aspect of personal hygiene daily. The nurse may need to shampoo the hair of those clients who cannot get out of bed for bathing and showering or who lack the strength or ability to independently care for their hair.

PURPOSES OF PROCEDURE

Shampooing the hair is done to

1. Cleanse the hair and scalp
2. Maintain or improve self-esteem
3. Treat conditions of the scalp with topical applications of medications
4. Remove substances, such as blood, body secretions, or electrode jelly (used when an electroencephalogram or other such study is done)

ASSESSMENT

OBJECTIVE DATA

- Examine the hair; note its distribution, cleanliness, texture, and any indications of parasitic infections, such as the nits of head lice on the hair shaft.
- Inspect the scalp for lacerations, dry scaley patches, scratches, lesions, and swollen areas.
- Observe the client for signs of an itchy scalp, such as scratching the head.
- Note signs of dandruff on the shoulders and back of clothing.
- Determine if the client is receiving toxic chemotherapy or radiation treatments that may cause loss of hair.
- Read the client's medical record to determine if the client has any pathology, such as hypothyroidism, or is receiving long-term steroid therapy that may alter the texture and distribution of hair.
- Identify if there are any sensory, cognitive, endurance, mobility, or motivational deficits that interfere with the client's ability to perform hygiene practices.

SUBJECTIVE DATA

- Ask the client to describe the usual routine for shampooing, including the frequency and types of hair care products routinely used.
- Inquire if the client experiences any itching, burning, or tenderness of the scalp.
- Note the client's history of hair or scalp problems and related treatments.

RELEVANT NURSING DIAGNOSES

Those clients who need assistance with shampooing are likely to have the following nursing diagnoses:

- *Self-Care Deficit*
- *Disturbance in Self-Concept*
- *Altered Health Maintenance*
- *Unilateral Neglect*

PLANNING

ESTABLISHING PRIORITIES

When blood or body fluids, such as emesis, collect in the hair, the nurse should thoroughly sponge the areas as soon as possible. Care of the scalp and accessory structures, such as the hair, helps maintain the integrity of the skin as a barrier to infection and trauma. Personal hygiene practices should always be considered an important aspect of preventive care. Since appearance is linked to self-esteem, regular shampooing also meets higher level needs.

SETTING GOALS	• The client's hair and scalp will be free of dirt, oil, and other substances.
	• The hair will be dried and combed free of tangles.
	• The client will express feelings of well-being and satisfaction about his appearance.
PREPARATION OF EQUIPMENT	The nurse should assemble the following items:

Several towels
Shampoo
Hair-care products, such as conditioner, mousse, setting gel, or petrolatum (optional)
Water pitcher
Shampoo trough
Bath blanket
Absorbent pad
Comb, hairbrush
Hair dryer (optional)

Technique for shampooing hair

ACTION	RATIONALE
1. Explain the procedure to the client.	An explanation facilitates understanding and cooperation.
2. Wash your hands.	Handwashing deters the spread of microorganisms.
3. Assemble the equipment near the client.	Organization is a form of appropriate time-management and prevents fatigue and frustration of the client.
4. Raise the bed to a height convenient for you and lower the nearer side rail.	Adjusting the bed helps to prevent muscle strain or fatigue.
5. Position the client on the back.	A supine position facilitates drainage away from the face, eyes, and head.
6. Comb or brush the client's hair.	Removing tangles before washing will prevent breaking strands of hair.
7. Place a folded bath blanket, several towels, or an absorbent pad under the client's head, shoulders, and back.	Layered material absorbs water and prevents the client from feeling wet and chilled. It also avoids saturating the bed linen.
8. Place a plastic tray or trough, like the one illustrated in Figure III-4-1, under the client's head.	Using a trough provides a method for collecting and draining the water away from the client and the bed.

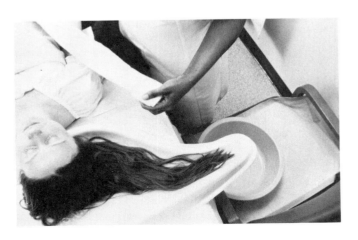

Figure III-4–1 This client's head is lying on a shampoo trough. A basin has been placed below the trough to catch the draining water.

9. Lay a towel or bath blanket over the client's chest and shoulders.

10. Wet the hair thoroughly with warm (40°C [105°F]) water and apply shampoo.

11. Work the shampoo into a lather, shown in Figure III-4-2.

12. Rinse the hair with clean, running water.

13. Wrap the client's head with dry towels, as shown in Figure III-4-3.

The edge can be used to wipe away any water that splashes the client's face or ears.

Wet hair dilutes the shampoo and helps to form suds.

Lathering helps distribute the shampoo throughout the entire head of hair for uniform cleansing.

Rinsing prevents leaving shampoo in the hair, which gives hair a dull appearance; if left on the scalp, shampoo could cause irritation for some people.

Towels absorb water, beginning the process of drying while allowing the client to assume a more comfortable position.

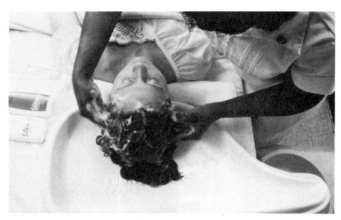

Figure III-4-2 The nurse lathers the shampoo from the front to the back of the head using the tips of the fingers. Fingernails are kept short to prevent scratching the scalp.

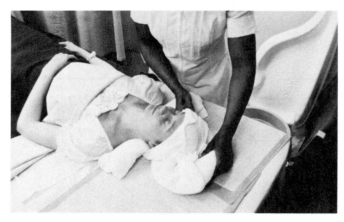

Figure III-4-3 Towels are used to remove as much moisture as possible from the scalp and hair.

14. Remove the equipment used for shampooing.

15. Fluff the hair with towels, and comb out the hair, as shown in Figure III-4-4.

Discarding the water and the equipment will prevent accidental spilling.

Loosening and combing the hair prepare it for styling.

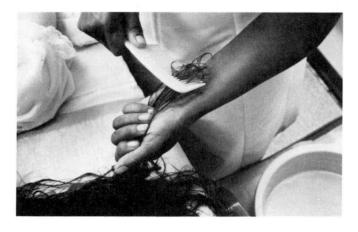

16. Braid, blow dry, or set the hair.

Figure III-4-4 A comb is gently worked through the hair to remove tangles.

Most clients prefer to style the hair in order to make it attractive as well as clean.

17. Raise the side rail and lower the bed when leaving the client.

Precautionary measures prevent falls and injury to the client.

18. Wash your hands.

Handwashing deters the spread of microorganisms.

19. Document the assessments, care provided, the client's ability to participate, and the client's response.

Careful recording is important for planning and individualizing the client's care.

SAMPLE DOCUMENTATION

Date	Time	Nurse's note
12/03	0600	Sleep-deprived EEG performed. Gel sponged from hair and then washed with shampoo. Hair towel dried and braided.
		D. Gibson, RN

EVALUATION

REASSESSMENT

Inspect the condition of the hair and scalp during daily physical assessment. Ask the client if the current plan for hygiene is satisfactory and meets expectations. Revise the plan for care when goals are unachieved.

EXPECTED OUTCOMES

The hair and scalp are clean.
The hair appears full-bodied and shiny.
The hair is styled to promote comfort and care.

UNEXPECTED OUTCOMES

The hair contains tangles that interfere with combing.
The client experiences scalp irritation from the shampoo.
Scalp or hair problems are not improved with the products used.
The hair shafts break or hair is lost in patchy areas about the scalp.

MODIFICATIONS IN SELECTED SITUATIONS

GENERAL VARIATIONS

The hair of a black person usually requires special attention. The hair is normally very dry and very curly, and becomes easily matted and tangled. Use a brush or select a comb with widely spaced teeth. Oil should be used after shampooing. White petrolatum or mineral oil is often recommended.

Apply dry shampoo or powder to the hair of clients too ill or incapacitated to have a wet shampoo. Comb or brush it from the hair. Dry shampoo or powder is not recommended for black clients because of their normally dry hair and scalp.

If a shampoo trough is not available and the client can sit up, shampoo the hair over the wash basin on the overbed table. If the client can sit in a chair, use the bathroom sink when shampooing.

Use specific medicated shampoos, such as Kwell soap, for treating head lice. Use antidandruff shampoos when indicated.

AGE-RELATED VARIATIONS

Nontearing shampoo may be used for children or place a towel or face cloth over the child's eyes when lathering and rinsing the shampoo.

HOME-HEALTH VARIATIONS

Use a hand-held sprayer in the shower or at the sink for wetting and rinsing the hair.

If a plastic tray or trough is unavailable, use a large, plastic trash bag to make a trough that empties into a wastepaper basket.

To prevent straining the back, lay a child on the kitchen counter, support the child's head over the sink, and shampoo the hair.

In lieu of using a dry shampoo, moisten cotton balls with alcohol. Place rows of alcohol-moistened cotton balls between the bristles of the client's hairbrush and brush through the hair.

RELATED TEACHING   Explain that a well-balanced diet consisting of a wide variety of foods from the basic four food groups can maintain the strength, texture, and appearance of hair.

Dispel the myth that shampooing the hair is unhealthy during menstruation.

Instruct male clients that there is no cure yet for hereditary baldness. One drug, minoxidil, is being used as a treatment for baldness. Its topical use causes fine, downy hair to grow for some, but not all, balding individuals. It works best on men who are just beginning to lose hair. The client must continue twice-daily applications to retain the hair growth. The long-term use of the drug is likely to be expensive.

Tell clients that pediculosis (lice) can be spread directly by contact with others who are infected or indirectly through contact with their clothing, bed linens, brushes, and combs. Children especially should be taught not to share personal items, such as hats and combs. Outbreaks of head lice in schools can be controlled by having all the children use a medicated shampoo on the same night. All members of a family may wish to use a medicated shampoo whether infected or not.

PERFORMANCE CHECKLIST

When assisting with a shampoo, the learner:

C	A	U	
[ ]	[ ]	[ ]	Greets and introduces self to the client
[ ]	[ ]	[ ]	Explains the purpose for the interaction
[ ]	[ ]	[ ]	Inspects the hair and scalp
[ ]	[ ]	[ ]	Determines the hygiene practices of the client
[ ]	[ ]	[ ]	Collaborates with the client in planning hair care
[ ]	[ ]	[ ]	Assembles equipment
[ ]	[ ]	[ ]	Raises the bed to an appropriate height to prevent back strain
[ ]	[ ]	[ ]	Lowers the nearer side rail
[ ]	[ ]	[ ]	Protects the bed and the client from becoming wet
[ ]	[ ]	[ ]	Places a shampoo trough on the bed or improvises an alternative method
[ ]	[ ]	[ ]	Locates a receptacle for collecting the water beneath the drain area of the trough
[ ]	[ ]	[ ]	Wets the hair
[ ]	[ ]	[ ]	Lathers the shampoo into the hair
[ ]	[ ]	[ ]	Massages the scalp with the fingertips
[ ]	[ ]	[ ]	Rinses the hair thoroughly
[ ]	[ ]	[ ]	Wipes any water and shampoo from the face
[ ]	[ ]	[ ]	Wraps the head in a towel
[ ]	[ ]	[ ]	Removes the shampoo trough
[ ]	[ ]	[ ]	Raises the side rail
[ ]	[ ]	[ ]	Discards the water and replaces reusable items in their proper location
[ ]	[ ]	[ ]	Changes any damp linen or bed clothing
[ ]	[ ]	[ ]	Combs, brushes, and styles the hair
[ ]	[ ]	[ ]	Washes hands
[ ]	[ ]	[ ]	Charts the assessments, procedure, and the client's response

Outcome: [ ] Pass   [ ] Fail

C = competent; A = acceptable; U = unsatisfactory

Comments: _____
_____
_____

_____   _____
Student's Signature   Date

_____   _____
Instructor's Signature   Date

A common North American hygiene practice is for men to remove, clean, or groom facial hair. Most men prefer to be clean shaven. Many prefer to shave at the time of bathing. The nurse may need to shave the client's face from time to time. Some clients may be unable to shave because they are too ill or because an arm is paralyzed or immobilized in a cast or traction.

PURPOSES OF PROCEDURE

The nurse assists with shaving to

1. Remove unwanted hair
2. Maintain or improve the client's self-concept
3. Promote comfort

ASSESSMENT

OBJECTIVE DATA

- Inspect the face of the male client, noting if he is clean shaven, has evidence of having neglected recent shaving, or prefers a beard or moustache.
- Examine the skin of the cheeks, chin, and neck for signs of elevated moles, warts, rashes, patchy skin lesions, or pustules.
- Review the medication Kardex for drugs that alter the clotting mechanisms, such as heparin.
- Read the client's medical record and be alert for laboratory tests, such as a complete blood count (CBC) and prothrombin time. Various tests reflect an individual's ability to control bleeding or the presence of a disease, such as a blood dyscrasia or liver disease, that can affect clotting.
- Determine if there are any sensory, cognitive, endurance, mobility, or motivational deficits that interfere with the client's ability to carry out personal hygiene practices.

SUBJECTIVE DATA

- Ask the client to describe his hygiene practices related to shaving; note his preference for using a safety or electric razor and any pre- or post-shaving products.
- Encourage the client to describe the characteristics of his beard and response of his skin to shaving.

RELEVANT NURSING DIAGNOSES

Clients who need assistance with shaving can have nursing diagnoses, such as

- *Altered Comfort*
- *Self-Care Deficit*
- *Disturbance in Self-Concept*
- *Unilateral Neglect*
- *Impaired Physical Mobility*

PLANNING

ESTABLISHING PRIORITIES

Grooming improves self-esteem and therefore the nurse may delay shaving until the client's more basic, or lower, needs, such as nourishment, elimination, safety, and so on, have been met. Nevertheless, this aspect of care should not be neglected even though its omission may not cause life-threatening consequences. The nurse considers the emotional needs of the client as important as his physical needs.

SETTING GOALS

- The client's shaving practices will be respected and followed on a regular basis.
- The client's facial hair will be removed.
- The client will indicate satisfaction with his appearance.

PREPARATION OF EQUIPMENT

The nurse may select items from the following list:

Safety razor or electric razor
Mirror (optional)
Wash basin
Washcloth and towels
Soap
Shaving cream (optional)
Aftershave or cologne (optional)

Technique for shaving facial hair

ACTION	RATIONALE
1. Introduce yourself to the client and explain the purpose for your presence.	An explanation provides the client with information and is more likely to facilitate his cooperation.
2. Assess the client and determine his usual shaving routine.	Gathering information provides a basis for planning individual care.
3. Note any problems that may interfere with the client's ability to perform his personal hygiene.	The nurse should assist the client with those aspects of care that cannot be performed independently.
4. Collaborate with the client on the time, frequency, and manner in which shaving will be performed.	The nurse respects the client's individuality and encourages him to become a partner in the care.
5. Gather shaving equipment if the client requires assistance.	Organizing the equipment helps the nurse complete the care efficiently.
6. Raise the bed and lower the side rail nearer to you.	Adjusting the bed prevents back strain.
7. Place the client in a sitting position, if possible.	Being upright is a similar position to one a client would assume himself when shaving. It also promotes eye contact and communication between the client and the nurse.
8. Wash the client's face with warm, soapy water.	Removing oil helps to raise the hair shaft, promoting its removal. Soap removes bacteria that can enter tiny cuts.
9. Inspect the face for elevated moles, birthmarks, or lesions.	Scraping or cutting can cause bleeding, irritation, or infection.
10. Lather the face with shaving cream or soap.	Lathering softens the beard and helps the razor slide over the skin without nicking or cutting.
11. Use short strokes with the razor in the direction of hair growth, as shown in Figure III-5-1. Start from the upper face and lip and extend to the neck. The client may tilt his head to help shave in hollow or curved areas.	Shaving in the direction of the hair will reduce irritation of the underlying skin.

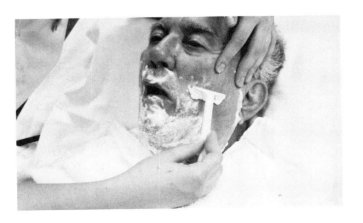

Figure III-5-1 Shaving cream has been applied to the client's face. The razor is gently pulled in the direction of the hair growth.

12. Use the hand without the razor to pull the skin below the area being shaved.

Pulling flattens and firms the skin surface, promoting uniform shaving.

13. Rinse the razor after each stroke.

Rinsing removes hair from between the blade and the blade guard so the cutting edge remains clean.

14. Rinse and dry the face when completely finished.

Final rinsing removes remnants of lather and shaved hair.

15. Apply the client's choice of lotion or cologne.

Most aftershave products contain scented alcohol. The alcohol acts as an antiseptic on the microabrasions. As the alcohol evaporates, it causes a cooling sensation that feels refreshing.

16. Reposition the client for comfort. Lower the bed and raise the side rail.

Adjusting the bed promotes the safety of the client.

17. Return all shaving equipment to its proper location. Discard any dulled disposable razors or razor blades in a puncture-proof container.

The nurse must take care that others will not be accidentally injured by sharp objects.

18. Wash your hands.

Handwashing deters the spread of infection.

19. Document assessments, the care provided, the extent of the client's participation, and the client's response.

The client's record represents a legal account of his individualized care.

SAMPLE DOCUMENTATION

Date	Time	Nurse's note
8/17	0800	Facial hair growth observed. Stated, "It's so hot. This stubble really itches and I feel like a bum." Shaved by nurse with a safety razor. States, "I feel like a new man."
		T. Riggs, RN

EVALUATION

REASSESSMENT

Reexamine the facial skin immediately after shaving. Control any bleeding. Discuss the frequency for repeating this aspect of the client's personal hygiene and any alterations in the manner in which it was performed.

EXPECTED OUTCOMES

The client's face is clean and free of hair.
The facial skin is smooth and intact.
The client feels more comfortable and self-confident about his appearance.

UNEXPECTED OUTCOMES

The hair is unevenly and incompletely removed.
The skin receives multiple abrasions or cuts.
The client experiences discomfort as the razor is used.
Elevated skin lesions become traumatized and bleed.

MODIFICATIONS IN SELECTED SITUATIONS

GENERAL VARIATIONS

Safety razors tend to give a closer shave, but the nurse may feel more confident using an electric razor. This may be the better alternative when the client is acutely ill and bedridden.
A very close shave can be achieved by drawing a safety razor counter to the direction of hair growth. This is likely to increase the potential for skin irritation as well.

Use an electric razor for any client who has a potential for bleeding. Also substitute the use of an electric razor if the client is confused or depressed.

Those clients receiving oxygen should use a safety razor or a battery-operated razor to reduce electrical hazards and the possibility of combustion.

Special preparations are available for softening the beard for easier shaving. If none is available, place a towel that has been soaked and wrung of hot water about the face for a few minutes before shaving.

The nurse may shave the leg or axillary hair for a dependent female client.

Women can have unwanted facial hair removed by tweezing, depilatory creams, or electrolysis.

AGE-RELATED VARIATIONS

Adolescent males may not require daily shaving until the beard has become well established.

HOME-HEALTH VARIATIONS

If an electric razor is used, drape the client to avoid irritation caused by loose whiskers that can fall onto the skin.

Offer praise to the family member or caregiver who shaves the client's face on a routine basis.

RELATED TEACHING

Explain that it has not been proven that repeated shaving causes excessive growth or coarseness of hair.

Tell female clients that bleaching facial hair is an inexpensive method for rendering it hardly noticeable.

Instruct a client that hair that extends from moles should not be plucked. The hair can be cut with small scissors.

(Performance checklist next page)

PERFORMANCE CHECKLIST

When assisting the client with shaving, the learner:

C	A	U	
[ ]	[ ]	[ ]	Reads the client's record and notes pertinent information
[ ]	[ ]	[ ]	Introduces self
[ ]	[ ]	[ ]	Explains the purpose for the interaction
[ ]	[ ]	[ ]	Washes hands
[ ]	[ ]	[ ]	Physically assesses the client's facial skin and hair
[ ]	[ ]	[ ]	Determines the client's preferences about shaving
[ ]	[ ]	[ ]	Assembles the equipment
[ ]	[ ]	[ ]	Adjusts the client's bed and position for proper use of body mechanics
[ ]	[ ]	[ ]	Cleans the face with soap and water
[ ]	[ ]	[ ]	Softens the beard with lathered soap
[ ]	[ ]	[ ]	Shaves the face in the direction of hair growth
[ ]	[ ]	[ ]	Rinses the lather and the razor
[ ]	[ ]	[ ]	Wipes the face and dries it after shaving
[ ]	[ ]	[ ]	Applies cosmetic products, if desired
[ ]	[ ]	[ ]	Lowers the bed and raises the side rails
[ ]	[ ]	[ ]	Removes the shaving equipment and discards the water
[ ]	[ ]	[ ]	Washes hands
[ ]	[ ]	[ ]	Makes pertinent entries on the client's record

Outcome: [ ] Pass   [ ] Fail

C = competent; A = acceptable; U = unsatisfactory

Comments: _____
_____
_____

_____   _____
Student's Signature   Date

_____   _____
Instructor's Signature   Date

III-6   *Providing foot and toenail care*

Toenails are an accessory structure of the integument and are composed of epithelial tissue. Healthy nails have a pink color and are convex, smooth, and evenly curved. Circulation and sensation to the feet tend to become compromised with certain diseases, such as diabetes mellitus and arteriosclerosis. Progressive vascular and neurologic changes occur with aging. The nurse may need to plan and implement the care of the feet and nails when the client can no longer do so safely by himself.

PURPOSES OF PROCEDURE

The nurse provides foot and nail care to

1. Cleanse and promote the comfort of the feet
2. Maintain the integrity of the integument
3. Stimulate circulation to the lower extremities
4. Prevent injury
5. Treat local infections by soaking the feet in a medicated solution

ASSESSMENT

OBJECTIVE DATA

- Read the chart to determine the client's predisposition to foot and nail problems due to aging, diabetes, and peripheral vascular disease.
- Review the agency's policy for cutting nails.
- Observe the client's standing posture and gait. Note whether the client limps or favors one foot.
- Note the color, temperature, and size of each foot; look for evidence of swelling, such as the imprint of the laces or the tongue of the shoe, an indentation at the shoe-top line, the impression of the stocking weave in the skin, or that the client is wearing slippers rather than shoes.
- Press the fingertips into the skin over the tibia. Observe if the skin rebounds immediately to its original contour.
- Feel and compare the quality, rhythm, and rate of the dorsalis pedis and posterior tibialis pulses bilaterally.
- Look for open lesions or scars from former lesions on the lower legs.
- Examine the nails for length, texture, contour, intactness, and cleanliness.
- Depress the nailbed of each great toe and observe the quality of capillary refill.
- Inspect the soft tissue around the nail; note if there is any redness, swelling, or drainage.
- Look between the toes for cracked skin, debris, or lesions that are not otherwise easily seen.
- Determine if there is an odor about the feet.
- Inspect the bottom of the foot for unhealed trauma or thickened areas that may be plantar warts.
- Look for foot problems that alter comfort, such as blisters, corns, calluses, bunions, or hammer toes.
- Determine if the client has adequate vision, strength, and coordination.

SUBJECTIVE DATA

- Ask the client to describe any history of nail or foot problems and their related treatments.
- Encourage the client to discuss his normal nail and foot care practices and preferences in foot wear.

• Inquire whether the client is experiencing any numbness or foot or nail discomfort. Also ask if he experiences stabbing leg pain with routine activity, such as walking, or leg cramps at night.

RELEVANT NURSING DIAGNOSES

The client in need of foot and nail care may have nursing diagnoses, such as

• *Altered Comfort*
• *Self-Care Deficit*
• *Altered Tissue Perfusion*
• *Potential for Infection*
• *Unilateral Neglect*
• *Impaired Skin Integrity*
• *Impaired Physical Mobility*
• *Knowledge Deficit*

PLANNING

ESTABLISHING PRIORITIES

Routine cleansing of the feet and periodic nail trimming can be performed when assisting the client with bathing. Since foot problems can lead to impaired mobility and inactivity, it is essential to maintain integrity and function of the feet. The nurse should inform the physician of the assessments indicating high-risk problems requiring other than nursing interventions. The client may be referred to a podiatrist, an individual with special training in the care of the feet.

SETTING GOALS

• The client's feet will be clean, warm, and dry.
• The client's toenails will be clean and short.
• The client's foot problems will show improvement with the daily implementation of the plan for care.
• The client will describe relief of soreness, itching, or discomfort.

PREPARATION OF EQUIPMENT

The nurse may select appropriate equipment from the following list:

Wash basin
Soap
Towels
Orange stick
Toenail clippers, manicuring scissors, emery board, or nail file
Lotion (optional)
Powder (optional)

Technique for providing foot and toenail care

ACTION	RATIONALE
1. Introduce yourself and state your purpose.	An explanation allays fears and aids in acquiring the client's cooperation.
2. Wash your hands.	Handwashing deters the spread of microorganisms.
3. Provide privacy.	Providing privacy demonstrates respect for the client's feelings.
4. Obtain objective and subjective data.	An appropriate plan for foot care cannot be individualized without pertinent data.
5. Discuss any identifiable foot and nail problems with the client.	The client should be informed of potential and actual health problems.
6. Present possible options involving foot and nail care.	The client is allowed the right to participate in the care plan.
7. Plan the foot and toenail care around the choices selected by the client.	Individualizing care can help ensure compliance.

8. Assemble the equipment.

Organization promotes efficient time management.

9. Protect the bed with towels beneath the feet or place a mat on the floor if the client can sit in a chair.

Towels absorb water and prevent damp linen or possible accidents due to falls.

10. Soak each foot separately in warm (40°C [105°F]) water for approximately 10 to 15 minutes, as the nurse in Figure III-6-1 is doing.

Soaking softens the nails and helps to loosen dry skin and debris. Warm water dilates blood vessels, which improves circulation and promotes comfort.

11. Wash each foot with liberal amounts of lathered soap.

Soap removes body oil, surface dirt, and microorganisms.

12. Change the water between the care of each foot.

The water should be clean and maintained at a temperature that promotes comfort.

13. Clean beneath the nail with an orange stick or nail file.

Dead cells and lint trapped between the nail and toe may require mechanical removal.

14. Cut the nail straight across and even with the tip of the toe, as shown in Figure III-6-2.

Cutting straight across is less likely to result in injury to adjacent tissue or potentiate the risk for ingrown nails.

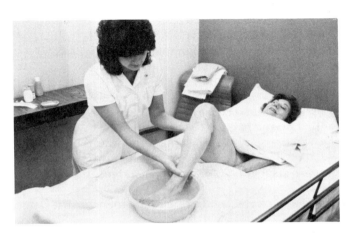

Figure III-6–1 The nurse helps the client place her foot into a basin of clean water prior to cleaning the feet and trimming the toenails.

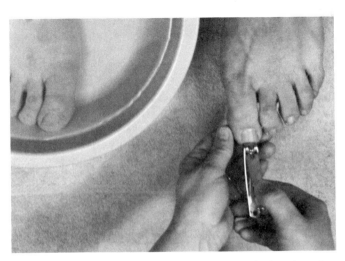

Figure III-6–2 The nurse cuts the toenail in a straight direction using nail clippers designed for trimming toenails rather than fingernails.

15. Dry each foot thoroughly.

Moisture supports the growth of fungi and can also tend to macerate skin if it cannot evaporate.

16. Apply lotion or powder to the legs or feet, if needed.

Lotion lubricates dry skin; powder absorbs perspiration.

17. Assist the client to don socks and shoes.

Socks absorb moisture and reduce friction from the shoe. Shoes provide support and prevent injury to the foot.

18. Dispose of the water and hygiene supplies; replace reusable equipment in its appropriate location.

Caring for soiled articles supports the principles of medical asepsis.

19. Wash your hands.

Handwashing deters the spread of microorganisms.

20. Chart the assessments, care given, and response of the client.

Written information is a permanent record of the care provided for the client.

SAMPLE DOCUMENTATION

Date	Time	Nurse's note
1/22	1430	Feet examined. Nails appear to extend $\frac{1}{4}''$ beyond toes. Client states, "I just can't bend over to cut them like I used to do." Feet are pink and warm. Skin is intact. Nails blanch and color returns immediately. Pedal and post. tibial pulses are strong and regular bilaterally. Feet soaked and nails trimmed. Client states, "I'm so glad that's taken care of."

O. McFee, RN

EVALUATION

REASSESSMENT

Observe the feet and nails daily when assisting the client with hygiene. If the feet are cold, pale, and pulseless, use a Doppler to verify that blood continues to circulate to the feet. Notify the physician immediately if assessments indicate an impairment in tissue perfusion.

EXPECTED OUTCOMES

The feet are clean, and the skin is intact.
The nails are clean and cut easily leaving no rough edges.

UNEXPECTED OUTCOMES

The nail clippers or scissors are not able to cut through tough, thick nails.
The toes appear cold, bluish, or dark black.
There are signs of trauma, inflammation, or infection.

MODIFICATIONS IN SELECTED SITUATIONS

GENERAL VARIATIONS

If the client is too restless to soak the feet in a basin of water, wrap the feet in damp towels and place each foot in a plastic bag for 10 to 15 minutes.
Rub calloused areas with a dry towel or use a pumice stone to remove the thickened outer layer of skin.
If the client cannot raise the foot for inspection of the plantar surface, the nurse can hold a mirror beneath the foot.
A miniature, electric, woodworking tool can be used to file tough toenails that cannot be trimmed by other means.
If the feet are sensitive to a water temperature of 40°C (105°F), first place each foot in tepid water and progressively add warmer water until the client can tolerate the desired temperature.
Chemicals, such as sodium bicarbonate, aluminum sulfate, calcium acetate, boric acid, magnesium sulfate, or potassium permanganate, can be prescribed as an additive to the water to sooth and relieve local infections and discomfort.

HOME-HEALTH VARIATIONS

Use a clean bucket or large plastic container, such as a dish pan, for a foot soak.
Test the temperature of the water by dripping it on the inner surface of the client's wrist or top of the foot before submerging the feet.
Follow the agency's policy and physician's order for cutting the toenails.

RELATED TEACHING

To control foot odor, instruct the client to wear clean socks daily. Rotating pairs of shoes provides time for moisture to evaporate.
Foot care products, such as arch supports and antifungal medications, can be purchased without a prescription. Tell the client that any condition that does not improve quickly with self-treatment warrants assessment by a physician or podiatrist.
Inform clients that the feet tend to swell as the day progresses. This could affect foot size and subsequent comfort when purchasing a new pair of shoes.
Wear newly purchased shoes for brief periods each day. This practice helps avoid blisters and discomfort from wearing unstretched shoes.
Leather shoes promote evaporation of foot moisture.
Explain that it is dangerous to go barefoot. Puncture wounds and other foot injuries can be avoided by wearing shoes.

Individuals with poor circulation should avoid the use of heating pads or electric blankets. The inability to perceive heat adequately makes them prone to burns. Advise these clients to wear socks to bed.

The dye or material used in the manufacture of socks and shoes can be an allergen for some hypersensitive individuals.

PERFORMANCE CHECKLIST

When providing care for the feet and toenails, the learner:

C	A	U	
[ ]	[ ]	[ ]	Greets the client and provides privacy
[ ]	[ ]	[ ]	Washes hands
[ ]	[ ]	[ ]	Obtains objective and subjective information
[ ]	[ ]	[ ]	Gathers equipment
[ ]	[ ]	[ ]	Positions the client either sitting or supine with the knees flexed
[ ]	[ ]	[ ]	Protects the area beneath the client's feet
[ ]	[ ]	[ ]	Fills the basin with warm water
[ ]	[ ]	[ ]	Places one foot at a time to soak approximately 10 minutes
[ ]	[ ]	[ ]	Washes the feet with soap and water
[ ]	[ ]	[ ]	Cleans beneath the nails
[ ]	[ ]	[ ]	Trims each nail straight and even with the toe
[ ]	[ ]	[ ]	Dries each foot, especially between the toes
[ ]	[ ]	[ ]	Massages the feet with lotion, if needed, or dusts the areas of the foot where skin surfaces touch with powder
[ ]	[ ]	[ ]	Assists the ambulatory client in donning socks and shoes
[ ]	[ ]	[ ]	Cares for soiled supplies
[ ]	[ ]	[ ]	Documents nursing assessments and care

Outcome: [ ] Pass   [ ] Fail

C = competent; A = acceptable; U = unsatisfactory

Comments: _____

_____

_____

_____   _____
Student's Signature   Date

_____   _____
Instructor's Signature   Date

III-7

Giving a back massage

A back massage is ordinarily given after a client is bathed. Most clients appreciate and enjoy this care. It is rare for a client to refuse a back massage. When this occurs, it is usually because the client feels that the massage will create an imposition on the nurse. The nurse should plan to provide adequate time so that the client does not feel that the nurse is rushed and needed elsewhere.

PURPOSES OF PROCEDURE

A back massage is given to

1. Nonverbally communicate a concern for the client's comfort
2. Stimulate blood flow to the skin and underlying tissues
3. Relax tense muscles
4. Promote rest or sleep

ASSESSMENT

OBJECTIVE DATA

- Review the client's chart to determine conditions that could be worsened if a back massage were provided. Examples are elevated blood pressure; tachycardia; increased intracranial pressure; back, rib, or neck injury; and surgery involving a flank incision.
- Read the medical orders to identify any restrictions in positioning the client.
- Inspect the skin integrity and color especially over bony prominences of the scapulae, vertebrae, or coccyx.

SUBJECTIVE DATA

- Inquire about any muscle tenderness or joint pain in the neck, shoulders, or vertebrae.
- Determine if the client would appreciate a back rub or prefers that it be omitted.

RELEVANT NURSING DIAGNOSES

Individuals who may benefit from a back massage are likely to have nursing diagnoses, such as

- *Anxiety*
- *Potential for Impaired Skin Integrity*
- *Sleep Pattern Disturbance*
- *Altered Comfort*
- *Impaired Physical Mobility*

PLANNING

ESTABLISHING PRIORITIES

The client who cannot turn and move about independently may need a massage over bony prominences each time his position is changed, which may be as frequently as every two hours. When the massage is provided as a comfort measure, it can be given just prior to periods of rest. Many find a back massage especially relaxing before bedtime.

SETTING GOALS

- The client's back will be massaged for a minimum of 4 to 6 minutes at least once each day.
- The blood flow to the skin of the back will increase.
- The client's muscles will feel less tense.

PREPARATION OF EQUIPMENT

The nurse is likely to need the following:

Massage lubricant or lotion
Powder
Bath blanket
Towel

Technique for giving a back massage

ACTION	RATIONALE
1. Explain the procedure and offer to give the client a back massage.	Offering rather than asking may make the client feel less reluctant to accept this aspect of care.
2. Wash your hands.	Handwashing deters the spread of microorganisms.
3. Close the curtain or door.	Privacy increases relaxation.
4. Assist the client to a prone or side-lying position with the back exposed. Use a bath blanket to drape the client. Raise the bed to a high position and lower the side rail closest to you.	Either of these positions exposes an adequate area for massage while maintaining privacy and warmth. Having the bed in high position reduces back strain for the nurse.
5. Warm the lubricant or lotion in the palm of your hand or place the container in warm water.	Cold lotion causes chilling and an uncomfortable sensation.
6. Using light strokes (*effleurage*), apply lotion to the client's shoulders, back, and sacral area.	Effleurage relaxes the client and lessens tension.
7. Place your hands beside each other at the base of the client's spine and stroke upward, as the nurse in Figure III-7-1 is doing, to the shoulders and back downward to the buttocks in slow, continuous strokes. Continue for 3 to 5 minutes.	Continuous hand contact is soothing and stimulates circulation and muscle relaxation.

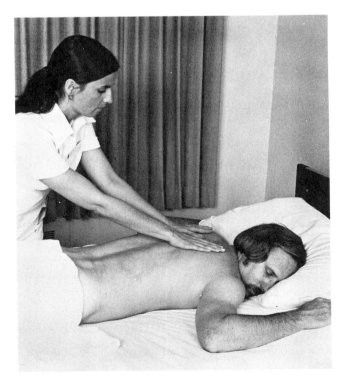

Figure III-7-1 The nurse uses long, firm strokes over the length of the back when giving a back rub. Note that she places her entire hand flat on the client's skin. The back massage should begin and end with this type of stroke.

8. Massage the shoulders, the entire back, areas over the iliac crests, and sacrum with circular stroking motions, shown in Figure III-7-2. Keep your hands in contact with the skin for 3 to 5 minutes, applying additional lotion as necessary.

Firmer strokes with continued hand contact promote relaxation.

9. Knead the skin, as shown in Figure III-7-3, by gently alternating grasping and compression motions, known as *pétrissage*.

Kneading increases circulation to areas.

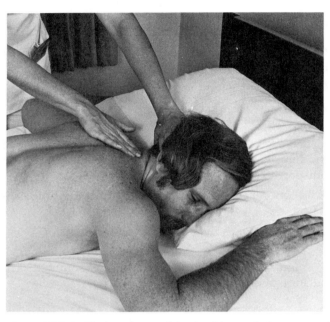

Figure III-7-2 The broad areas of the shoulders are being massaged using circular strokes.

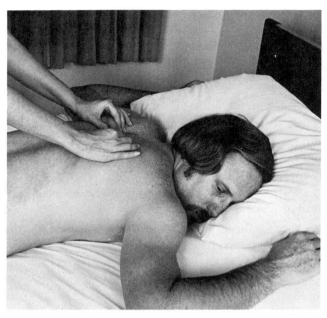

Figure III-7-3 Using the fingers to grasp and compress the skin is effective for stimulating the integument by increasing the blood flow to the skin.

10. Complete the massage with additional long stroking movements.

Long stroking motions are soothing and promote relaxation.

11. During the massage, observe the skin for reddened or open areas. Pay particular attention to skin over bony prominences. Avoid rubbing any areas that remain red after pressure has been relieved.

Pressure may interfere with circulation and lead to the development of decubitus ulcers. A back massage stimulates circulation to these areas. Rubbing skin that remains reddened can contribute to additional injury.

12. Use a towel to pat dry and remove excess lotion. Apply powder if the client requests it.

Removing excess lotion and applying powder provide additional comfort for the client.

13. Wash your hands.

Handwashing deters the spread of microorganisms.

14. Assess the client's response and record observations on the chart.

Accurate documentation provides a legal record of the care provided and the condition of the client.

SAMPLE DOCUMENTATION

Date	Time	Nurse's note
6/09	2100	Restlessness noted. Turned from supine to lateral position. Skin over scapulae and skin over coccyx appear red but blanch when pressure is relieved. Back massaged for 10 minutes. Presently sleeping.
		P. Swaboda, RN

EVALUATION

REASSESSMENT

During the massage, the nurse is likely to observe objective, beneficial effects to the skin and muscles. The nurse can infer from the client's rested appearance and relaxation in muscle tone that the massage promoted comfort and relief of tension. The client is likely to verbalize appreciation.

EXPECTED OUTCOMES

The client's skin is intact.
The client's state of arousal decreases and the client becomes relaxed.

UNEXPECTED OUTCOMES

The skin remains reddened over bony prominences despite the relief of pressure and therefore some areas are not massaged.
The client feels chilled.
The client remains tense and restless.

MODIFICATIONS IN SELECTED SITUATIONS

GENERAL VARIATIONS

Offer the client the opportunity to use the toilet, bedpan, or urinal to ensure that the massage and the relaxed feeling will be uninterrupted.
Pressure areas that are red and do not blanch should not be massaged since this may further separate the tissue layers and cause additional trauma to the skin.
The nurse may use *tapotement,* a massage stroke in which the skin is stimulated by lightly striking the skin with the side of the hands. It is not recommended for debilitated clients.
Include massaging the neck area up to the hairline when the client is unusually tense.
Alcohol can be used in lieu of lotion. It causes a cooling sensation because it promotes heat loss through evaporation. However, it dries the skin, which may be an undesirable effect for some clients.
Limit environmental stimuli, such as bright lights and loud noises, to promote relaxation.
If the massage is intended to relieve tension, avoid talking. The effect of the back massage can be further enhanced by playing recorded music or providing the client with headphones and a relaxation tape.

AGE-RELATED VARIATIONS

Touch is the primary source by which an infant perceives his environment. An infant who is irritable may be calmed by gently stroking the skin.
An infant's back can be massaged by positioning him on his abdomen over the nurse's lap.

HOME-HEALTH VARIATIONS

Intact skin is an indication that good circulation has been maintained. Encourage and praise family members and caregivers who provide back massage to the client on a routine basis.

RELATED TEACHING

Tell parents to avoid applying powder after an infant's skin has been bathed and massaged. The talc in the powder can be inhaled into the respiratory passages.
Explain that reddened skin over bony prominences that does not blanch should not be massaged. Instruct the client to avoid lying in positions that put pressure on the reddened areas.

(Performance checklist next page)

PERFORMANCE CHECKLIST

When a back massage is given, the learner:

C	A	U	
[ ]	[ ]	[ ]	Introduces self and explains the purpose of the procedure
[ ]	[ ]	[ ]	Provides privacy
[ ]	[ ]	[ ]	Assesses the client for objective and subjective information
[ ]	[ ]	[ ]	Raises the bed and lowers the nearer side rail
[ ]	[ ]	[ ]	Positions the client on the abdomen or side
[ ]	[ ]	[ ]	Exposes the client's back to the hip area
[ ]	[ ]	[ ]	Warms the lotion
[ ]	[ ]	[ ]	Applies the lotion to the back with light strokes
[ ]	[ ]	[ ]	Distributes the lotion across the surface of the back with long strokes from the sacrum to the shoulders and back again
[ ]	[ ]	[ ]	Administers firmer strokes over bony prominences
[ ]	[ ]	[ ]	Kneads areas that are especially affected by the pressure of body weight against the mattress
[ ]	[ ]	[ ]	Removes excess lotion with a towel
[ ]	[ ]	[ ]	Covers the client with bed clothes and linens
[ ]	[ ]	[ ]	Lowers the bed and raises the side rail
[ ]	[ ]	[ ]	Observes the response of the client
[ ]	[ ]	[ ]	Charts the care and any alterations that may affect a revision of the nursing care plan

Outcome: [ ] Pass   [ ] Fail

C = competent; A = acceptable; U = unsatisfactory

Comments: _____

_____

_____

_____   _____

Student's Signature   Date

_____   _____

Instructor's Signature   Date

III-8 *Providing perineal care*

The perineum is located in the area of the genitals and rectum. The area is dark, warm, and often moist, conditions that favor the production of odors and bacterial growth. Regular bathing promotes cleanliness. When a client cannot wash his or her own genitals and anal area, or this type of hygiene requires more skill than the client can provide, the nurse provides perineal care.

PURPOSES OF PROCEDURE

Perineal care is provided to

1. Cleanse the area of secretions and excretions
2. Reduce unpleasant odors
3. Prevent skin irritation and excoriation
4. Control the potential for infection
5. Promote comfort

ASSESSMENT

OBJECTIVE DATA

- Note any history of genital, urinary, or rectal pathology.
- Read the client's chart and review the laboratory data to determine the potential for transmitting pathogens.
- Using gloves, examine the genitalia for lesions, swelling, inflammation, excoriation, or discharge.
- Inspect the anal area for cracks, nodules, distended veins, masses, or polyps.
- Note the existence of unpleasant odor.
- Identify factors that indicate a greater potential for needing special perineal care, such as an indwelling urinary catheter.
- Determine if there are any sensory, cognitive, endurance, mobility, or motivational deficits that interfere with the client's ability to carry out personal hygiene measures independently.

SUBJECTIVE DATA

- Question the client about pain, soreness, tenderness, itching, or burning that he or she may be experiencing in the perineal area.
- Ask the client to discuss any special perineal hygiene practices performed, such as douching or sitz baths, the frequency of the practices, and the products used.
- Request that the client describe usual patterns of bowel and bladder elimination.
- Ask a female client to identify her reproductive history, such as the date of the last menstrual period and the pattern of her menstrual cycles. Obtain the approximate date of the last pelvic and Pap examinations.
- Inquire of male clients if they are familiar with the techniques for performing testicular self-examination.

RELEVANT NURSING DIAGNOSES

Depending on the information gathered by the nurse, the client needing perineal care may have nursing diagnoses, such as

- *Altered Bowel Elimination*
- *Altered Patterns of Urinary Elimination*
- *Total, Urge, or Stress Incontinence*
- *Self-Care Deficit*
- *Disturbance in Self-Concept*
- *Altered Sexuality Patterns*

301

- *Potential for Infection*
- *Knowledge Deficit*

PLANNING

ESTABLISHING PRIORITIES

The nurse should plan daily or more frequent measures with the client that will maintain or restore optimal cleanliness, integrity of the tissue, and the client's sense of well-being.

SETTING GOALS

- The client's perineal area will be clean and intact.
- Signs of skin impairment, inflammation, and infection will become decreased or absent.
- The client will perform appropriate perineal hygiene independently.

PREPARATION OF EQUIPMENT

When providing perineal care, the nurse will need items from the following list:

Wash basin
Soap
Washcloth, cotton balls (optional)
Towels
Bath blanket
Protective bed pad
Bedpan
Paper tissues
Disposable gloves

Technique for providing perineal care

ACTION	RATIONALE
1. Introduce yourself and explain your intentions.	Exchanging information allays fears and promotes co-operation.
2. Wash your hands.	Handwashing deters the spread of microorganisms.
3. Provide for privacy and ask questions that enable the acquisition of subjective data.	Most individuals are especially sensitive in discussing information about anal and genital structures.
4. Position the client in a supine position.	A supine position facilitates inspection of the genitalia.
5. Don gloves to examine the perineal structures.	Gloves act as a transmission barrier to pathogens.
6. Reposition the client in a side-lying position.	A side-lying position provides better inspection of the anal area.
7. Remove gloves, discard them in a lined receptacle, and assist the client to a position of comfort.	To control the spread of pathogens, the gloves should be removed before handling clean equipment.
8. Wash your hands.	Handwashing deters the spread of microorganisms.
9. Bring equipment and supplies to the bedside.	Organization promotes efficient time management.
10. Protect the bed with an absorbent pad.	Cleansing may wet or soil an unprotected bed.
11. Place the client on a bedpan in a dorsal recumbent position.	A bedpan will collect the water used during perineal cleansing.
12. Drape the client with a bath blanket to permit exposing just the perineal area.	The nurse provides warmth and is respectful of the client's modesty.
13. Don clean gloves.	Gloves prevent transferring microorganisms from the client to the nurse and other susceptible clients.
14. Flush the area with warm (40°C [105°F]) water or a soapy solution until the area is clean.	Water dissolves or dilutes dried secretions. Soap emulsifies fatty substances on the skin and reduces the ability of microbes to grow and multiply.

15. Wash the area with a washcloth or cotton balls if the area is not sufficiently cleansed, as shown in Figures III-8-1 and III-8-2.

Manual cleansing may be required to remove debris and secretions from the skin.

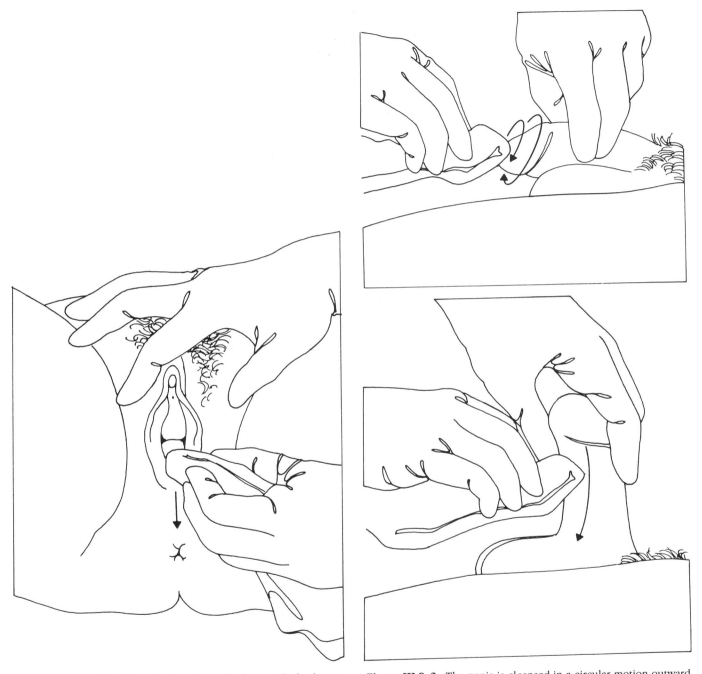

Figure III-8–1 The client is placed on a bedpan with the knees flexed to expose the vulva and perineum. A separate cotton ball or corner of the washcloth is used for each stroke. The area is cleansed from the pubis toward the anal area to avoid introducing intestinal organisms into the urinary meatus or vagina.

Figure III-8–2 The penis is cleansed in a circular motion outward from the meatus. The foreskin of an uncircumcized male should be retracted prior to cleaning and replaced afterward.

16. Move the cotton balls with sufficient firmness.

Light stroking may cause tickling and do little to remove soiled material.

17. Use a clean cotton ball or area of the washcloth for each stroke.

Using a clean surface prevents redistributing secretions and organisms from one area to another.

18. Wash away from the area of the urinary meatus. For a female, wash from the pubic area toward the anus. For a male, wash in a circle from the tip of the penis, taking care to retract the foreskin of an uncircumcised client.

Care is taken to avoid introducing secretions and bacteria into the opening through which urine is released. Contamination of this area can lead to a urinary tract infection.

19. Rinse the scrubbed areas well with plain water. Remove the client from the bedpan.

Rinsing removes loosened secretions, organisms, and cleaning solution.

20. Dry the area with a towel.

Moisture supports the growth of microorganisms and contributes to discomfort.

21. Replace the foreskin over the glans penis of an uncircumcised male.

Failure to replace the foreskin can cause injury to the penis.

22. Wash, rinse, and dry the male client's scrotum and the groin areas of both male and female clients.

Secretions may accumulate in the folds of skin beneath and surrounding the genitals.

23. Turn the client to the side; wash, rinse, and dry the anal area, as shown in Figure III-8-3.

The anus is washed last because it has the highest potential for the presence of microorganisms.

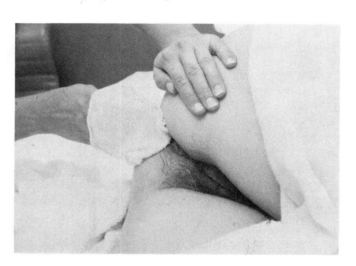

Figure III-8-3 The client is turned to a side-lying position to finish cleaning the anal area. Washing from a cleaner area to one that is more soiled follows the principles of medical asepsis.

24. Apply lotion as needed.

An emollient helps to soothe excoriated tissue.

25. Discard the soiled water; clean the equipment; dispose of soiled gloves.

Controlling the spread of pathogens is a primary principle of asepsis.

26. Wash your hands.

Handwashing deters the spread of microorganisms.

27. Document objective and subjective findings, the implemented nursing orders, and the client's response.

Written information documents the individualized care of the client.

SAMPLE DOCUMENTATION

Date	Time	Nurse's note
8/21	1000	Mod. amt. of pink drainage noted on peri-pad. Episiotomy and perineum are swollen. External hemorrhoids noted. Perineal care provided. Client states, "That warm water makes me feel so much better." *E. Pappas, RN*

EVALUATION

REASSESSMENT

Utilize the time when assisting the client with bathing or elimination to reexamine perineal structures. If the goals are not being met or new problems are identified, the nurse should revise the plan for care.

EXPECTED OUTCOMES

The client's perineum is cleansed daily, at the time of bathing, after elimination, and when secretions are apparent.

The client learns and performs perineal care.

UNEXPECTED OUTCOMES

The perineal area is continuously soiled, causing the skin to become reddened and macerated.

There is a persistent, unpleasant odor about the client.

MODIFICATIONS IN SELECTED SITUATIONS

GENERAL VARIATIONS

Provide the client the opportunity for bowel and bladder elimination prior to the perineal care.

A portable sitz bath may be used for cleansing the perineal area rather than positioning the client on a bedpan.

Medication, such as aerosol antiseptics or pads saturated with witch hazel, may be applied to perineal or rectal incisions.

Perineal pads may be used to absorb drainage after the area has been cleansed and dried.

HOME-HEALTH VARIATIONS

Instruct and demonstrate how to provide perineal care to the client's caregivers. Emphasize the importance of performing this daily or more frequently if needed.

Obtain an order from the physician if a douche, a vaginal irrigation, would promote further cleanliness of the area.

RELATED TEACHING

Stress the importance of good handwashing to the client following urinary or bowel elimination.

Explain that ovulating women secrete an odorless, clear, mucoid discharge midway in the menstrual cycle. This is normal and should not be confused with a vaginal infection. Any vaginal drainage that has an unpleasant odor or causes itching or skin irritation should be assessed by a physician.

Explain that routine vaginal irrigation, also known as a *douche,* is unnecessary and, in fact, can be harmful. The vagina is protected from infection by helpful microbes that maintain an acid environment within that cavity. Irrigation can reduce the number of these organisms.

Instruct women that regular bathing is usually sufficient for controlling odors. Use of feminine hygiene products has caused tissue irritation and allergic reactions in some individuals.

(Performance checklist next page)

PERFORMANCE CHECKLIST

When providing perineal care, the learner:

C   A   U

C	A	U	
[ ]	[ ]	[ ]	Introduces self and identifies the purpose of the interaction
[ ]	[ ]	[ ]	Provides privacy
[ ]	[ ]	[ ]	Asks the client questions that provide subjective data
[ ]	[ ]	[ ]	Dons gloves
[ ]	[ ]	[ ]	Examines the client's genitalia, perineum, and rectal areas
[ ]	[ ]	[ ]	Removes and discards gloves
[ ]	[ ]	[ ]	Washes hands
[ ]	[ ]	[ ]	Assembles equipment
[ ]	[ ]	[ ]	Raises the bed and lowers the nearer side rail
[ ]	[ ]	[ ]	Positions the client
[ ]	[ ]	[ ]	Drapes the client with a bath blanket
[ ]	[ ]	[ ]	Protects the bed
[ ]	[ ]	[ ]	Places the client on the bedpan
[ ]	[ ]	[ ]	Dons gloves if there is the possibility that contact will be made with blood or body secretions
[ ]	[ ]	[ ]	Cleanses the perineum with poured solution, soapy water, and washcloth or cotton balls
[ ]	[ ]	[ ]	Rinses and dries the cleansed areas
[ ]	[ ]	[ ]	Removes the bedpan
[ ]	[ ]	[ ]	Turns the client to the side
[ ]	[ ]	[ ]	Cleans, rinses, and dries the anal area
[ ]	[ ]	[ ]	Repositions the client
[ ]	[ ]	[ ]	Lowers the bed and raises the side rail
[ ]	[ ]	[ ]	Removes soiled equipment
[ ]	[ ]	[ ]	Washes hands
[ ]	[ ]	[ ]	Charts pertinent information

Outcome: [ ] Pass   [ ] Fail

C = competent; A = acceptable; U = unsatisfactory

Comments: _____
_____
_____

_____
Student's Signature   Date

_____
Instructor's Signature   Date

III-9

Shaving the skin of the preoperative client (dry shave and wet shave)

Intact skin is the body's first line of defense against microorganisms. An alteration in skin integrity provides a potential risk of infection. Because surgery involves opening the skin, precautions are taken to prevent the entry of microorganisms. Body hair serves as a reservoir for bacteria and therefore is removed from a wide area of the skin before surgery. The hair may be removed by shaving with a razor, hair clippers, or use of depilatory cream. Shaving with a razor has been found to cause microabrasions that can be colonized by bacteria, thus increasing the potential for infection.

PURPOSES OF PROCEDURE

The skin of the preoperative client is shaved to

1. Reduce the potential for postoperative infection
2. Provide comfort when removing tape used to secure the dressing over the surgical wound

ASSESSMENT

OBJECTIVE DATA

- Consult the surgical schedule to determine the specific operative procedure that has been scheduled for the client.
- Review the agency's policy concerning preoperative skin preparation.
- Determine any alterations in policy that have been written by the client's surgeon.
- Consult the agency's diagram, such as that shown in Figure III-9-1, indicating the anatomical area from which hair is removed for certain surgical procedures.
- Inspect the skin; note the integrity of the skin and the presence of a rash, moles, or lesions.

SUBJECTIVE DATA

- Determine if the client has ever had surgery before and his recollection of the experience.
- Ask if the client's skin was shaved prior to previous surgical procedures and any positive or negative aspects that resulted from this.

RELEVANT NURSING DIAGNOSES

The client whose skin is being prepared preoperatively may have nursing diagnoses, such as

- *Anxiety*
- *Fear*
- *Altered Comfort*
- *Potential for Infection*
- *Knowledge Deficit*
- *Potential for Impaired Skin Integrity*

PLANNING

ESTABLISHING PRIORITIES

Wet shaving the skin was once done routinely the evening before surgery. It is now most often done immediately before the operation, often in the surgical holding area. Since a dry shave is less likely to cause an impairment in the integrity of the skin, the agency's protocol should be followed for planning and performing the procedure.

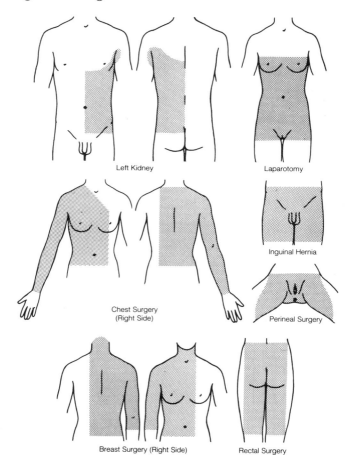

Left Kidney

Laparotomy

Chest Surgery
(Right Side)

Inguinal Hernia

Perineal Surgery

Breast Surgery (Right Side)

Rectal Surgery

Figure III-9–1 Areas that are ordinarily shaved preoperatively for various types of surgery. Follow the physician's order or local policy, which may differ slightly at times from the areas designated here.

SETTING GOALS

- The client's hair will be removed in a wide distance surrounding the potential incision site.
- The client's skin will remain intact.

PREPARATION OF EQUIPMENT

The nurse will need selected items from either of the two lists below:

WET SHAVE
Adequate lighting
Bath blanket
Prep kit containing
    Razor
    Sponge soaked with antiseptic soap
    Waterproof pad
    Basin
    Cotton-tipped applicator

DRY SHAVE
Adequate lighting
Bath blanket
Electric clippers
Scissors
Antiseptic solution and applicator (if ordered)

Technique for dry shaving the skin of the preoperative client

ACTION	RATIONALE
1. Explain the procedure to the client.	An explanation facilitates cooperation and provides reassurance for the client.
2. Assemble the equipment. Expose the area to be shaved, and drape the client appropriately.	Having equipment in readiness saves time. Draping the client provides for privacy.
3. Wash your hands.	Handwashing deters the spread of microorganisms.
4. Shave with the clippers.	Clipping hair minimizes the risk of abrasions in the operative area.
5. Move the drape and continue shaving until the entire area is shaved.	Draping provides for the client's privacy.
6. Brush off the remaining hair with a towel.	Brushing minimizes skin irritation and improves the client's comfort.
7. If an antiseptic solution is ordered, use cotton-tipped applicators to clean in skin crevices, such as the groin or umbilicus.	This is an additional protection against microorganisms that may accumulate in crevices.
8. Discard equipment according to agency policy. Cleanse electric clippers by wiping them with antiseptic solution.	Discarding disposable equipment prevents transmitting microorganisms. Antiseptic solution retards the growth of microbes.
9. Wash your hands.	Handwashing deters the spread of microorganisms.
10. Record the completion of the skin preparation.	Charting provides documentation of the care that was provided for the client.

Technique for wet shaving the skin of the preoperative client

ACTION	RATIONALE
1. Follow Steps 1, 2, and 3 for a dry shave.	
2. Place a waterproof pad under the area to be shaved.	Waterproof material protects the bed linens from becoming damp.
3. Apply the soap solution to small areas of the skin and work up a lather.	Soap emulsifies normal fatty substances on the skin and loosens dirt so that water can penetrate and soften the hair.
4. Shave with one hand while gently stretching the skin taut with the other hand, as shown in Figure III-9-2. Hold the razor at an angle between 30 degrees and 45 degrees, and take long, gentle strokes in the direction of hair growth. Rinse the hair and soap from the razor as necessary.	Stretching the skin eliminates wrinkles and smooths the skin so that the nurse can accomplish a close shave. Gentle, long strokes with the razor held at a 30-degree to 45-degree angle help prevent nicking and cutting the skin. Shaving in the direction of hair growth helps minimize skin irritation.
5. Continue moving the drape until the entire area is shaved. Replace the razor if it becomes dull.	Moving the drape provides for the client's privacy. A sharp edge on the razor reduces the risk of injury.
6. Use a washcloth and warm water to remove any excess soap and remaining hair. Dry the skin carefully.	Removing excess soap and hair minimizes skin irritation.

7. Stoop, as the nurse in Figure III-9-3 is doing, so that your eyes are at the level of the shaven area to check for isolated hairs that may have been missed by the razor.

Looking at the area with the eyes at the level of the skin helps in checking whether all the hair has been removed.

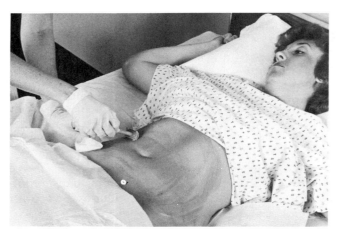

Figure III-9-2 Note that the nurse holds the razor at an angle of approximately 45 degrees. The skin is pulled sufficiently to remove any wrinkles and to provide a smooth area over which to move the razor. This nurse wears gloves as a transmission barrier in case there may be contact with the client's blood.

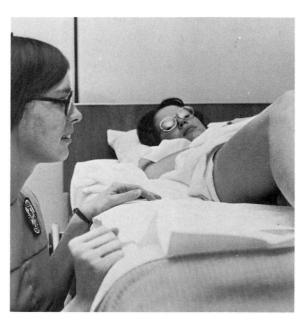

Figure III-9-3 After completing the shave, the nurse stoops so that her eyes are at the level of the area that was shaved. She then inspects the skin carefully to be sure that all the hair has been removed.

8. Report any cuts in the skin to the physician or charge person.

Cuts in the skin may be a potential source of infection.

9. Follow Steps 8, 9, and 10 of the dry shave procedure.

SAMPLE DOCUMENTATION

Date	Time	Nurse's note
2/25	0630	Appendectomy scheduled for 0800. Skin wet shaved from nipple line to pubis. Skin remains intact. No evidence of hair remaining in shaved area. *A. Timm, RN*

EVALUATION

REASSESSMENT

After shaving it is helpful to examine the shaved area closely to determine if the skin is free of hair. A flashlight or other light source may be held close to the skin to improve the ability to evaluate the success of hair removal.

EXPECTED OUTCOMES

No hair can be seen in the shaved area.
The skin shows no evidence of bleeding.
The client is warm and dry.

UNEXPECTED OUTCOMES

Hair remains in patchy areas across the shaven skin.

There are obvious cuts and bleeding caused by the razor.

The client experiences discomfort when hair is caught in the clippers.

MODIFICATIONS IN SELECTED SITUATIONS

GENERAL VARIATIONS

Shorten the length of long hair with scissors before attempting to shave the client's skin.

The client may bathe or shower before the shave using an antibacterial soap. In some cases, the client can be instructed to scrub the potential operative area for a specific number of minutes.

A shower can be taken after the skin is shaved.

Following the skin shave before an orthopedic operative procedure, the area may be wrapped with sterile roller gauze, as shown in Figure III-9-4. The gauze is secured, as illustrated in Figure III-9-5, by taping sterile towels about the area. These rigid precautions are followed because infections within bone and joint structures are extremely difficult to treat and cure.

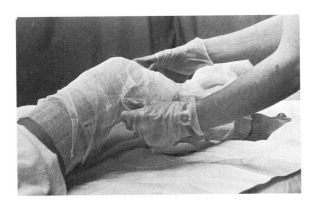

Figure III-9-4 Sterile gauze dressings are applied to the entire area that has been shaved before orthopedic surgery.

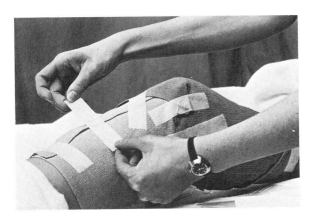

Figure III-9-5 The nurse completes the preoperative skin preparation before orthopedic surgery by securing the sterile gauze dressings with sterile towels. Notice how strips of tape are used along the long axis of the leg to hold the sterile materials in place.

When cranial surgery or surgery about the ears will be performed, it is a common practice to require written permission from the client to cut and shave the hair. Some may want the hair as a keepsake, especially when the client is a child, or use the hair for wig construction.

AGE-RELATED VARIATIONS

To reduce anxiety and fear, let a child hear the sound that electric clippers produce before using them to shave the hair.

Let the child feel the vibration produced by the clippers.

HOME-HEALTH VARIATIONS

If the client is scheduled for outpatient surgery, teach the client or a family member when and how the skin should be prepared prior to coming for the surgical procedure.

RELATED TEACHING   Inform the client that the hair will grow back in the same texture and distribution as it appeared before shaving.

PERFORMANCE CHECKLIST

When shaving the skin of the preoperative client, the learner:

C	A	U	
[ ]	[ ]	[ ]	Introduces self and identifies the purpose for the interaction
[ ]	[ ]	[ ]	Checks the identity of the client by reading the name on the wristband
[ ]	[ ]	[ ]	Provides privacy
[ ]	[ ]	[ ]	Assesses the client
[ ]	[ ]	[ ]	Assembles the equipment
[ ]	[ ]	[ ]	Washes hands
[ ]	[ ]	[ ]	Raises the bed and lowers the nearer side rail
[ ]	[ ]	[ ]	Drapes the client for warmth and modesty
[ ]	[ ]	[ ]	Exposes the skin that requires shaving
[ ]	[ ]	[ ]	Lathers the skin (omit for dry shave)
[ ]	[ ]	[ ]	Removes hair with razor or hair clippers
[ ]	[ ]	[ ]	Rinses shaved skin, or brushes off hair if dry shave was performed
[ ]	[ ]	[ ]	Applies antiseptic (if ordered)
[ ]	[ ]	[ ]	Inspects shaved skin
[ ]	[ ]	[ ]	Lowers the bed and raises the side rail
[ ]	[ ]	[ ]	Cares for the used equipment
[ ]	[ ]	[ ]	Washes hands
[ ]	[ ]	[ ]	Charts pertinent information

Outcome: [ ] **Pass**   [ ] **Fail**

C = competent; A = acceptable; U = unsatisfactory

Comments: _____

_____

_____

_____   _____

Student's Signature   Date

_____   _____

Instructor's Signature   .   Date

III-10   *Applying binders*

Binders are designed for covering a specific body part. Binders may be made of cloth, such as flannel or muslin, or of elasticized material that fastens together with Velcro. Examples of binders include slings, abdominal binders, chest binders, and T-binders.

PURPOSES OF PROCEDURE

Binders are applied to

1. Hold dressings in place
2. Support a part of the body
3. Protect an injured area
4. Prevent additional injury
5. Promote comfort and a sense of security

ASSESSMENT

OBJECTIVE DATA

- Note the client's level of activity and posture.
- Observe if the client uses another part of the body, like a hand or arm, to protect or support a painful part of the body.
- Inspect the client's incision, if there is one, for separation, swelling, and characteristics of any drainage.
- Percuss or palpate the abdomen for distention. Auscultate the location and quality of bowel sounds.
- Examine areas where tape has been used for signs of redness, rash, or injured skin.
- Examine an injured area for color, swelling, and signs of ecchymosis.

SUBJECTIVE DATA

- Ask the client to describe any pain he or she is experiencing about the injured area.
- Touch the area lightly so as not to cause pain and ask the client to indicate ability to perceive the sensation.

RELEVANT NURSING DIAGNOSES

The client in need of a binder may have nursing diagnoses, such as

- *Activity Intolerance*
- *Altered Comfort*
- *Impaired Physical Mobility*
- *Ineffective Breathing Patterns*
- *Impaired Skin or Tissue Integrity*

PLANNING

ESTABLISHING PRIORITIES

A binder should be applied as soon as possible to relieve swelling, pain, or other conditions that interfere with the client's basic needs for effective breathing, comfort, and movement.

SETTING GOALS

- The affected body part will be supported above and below the injury.
- The bound area will have adequate circulation and manifest progressive healing.
- The client's activity will be accompanied by decreased discomfort.

PREPARATION OF EQUIPMENT

The nurse should gather the following:

Binder (The type will vary depending on the body area that will be covered.)
Safety pins
Wash basin, soap, washcloth, and towel (optional)
Gauze pads (optional)

Technique for applying binders

ACTION	RATIONALE
1. Introduce yourself, provide privacy, and explain your purpose.	Explanation is more apt to allay the client's fears and promote cooperation.
2. Gather assessment data.	Assessment is the essential first step for identifying the client's problems.
3. Wash your hands.	Handwashing deters the spread of microorganisms.
4. Select a binder designed for covering a particular body part.	Binders are available in a variety of sizes and shapes depending on the client's individual needs.
5. Assist the client to assume a comfortable position that facilitates application of the binder; for most clients this will be a supine or dorsal recumbent position.	Applying a binder while the client is lying down prevents its slipping out of place.
6. Place the body part in a neutral position.	Avoiding extreme flexion or hyperextension prevents deformities and discomfort, and enhances circulation.
7. Clean and dry the area thoroughly.	Prolonged heat and moisture on the skin may cause epithelial cells to deteriorate.
8. Use absorbent material to separate any two skin surfaces that touch one another.	Padding absorbs moisture and reduces skin irritation or breakdown. It also promotes separate healing for surfaces that may each contain an open wound.
9. Pad body prominences over which the binder is placed. Fill hollows in the body contour with padding.	Padding cushions and distributes pressure equally over all skin surfaces. It promotes comfort and prevents skin breakdown.
10. Begin enclosing the lowest point of the body part moving upward, as shown in Figure III-10-1.	Proceeding from lower areas to higher ones promotes venous circulation.

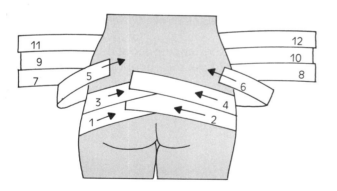

Figure III-10–1 This scultetus, or many-tailed binder, is used to support the abdomen. Each tail crisscrosses the abdomen from side to side.

ACTION	RATIONALE
11. Apply the binder with sufficient pressure, using neither too little nor too much. Avoid applying a binder on the chest too snugly.	Sufficient pressure provides for adequate support and ensures that the binder will remain in place. Too much pressure may interfere with circulation or breathing, and may cause discomfort.
12. Ask the client to breathe deeply or indicate level of comfort before securing the binder.	Adjustments can be made if the binder is too tight or too loose.
13. Place pins used to secure the binder well away from the wound or sensitive area.	A pin is rigid and may cause additional discomfort in an area that is already painful.
14. Tie knots so as not to cause pressure on a bony prominence.	Pressure from a knot may interfere with circulation and can cause injury to skin and underlying nerves.
15. Wash your hands.	Handwashing deters the spread of microorganisms.

16. Record your assessments, the care provided, and the client's response.

Written documentation provides a narrative of the client's care and treatment.

SAMPLE DOCUMENTATION

Date	Time	Nurse's note
7/14	1300	Abdominal incision cleansed with Betadine swabs. Edges are clean with sm. amt. of serous drainage. Skin in areas where tape has been used to secure the dressing is red. Patchy areas of skin have separated with tape removal. Dry sterile dressing secured with an abdominal binder.

C. Gilroy, RN

EVALUATION

REASSESSMENT

A severely swollen area should be evaluated at frequent intervals. The nurse documents the color, sensation, temperature, and presence of a peripheral pulse. A binder that covers a wound should be inspected for wrinkles, loosening, slipping, and drainage several times during the shift, especially after the client has been ambulating.

EXPECTED OUTCOMES

The binder is clean and free of wrinkles.
The client can breathe and move adequately.
The injured area retains adequate blood supply and venous return is not restricted.
Wound edges remain approximated.
The client expresses feeling comfortable.

UNEXPECTED OUTCOMES

The binder is loose, tight, or wrinkled.
The client's chest expansion is restricted.
The area below the binder becomes pale, cyanotic, or more swollen.
The client states that the binder increases discomfort.

MODIFICATIONS IN SELECTED SITUATIONS

GENERAL VARIATIONS

Tucks may need to be formed into the fabric of a breast or abdominal binder with safety pins to accommodate curves in various body areas.
Place additional absorbent dressings under the binder at the bottom of an incision where drainage is likely to accumulate when the client ambulates.
A binder can be reused until it becomes soiled or wet.
A supportive bra can be used as a breast binder.
Different T-binders are designed for male and female use. Figure III-10-2 shows a single T-binder used for women and a double T-binder as it would be used for men.

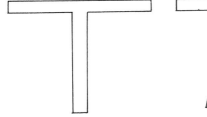 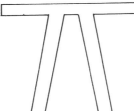

Figure III-10-2 These binders resemble the letter **T**. They are used to hold a perineal dressing in place. The double T-binder is more useful for elevating and supporting the scrotum.

AGE-RELATED VARIATIONS

Stretchable, tubular stockinet can be used as a binder for an infant or child. Select the width that will best encircle the youngster's body part without becoming loose.

HOME-HEALTH
VARIATIONS

A towel or discarded sheeting material can be substituted for commercially manufactured binders.

Periodically reinforce prior teaching to include removing the binder, inspecting the condition of the skin, bathing the area, and reapplying the binder.

RELATED TEACHING

Inform the client that sutures ordinarily are of sufficient strength to maintain wound closure.

Explain that swelling and discomfort are expected immediately following trauma or surgery. Using a binder for elevation or support can promote circulation that will relieve these problems.

PERFORMANCE CHECKLIST

When applying a binder, the learner:

C	A	U	
[ ]	[ ]	[ ]	Washes hands
[ ]	[ ]	[ ]	Explains the intention of the interaction
[ ]	[ ]	[ ]	Provides privacy
[ ]	[ ]	[ ]	Gathers assessment data
[ ]	[ ]	[ ]	Provides the client with an explanation for the purpose of using a binder
[ ]	[ ]	[ ]	Obtains the appropriate type of binder
[ ]	[ ]	[ ]	Raises the bed and lowers the nearer side rail
[ ]	[ ]	[ ]	Places the client in an appropriate position for applying the binder
[ ]	[ ]	[ ]	Utilizes padding for comfort and protection
[ ]	[ ]	[ ]	Secures the binder from lower to upper body areas
[ ]	[ ]	[ ]	Avoids pinning or tying knots where they will cause discomfort or potentiate circulatory or respiratory complications
[ ]	[ ]	[ ]	Determines the client's state of comfort
[ ]	[ ]	[ ]	Lowers the bed and raises the side rail
[ ]	[ ]	[ ]	Washes hands
[ ]	[ ]	[ ]	Charts pertinent information

Outcome: [ ] Pass [ ] Fail

C = competent; A = acceptable; U = unsatisfactory

Comments: _____

_____

_____

_____

_____   _____
Student's Signature   Date

_____   _____
Instructor's Signature   Date

III-11 *Applying a roller bandage*

A roller bandage is a continuous strip of woven cloth, gauze, or elastic fabric wound on itself to form a cylinder or roll. Roller bandages are available in various widths and lengths.

PURPOSES OF PROCEDURE

A roller bandage is used to

1. Maintain a thick, bulky dressing in place
2. Aid in attaching mechanical immobilizing devices, such as splints or traction
3. Limit motion in a sore or injured area of the body
4. Reduce pain and promote comfort

ASSESSMENT

OBJECTIVE DATA

- Examine and compare the appearance of the injured body part with a comparable uninjured area; note color, temperature, size, and alignment.
- Bilaterally depress the nailbed of an injured extremity and observe the quality of blood refill.
- Palpate the rate and quality of all peripheral pulses below the injury.
- Inspect the skin or wound for color and characteristics of any drainage.
- Note any restriction in movement.
- Estimate the area that will require bandaging.

SUBJECTIVE DATA

- Ask the client to describe any pain or numbness he or she may be experiencing.

RELEVANT NURSING DIAGNOSES

The client who requires the application of a roller bandage may have nursing diagnoses, such as

- *Altered Comfort*
- *Impaired Physical Mobility*
- *Self-Care Deficit*
- *Impaired Skin or Tissue Integrity*
- *Altered Tissue Perfusion*

PLANNING

ESTABLISHING PRIORITIES

Pain and additional injury can be prevented by the application of a roller bandage. The skin should be cleaned and dressed before any roller bandage is applied. Since a dependent position can interfere with venous return, the nurse should plan, if at all possible, to apply a roller bandage before a client assumes an upright position in the morning. If this is not possible, elevate the area higher than the heart for about 15 to 20 minutes.

SETTING GOALS

- The client's dressing will be covered and maintained in place over the wound.
- The client's localized swelling will be reduced.
- Circulation will remain adequate.
- The client will indicate a reduction in pain or discomfort.

PREPARATION OF EQUIPMENT

The nurse will need

Roller bandages (The type, number, and width depend on the purpose for its use and the body part that will be covered.)

Clips, safety pins, or tape
Wash basin, soap, washcloth, and towels
Gauze padding (optional)
Dressing supplies, including clean and sterile gloves (optional if there is a wound)

Technique for applying a roller bandage

ACTION	RATIONALE
1. Introduce yourself and state your purpose.	Providing information reduces fear and promotes co-operation.
2. Provide privacy.	The nurse protects the client from the view of others.
3. Wash your hands.	Handwashing deters the spread of microorganisms.
4. Gather assessment data.	Assessment is the essential first step for identifying the client's problems.
5. Bring supplies to the bedside.	Organization promotes efficient time management.
6. Wash and dry the skin that will be covered by the roller bandage.	Prolonged heat and moisture on the skin may cause epithelial cells to deteriorate.
7. Change any preexisting dressing following the description in Procedure III-17.	Warm, soiled dressings support the growth of microorganisms.
8. Separate skin surfaces that touch one another with absorbent gauze padding.	Absorbing moisture reduces skin irritation or breakdown. It also prevents the two surfaces from adhering to each other during healing.
9. Elevate and support the area so that the roller bandage can be easily wrapped around the body part.	Elevation promotes venous return. Support reduces muscle fatigue.
10. Place joints in a slightly flexed, neutral position.	Slight flexion promotes comfort and functional use.
11. Hold the free end of the roll in place with one hand while the other hand passes the roll around the body part, as shown in Figure III-11-1.	Encircling the free end of the roll anchors the bandage.

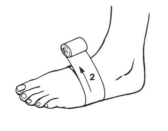

Figure III-11–1   A circular turn helps secure the beginning end of the roller bandage.

12. Leave a small portion of an extremity, such as the fingers or toes, exposed.	The fingers or toes provide an accessible area for assessing the circulation through the bandaged area.
13. Cover the heel when bandaging the foot.	Leaving the heel exposed is likely to impede circulation in that one area because there would be a difference in the pressure gradient.
14. Use equal tension and continue overlapping one half to two thirds of the width of the roller bandage in various patterns, such as the spiral turn in Figure III-11-2.	Maintaining the same amount of tension helps promote the unencumbered flow of blood back to the heart. Pockets of edematous tissue are not likely to form. The client is less likely to experience discomfort.
15. Wrap from the distal to the proximal direction of a body part.	Wrapping in a distal to proximal direction helps prevent venous blood from pooling and becoming trapped in the lower wrapped areas.

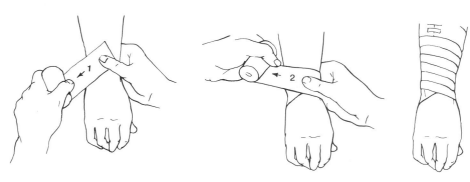

Figure III-11-2 A spiral turn is made by wrapping the roller bandage in an oblique angle about the area.

16. Secure the roller bandage with metal clips, tape, or safety pins well away from a bony prominence, where the client is likely to lie on it, or a tender and inflamed area.

Pressure from clips or pins is uncomfortable, may interfere with circulation, and may cause injury to the skin and nerve tissue.

17. Reassess the client's level of comfort.

The client's response is a good indication that the bandage is not being applied too tightly.

18. Wash your hands.

Handwashing deters the spread of microorganisms.

19. Document the assessments, care given, and the client's response.

A written summary describes the progress of the client.

SAMPLE DOCUMENTATION

Date	Time	Nurse's note
9/10	1115	Ace bandages removed from the R and L legs. Sterile dressings over vein-stripping incisions changed. Small amount of serosanguineous drainage noted. Incisions are clean and intact bilaterally. Feet are not edematous. Toes are warm with strong pedal pulses. Ace bandages reapplied. Nails blanch with compression and fill immediately after release.
		F. Hooley, RN

EVALUATION

REASSESSMENT

The circulation should be assessed and tested every 1 to 2 hours. Always compare the bandaged area with one that is unbandaged. Report any coldness, numbness, swelling, pallor, or flushed or cyanotic skin. Ask the client if he feels throbbing, tingling, or pain.

EXPECTED OUTCOMES

Dressings remain in place.
The roller bandage contiguously covers an area of the body.
The roller bandage is free of wrinkles.
The tissue is evenly compressed with signs of adequate circulation.
The client feels more comfortable with the additional support provided by the bandage.

UNEXPECTED OUTCOMES

The roller bandage loosens, causing underlying dressings to shift out of place.
Portions of the skin are exposed between wraps of the bandage.
The bandage is wrinkled.
The client's feet are cold or swollen, indicating impaired circulation.
The client reports pain and throbbing that he associates with the bandage.

MODIFICATIONS IN SELECTED SITUATIONS

GENERAL VARIATIONS

Use more than one roller bandage when a large area of the body must be covered. Tube dressings of gauze or stockinet may be used to retain dressings or cover the circumference of an area of the body.

For wrapping a cone-shaped body part, use the spiral reverse turn, shown in Figure III-11-3.

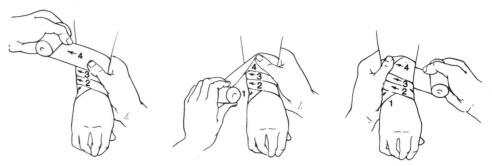

Figure III-11-3 The spiral reverse turn is wrapped similarly to a spiral except that each layer is reversed halfway through the turn.

Use the figure-of-eight turn, shown in Figure III-11-4, for wrapping around joints, such as the knee, elbow, ankle, or wrist.

The spica wrap, shown in Figure III-11-5, is useful in bandaging the thumb, breast, shoulder, groin, and hip.

A recurrent turn, shown in Figure III-11-6, is used to bandage a stump or the head.

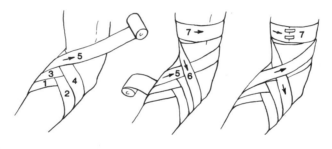

Figure III-11-4 A figure-of-eight turn consists of oblique overlapping turns that ascend and descend alternately. Each turn crosses the one preceding it so that it resembles the number 8.

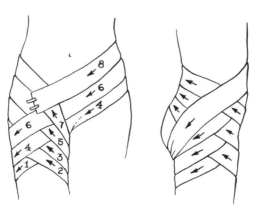

Figure III-11-5 A spica turn is an adaptation of the figure-of-eight turn. The turn consists of ascending and descending turns overlapping and crossing each other to form a sharp angle.

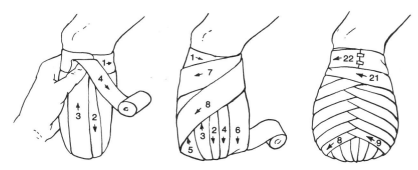

Figure III-11-6 A recurrent turn is formed by passing the roll back and forth over the tip of the body part from one side to the other after the free end has been anchored. To hold the recurrent turns in place, the bandaging may be completed using a figure-of-eight turn.

Remove gauze roller bandages with scissors to prevent excessive manipulation of the area. Cutting should be done on the side opposite the injury or wound, from one end to the other, so that the bandage can be opened its entire length.

When planning to reuse an elastic roller bandage, unwind the loose end and pass it as a ball from one hand to the other.

AGE-RELATED VARIATIONS	Use small widths, 1 to 2 inches, when wrapping a roller bandage on an infant or small child.
HOME-HEALTH VARIATIONS	If an elastic roller bandage becomes soiled, it may be washed according to usual laundering practices. However, a roller bandage should be laid flat for drying. Stretching the weave during hanging causes the bandage to lose its elasticity.
RELATED TEACHING	Tell the client that elevating the wrapped body part periodically can relieve swelling. Identify the signs of complications to the client, such as swelling unrelieved by elevation, numbness, coldness, or white or dusky color to the skin.

(Performance checklist next page)

PERFORMANCE CHECKLIST

When applying a roller bandage, the learner:

C	A	U	
[ ]	[ ]	[ ]	Washes hands
[ ]	[ ]	[ ]	Provides the client with an explanation
[ ]	[ ]	[ ]	Assesses pertinent data
[ ]	[ ]	[ ]	Explains the procedure
[ ]	[ ]	[ ]	Obtains appropriate supplies and equipment
[ ]	[ ]	[ ]	Cleans and dries the skin
[ ]	[ ]	[ ]	Changes any dressings, if needed
[ ]	[ ]	[ ]	Supports the body part in a functional position
[ ]	[ ]	[ ]	Pads areas of potential pressure or where skin surfaces touch one another
[ ]	[ ]	[ ]	Anchors the bandage with a circular turn
[ ]	[ ]	[ ]	Wraps from a distal to proximal direction
[ ]	[ ]	[ ]	Applies even pressure throughout
[ ]	[ ]	[ ]	Overlaps each turn at least one-half to two-thirds the width of the bandage
[ ]	[ ]	[ ]	Uses an appropriate wrapping pattern for the area being bandaged
[ ]	[ ]	[ ]	Checks the circulation and comfort after the area is wrapped
[ ]	[ ]	[ ]	Secures the bandage in an area where there will be less potential for discomfort or injury
[ ]	[ ]	[ ]	Washes hands
[ ]	[ ]	[ ]	Charts significant information

Outcome: [ ] Pass   [ ] Fail

C = competent; A = acceptable; U = unsatisfactory

Comments: _____

_____

_____

_____   _____
Student's Signature   Date

_____   _____
Instructor's Signature   Date

III-12 *Applying transdermal medication*

The prefix *trans-* means across or through. The word *transdermal* means through the skin. A drug intended for application by this route enters the bloodstream after being absorbed through the skin's hair follicles and sweat glands. Several drugs, such as nitroglycerin, scopolamine, and estrogen, are being manufactured for transdermal application. The medications are applied with a skin patch or disc. Nitroglycerin is also prepared as an ointment that is spread on a dose-calibrated paper and taped to the skin.

PURPOSES OF PROCEDURE

Transdermal medication is applied to

1. Administer medication for slow absorption
2. Maintain a sustained blood level of a drug with one application lasting several hours or days depending on the specific medication
3. Facilitate ease and comfort of drug administration

ASSESSMENT

OBJECTIVE DATA

- Read the physician's order.
- Compare the transcribed information on the medication card with the written order.
- Review the action of the drug, side-effects, contraindications, usual dosage, and other pertinent information in an appropriate pharmacology reference if unfamiliar with the medication.
- Read the client's chart and note any condition; such as pregnancy, allergy, or potential drug interactions, that would contraindicate the administration of the prescribed medication.
- Read the medication label to verify that the correct medication, in an appropriate supply dose prepared for transdermal application has been delivered for the intended client.
- Examine the skin to determine that the area intended for drug application is clean, nonhairy, and intact.

SUBJECTIVE DATA

- Interview the client to determine any prior experience in receiving transdermal medication.
- Ask the client about any history of drug allergies and a description of the types of symptoms experienced during prior allergic reactions.

RELEVANT NURSING DIAGNOSES

Depending on the gathered data, the client receiving a transdermal application of medication may have nursing diagnoses, such as

- *Anxiety*
- *Fear*
- *Altered Comfort*
- *Knowledge Deficit*
- *Potential for Injury*

PLANNING

ESTABLISHING PRIORITIES

Medications should be administered with relative regularity and continuity according to the agency's established schedule. With the exception of stat medication orders, which should be given as soon as possible, the nurse should strive to administer medication within a half hour of the established timetable.

SETTING GOALS
- The client will receive the right medication, the right dosage, by the right route, at the right time.
- The client will experience the expected results and no side-effects of the medication.
- The application system will adhere to the skin until the next dose is administered.

PREPARATION OF EQUIPMENT

The nurse will need the following for applying medication by the transdermal route:

Medication
Medication card or Kardex
Washcloth, soap and water, and towel
Scissors (optional)
Tape (if ointment is applied to paper)

Technique for applying transdermal medication

ACTION	RATIONALE
1. Assemble the equipment and check the physician's order.	Checking the order with the drug label ensures that the client receives the right medication at the right time by the proper route.
2. Explain the procedure to the client.	An explanation reduces apprehension and facilitates cooperation.
3. Wash your hands.	Handwashing deters the spread of microorganisms.
4. Select an area somewhat distant from one where a current transdermal application is located.	Skin irritation may occur with repeated application at the same site.
5. Choose from areas such as the upper arm, chest, back, or abdomen; small scopolamine discs are usually placed behind the ear.	Avoiding an area that is involved in frequent muscle activity and friction with clothing prevents loosening once the application is attached to the skin. Areas close to the trunk are less likely to be noticed by others. Distal areas may provide slower absorption of medication.
6. Clean the area where the medication will be applied with soap and water.	Body oil may interfere with the adhesive properties of the patch, disc, or tape.
7. Clip hair from the area if there is an unusual amount. Avoid shaving the area.	Hair may interfere with the ability of the patch to stick to the skin. Pulling an adhesive from body hair causes discomfort. Shaving can impair skin integrity and alter the rate of drug absorption.
8. Pull the protective backing from the patch or disc exposing the drug. OR Squeeze a thin, uniform ribbon of ointment, the prescribed length, on the application paper.	The drug is kept covered to prevent deterioration until it is ready for application to the skin. The absorption of the ointment is related to the size of the skin area exposed to the drug.
9. Place the paper, patch, or disc to the skin, as the nurse in Figure III-12-1 is doing, without touching the drug.	The drug must be in direct contact with the skin in order to be absorbed. Touching the drug surface can lead to accidental absorption through the nurse's skin.
10. Press the adhesive patch or disc firmly for about 10 seconds.	Making contact on all sides of the patch or disc promotes adherence to the skin.
11. Tape the paper to the skin if the medication is in ointment form.	Tape secures the paper to the skin.
12. Date and initial the patch or paper.	Identifying the date and adding initials aid in establishing that an application is current.
13. Wash your hands.	Handwashing deters the spread of microorganisms.
14. Chart the time, drug, dosage, and site of application.	Accurate medication recording prevents errors in drug administration.

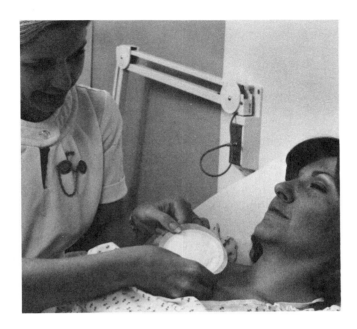

Figure III-12–1 The nurse applies a transdermal patch to the upper chest wall of this client.

15. If the client has received a prior dose, remove the old patch or paper 30 minutes after the current application.

The most recent application may take 30 minutes before its blood level matches that achieved with the previous application.

16. Evaluate the response of the client to medication within an appropriate period of time.

Transdermal medication is absorbed slowly, but the effects and side-effects may be observed in 30 minutes.

SAMPLE DOCUMENTATION

Date	Time	Nurse's note
5/23	0900	No chest pain in past 24 hrs. Transdermal nitroglycerin 5-mg patch applied to R upper arm
	0930	Transdermal patch dated 5/22 removed.
		L. Fowler, RN

EVALUATION

REASSESSMENT

The date on the transdermal application should be noted by each nurse when performing routine physical assessments. The nurse who applied the patch, disc, or paper should inspect the area at frequent intervals to determine the status of its contact with the skin. Periodic observation is indicated for determining the client's response to desired and undesirable effects of the drug.

EXPECTED OUTCOMES

The patch, disc, or paper maintains firm contact with the skin.
The client's symptoms are relieved or controlled by the medication.

UNEXPECTED OUTCOMES

The patch, disc, or paper becomes loose or falls off the skin.
The client does not experience relief or control of symptoms.
The client manifests adverse or undesirable side-effects.

MODIFICATIONS IN SELECTED SITUATIONS

GENERAL VARIATIONS

Bathing, showering, or swimming should not affect the adhesion and drug absorption from a firmly applied patch or disc. Ointment applied with paper should be made water tight by covering the area with plastic secured with tape.

HOME-HEALTH
VARIATIONS

Establish a system that will remind the client when to change other than daily applications of transdermal medications. Scopolamine discs can be worn for 3 days; estrogen patches are changed twice weekly.

RELATED TEACHING

Explain what kinds of effects and side-effects the client is likely to experience.

Instruct the client and family on the technique for applying transdermal medication if the client will continue this form of medication at home. Plan occasions for practicing the technique.

Advise the client to keep transdermal medication out of the reach of children.

Explain that a patch, disc, or paper should be replaced at another location if it becomes lost or loose.

Inform the client to report any symptoms related to the drug. The client should be cautioned against abruptly discontinuing its application without consulting the physician.

PERFORMANCE CHECKLIST

When applying transdermal medication, the learner:

C	A	U	
[ ]	[ ]	[ ]	Compares the medication order with its transcription on the medication kardex or medication card
[ ]	[ ]	[ ]	Reviews an authoritative reference for pertinent information about the drug, if unfamiliar with the medication
[ ]	[ ]	[ ]	Reads the client's record for significant information related to the drug administration
[ ]	[ ]	[ ]	Interviews the client to obtain objective and subjective information
[ ]	[ ]	[ ]	Reads the drug label at least three times
[ ]	[ ]	[ ]	Washes hands
[ ]	[ ]	[ ]	Assembles equipment
[ ]	[ ]	[ ]	Takes supplies to the bedside
[ ]	[ ]	[ ]	Identifies the client by checking the wristband
[ ]	[ ]	[ ]	Explains the procedure
[ ]	[ ]	[ ]	Washes and dries the skin
[ ]	[ ]	[ ]	Clips hair from a site, if necessary
[ ]	[ ]	[ ]	Peels the adhesive backing from the drug or applies ointment to the paper
[ ]	[ ]	[ ]	Avoids touching the drug surface
[ ]	[ ]	[ ]	Presses the application to the skin
[ ]	[ ]	[ ]	Determines that there is uniform adherence
[ ]	[ ]	[ ]	Dates and initials the application on the outside of the patch, disc, or paper
[ ]	[ ]	[ ]	Washes hands
[ ]	[ ]	[ ]	Charts significant information
[ ]	[ ]	[ ]	Returns in 30 minutes to remove the older application and reassess the client

Outcome: [ ] Pass   [ ] Fail

C = competent; A = acceptable; U = unsatisfactory

Comments: _____

_____

_____

_____   _____
Student's Signature   Date

_____   _____
Instructor's Signature   Date

III-13

Giving a sitz bath

To give a sitz bath, a client is placed in a shallow tub or basin containing warm water. Just the client's pelvic area is submerged while the legs and feet remain out of the water. Portable models, like the one in Figure III-13-1, have been adapted to fit into the toilet.

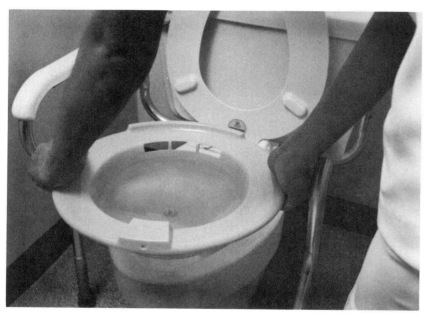

Figure III-13–1 This portable sitz basin fits within the bowl of the toilet. Water must be added and changed periodically from another source.

PURPOSES OF PROCEDURE

1. Apply heat to the perineal area of the body.
2. Increase local circulation.
3. Reduce swelling.
4. Promote healing.
5. Soothe irritated or impaired tissue.

ASSESSMENT

OBJECTIVE DATA

- Read the physician's written order.
- Consult the agency's policy for the amount of time and temperature recommended for a sitz bath.
- Read the client's record to determine the reason for the sitz bath, such as promoting healing of a perineal incision.
- Assess the client's mental status and any evidence of sensory or cardiovascular disease.
- Inspect the perineum for color, swelling, discharge, integrity, evidence of external hemorrhoids, drains, packing, or dressing material.

- Observe the client's ability to sit directly on the buttocks; note signs that the client distributes body weight to relieve pressure on this area.
- Take the client's vital signs and compare them with the recommended range for the client's age; determine the pattern of the vital sign recordings.

SUBJECTIVE DATA

- Ask the client to describe the sensations he experiences in the perineum and rectum especially with sitting, walking, and when eliminating urine or stool.

RELEVANT NURSING DIAGNOSES

A client for whom a sitz bath is given is likely to have nursing diagnoses, such as

- *Altered Comfort*
- *Impaired Skin or Tissue Integrity*
- *Potential for Injury*
- *Potential for Infection*
- *Altered Bowel Elimination*
- *Altered Patterns of Urinary Elimination*
- *Potential Sexual Dysfunction*
- *Knowledge Deficit*

PLANNING

ESTABLISHING PRIORITIES

The nurse should implement the plans for the care of assigned clients so as to allow approximately 15 to 30 minutes for the sitz bath. Although intended to cause vasodilation, prolonged heat may produce the reverse effect if the warm temperature is sustained. By coordinating the preparation of the equipment with the client's readiness, the maximum effects of the procedure are likely to be achieved.

SETTING GOALS

- The tissue in the pelvic area will be clean and free of secretions or excretions.
- The pelvic area will not be injured by heat.
- The client will indicate that his level of comfort is improved.

PREPARATION OF EQUIPMENT

Before giving a sitz bath, the nurse will need to gather items from the following list:

Portable or stationary sitz tub
IV pole to support the container for filling a portable sitz tub
Bath thermometer
Bath mat, towels, and clean bed clothes
Bath blankets
Sterile dressings and T-binder (optional)

Technique for giving a sitz bath

ACTION	RATIONALE
1. Check the physician's order.	Reading the order ensures that it is implemented according to the physician's directions.
2. Explain the procedure to the client.	An explanation relieves apprehension and promotes cooperation.
3. Wash your hands.	Handwashing deters the spread of microorganisms.
4. Gather objective and subjective data from the client.	The client is the main source for information.
5. Obtain supplies.	Organization promotes efficient time management.
6. Fill the tub one-third full.	When the client's hips are submerged, the water will be displaced and the level of the water will be increased.
7. Test the temperature of the water with a thermometer.	Using a thermometer is the most reliable method for determining the actual temperature.
8. Circulate and maintain the water temperature at 43°C to 46°C (110°F to 115°F). A temperature of 34°C	Fluctuations in temperature may burn or chill the client.

to 37°C (94°F to 98°F) may be used to produce relaxation or cleanse the area of discharge or debris.

9. Provide privacy by closing the door to the bathroom and posting an "in-use" sign on the door.

The client's right to privacy is protected.

10. Remove clothing from below the waist.

Leaving the upper part of the body covered maintains modesty and warmth.

11. Assist the client to sit in the tub without pressure on the perineum and with the feet flat on the floor.

Direct pressure may heighten discomfort.

12. Cover the client's back, shoulders, and lower legs with a cotton bath blanket, as shown in Figure III-13-2.

Covering the client maintains body warmth and prevents chilling.

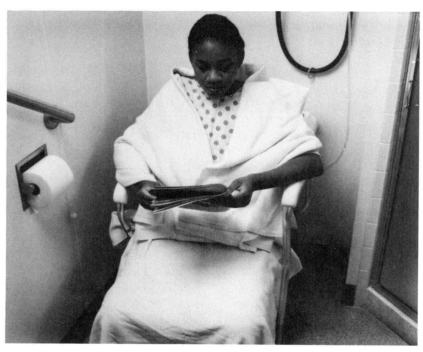

Figure III-13–2 This client has been made warm and comfortable while taking a sitz bath.

13. Observe the client closely for signs of weakness, vertigo, pallor, tachycardia, and nausea.

Changes in the distribution of blood and external heat can increase the potential for adverse effects.

14. Test the temperature of the water midway through the procedure.

For the best therapeutic effect, the warmth of the water should be maintained at the target temperature.

15. Agitate the water when adding more volume to the sitz tub.

Circulating the water equalizes the temperature and prevents burning the client.

16. Stay with the client or provide a signal device.

The nurse should not leave the client alone unless absolutely certain that it is safe to do so. The client should be provided with a means of seeking assistance.

17. Help the client out of the tub when it is completed.

The client may feel faint with changes in posture and the redistribution of blood volume to the pelvic region.

18. Assist the client to dry and dress in clean bed clothes.

Being clean and dry promotes a refreshed feeling.

19. Help the client return to bed and reassess the objective and subjective data.

The nurse compares baseline data with changes in order to evaluate the response of the client to the treatment and care.

20. Replace a sterile, perineal dressing, if needed.

A sterile dressing should be applied to any open, draining area.

21. Empty the sitz tub and wipe away water that may have dripped on the floor.

Water left on the floor can lead to falls and injury.

22. Disinfect a stationary sitz tub; clean and dry a portable unit before returning it to the client's bedside.

Permanent porcelain basins should be disinfected between uses to control the spread of microorganisms. Individual equipment stored at the bedside should be clean and dry.

23. Wash your hands.

Handwashing deters the spread of microorganisms.

24. Document your observations, the pertinent information about the procedure, and the response of the client.

Accurate written accounts provide a permanent record of the individual's care.

SAMPLE DOCUMENTATION

Date	Time	Nurse's note
11/1	2000	Sm. amt. of bloody drainage noted on peri-pad from the area of hemorrhoidectomy. States that the area is tender and finds sitting difficult. Has not felt the urge to have a BM since surgery. Tap-water sitz bath provided at 105°F for 20 minutes according to agency policy. States, "I look forward to this because I feel so much better afterwards." Dry, sterile dressing applied.

T. Coppen, RN

EVALUATION

REASSESSMENT

The nurse reinspects the client's perineal area after terminating the procedure. Questioning the client provides comparisons of subjective data. Examining the skin well after the procedure can be helpful in determining if there are any ill-effects from the application of the heat.

EXPECTED OUTCOMES

The skin in the pelvic area appears slightly pink immediately after the sitz bath.
Debris and drainage are eliminated from the area.
The client remains alert and normotensive.
The client expresses feelings of increased comfort.

UNEXPECTED OUTCOMES

The skin is painful, reddened, and blanches in response to finger compression (superficial, partial-thickness burn).
The client's blood pressure falls, heart rate increases, or fainting occurs.
The client indicates that the sitz bath causes an increase in discomfort.

MODIFICATIONS IN SELECTED SITUATIONS

GENERAL VARIATIONS

Use a sterile basin if the tissue is likely to become infected.
An antiseptic solution may be ordered to inhibit the growth of microorganisms in a wound or incision.

AGE-RELATED VARIATIONS

Young children, elderly clients, diabetic clients, and individuals with circulatory or sensory alterations have a lower tolerance for heat. The temperature of the bath water in relation to the client's responses needs to be monitored closely in order to ensure safety.

HOME-HEALTH VARIATIONS

A sitz bath may be improvised using a bath tub. However, sitting in a porcelain tub is not as satisfactory as using a disposable, portable type of basin because in the tub the heat is also applied to the legs. This reduces the amount of blood that is drawn to the perineal area. If the client can tolerate, elevate the lower extremities by positioning the client's legs over an inverted dishpan or a large mixing bowl.

Place a skid-proof mat or towels in the tub to prevent falls when getting in and out.

RELATED TEACHING

Explain the purpose and frequency for giving a sitz bath.

Inform the client that heat receptors in the skin adapt quickly. This may reduce the sensation of warmth that is experienced. However, adding more hot water may increase the temperature beyond safe limits, causing the potential for sustaining a burn. Tell the client to always check the temperature of the water at home before immersing the body. If there is no thermometer available, drip water on a part of the body where the skin is thinner, such as the inner forearm. This area is likely to be a more sensitive indicator of the effect of the heat on the skin.

Instruct the client who performs this procedure at home that manufactured disinfectants, such as Lysol, or dilute solutions of bleach are appropriate to use for cleaning the bath tub, if the client has an open, draining wound.

Explain that to control the spread of microorganisms, soiled dressings should be placed in a paper bag and burned. If incineration is prohibited, the paper bag should be secured within a plastic bag.

Demonstrate proper handwashing technique before and after touching areas of the body, especially those that contain secretions or excretions.

PERFORMANCE CHECKLIST

When giving a sitz bath, the learner:

C	A	U	
[ ]	[ ]	[ ]	Checks the physician's order
[ ]	[ ]	[ ]	Reviews the agency's policy and procedure manual for the recommended time and temperature
[ ]	[ ]	[ ]	Requisitions the necessary supplies
[ ]	[ ]	[ ]	Inspects the cleanliness of the bathroom or stationary sitz bath tub
[ ]	[ ]	[ ]	Explains the procedure to the client
[ ]	[ ]	[ ]	Washes hands
[ ]	[ ]	[ ]	Examines and interviews the client to obtain pertinent objective and subjective data
[ ]	[ ]	[ ]	Assembles equipment and fills the sitz tub
[ ]	[ ]	[ ]	Checks the temperature of the water
[ ]	[ ]	[ ]	Provides privacy and protection from drafts
[ ]	[ ]	[ ]	Assists the client into the sitz tub
[ ]	[ ]	[ ]	Provides the client with a means to call for assistance
[ ]	[ ]	[ ]	Observes the response of the client frequently
[ ]	[ ]	[ ]	Adds more warm water safely, if it cools below the therapeutic range
[ ]	[ ]	[ ]	Observes the time so as to maintain the bath for a minimum of 15 minutes, but not exceeding 30 minutes
[ ]	[ ]	[ ]	Assists the client to dry, dress, and return to bed
[ ]	[ ]	[ ]	Inspects the skin and assesses the client's level of comfort
[ ]	[ ]	[ ]	Washes hands and applies a fresh dressing, if needed
[ ]	[ ]	[ ]	Empties the water and cleans the area where the sitz bath was given
[ ]	[ ]	[ ]	Replaces reusable equipment
[ ]	[ ]	[ ]	Charts significant information
[ ]	[ ]	[ ]	Reassesses the response of the client

Outcome: [ ] Pass   [ ] Fail

C = competent; A = acceptable; U = unsatisfactory

Comments: _____

_____ Student's Signature   Date

_____ Instructor's Signature   Date

III-14 *Preventing pressure sores*

Intact skin is a barrier to microorganisms. It also helps to retain fluids and proteins within cells and tissue. Skin can become impaired when there is inadequate blood flow to an area. Pressure can interfere with adequate circulatory perfusion to the integument, causing a pressure sore to form. Sites that are prone to skin breakdown are shown in Figure III-14-1. The terms *pressure sore, decubitus ulcer,* and *pressure ulcer* are used interchangeably. Figure III-14-2 illustrates the progression of damage that can occur.

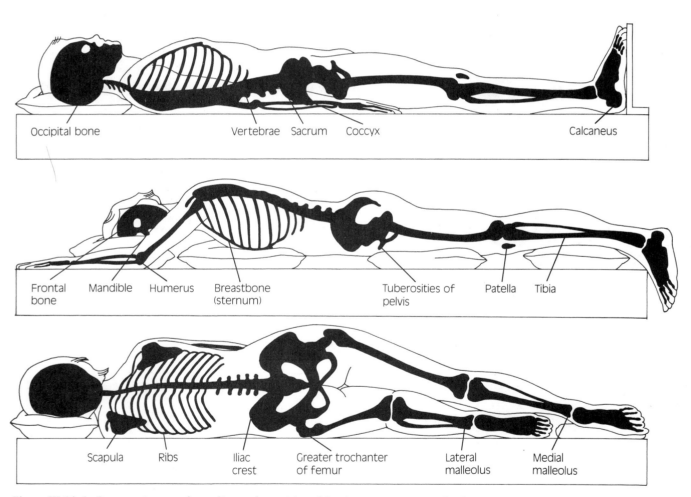

Figure III-14-1 Pressure sites vary depending on the position of the client. Common sites for developing pressure sores are identified here for the supine, prone, and side-lying positions. Since literally any position that is maintained for a relatively prolonged period of time is likely to impair circulation to the skin over bony prominences, the inactive client's position should be changed at least every 2 hours.

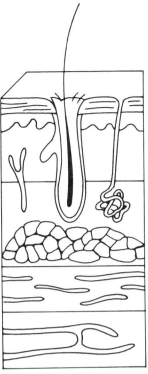

Stage 1
The primary sign is redness. The skin doesn't return to a normal color when the pressure is relieved, but there is no induration—the skin and underlying tissues remain soft.

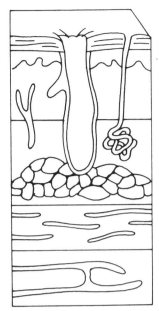

Stage 2
Redness persists, usually accompanied by edema and induration. The epidermis may blister or erode.

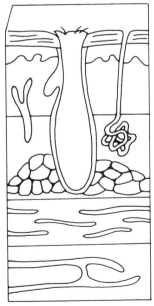

Stage 3
There is an open lesion and a crater exposing subcutaneous tissue. You may be able to see fascia at the base of the ulcer.

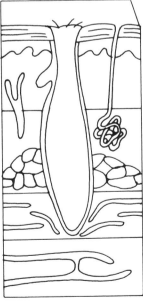

Stage 4
Necrosis will extend through the fascia and may even involve the bone. Eschar is a common finding. Bone destruction can lead to periosteitis, osteitis, and osteomyelitis.

Figure III-14-2 The characteristics of a pressure sore.

PURPOSES OF PROCEDURE	1. Promote skin integrity. 2. Relieve pressure. 3. Improve local circulation.

ASSESSMENT

OBJECTIVE DATA

- Determine the client's level of consciousness.
- Note the client's patterns of bowel and bladder continence.
- Identify any deficits in physical mobility.
- Review the client's record for restrictions in activity.
- Evaluate the client's nutritional and metabolic pattern; note his appetite, weight, ability to consume an adequate caloric and fluid intake, and the amount of tissue that covers bony prominences.
- Inspect the skin for color, turgor, moisture, and integrity, especially in areas subject to compression.
- Obtain data related to the client's circulatory status; note the client's red cell and hemoglobin levels, heart rate, cardiovascular pathology, evidence of edema, and peripheral circulation.
- Review the client's temperature pattern; be attentive to recent fever with or without diaphoresis.
- Scan the medication Kardex for drugs that can alter activity or fluid distribution, such as narcotics or steroids.
- Investigate the effect of immobilizing devices, such as restraints, splints, traction, and casts, to the skin.
- Review the agency's protocols for preventing pressure sores.

SUBJECTIVE DATA

- Ask the client to indicate any areas where he experiences pressure, friction, or tenderness.

RELEVANT NURSING DIAGNOSES

The client for whom the nurse plans measures for preventing pressure sores may have nursing diagnoses, such as

- *Potential for Impaired Skin Integrity*
- *Altered Tissue Perfusion*
- *Self-Care Deficit*
- *Impaired Physical Mobility*
- *Unilateral Neglect*
- *Altered Nutrition: Less than Body Requirements*
- *Fluid Volume Deficit*
- *Hyperthermia*
- *Altered Bowel Elimination: Incontinence*
- *Total Incontinence*

PLANNING

ESTABLISHING PRIORITIES

To prevent impairment of the skin from developing, the nurse should order pressure-relieving measures at least every 2 hours. Relieving factors that contribute to skin breakdown, such as keeping the client free of urine or stool, may be performed more frequently.

SETTING GOALS

- The client's skin will remain intact throughout the care.
- The dependent client's position will be changed at least every 2 hours.
- Factors contributing to the development of a pressure sore will be alleviated.

PREPARATION OF EQUIPMENT

The nurse uses a variety of approaches to promote skin integrity depending on the client's potential risk factors. Some suggestions include items in the following list:

Pillows
Cleansing supplies, such as soap, water, basin, washcloth, and towels
Pressure-relieving pads or mattress
Friction-reducing supplies, such as corn starch or a turning sheet
Massage lotion

Technique for preventing pressure sores

ACTION	RATIONALE
1. Change the client's position as often as every hour or two if the person is at risk for developing pressure sores.	Changing positions helps relieve pressure and restore circulation.
2. Alternate between side-lying and prone positions. Use the supine position as infrequently as possible.	The back-lying position causes pressure to many vulnerable areas on the body.
3. Try not to raise the head of the bed more than 30 degrees when in a supine position.	Pressure and shearing forces, illustrated in Figure III-14-3, increase in proportion to the head elevation of the body.

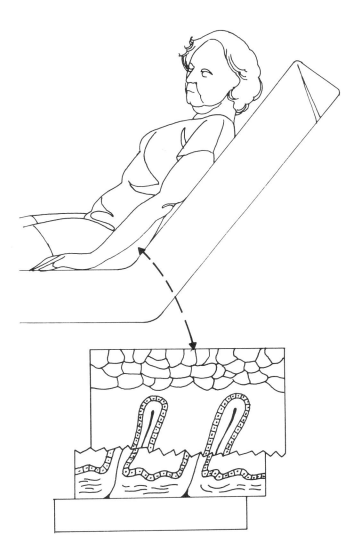

Figure III-14–3 Shearing force can occur when capillaries in the underlying tissue are stretched and torn in pressure areas by the opposing forces of movement. Conditions that result in shearing force include moving a client carelessly or sliding down in bed. Friction causes resistance on the surface layers of the skin while underlying tissue moves in the direction of the body movement.

ACTION	RATIONALE
4. Keep the skin clean and dry.	Dampness and uncleanliness predispose to skin breakdown.
5. Use skin cleansers that do not destroy the natural acid condition of the skin.	Bathing with alkaline soaps destroys the ability of the skin to retard the growth of bacteria and fungi.
6. Rinse off soap, detergent, or skin cleansers well with water.	Residues left on the skin can be irritating and predispose to skin impairment.

7. Avoid using waterproof materials on the client's bed.

Waterproof materials tend to cause the client to perspire and prevent evaporation. Moisture and heat can contribute to skin maceration.

8. Keep bed linens clean, dry, and free of wrinkles and debris.

Damaged skin is more susceptible to breakdown.

9. Apply top linens loosely and use a toe pleat.

Restricting the freedom of movement contributes to prolonged, continuous pressure.

10. Massage areas carefully and frequently where there is pressure on the body except when redness is already present.

Massage stimulates circulation but may cause separation of skin layers once damage has begun to occur.

11. Protect areas especially prone to friction, shearing forces, and pressure, such as the heels and elbows.

Reducing friction and providing a cushioning effect protect the skin when turning, moving, and positioning the client.

12. Use a mattress that reduces the pounds per square inch of body weight. Such devices as a water mattress, alternating air-pressure mattress, eggcrate mattress, shown in Figure III-14-4, and Clinitron bed function on this principle.

The even distribution of the client's weight helps improve circulation and prevent injury to the skin.

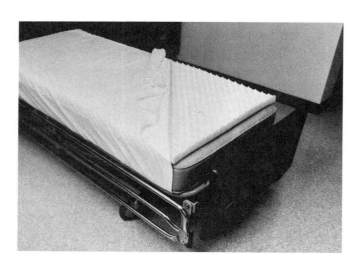

Figure III-14-4 This eggcrate mattress adds to comfort and helps distribute body weight evenly to reduce the risk of pressure sores.

13. Use cornstarch if the client's skin sticks to the bed, chair, or bedpan.

Cornstarch reduces friction and absorbs moisture from the skin.

14. Lift or use a turning sheet rather than slide the client when he is moved.

Reducing friction can promote and maintain skin integrity.

15. Avoid using doughnuts and air-inflated rings or use them only with the greatest of care and for very short periods of time.

Rings may relieve pressure over an area but they restrict circulation where the body part rests on the ring, causing more problems than they solve.

16. Do everything possible to help keep the client in the best possible physical condition. This includes ensuring that the client eats a nutritious diet and takes plenty of fluids.

Healthy, well-nourished, hydrated clients are less prone to injury and deterioration.

SAMPLE DOCUMENTATION

Date	Time	Nurse's note
2/04	0730	Red area noted over coccyx. Area blanches when pressure is relieved. Skin over back and buttocks massaged with lotion. Eggcrate mattress applied to bed. Position alternately changed from R to L side. Skin over coccyx compares with that of adjacent tissues now and remains intact.
		D. Vogt, RN

EVALUATION

REASSESSMENT

The skin over the entire body should be assessed daily. The skin of the client who is prone to developing a pressure sore should be inspected each time the client's position is changed. Once there is evidence of a pressure sore, the nurse should strive to compare its characteristics with the stages described earlier. Increased impairment warrants additions and changes in the nursing orders to aggressively prevent further breakdown.

EXPECTED OUTCOMES

The client's skin is clean and dry.
The client's skin shows no sign of irritation, induration, or breakdown.
Variations in skin color and temperature are relieved when pressure is reduced.

UNEXPECTED OUTCOMES

The skin is damp and soiled.
The skin is warmer and darker in appearance over an area subjected to pressure even after the pressure is relieved.
The skin is irritated over bony prominences with signs of blisters or open lesions.

MODIFICATIONS IN SELECTED SITUATIONS

GENERAL VARIATIONS

When there is a need to use tape, substitute paper tape for individuals who have thin, fragile skin in order to avoid removing the upper layer of epidermis and dermis.
If skin breakdown occurs, follow agency guidelines for treatment. The recommended practices vary according to the stage of the pressure sore. If no protocols exist, nursing management and wound care guides have been described by the skin task force of Beth Israel Hospital in Boston, Massachusetts. Their recommendations have been published in the August 1984 issue of the American Journal of Nursing.

HOME-HEALTH VARIATIONS

For high-risk clients, instruct the family on the need for routine systematic inspection of all bony prominences.
An eggcrate mattress and other pressure-relieving devices are available to the public from medical-supply distributers.
Hand and body lotion can be substituted for the massage lotion used in health-care agencies.
Assist the client's family to improvise ways of keeping the client dry, such as using an external catheter, if urinary incontinence is a problem. Plastic sheets should be avoided because they interfere with heat regulation and moisture evaporation.
Maintaining a debilitated client's nutrition can be achieved by providing liquid dietary supplements sold in most drug stores.
Help the family develop a schedule for alternating the client's position.
Child-size swimming flotation devices normally worn around a youngster's arms could be padded with absorbent fabric and placed around the elbow or ankle areas of an adult. Stress the necessity for removing these devices every 2 hours for lotion and massage. Advise clients that if these devices cause extreme heat and moisture to accumulate, their use should be discontinued.

RELATED TEACHING   Instruct the client on the purpose and need for changing positions frequently. Some may protest because the movement temporarily interferes with comfort.

Emphasize that once an area remains reddened, it should not be massaged anymore. Rubbing can lead to separation of the skin layers and further breakdown.

Teach a home-bound client's family how to use proper body mechanics as well as lifting, turning, and positioning techniques.

Explain that alcohol dries the skin but tends to toughen it. Excess lotion should be removed or it may soften the skin, adding moist conditions that can predispose to breaks in the skin.

PERFORMANCE CHECKLIST

When preventing pressure sores, the learner:

C	A	U	
[ ]	[ ]	[ ]	Assesses the factors that increase a client's potential for developing pressure sores
[ ]	[ ]	[ ]	Examines the skin from head to toe, especially noting areas over bony prominences like the sacrum, coccyx, trochanters, ischial tuberosities, ankles, elbows, scapulae, and ears
[ ]	[ ]	[ ]	Keeps the client clean and dry
[ ]	[ ]	[ ]	Changes bed linen when it becomes soiled, damp, or wrinkled
[ ]	[ ]	[ ]	Changes the inactive client's position at least every 2 hours
[ ]	[ ]	[ ]	Massages all intact bony prominences that blanch when pressure is relieved
[ ]	[ ]	[ ]	Straightens wrinkled linen
[ ]	[ ]	[ ]	Uses a turning sheet when moving the client about in bed
[ ]	[ ]	[ ]	Obtains and uses pressure-relieving devices when indicated
[ ]	[ ]	[ ]	Promotes adequate hydration and nutrition
[ ]	[ ]	[ ]	Records significant observations
[ ]	[ ]	[ ]	Evaluates the effectiveness of the nursing orders

Outcome: [ ] Pass   [ ] Fail

C = competent; A = acceptable; U = unsatisfactory

Comments: _____

_____

_____

_____   _____
         Student's Signature   Date

_____   _____
        Instructor's Signature   Date

III-15 *Applying an external heating device*

Heat is applied by both dry and moist methods. Moist applications of heat include compresses or packs, sitz bath, and soaks. Hot water bottles, electric heating pads, chemical heat packs, and the Aquathermia pad, shown in Figure III-15-1, are forms of dry heat that release warmth by conduction. Conduction is the transfer of heat by direct contact between one source that is warmer than another. Heat lamps or heat cradles also produce dry heat. However, this form of heat is transferred by radiation, the dissemination of heat by electromagnetic waves.

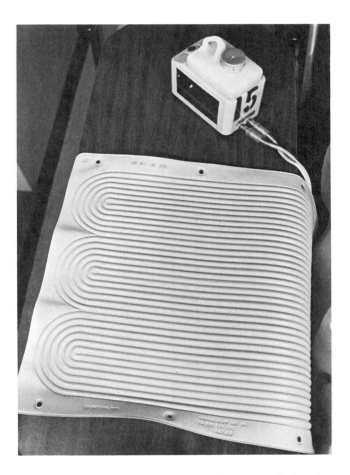

Figure III-15-1 An example of an Aquathermia pad. It can be electronically set to maintain water at a constant temperature and circulate it through the coils of the plastic pad.

PURPOSES OF PROCEDURE

External heating devices are used to provide local warmth to

1. Dilate blood vessels in the area of application
2. Relax muscles
3. Relieve swelling
4. Increase joint flexibility
5. Reduce pain
6. Promote comfort
7. Accelerate healing

341

ASSESSMENT

OBJECTIVE DATA

- Read the physician's order written on the client's record.
- Consult the agency's policy for the recommended temperature setting if it has not been specified by the physician.
- Read the chart to determine the reasons for which the application of heat has been prescribed.
- Review the client's history for conditions that place him at risk for burning, such as peripheral vascular disease and diabetes mellitus.
- Observe the client's posture and positioning; flexion, guarding, or resisting movement may indicate a high level of discomfort in a specific area.
- Inspect the skin where the heat will be applied; note its integrity, color, and temperature, and the client's ability to interpret tactile and thermal stimulation.
- Note the circulatory status of an extremity by palpating peripheral pulses, compare the responses when nailbeds are compressed, and observe for local edema.
- Check the equipment, making sure that all components are intact, no fluid leaks, electrical systems are grounded, and plugs do not contain loose or exposed wires.

SUBJECTIVE DATA

- Ask the client to describe his pain, muscle tenderness, and any abnormal sensations, such as heaviness, tingling, or numbness.

RELEVANT NURSING DIAGNOSES

Clients for whom applications of heat are prescribed likely have nursing diagnoses, such as

- *Altered Comfort*
- *Potential for Injury*
- *Impaired Physical Mobility*
- *Altered Tissue Perfusion*
- *Knowledge Deficit*

PLANNING

ESTABLISHING PRIORITIES

The application of heat is a therapeutic measure that is generally implemented intermittently several times a day. The nurse should adapt the client's care to allow adequate time for applying the heating device and removing it after the recommended amount of time. Maximum vasodilation occurs within a half hour; applications of heat lasting longer than this are likely to promote tissue congestion followed by rebound vasoconstriction.

SETTING GOALS

- The client's skin will be warmed and manifest signs of reduced swelling.
- The client will be able to demonstrate less restrictive movement.
- The client will describe an improved level of comfort.

PREPARATION OF EQUIPMENT

The nurse will need selected items from the following list:

Hot water bag
   Cover for bag
   Water at the appropriate temperature: 46.1°C to 51.5°C (115°F to 125°F) for older children and adults or 40.5°C to 43.3°C (105°F to 110°F) for infants, young children, elderly, diabetics, and unconscious clients
   Bath thermometer
Aquathermia pad
   Electrically controlled unit
   Distilled water
   Cover for pad
   Gauze bandage or tape (to secure the pad)

Technique for applying an external heating device

ACTION	RATIONALE
1. Explain the procedure to the client.	An explanation provides reassurance for the client and facilitates cooperation.
2. Assess the condition of the skin where heat is to be applied.	Impaired circulation may affect the sensitivity to heat. The elderly and very young children have the least tolerance to applications of heat.
3. Assemble necessary equipment and close the door or curtain.	Organization promotes efficient time management. Providing privacy shows respect for the client and maintains warmth.
4. Wash your hands.	Handwashing deters the spread of microorganisms.

HOT WATER BAG

ACTION	RATIONALE
5. Check the temperature of the water with a bath thermometer or test on the inner wrist. Rinse the bag with water, empty, and then fill again.	Testing ensures that the application within the acceptable temperature range for the individual. Rinsing the bag warms the rubber.
6. Fill the hot water bag one-half to two-thirds full.	A hot water bag that is not filled to the maximum capacity molds more easily to the area and puts less pressure on the site.
7. Expel any remaining air from the bag by compressing the bag until the water reaches the top. Fasten the top securely. Check for leaks.	Air reduces the pliability of the bag. Securing the top prevents leakage of water and discomfort for the client.
8. Cover the bag with a towel or other protector and apply the hot water bag to the prescribed area.	Covering protects the skin from direct contact with the rubber. Heat travels by conduction from one object to another.
9. Assess the condition of the skin and the client's response to the heat at frequent intervals. Do not exceed the prescribed length of time for application of the heat. Remove the hot water bag if excessive swelling, redness, or pain occurs and report the findings to the physician.	Maximum therapeutic effects from the application of heat occur within 20 to 30 minutes. Extended use of heat (beyond 45 minutes) results in tissue congestion and vasoconstriction. This rebound phenomenon results in increased risk to the client from application of heat.
10. After removal, record the client's response and dispose of equipment appropriately.	Written records provide an accurate documentation of the procedure.
11. Wash your hands.	Handwashing deters the spread of microorganisms.

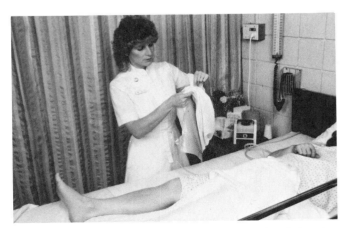

Figure III-15-2 This Aquathermia pad is covered with a cloth casing before being placed in contact with the client's skin.

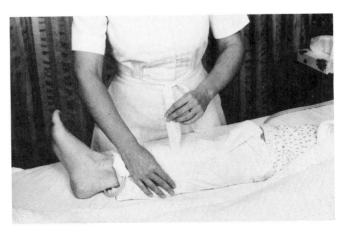

Figure III-15-3 The nurse covers the leg of the client with an Aquathermia pad and secures it in place.

AQUATHERMIA PAD

12. Check that the distilled water is at the appropriate level. Use the key to adjust the temperature at 40.5°C (105°F) if it has not already been preset. Plug in the unit and warm the pad before use if recommended by the manufacturer.

The water temperature is regulated by the key. Presetting the temperature eliminates the risk of the client adjusting the temperature.

13. Cover the pad with a pillow case or other protector, as shown in Figure III-15-2, and apply it to the prescribed area. Do not allow the client to lie on the pad.

Covering protects the skin from direct contact with rubber or other source of heat. Pressure reduces the dissipation of heat.

14. Secure the pad with a gauze bandage or tape as shown in Figure III-15-3. Never use safety pins to hold the pad in place.

Using gauze or tape holds the pad in position on the client. Pins may puncture and damage the pad.

15. Follow Steps 9, 10, and 11.

Rationales remain the same.

SAMPLE DOCUMENTATION

Date	Time	Nurse's note
2/05	1600	R leg 1½ larger around calf than L. States L leg feels "heavy and aches." Color return is slower in nailbed of R great toe. Homan's sign is positive. R leg wrapped in Aquathermia pad for 30 min. at a temp. of 105°F.

B. Coy, RN

EVALUATION

REASSESSMENT

The response to heat may be gradual after frequent applications. Continue to assess both objective local signs and the cumulative, subjective effect described by the client.

EXPECTED OUTCOMES

Swelling is relieved in the affected area.
The color, temperature, and sensation indicate improved perfusion.
The client experiences less pain and discomfort with movement.

UNEXPECTED OUTCOMES

The skin is red and painful, indicating a superficial, partial-thickness burn has occurred.
The client indicates that the temperature feels too warm or cool.
The client experiences discomfort from the weight of the heating device.

MODIFICATIONS IN SELECTED SITUATIONS

GENERAL VARIATIONS

Chemically filled containers that release heat when activated may be substituted for a hot water bottle. These products are disposable after one use.
Besides earlier mentioned forms of heat applications, areas of the body may be warmed using paraffin, chemical counterirritants applied directly to the skin, and diathermy.
Provide the client with a watch, clock, or timer to ensure that the application will not be excessively prolonged.

AGE-RELATED VARIATIONS

Infants, children, and the elderly tolerate temperature changes less well than adults. Use lower therapeutic levels of heat when applying external heating devices. Check the effect of heat to the skin with greater frequency.

HOME-HEALTH VARIATIONS

Any container that can be tightly sealed could be substituted as an external heating device. Some are less pliable than a flexible rubber bag.
If an electrical heating device is used, set a kitchen timer to remind the client when to remove and unplug the source of heat.
A heat lamp can be constructed by placing a small lamp with a low-wattage bulb inside a cardboard box.

RELATED TEACHING
As with any other procedure, the nurse explains the purpose, the steps of the procedure, and the sensations that the client will experience.

Tell the client not to move the device or adjust the controls. A client who suspects malfunction or experiences discomfort should summon the nurse immediately.

Instruct the client to avoid applying heat if an injury is recent. Heat will increase the congestion of blood in the area and intensify the pain due to the pressure from expanding trapped fluid. Elevation and cold applications are preferred immediately after trauma is experienced.

Explain that heat is not recommended when there is a possibility of appendicitis, which is characterized by right lower quadrant pain. The promotion of blood to this area could precipitate its rupture.

A client should be cautioned about lying on a heating device. The heat may not dissipate and can potentiate the risk for burning.

PERFORMANCE CHECKLIST

When applying an external heating device, the learner:

C	A	U	
[ ]	[ ]	[ ]	Checks the written order
[ ]	[ ]	[ ]	Reviews the agency policies concerning heating devices
[ ]	[ ]	[ ]	Explains the procedure
[ ]	[ ]	[ ]	Provides privacy
[ ]	[ ]	[ ]	Washes hands
[ ]	[ ]	[ ]	Assesses the client
[ ]	[ ]	[ ]	Gathers equipment
[ ]	[ ]	[ ]	Checks or regulates the temperature
[ ]	[ ]	[ ]	Applies a fabric cover over the device
[ ]	[ ]	[ ]	Positions the client for comfort
[ ]	[ ]	[ ]	Places the device so that it is superior or lateral to the affected body part
[ ]	[ ]	[ ]	Reassesses the client's response to the heat
[ ]	[ ]	[ ]	Removes the device at the prescribed time
[ ]	[ ]	[ ]	Replaces the equipment where it is usually stored
[ ]	[ ]	[ ]	Washes hands
[ ]	[ ]	[ ]	Documents significant information
[ ]	[ ]	[ ]	Repeats observations to determine the client's overall response to the application of heat

Outcome: [ ] Pass   [ ] Fail

C = competent; A = acceptable; U = unsatisfactory

Comments: _____
_____
_____

_____   _____
Student's Signature   Date

_____   _____
Instructor's Signature   Date

III-16

Applying warm sterile compresses to an open wound

One form of moist heat is the application of compresses. This requires warming material, such as gauze pads, cotton towels, or flannel, and placing them directly to the skin. Moist heat evaporates, radiating warmth into the cooler environment. For this reason compresses are often covered with folded layers of a towel, covered with plastic wrap, and topped with an external heating device. Compresses may need to be changed frequently to maintain the warmth.

PURPOSES OF PROCEDURE

Warm sterile compresses are applied to

1. Dilate blood vessels in the area of application
2. Promote wound suppuration
3. Relieve swelling
4. Relax muscles
5. Reduce pain
6. Accelerate healing
7. Promote comfort

ASSESSMENT

OBJECTIVE DATA

Refer to Procedure III-15, with the following additions:

- Consult the chart for a cluster of signs and symptoms that indicate sepsis, such as elevated temperature and pulse rate, low blood pressure, malaise, poor appetite, elevated white blood count, and positive wound culture.
- Review the agency's policies concerning drainage and secretion precautions if the wound contains purulent exudate or a wound culture indicates an infectious process.
- Inspect the wound, as the nurse in Figure III-16-1 is doing. Note its size, color, and characteristics of drainage.
- Observe for relative swelling when compared with other similar tissue.

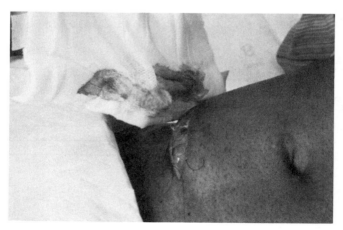

Figure III-16–1 The nurse examines the wound and the dressing that has been covering it. By comparing the data with what has been noted previously, the nurse can determine the response of the client to the effects of the treatment.

RELEVANT NURSING DIAGNOSES

Examples of nursing diagnoses that may be applicable to a client with an open wound needing warm, sterile compresses are

- *Impaired Skin Integrity*
- *Altered Comfort*
- *Potential for Infection*
- *Potential for Injury*

PLANNING

ESTABLISHING PRIORITIES

The nurse must organize the many aspects of the client's care to provide adequate time for the application of the compress. The nurse will want to utilize a time when the client can maintain bedrest for at least 30 minutes. It is wise to encourage the use of the toilet before the compresses are applied.

SETTING GOALS

- The client's wound margins will show evidence of granulation, eventually becoming intact.
- Swelling in the area will be reduced.
- Drainage will subside.
- The client will experience reduced discomfort.

PREPARATION OF EQUIPMENT

The nurse will need selected items from the following list:

Prescribed solution (warmed to approximately 40°C to 43°C [105°F to 110°F])
Sterile container for solution
Sterile gauze dressings or compresses
Sterile gloves
Clean disposable gloves
Waterproof pad
Dry bath towel
Bath blanket
Tape or ties
Aquathermia or external heating device (optional)
Sterile bath thermometer (if available, to check the temperature of the solution)

Technique for applying warm sterile compresses to an open wound

ACTION	RATIONALE
1. Assess the client for any circulatory impairment to the area where the compress is to be applied (numbness, tingling, impairment in temperature sensation, or cyanosis).	Circulatory impairment may interfere with the client's ability to perceive heat and place him at risk of injury from the application of heat.
2. Check the physician's order for warm compresses. Explain the procedure to the client.	An explanation encourages the client's cooperation and reduces apprehension.
3. Gather equipment.	Organization promotes efficient time management.
4. Wash your hands.	Handwashing deters the spread of microorganisms.
5. Close the door or curtain. Use a bath blanket as needed when exposing an area for the application of warm compresses. Position a waterproof pad under the client.	These measures provide for privacy and warmth.
6. Assist the client to a comfortable position that provides easy access to the area.	Positioning provides for comfort and ease when applying compresses.

7. Place an opened, cuffed plastic bag near the working area.

8. Prepare the Aquathermia pad or external heating device, if it will be used.

9. Using sterile technique, open the dressings and warmed solution. Pour the solution into the sterile container, as the nurse in Figure III-16-2 is doing. Carefully drop the gauze for compresses into the sterile solution, as shown in Figure III-16-3.

Soiled dressings may be placed in a disposal bag without contaminating the outside surfaces of the bag.

An external heating device allows the compress to retain heat for a longer interval.

Sterile technique is used for warm moist compresses applied to an open wound.

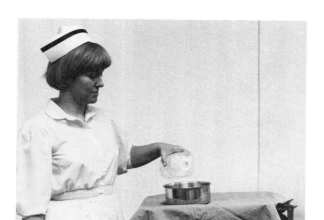

Figure III-16–2   The nurse pours sterile solution into a sterile basin. She holds the bottle close to the basin while pouring so that the solution will not splash and wet the sterile field.

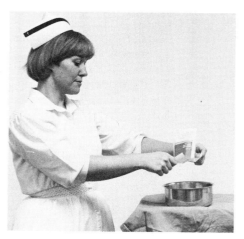

Figure III-16–3   This nurse pulls apart the edges of a package of sterile gauze that will be used as compress material on a wound.

10. Don a clean disposable glove and remove any dressing carefully. Discard the dressing in a disposable plastic bag. Pull off the soiled glove inside out and drop in the bag.

11. Assess the status of wound healing or presence of infection.

12. Don sterile gloves. Refer to Procedure I-12.

13. Retrieve the sterile compress from the warmed solution and squeeze the moisture from it. Apply it carefully, gently molding it around the wound. Be alert for the client's response to the heat.

14. Cover the gauze compresses with a dry bath towel and tie it in place if necessary.

15. Apply an Aquathermia pad or other external heating device over the towel (optional).

16. Monitor the condition of the skin and the client's response to the warm compress at frequent intervals.

17. After 30 minutes (or the time ordered by the physician) remove the warm compress. Carefully observe the condition of the skin around the wound and the client's response to the application of the heat.

18. Apply a dry sterile dressing to the wound.

Enclosing soiled material prevents the spread of microorganisms by means of contaminated dressings.

Noting the characteristics of the wound aids in determining the eventual effectiveness of treatment and acts as a baseline for future comparisons.

Sterile gloves are needed to maintain surgical asepsis.

Excess moisture may contaminate the surrounding area and is uncomfortable for the client. Molding the compress to the skin promotes the retention of warmth around the wound site.

Using a towel provides additional insulation.

An external heating device controls the temperature and extends the therapeutic effect of the compress.

Impaired circulation may affect the sensitivity to heat.

Maximum therapeutic effects of heat occur within 20 to 30 minutes. Extended use of heat (beyond 45 minutes) results in tissue congestion and vasoconstriction. This rebound phenomenon results in increased risk of burns from the application of heat.

A dressing protects the wound from microorganisms in the environments.

19. Dispose of equipment appropriately. Wash your hands.

These techniques support the principles of asepsis.

20. Record the client's response and the condition of the wound and the surrounding skin area.

Written records provide accurate documentation of the procedure.

SAMPLE DOCUMENTATION

Date	Time	Nurse's note
12/20	1115	Dressing on R leg removed. Small $\frac{1}{4}$″ round, red area over tibia draining purulent matter. Client experiences an increase in pain with movement. R calf is swollen; the skin is shiny; hair growth is sparse in comparison with L leg. Warm saline compress applied, wrapped with plastic wrap. Aquathermia pad applied over area for 30 minutes.
		G. Briosi, RN

EVALUATION

REASSESSMENT

The nurse can compare the effect that moist heat produces in the area by noting any skin color changes. Wound healing and swelling reduction are likely to be insidious and take several days of treatment before clinical improvement is noticed. The client may be able to experience beneficial effects with each application.

EXPECTED OUTCOMES

The compress remains warm and moist.
There is no evidence of burning to the skin.
The area and depth of the wound are reduced.
The client's analgesic use is reduced.

UNEXPECTED OUTCOMES

The temperature of the compress rises or falls below a therapeutic range.
The client feels chilled or becomes diaphoretic.
The skin shows evidence of thermal injury.

MODIFICATIONS IN SPECIAL SITUATIONS

GENERAL VARIATIONS

Warm compresses can be applied to intact areas of the body without maintaining sterile conditions.

Possible solutions for sterile compresses include sterile distilled water, sterile normal saline, and sterile sodium hypochlorite solution, also known as Dakin's solution.

Cold compresses can be used to relieve swelling and reduce pain. The use of cold is more effective when applied immediately after an injury to limit the effects of trauma to surrounding tissue.

If the skin around the wound shows signs of maceration from prolonged moisture, it may be protected by applying petroleum jelly or zinc oxide directly to the skin before applying the compress.

AGE-RELATED VARIATIONS

Use a roller bandage or binder to retain a compress on an active child or confused adult.

HOME-HEALTH VARIATIONS

Sterile compresses can be prepared by boiling towels or using a pressure cooker. The cloth fabric must be cooled and wrung before actually applying it to the skin.

Use plastic food bags or trash bags as a waterproof cover around the compress material.

PERFORMANCE CHECKLIST

When applying a warm sterile compress to an open wound, the learner:

C	A	U	
[ ]	[ ]	[ ]	Confirms the written physician's order
[ ]	[ ]	[ ]	Reviews the agency's policy concerning compresses
[ ]	[ ]	[ ]	Explains the procedure
[ ]	[ ]	[ ]	Assembles the equipment
[ ]	[ ]	[ ]	Provides privacy
[ ]	[ ]	[ ]	Adjusts the bed and position of the client
[ ]	[ ]	[ ]	Washes hands
[ ]	[ ]	[ ]	Dons a clean glove and removes the soiled dressing
[ ]	[ ]	[ ]	Washes hands after glove removal
[ ]	[ ]	[ ]	Protects the bed from becoming wet
[ ]	[ ]	[ ]	Prepares sterile supplies
[ ]	[ ]	[ ]	Warms the solution
[ ]	[ ]	[ ]	Saturates the compress material
[ ]	[ ]	[ ]	Wrings excess moisture without contamination
[ ]	[ ]	[ ]	Applies compress material to the area
[ ]	[ ]	[ ]	Covers the compress with a thick dry towel or plastic wrap
[ ]	[ ]	[ ]	Maintains warmth by applying an external heating device, if necessary
[ ]	[ ]	[ ]	Assesses the response of the client to the heat
[ ]	[ ]	[ ]	Removes the compress after 30 minutes or the time prescribed by the physician
[ ]	[ ]	[ ]	Observes the effect of the heat to the skin and wound
[ ]	[ ]	[ ]	Applies a sterile dressing
[ ]	[ ]	[ ]	Replaces wet linen
[ ]	[ ]	[ ]	Assists the client to a safe, comfortable position
[ ]	[ ]	[ ]	Disposes of equipment and supplies appropriately
[ ]	[ ]	[ ]	Washes hands
[ ]	[ ]	[ ]	Charts significant information

Outcome: [ ] Pass   [ ] Fail

C = competent; A = acceptable; U = unsatisfactory

Comments: _____

_____

_____

_____   _____
Student's Signature   Date

_____   _____
Instructor's Signature   Date

III-17

Cleaning a wound and applying a clean dressing

A wound is a disruption in the normal integrity of the skin and underlying tissues. The wound may be caused accidentally or intentionally. Trauma may produce a wound that is open or closed, clean or contaminated, superficial or deep. Care of the client with a wound is a fundamental aspect of nursing care that requires knowledge and skill.

PURPOSES OF PROCEDURE

The nurse cleanses a wound and applies a clean dressing to

1. Remove drainage, debris, and microorganisms from the wound
2. Promote wound healing
3. Absorb drainage as it accumulates
4. Provide a barrier against the entry of contaminants into the wound
5. Protect the wound from additional injury

ASSESSMENT

OBJECTIVE DATA

- Read the physician's order to determine that the nurse has been designated to assume responsibility for changing the dressing.
- Determine if the physician has a preferred protocol for dressing changes, such as using a particular skin antiseptic or antimicrobial ointment.
- Read the chart for information that reflects the development of possible complications, such as elevated temperature, pulse rate, white blood cell count, or positive wound culture.
- Scan the client's medical history noting conditions that can contribute to poor healing, such as a malignancy, diabetes mellitus, obesity, or low red cell or hemoglobin levels.
- Consult with colleagues or the documentation on the chart for wound descriptions made during prior dressing changes.
- Inspect the wound; note its color, approximation, characteristics of drainage, odor, appearance of sutures or staples, and presence of drains.
- Gently palpate the area surrounding the wound; feel for warmth and swelling.
- Observe the client's reactions during the assessment. Watch to see if the client looks at the wound. Analyze the significance of verbal and nonverbal communication.
- Be aware of the client's level of activity, effort to move, appetite, and hydration.
- Note the client's pattern for requiring analgesia.

SUBJECTIVE DATA

- Ask the client to describe any pain or other sensations experienced in or near the wound.

RELEVANT NURSING DIAGNOSES

The client with a wound may have nursing diagnoses, such as

- *Impaired Skin or Tissue Integrity*
- *Altered Comfort*
- *Potential for Infection*
- *Anxiety*

- *Fear*
- *Disturbance in Self-Concept*
- *Knowledge Deficit*

PLANNING

ESTABLISHING PRIORITIES

A wound must be cleaned and a fresh dressing applied whenever it becomes damp with drainage. A wet dressing acts as a wick pulling organisms on the outer surface of the dressing into the wound. Wound drainage combined with a dark, warm environment promotes the growth of pathogens. Changing a dressing should be done on a regular basis in order to obtain a current appraisal of healing.

SETTING GOALS

- The client's wound edges will be approximated and of similar appearance to the surrounding tissue within 1 week.
- The client's vital signs will remain within normal ranges for his age and there will be no local evidence of an infectious process within the wound.
- The client will experience reduced discomfort at and about the wound as evidenced by a reduced need for analgesia and increased activity.

PREPARATION OF EQUIPMENT

The nurse will need selected items from the following list:

Sterile gloves
Gauze dressings or squares
Sterile dressing set or suture set (contains scissors and forceps)
Cleansing solution
Clean disposable gloves
Sterile basin (optional)
Sterile drape (optional)
Plastic bag for soiled dressings
Waterproof pad
Bath blanket
Tape or ties
Assorted dressings
Acetone or adhesive remover (optional)
Sterile normal saline (optional)

Technique for cleaning a wound and applying a clean dressing

ACTION	RATIONALE
1. Check the physician's order.	Reading the order clarifies the procedure and the type of supplies required.
2. Explain the procedure to the client.	An explanation encourages the client's cooperation and reduces apprehension.
3. Gather the equipment.	Organization promotes efficient time management.
4. Wash your hands.	Handwashing deters the spread of microorganisms.
5. Close the door or curtain. Use a bath blanket as needed when exposing the area to be redressed. Position a waterproof pad under the client if desired.	Closing the door or curtain provides privacy and warmth.
6. Assist the client to a comfortable position that provides easy access to the wound area.	Consideration for the comfort of the client is a primary concern. The nurse promotes good body mechanics to avoid muscle strain.
7. Place an opened, cuffed, plastic bag near the working area.	Soiled dressings may be placed in a disposal bag to control the transmission of microorganisms.

8. Loosen the tape on the dressing, as shown in Figure III-17-1. Use adhesive remover if necessary.

It is easier to loosen tape before putting on gloves.

9. Don a clean, disposable glove and remove soiled dressings carefully, as the nurse in Figure III-17-2 is doing. Check the position of a drain before removing the dressing. If a dressing is not a wet-to-dry application and is adhering to the skin surface, it may be moistened by pouring a small amount of sterile saline onto it.

A glove protects the nurse when handling a contaminated dressing. Using caution in removing a dressing promotes comfort and ensures that a drain will not be removed if one is present. Sterile saline loosens the dressing for easier removal.

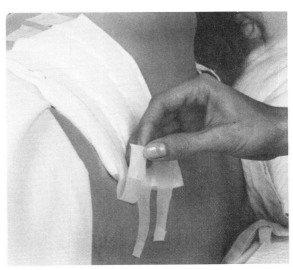

Figure III-17-1 The nurse removes tape that is securing the client's dressing. Notice that the tape is being pulled toward the wound and held parallel to the client's skin to reduce discomfort.

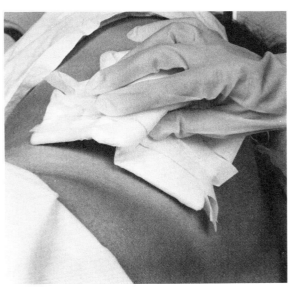

Figure III-17-2 The nurse is using gloves to remove and handle a dressing from a wound. The dressing is then placed in a moisture-proof bag for eventual incineration. Fresh, sterile gloves will be donned to apply the new dressing.

10. Assess the amount, type, and odor of drainage.

Assessment documents the wound-healing process or presence of infection.

11. Discard the dressing in the plastic disposable bag, as shown in Figure III-17-3. Pull off the glove inside out and drop it in the bag. Wash hands.

Placing contaminated objects in a bag prevents the spread of microorganisms.

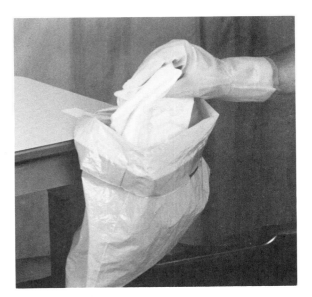

Figure III-17-3 The soiled dressing, gloves, and contaminated disposable equipment and supplies are placed in a waterproof bag. In this case a plastic bag has been attached to the overbed table.

12. Using aseptic technique, open the sterile dressings and supplies on the work area.

Supplies should be within easy reach to maintain sterility.

13. Open the sterile cleansing solution and pour it over the gauze sponges in a plastic container or over sponges placed in a sterile basin.

Pouring sterile solution over sterile dressings supports principles of aseptic technique.

14. Don sterile gloves. Refer to Procedure I-12.

Using sterile gloves prevents contaminating sterile equipment and introducing microorganisms within the wound.

15. Cleanse the wound or surgical incision as the nurse in Figure III-17-4 is doing. Follow the options illustrated in Figure III-17-5. Use sterile forceps if desired.

Cleansing removes drainage, debris, and microorganisms.

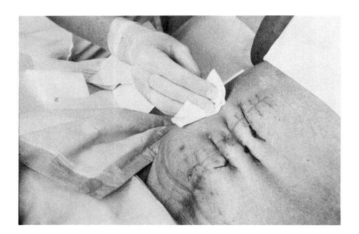

Figure III-17–4 The nurse is using a sterile gauze square to cleanse the wound and adjacent skin area. Using gauze moistened with an antiseptic removes accumulated drainage and reduces the growth of microorganisms that are present on the skin.

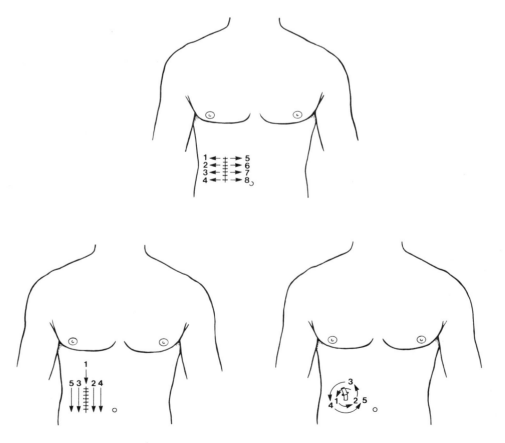

Figure III-17–5 The arrows in these diagrams show options for maintaining medical asepsis when cleaning a wound or around a drain. It is important that cleansing procedures start at the cleaner area and move outward.

a. Clean from top to bottom or from the center outward.

b. Use one gauze square for each wipe, discarding each square by dropping it into the plastic bag. Do not touch the bag with the forceps.

c. Clean around a drain, if present, moving from the center outward in a circular motion. Use one gauze square for each circular motion.

d. Dry the wound using a gauze square in the same motion.

16. Apply a layer of dry, sterile dressings over the wound as shown in Figure III-17-6. Use sterile forceps if desired.

17. Place sterile gauze under and around the drain if one is present.

Aseptic principles direct that an area be cleaned from the least contaminated to the most contaminated area.

Using a separate gauze square prevents recontaminating previously cleaned areas.

Wiping in a circular manner moves debris, drainage, and pathogens from the least contaminated to the most contaminated areas.

Moisture provides a medium for growth of microorganisms.

The primary dressing serves as a wick for drainage.

The gauze absorbs drainage and protects the surrounding skin area.

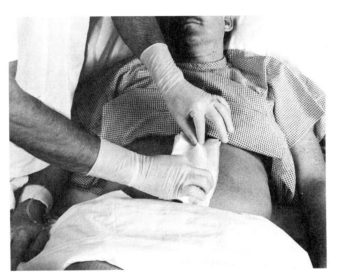

Figure III-17-6   The nurse is placing the first layer of gauze over a wound.

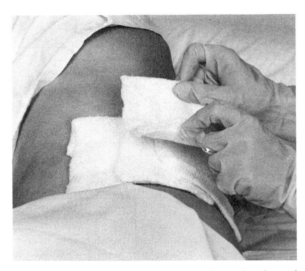

Figure III-17-7   Layers of thick gauze pads are placed over the wound to absorb drainage while keeping the exposed surface of the dressing dry. Use only the minimum amount of dressings because excess bulk can cause discomfort.

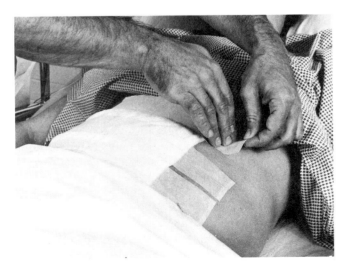

Figure III-17-8   Strips of tape are used to secure the dressing. Note that the dressing is not entirely covered with tape. This technique allows for the dissipation of moisture and heat.

18. Apply a second gauze layer to the wound site.

The second layer provides for increased absorption of drainage.

19. Place a Surgi-pad or ABD dressing over the wound as the outermost layer, as shown in Figure III-17-7.

The last layer of the dressing protects the wound from microorganisms in the environment.

20. Remove the gloves from the inside out and discard them in the plastic waste bag. Apply tape, as shown in Figure III-17-8, or secure ties to maintain the dressing in place.

Tape is easier to apply after gloves have been removed.

21. Wash your hands. Remove all the equipment and make the client comfortable.

These actions prevent the spread of microorganisms.

22. Check the dressing and wound site every shift. Record the dressing change and appearance of the wound, and describe any drainage in the chart.

Recording observations provides an accurate documentation of the care of the client.

SAMPLE DOCUMENTATION

Date	Time	Nurse's note
6/13	1000	Dressing saturated with 2″ area of serosanguineous drainage. Wound appears intact. Edges are pink and slightly swollen. Incision cleansed with povidone iodine solution and covered with Telfa gauze, fluffs, and ABD pads. Does not express the need for pain medication.

W. Zonyk, RN

EVALUATION

REASSESSMENT

The dressing over a fresh wound should be assessed frequently, every 15 minutes in the first few hours after it has occurred, to detect signs of hemorrhage. The nurse may reinforce a dressing if it becomes saturated. Once it has been determined that the client's condition has stabilized, the nurse may use judgment in determining how often the dressing and wound should be inspected. It is expected that the nurse would evaluate the condition of the dressing and the wound at least once per shift. It is customary for the physician to perform the first dressing change following surgery. The nurse is likely to be responsible for subsequent dressing changes on an "as needed" or daily basis after 24 to 48 hours.

EXPECTED OUTCOMES

The drainage and debris are removed from the wound.
The edges of the wound are pink and uniformly close together.
The dressing covers the wound completely and remains secured to the skin.

UNEXPECTED OUTCOMES

The wound edges are red, swollen, hot, and tender.
Parts of the wound are gaping.
Purulent, foul-smelling drainage is released from the wound.

MODIFICATIONS IN SELECTED SITUATIONS

Some hospital units have special dressing carts containing a variety of dressing and wound care supplies. The mobile cart is wheeled down the hallway when there is a need to change one or several dressings. This avoids extra trips to a supply room if the wound care involves unexpected modifications in cleansing or dressing techniques.

The number and types of dressings used depend on the location and size of the wound.

There are many possible antiseptic cleansing agents that can be used to cleanse a wound. Some commonly used are povidone–iodine (Betadine), 70% alcohol, 3% hydrogen peroxide, and sterile normal saline. Some authorities feel saline is the only agent that avoids a caustic effect to the wound.

Transparent dressings, such as Op-Site, can be applied directly over a small wound or tube. This type of covering is air-occlusive and allows visualization of the wound.

Use Montgomery straps, shown in Figure III-17-9, when a dressing must be changed frequently.

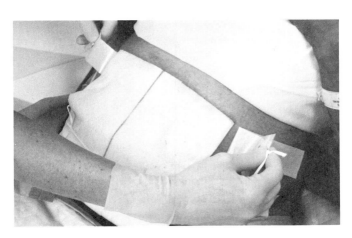

Figure III-17–9 When the nurse uses Montgomery straps, the need for removing and reapplying adhesive tape to the skin can be avoided each time the dressing is changed.

AGE-RELATED VARIATIONS

Use paper tape for individuals who are allergic to adhesive or whose skin is thin and fragile, as may be the case in infants and elderly adults.

To keep a dressing intact or to prevent contamination of a wound and dressings on an infant or small child, it may be necessary to restrain the child's hand. An old stocking or piece of stockinet may be used to encircle the child's hand and then secured to the bed or crib with a tie or safety pin. Care must be taken not to compromise circulation to that extremity.

To gain a child's cooperation, use large decorated Band-Aids to cover a small wound. Let the child apply a similar dressing to a doll or stuffed animal to promote the ability to cope with the procedure.

HOME-HEALTH VARIATIONS

Metal instruments needed for wound care can be first rinsed in cool water, then washed in warm soapy water, and boiled for 10 minutes to ensure sterility.

Inform the client and family about the availability of disposable wound care supplies.

The American Cancer Society is a source for free dressings when the client has a draining wound caused by a malignancy.

Soiled dressings can be wrapped in old newspapers and placed in a plastic bag for disposal.

RELATED TEACHING

Explain the purpose for cleaning and applying fresh dressings.

Describe the normal, expected appearance of a wound according to the stage of its healing.

Encourage splinting the wound during activity, such as coughing, sneezing, sudden movement, or change in position.

When preparing a client or family member for home care, reinforce the need for thorough handwashing before and after removing a soiled dressing and again after the fresh dressing has been applied.

Instruct the client that any break or interruption in the suture line may require immediate intervention and the surgeon should be notified immediately. Inform the client and family about significant changes that need to be reported to the nurse or physician.

PERFORMANCE CHECKLIST

When cleaning a wound and applying a dressing, the learner:

C	A	U	
[ ]	[ ]	[ ]	Checks the physician's order
[ ]	[ ]	[ ]	Gathers information from the chart
[ ]	[ ]	[ ]	Informs the client concerning the purpose for the assessment and procedure
[ ]	[ ]	[ ]	Provides privacy
[ ]	[ ]	[ ]	Washes hands
[ ]	[ ]	[ ]	Assists the client to a comfortable position
[ ]	[ ]	[ ]	Drapes the client
[ ]	[ ]	[ ]	Prepares a receptacle for the soiled dressing
[ ]	[ ]	[ ]	Dons a clean, disposable glove
[ ]	[ ]	[ ]	Removes and discards the soiled dressing and glove
[ ]	[ ]	[ ]	Washes hands
[ ]	[ ]	[ ]	Opens sterile supplies, instrument wrappers, and antiseptic containers
[ ]	[ ]	[ ]	Dons sterile gloves
[ ]	[ ]	[ ]	Cleans the wound from the least contaminated to the most contaminated areas
[ ]	[ ]	[ ]	Uses a separate gauze square for each wiping of the wound
[ ]	[ ]	[ ]	Covers the wound with various dressing supplies in an appropriate sequence
[ ]	[ ]	[ ]	Removes gloves
[ ]	[ ]	[ ]	Secures the dressing with tape, ties, roller bandage, or binder
[ ]	[ ]	[ ]	Removes and disposes of soiled objects
[ ]	[ ]	[ ]	Washes hands
[ ]	[ ]	[ ]	Replaces unopened sterile supplies
[ ]	[ ]	[ ]	Charts significant information

Outcome: [ ] Pass   [ ] Fail

C = competent; A = acceptable; U = unsatisfactory

Comments: _____
_____
_____

_____   _____
Student's Signature   Date

_____   _____
Instructor's Signature   Date

III-18 *Irrigating a wound and inserting packing*

Normal healing is promoted when the wound is free of debris and foreign materials. Excessive exudate, dead or damaged tissue cells, pathogenic organisms, or embedded fragments of bone, metal, glass, or other substances can interfere with healing until they are removed. The body's own restorative processes, such as localization and suppuration, aid the natural removal of this material. However, sometimes mechanical means, such as irrigation and packing, may be necessary.

PURPOSES OF PROCEDURE

A wound is irrigated and packed to

1. Assist in removing debris from a wound
2. Promote healing from the internal areas of the wound toward its surface
3. Shorten the time required for wound healing
4. Prevent abscess formation
5. Reduce discomfort

ASSESSMENT

Refer to the assessments in Procedure III-17, with the following additions:

- Estimate the length and depth of the open wound.
- Consult the agency's infection-control policy concerning drainage and secretion precautions.
- Review the agency's procedure manual for the recommended volume, temperature, and type of irrigation solution if unspecified by the physician.
- Note the identity of any pathogens in the wound culture report.

RELEVANT NURSING DIAGNOSES

In addition to the nursing diagnoses listed with Procedure III-17, the client who requires a wound irrigation and insertion of packing can have nursing diagnoses, such as

- *Altered Body Temperature*

PLANNING

ESTABLISHING PRIORITIES

The body responds systemically to trauma and the use of its reserves for healing. Therefore, the nurse must attend to basic needs, such as adequate rest, supplying sufficient quality and amounts of nutrition and fluids, and so on. The specification for the frequency of a wound irrigation and packing is prescribed by the physician. The nurse is held accountable for implementing those directives. It may be that this procedure will be repeated more than once each day.

SETTING GOALS

- Drainage and debris will be removed from the wound.
- The client's wound will heal by second intention.

PREPARATION OF EQUIPMENT

The nurse will need selected items from the following list:
Sterile irrigation set (basin, container for irrigant, irrigating syringe)
Prescribed irrigating solution (warmed to body temperature or 34°C to 37°C)
Sterile soft catheter (optional)

Sterile gloves
Clean disposable gloves
Sterile dressing set or suture set (contains scissors and forceps)
Waterproof pad
Assorted sterile dressings
Packing gauze (as specified by physician)
Gown (optional)
Bath blanket
Tape

Technique for irrigating a wound and inserting packing

ACTION	RATIONALE
1. Check the physician's order for irrigation and packing of the wound.	Reading the written order clarifies the procedure and type of supplies.
2. Explain the procedure to the client.	An explanation reduces the client's apprehension and facilitates cooperation.
3. Gather the equipment.	Organization promotes efficient time management.
4. Wash your hands.	Handwashing deters the spread of microorganisms.
5. Close the door or curtain. Use a bath blanket as needed when exposing the wound site.	Covering and protecting the client from the view of others provides privacy and warmth.
6. Position the client so the irrigating solution will flow from the upper end of the wound toward the lower end. Place a waterproof pad under the client.	Gravity directs the flow of liquid from the least contaminated to the most contaminated area. A waterproof pad protects the client and bed linens.
7. Warm sterile irrigating solution to body temperature.	Warmed solution is more comfortable for the client and promotes vasodilation.
8. Place an opened, cuffed plastic bag near the working area. Don a gown if recommended.	Soiled dressings and packing may be placed in a disposal bag without contaminating outside surfaces of the bag. The gown protects the uniform from contamination should splashing occur.
9. Loosen the tape on the dressing and put on a clean glove to remove soiled dressings and packing, as shown in Figure III-18-1.	A glove acts as a transmission barrier and protects the nurse when handling contaminated objects.

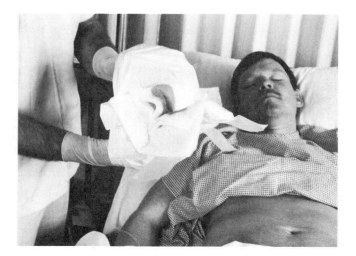

Figure III-18–1   The nurse is using gloves to remove a soiled dressing. All contaminated items are placed in a moisture-proof bag.

10. Assess the amount, type, and odor of drainage. Observe the condition of the wound.	Assessment provides information about the wound-healing process or presence of infection.

11. Discard the dressings in the plastic disposal bag. Remove the glove inside out and drop it in the bag also.

Enclosing contaminated objects prevents the spread of microorganisms.

12. Wash your hands.

Handwashing deters the spread of microorganisms.

13. Using aseptic technique, open sterile dressings and supplies on a work area.

Supplies that are within easy reach are likely to remain sterile.

14. Pour warmed sterile irrigating solution into a sterile container. The amount may vary from 200 ml to 500 ml depending on the size and depth of the wound.

Filling a container facilitates wound irrigation.

15. Don sterile gloves.

Sterile gloves maintain surgical asepsis.

16. Hold the sterile basin with the nondominant hand below the wound to collect the irrigation fluid.

Positioning the basin below the wound protects the client and the bed linens from contaminated fluid.

17. Use the dominant hand to fill a syringe with irrigant. Gently direct a stream of solution into the wound keeping the tip of the syringe 1 inch (2.5 cm) above the upper area of the wound, shown in Figure III-18-2. If using a catheter tip on a syringe, insert it gently into the wound to the point of resistance.

Debris and contaminated solution flow from the least contaminated to the most contaminated area. A catheter tip allows introduction of the irrigant into a wound with a small opening or one that is deep.

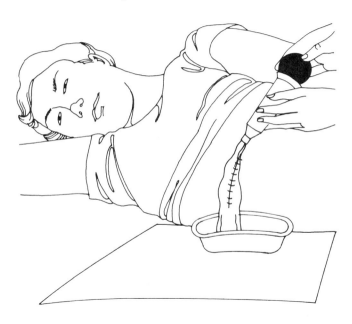

Figure III-18–2 Sterile solution is instilled into the wound to remove accumulated exudate and debris.

18. Continue the irrigation until the solution returns clear. Try to maintain a steady flow of solution.

The purpose of the irrigation is to remove exudate and debris.

19. Use sterile forceps to gently insert sterile packing into the wound. Be careful not to pack the wound excessively. Cut the packing, if necessary, with sterile scissors. Allow a small strip of packing to protrude from the wound for easier removal.

Packing is used to absorb drainage and promote healing. Excessive packing of a wound may impede blood flow and delay the healing process.

20. Dry the area around the wound with a sterile gauze square.

Moisture provides a medium for the growth of microorganisms.

21. Apply layers of sterile dressing material.

Dressings absorb drainage and protect the wound and surrounding skin.

22. Remove the gloves and discard them in the plastic disposal bag. Apply tape to secure the dressing.

The gloves are disposed after one use. Tape is easier to apply after the gloves have been removed.

23. Wash your hands. Remove all equipment and make the client comfortable.

These practices prevent the spread of microorganisms.

24. Check the dressing and wound site every shift. Record the length and depth of the wound, irrigation, insertion of packing, appearance of the wound, and a description of the drainage.

The written record provides an accurate documentation of the client's care and treatment.

SAMPLE DOCUMENTATION

Date	Time	Nurse's note
10/02	1800	Tylox i cap. for continuous "throbbing" in abdominal wound.
		T. Hensley, RN
	1830	Dressing and gauze packing removed. Inner area of wound is red. Packing saturated with purulent and bloody drainage which is foul-smelling. Holds body rigid and winces when wound is examined. Wound irrigated with 200 ml of warmed 3% hydrogen peroxide solution. Iodoform gauze packed into wound and covered with a sterile dressing.
		T. Hensley, RN

EVALUATION

REASSESSMENT

Inspect the dressing and the wound at least once per shift.
Compare the observations with those recorded by other nurses.
Evaluate signs of overall well-being, such as lifting of malaise, improved appetite, increased activity, a more positive attitude, and so forth, as correlated with progressive healing.

EXPECTED OUTCOMES

Drainage and debris are washed from the wound.
The wound is moist and does not bleed during the removal or insertion of the packing.

UNEXPECTED OUTCOMES

The packing sticks within the wound.
The length or depth of the wound increases.
The wound continues to produce large amounts of drainage.
The client experiences pain.

MODIFICATIONS IN SELECTED SITUATIONS

GENERAL VARIATIONS

The nurse may choose to wear a gown over the uniform at any time that soiling is likely. However, if a wound is infected with *Staphylococcus aureus,* beta-hemolytic *Streptococcus,* or *Clostridium perfringens,* the Centers for Disease Control recommend that a gown and mask should be worn. Furthermore, forceps should be used rather than a gloved hand to remove soiled dressings. The soiled dressing, packing, instruments, gown, and mask should be double wrapped in a labeled bag and disposed according to the agency's infection-control policies.
Sterile normal saline, an antiseptic, or an antibiotic solution may be used for a wound irrigation. Hydrogen peroxide is often prescribed because its oxygen-releasing ability has an effective cleansing effect.
A sterile intravenous solution and tubing may be substituted for an irrigating syringe when a large volume is necessary for irrigation.
Consider using Montgomery straps, shown in Figure III-18-3, to avoid irritating the skin with frequent removal of tape.
Supply the debilitated client with nutritional supplements at frequent times throughout the day. Undernourished individuals have difficulty in achieving wound healing when they lack the basic components for energy and cellular repair.

AGE-RELATED VARIATIONS

Expect that a wound may take longer than usual to heal when a person is very old.
Provide a school-age or older child with a radio head set for distraction while caring for a wound.

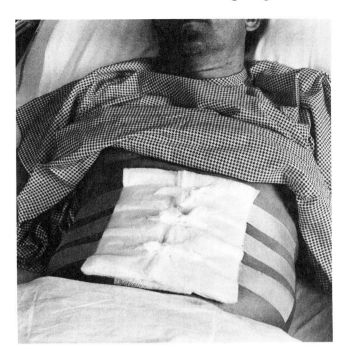

Figure III-18–3 Montgomery straps make it possible to care for a wound without removing tape each time the soiled dressing is removed and reapplied.

HOME-HEALTH VARIATIONS

Advise a parent to cover an infant or child's hands with a cotton anklet or kneesock to prevent the child from removing a dressing and packing.

Instruct the client and family never to use cotton as packing material.

Use large, plastic trash bags to protect the bed and linen from becoming wet when the wound is irrigated.

RELATED TEACHING

Always help the client understand the sequence of steps in the procedure and their purpose.

Identify the signs associated with healing and those indicating complications.

Teach the client who will be discharged needing self-care how to construct homemade Montgomery straps.

Advise the client to stoop from the knees and avoid heavy lifting if the wound edges are not approximated.

Explain why a gown, mask, or gloves are worn using language that will not frighten a client or the family.

(Performance checklist next page)

PERFORMANCE CHECKLIST

When irrigating a wound and inserting packing, the learner:

C	A	U	
[ ]	[ ]	[ ]	Checks the physician's written order
[ ]	[ ]	[ ]	Reviews the agency's policies and procedures, if unknown
[ ]	[ ]	[ ]	Gathers data
[ ]	[ ]	[ ]	Provides the client with an explanation of the procedure
[ ]	[ ]	[ ]	Assembles equipment
[ ]	[ ]	[ ]	Warms the solution
[ ]	[ ]	[ ]	Brings the equipment to the bedside
[ ]	[ ]	[ ]	Provides privacy
[ ]	[ ]	[ ]	Positions the client so that the solution will flow from the least contaminated to the most contaminated areas
[ ]	[ ]	[ ]	Washes hands
[ ]	[ ]	[ ]	Protects the linen and the client's bed clothing from becoming wet
[ ]	[ ]	[ ]	Prepares a bag for holding soiled objects
[ ]	[ ]	[ ]	Dons a clean glove and removes the soiled dressing
[ ]	[ ]	[ ]	Places soiled glove in refuse bag
[ ]	[ ]	[ ]	Washes hands
[ ]	[ ]	[ ]	Opens sterile equipment and packages
[ ]	[ ]	[ ]	Dons sterile gloves
[ ]	[ ]	[ ]	Holds a drainage basin below the wound
[ ]	[ ]	[ ]	Instills solution into the wound
[ ]	[ ]	[ ]	Regulates the rate and volume of administration so as to remove accumulated drainage and debris
[ ]	[ ]	[ ]	Dries the skin
[ ]	[ ]	[ ]	Packs gauze loosely and gently within the wound
[ ]	[ ]	[ ]	Applies a dressing
[ ]	[ ]	[ ]	Removes and discards gloves
[ ]	[ ]	[ ]	Secures the dressing
[ ]	[ ]	[ ]	Washes hands
[ ]	[ ]	[ ]	Disposes of equipment appropriately
[ ]	[ ]	[ ]	Charts significant information

Outcome: [ ] Pass   [ ] Fail

C = competent; A = acceptable; U = unsatisfactory

Comments: _____
_____
_____

_____   _____
Student's Signature   Date

_____   _____
Instructor's Signature   Date

III-19   *Removing sutures or staples*

Optimum healing takes place by primary intention. This occurs when there is no infection present and the edges of a wound are well approximated. Sutures or metal staples may be used to keep the edges of the wound together until the body can repair the area. Primary intention healing is illustrated in Fig. III-19-1. This type of wound closes rapidly and leaves minimal scarring. Eventually the sutures or staples must be removed.

First Intention (Primary union)

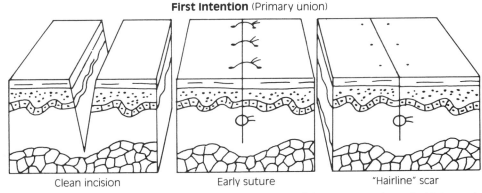

Clean incision   Early suture   "Hairline" scar

Figure III-19-1   This series of drawings shows how tissue and skin are approximated with internal and skin sutures so that healing takes place with minimal inflammation and scarring.

PURPOSES OF PROCEDURE

Sutures and staples are removed to:

1. Prevent a reaction to foreign material used for temporary wound approximation.
2. Facilitate complete natural repair of the wound.
3. Avoid a pathway for microorganisms to enter the deeper areas of a healing wound.

ASSESSMENT

Refer to Procedure III-17, with the following additions:
- Determine the method used for suturing. Examples are shown in Fig. III-19-2.
- Note if retention sutures, illustrated in Fig. III-19-3, are present.

RELEVANT NURSING DIAGNOSES

The client who is about to have sutures or staples removed may have nursing diagnoses, such as:

- *Fear*
- *Altered Comfort*
- *Potential for Infection*
- *Potential for Injury*
- *Potential for Impaired Skin Integrity*
- *Knowledge Deficit*

Types of sutures

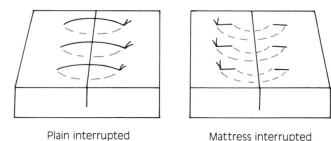

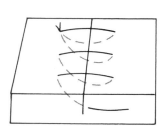

Plain interrupted

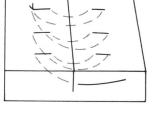

Mattress interrupted

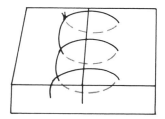

Plain continuous

Mattress continuous

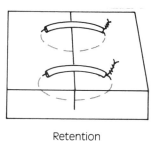

Blanket continuous

Figure III-19–2 The surgeon may select any of the following methods for closing a wound: plain interrupted sutures, mattress interrupted sutures, plain continuous sutures, mattress sutures, and blanket continuous sutures.

Retention

Figure III-19–3 Retention sutures are used to add reinforcing strength to an area subject to stress. To avoid cutting into the skin, the external portion of the suture is threaded through flexible tubing. Retention sutures are usually left in place longer than skin sutures.

PLANNING

ESTABLISHING
PRIORITIES

Sutures and staples are removed when the surgeon specifies. The nurse may encourage the client to shower before their removal. The water may tend to soften the incision line and partially separate the upper layers of skin. Alternating sutures or staples may be removed to test the integrity of the wound closure. It is not unusual for every other suture or staple to be removed initially. Be sure to read the written orders closely so there is no misunderstanding.

SETTING GOALS
- The client's wound edges will remain closed.
- The adjacent skin will not be injured.
- The client will experience minimal discomfort.

PREPARATION OF EQUIPMENT

The nurse will need selected items from the following list:

Suture removal set, shown in Fig. III-19-4, or staple remover
Portable lamp, if available lighting is poor
Antiseptic swabs
Sterile dressing supplies
Refuse bag
Steri-strips (optional)

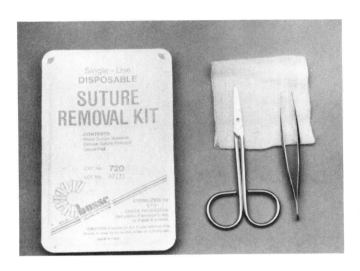

Figure III-19-4 Disposable suture removal sets are available in most hospitals. They contain sterile forceps and scissors. (Photo © Ken Kasper)

Technique for removing sutures or staples

ACTION	RATIONALE
1. Read the physician's written order.	Checking the order aids in clarifying specific directions.
2. Explain the procedure to the client.	An explanation reduces apprehension and promotes cooperation.
3. Gather equipment and bring supplies to the bedside.	Organization promotes efficient time management.
4. Open the bag that will be used for soiled material.	The bag acts as a transmission barrier by preventing pathogens from contact with clean areas.
5. Raise the bed to a high position and lower the nearer side rail.	Adjusting the bed prevents straining muscles.
6. Provide privacy by pulling the curtain and closing the door.	The nurse protects the client from being exposed to the view of others.
7. Wash your hands.	Handwashing deters the spread of microorganisms.
8. Don a clean glove, and remove the soiled dressing.	A glove acts as a transmission barrier to pathogens that may be spread by direct contact.
9. Discard the soiled dressing and glove by turning it inside out.	Enclosing the contaminated surface to the inside acts to restrict the transmission of pathogens.
10. Wash your hands.	Handwashing deters the spread of microorganisms.
11. Open sterile packages.	Packages can be opened without contaminating the contents.

12. Don sterile gloves.

Using sterile gloves maintains the sterility of equipment and prevents introducing pathogens into the area.

13. Cleanse the suture line with an antiseptic from the least to the most contaminated areas.

Swabbing mechanically moves organisms from the surface. Antiseptics inhibit the growth of microorganisms.

14. Grasp the knotted end of the suture with the forceps.

The knot is easier to grasp and hold than a single thread.

15. Pull and elevate the knot enough to provide room to insert the point of the scissors, as shown in Fig. III-19-5.

Freeing the suture prevents injuring the skin with the sharp point of the scissors.

16. Cut the suture beneath the knot, and remove it by pulling on the knotted end, as shown in Figure III-19-6.

This prevents pulling the portion of suture on the skin surface through underlying layers where pathogens could be transferred.

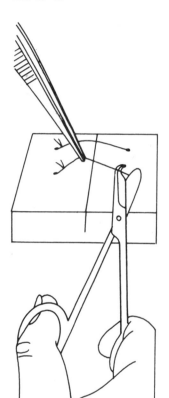

Removing interrupted sutures

Figure III-19-5 After cleansing the incision, a forceps is used to grasp and elevate the knot. The tip of the scissors is carefully inserted just under the knot. If the suture sticks, making insertion unsafe, it can be loosened by moistening the area with a wet, sterile gauze square placed over the wound for a few minutes.

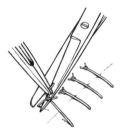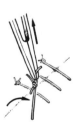

Figure III-19-6 The suture is cut just below the knot as close to the skin as possible. The knot is pulled gently in one continuous motion to remove the suture.

17. For staples, place the remover under the center of the staple, as shown in Fig. III-19-7.

Centering provides the ability to exert equal force to both buried ends of the staple.

18. Compress the staple remover.

As the instrument bends the bridge of the staple, the embedded teeth are released from the skin.

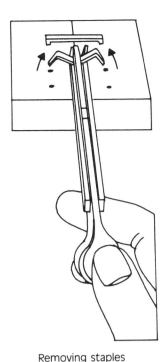

Removing staples

Figure III-19–7 Staples do not encircle the wound. A special instrument is used to release them from the skin.

19. Remove every other suture or staple.

To be sure the wound remains intact, half of the sutures are removed.

20. Drop each removed suture or staple into the refuse bag.

The bag contains objects that are a potential source of pathogens.

21. Cleanse the incision again with antiseptic as described in step 13.

Swabbing cleanses the tracks opened in the skin when the sutures and staples were removed.

22. Apply steri-strips across the incision, if indicated.

Small strips of adhesive keep a potentially weak wound closed after sutures have been removed.

23. Cover the area with a dry sterile dressing, if necessary.

Only a light dressing may be necessary to protect clothing from slight bleeding that may occur.

24. Remove gloves by turning them inside out, and discard them within the refuse bag.

Containing pathogens prevents their transmission to other susceptible hosts.

25. Remove soiled articles for proper disposal or disinfection.

Instruments can be cleaned and sterilized. Sharp disposable equipment should be placed in a puncture-resistant container to avoid injuring others.

26. Wash your hands.

Handwashing deters the spread of microorganisms.

27. Document assessments, the procedure as it was performed, and the response of the client.

The chart is a legal record of the care provided for the client.

SAMPLE DOCUMENTATION

Date	Time	Nurse's note
3/09	1400	Wound cleansed with betadine. Incision is dry with a thin pink margin. Every other suture removed at this time. Wound edges remain approximated.
		S. Pope, RN

EVALUATION REASSESSMENT	Note the integrity of the skin during the procedure. If the wound edges appear to separate, discontinue the removal and inform the physician. Inspect the wound again after physical activity.
EXPECTED OUTCOMES	The incision line is clean and dry. The sutures or staples are withdrawn easily with no additional trauma. The wound is securely closed.
UNEXPECTED OUTCOMES	The incision separates. Sutures or staples resist removal. Fragments of suture remain beneath the closed incision. The skin is traumatized with the instruments or tips of removed staples.
MODIFICATIONS IN SELECTED SITUATIONS GENERAL VARIATIONS	If there are indications that the client is prone to poor healing, remove random sutures in various areas of the incision to evaluate the integrity of the wound. The client may feel more secure with a binder supporting the incision line after sutures have been removed. Use an alternative skin cleanser, like 3% hydrogen peroxide, rather than betadine, if the client is allergic to iodine. Chart the number of sutures or staples removed.
HOME-HEALTH VARIATIONS	Instruct the client or his family on emergency procedures to follow if the incision should separate following the removal of sutures or staples.
RELATED TEACHING	Explain the body's normal responses to injury and healing processes to overcome misconceptions and fears about reopening a healed incision. Discharge planning should include informing the client of the signs indicating wound complications. Warn the client with a healing thoracic or abdominal incision to avoid situations that increase intrathoracic and intra-abdominal pressure, such as straining while having a bowel movement, sneezing, and coughing. A stool softener may be recommended as well as splinting the incisional area.

PERFORMANCE CHECKLIST

When removing sutures or staples, the learner:

C	A	U	
[ ]	[ ]	[ ]	Reads the written medical order.
[ ]	[ ]	[ ]	Reviews the client's hospital record for pertinent information.
[ ]	[ ]	[ ]	Assembles supplies.
[ ]	[ ]	[ ]	Explains the procedure to the client.
[ ]	[ ]	[ ]	Washes hands.
[ ]	[ ]	[ ]	Provides privacy.
[ ]	[ ]	[ ]	Dons a clean, disposable glove.
[ ]	[ ]	[ ]	Removes the current dressing, if one exists, and deposits it with the glove in a refuse bag.
[ ]	[ ]	[ ]	Examines the wound.
[ ]	[ ]	[ ]	Washes hands.
[ ]	[ ]	[ ]	Opens sterile supplies.
[ ]	[ ]	[ ]	Dons sterile gloves.
[ ]	[ ]	[ ]	Cleans the wound according to principles of asepsis.
[ ]	[ ]	[ ]	Cuts and removes sutures or uses a staple remover to bend and release metal clips.
[ ]	[ ]	[ ]	Swabs the incision line with antiseptic.
[ ]	[ ]	[ ]	Applies steri-strips or a dry sterile dressing, if needed.
[ ]	[ ]	[ ]	Removes and discards gloves.
[ ]	[ ]	[ ]	Makes the client comfortable.
[ ]	[ ]	[ ]	Removes soiled material and instruments according to agency policy.
[ ]	[ ]	[ ]	Washes hands.
[ ]	[ ]	[ ]	Charts significant information.

Outcome: [ ] **Pass** [ ] **Fail**

C = competent; A = acceptable; U = unsatisfactory

Comments: _____

_____

_____

_____   _____
　　　　Student's Signature　　　　　　　　**Date**

_____   _____
　　　　Instructor's Signature　　　　　　　**Date**

III-20

Maintaining and removing a wound drain

A drain is a hollow tube through which liquid secretions are removed from the cavity of a wound. Drains may be closed (*i.e.,* have a collection reservoir) or open. An open drain deposits exudate onto an absorbent gauze dressing. A closed drain pulls exudate into a container with the aid of gravity, portable suction shown in Fig. III-20-1, or electric suction machine. Some studies show that the infection rate is cut nearly in half when drains are placed only when necessary and through a separate stab wound rather than in the incision itself.

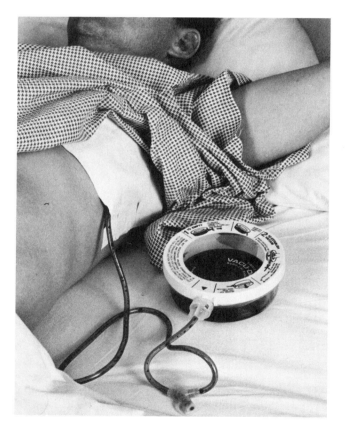

Figure III-20–1 The portable vacuum suction apparatus pulls drainage from the wound into a collection reservoir.

PURPOSES OF PROCEDURE

A drain is used to:

1. Remove wound drainage.
2. Promote accelerated healing.
3. Relieve discomfort from the pressure of accumulating secretions.
4. Reduce tension on sutures or staples.
5. Prevent or relieve an infection.

ASSESSMENT

OBJECTIVE DATA

- Inspect the wound, identifying the type of drain, its location either within or beside the wound, and whether the drain has been secured in place with sutures.
- Identify if drainage is promoted by gravity, electric suction, or portable vacuum.
- Examine the skin around the drain; observe for maceration, excoriation, or inflammation.
- Look at the characteristics of the drainage, specifically its volume, color, consistency, and odor.
- Read the chart to determine where the distal end of the drain is located. For example, a T-tube is located within the common bile duct. Also, note if the doctor has indicated that the drain should be shortened a certain amount.
- Check the laboratory reports for the results of cultures taken from the wound and white blood cell count.
- Assess and check the trends in the client's vital signs for indications of infection.

SUBJECTIVE DATA

- Ask the client to indicate his level of comfort and describe sensations associated with the drain's location or placement.

RELEVANT NURSING DIAGNOSES

A client with a drain is likely to have nursing diagnoses, such as:

- *Altered Comfort*
- *Potential for Infection*
- *Impaired Skin and Tissue Integrity*
- *Potential for Injury*

PLANNING

ESTABLISHING PRIORITIES

The collector attached to a closed drain must be emptied at least once per shift. This is generally done at the end of the shift when the volume is recorded on the client's intake and output sheet. The dressing covering a drain is changed at the same time the wound is assessed and redressed.

SETTING GOALS

- The drain will remain patent.
- The skin will not be further impaired through contact with secretions, pulling, or displacement of the drain.
- The wound will be free of infection and heal from deeper areas toward the surface.

PREPARATION OF EQUIPMENT

The nurse will need items from the following list:

Sterile instrument set
Sterile dressing supplies
Refuse bag
Clean disposable glove
Sterile gloves
Antiseptic swabs
Sterile safety pin (if the client has a Penrose drain)
Graduate pitcher

Technique for maintaining and removing a drain

ACTION	RATIONALE
1. Read the written medical order.	Checking clarifies the directions prescribed by the physician.
2. Gather supplies.	Organization promotes efficient time management.
3. Explain the procedure to the client.	An explanation relieves apprehension and promotes cooperation.

4. Shut the door and pull the curtain.

The nurse shows concern by maintaining privacy and warmth.

5. Raise the bed and lower the near side rail.

Placing the client at an appropriate height prevents back strain and muscle fatigue.

6. Open the refuse bag.

Using a bag to contain soiled objects prevents the transmission of pathogens.

7. Loosen the tape securing the dressing.

Loosening the tape facilitates removing the dressing.

8. Wash your hands.

Handwashing deters the spread of microorganisms.

9. Don a clean glove.

A glove acts as a transmission barrier against the direct contact with pathogens.

10. Remove the soiled dressing and pull the glove off by turning it inside out. Discard the soiled material within the bag.

Containing soiled articles supports principles of medical asepsis by restricting the presence of contaminated objects to one location.

11. Wash your hands.

Handwashing deters the spread of microorganisms.

12. Open sterile supplies.

Opening supplies without touching the contents maintains their sterility.

13. Don sterile gloves.

Gloves act as a transmission barrier protecting the wound from any pathogens on the nurse's skin and vice versa.

14. Use an antiseptic swab to cleanse the area around the drain. Use a separate swab for each circular rotation.

Pathogens and secretions are moved from least to most contaminated areas.

TO SHORTEN A DRAIN:

15. Grasp the drain with forceps and pull the drain the specified length.

The drain is less likely to slip with a secure grasp of forceps than with latex gloves.

16. Place a sterile safety pin crossways through the drain as it exits near the skin surface.

A safety pin prevents the drain from slipping back within the wound.

17. Cut a portion of the drain above the safety pin, leaving no more than 2 inches protruding.

Excess length is likely to retain moisture and lead to skin maceration.

18. Place gauze that has been presplit to the center by the manufacturer to prevent fraying, as shown in Fig. III-20-2, or unfold and refold two gauze squares to fit around the circumference of the drain, as shown in Fig. III-20-3.

The gauze lifts and suspends secretions away from the skin. If secretions remain in contact with the skin, it may become irritated.

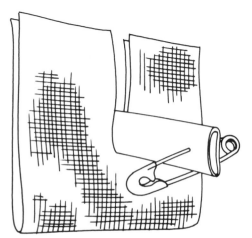

Figure III-20-2 This manufactured drain gauze is designed to fit completely around the base of a drain.

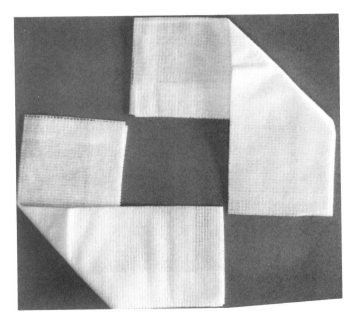

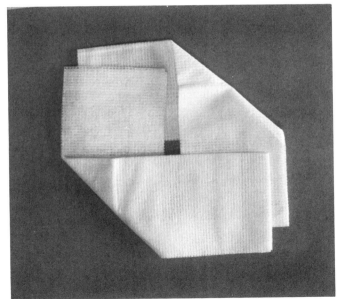

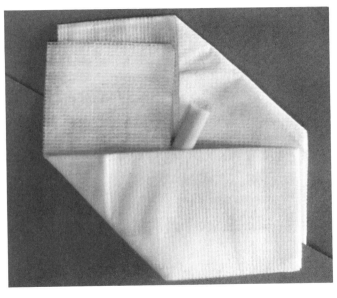

Figure III-20-3 Two 2 × 2 gauze squares can be opened and folded lengthwise. By positioning each at opposing right angles, the skin around the drain is protected from accumulating secretions.

TO REMOVE A DRAIN:

19. Grasp the drain with forceps and exert gentle traction to pull the drain from the wound.

The drain is compressed and folded beneath the skin. Pulling with force may injure tissue.

20. Deposit the entire drain within the refuse bag.

All soiled objects should be enclosed and kept separate from clean work areas to control the spread of pathogens.

21. Dress the wound with layers of absorbent gauze.

The cotton fibers within the gauze act as a wick to pull drainage away from the wound.

22. Discard gloves, turning them inside out.

The gloves are a possible source of organisms.

23. Secure the dressing with tape.

Tape keeps the dressing in place covering the drain and wound.

24. Return the client to a position of comfort. Lower the bed, raise the side rail.

The nurse maintains the client's comfort and safety.

25. Dispose of soiled equipment according to agency policy.

Disposable contaminated items should be incinerated. Reusable instruments are disinfected and resterilized to prevent the transmission of pathogens.

26. Wash your hands.

Handwashing deters the spread of microorganisms.

27. Document assessments, the procedure, and the outcomes.

The client's record is an accurate summary of care.

SAMPLE DOCUMENTATION

Date	Time	Nurse's note
7/18	1400	Dressing removed. Sm. amt. of clear serous drainage noted. Penrose drain shortened 1 inch. Skin around the drain appears normal in color and intact. States, "It's much less tender than before."
		V. Casper, RN

EVALUATION

REASSESSMENT

The status of the drain and the skin surrounding it is assessed daily. Periodically the nurse should note that the volume in a collection reservoir continues to increase verifying that the system is patent. The nurse can consult the written records or personally communicate with others who have cared for the client to determine the progress. Changes in the volume and characteristics of the drainage, an increase in body temperature, and other signs indicating an infection are significant observations. The nurse must collaborate with the physician to modify the plan for care if complications develop.

EXPECTED OUTCOMES

The drainage collects on the dressing or within the collection reservoir.
The drain remains within the wound or pulls easily during shortening or removal.
The wound edges remain approximated.
The client experiences diminished discomfort.

UNEXPECTED OUTCOMES

The wound bulges; drainage is absent or reduced.
The client experiences tenderness and pain around the area of the drain.
The drain is accidentally pulled from the wound.
The drain slips within the wound leaving no free end for removal.

MODIFICATIONS IN SELECTED SITUATIONS

GENERAL VARIATIONS

Empty a drainage container once per shift and record the volume and the characteristics of the exudate. Avoid touching the opening from which the fluid is removed.
To create vacuum suction, compress the reservoir, as shown in Fig. III-20-4, to empty the container of atmospheric air. Cap the container while it is still compressed.
A specially designed drain clip may be used in lieu of a sterile safety pin to maintain the location of the drain.
Irrigate a collection reservoir that has become obstructed with thick drainage. Take care to protect the sterility of the drain and the connection area. Record the volume used as irrigation so it is not calculated as wound drainage. The drain itself should not be irrigated unless the physician so orders.
Wear a gown and mask if the wound is infected with virulent pathogens. Double-bag and label all soiled wound articles from clients on drainage and secretion precautions.

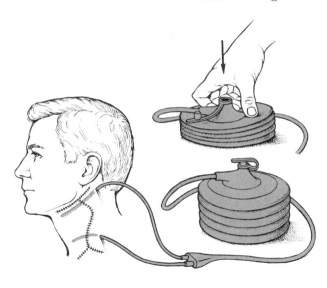

Figure III-20–4 This closed drain facilitates wound drainage by creating a vacuum when it is flattened and sealed.

Tape connections when a drain is attached to an extension piece of tubing.

Relieve the weight of a portable vacuum suction container before a client begins ambulating so it does not become displaced. This can be done by emptying the drainage reservoir and supporting the collector while the client is up and about.

HOME-HEALTH VARIATIONS

Advise the client to avoid wearing tight clothing at home which may restrict the flow of drainage.

Develop a written schedule with the caregiver for measuring and recording the drainage.

Instruct the client or caregiver to empty the reservoir into the toilet. Advise that the head should be held to one side to avoid contact with splashed pathogens or inhalation of droplets.

RELATED TEACHING

Explain the purpose for the drain and the rationale for shortening it a little at a time.

Discuss the significance of the client's drainage and inform him of signs that indicate an infection.

Demonstrate wound care which includes caring for the drain. Provide the client or family member the opportunity to return the demonstration, if the client will be discharged needing this skill.

(Performance checklist next page)

PERFORMANCE CHECKLIST

When maintaining or removing a drain, the learner:

C	A	U	
[ ]	[ ]	[ ]	Checks the written order.
[ ]	[ ]	[ ]	Assembles equipment.
[ ]	[ ]	[ ]	Provides the client with an explanation.
[ ]	[ ]	[ ]	Maintains privacy.
[ ]	[ ]	[ ]	Positions the client and adjusts the bed to provide access to the wound.
[ ]	[ ]	[ ]	Prepares a bag for collecting soiled articles.
[ ]	[ ]	[ ]	Loosens tape that secures the dressing.
[ ]	[ ]	[ ]	Washes hands.
[ ]	[ ]	[ ]	Dons a clean glove.
[ ]	[ ]	[ ]	Removes the dressing.
[ ]	[ ]	[ ]	Removes the glove discarding it with the soiled dressing.
[ ]	[ ]	[ ]	Washes hands.
[ ]	[ ]	[ ]	Opens sterile supplies without contamination.
[ ]	[ ]	[ ]	Dons sterile gloves.
[ ]	[ ]	[ ]	Uses forceps to lift and hold the drain away from the skin.
[ ]	[ ]	[ ]	Cleans around the drain according to aseptic principles.
[ ]	[ ]	[ ]	Withdraws the drain completely or just the prescribed distance, when indicated.
[ ]	[ ]	[ ]	Reinserts a safety pin or clip at the lower area of the drain, if a portion remains.
[ ]	[ ]	[ ]	Cuts all but 2 inches of the exposed drain.
[ ]	[ ]	[ ]	Dresses the wound.
[ ]	[ ]	[ ]	Removes gloves.
[ ]	[ ]	[ ]	Encloses all soiled disposables within the refuse bag.
[ ]	[ ]	[ ]	Disposes of items according to agency policy.
[ ]	[ ]	[ ]	Washes hands.
[ ]	[ ]	[ ]	Charts significant information.

Outcome: [ ] Pass   [ ] Fail

C = competent; A = acceptable; U = unsatisfactory

Comments: _____
_____
_____

_____   _____
Student's Signature   Date

_____   _____
Instructor's Signature   Date

III-21   *Collecting a wound culture*

When a wound begins draining purulent exudate, it is likely that an infection exists. To validate the suspicion, a culture must be collected. It is important to obtain an adequate sample, to avoid coincidental contamination from another source containing microbes, and to sustain the living microorganisms once they have been collected.

PURPOSES OF PROCEDURE

A wound culture is collected to:

1. Identify specific pathogens present in a wound.
2. Aid in selecting appropriate drug therapy.
3. Guide the type and use of medical asepsis procedures.
4. Protect others from the transmission of infectious organisms.
5. Evaluate the success of antibiotic therapy.

ASSESSMENT

OBJECTIVE DATA

- Verify the type of wound culture specified in the medical order.
- Review the infection control policy concerning institution of isolation precautions when an infection is suspected.
- Consult laboratory personnel or an authoritative manual if there are questions about the collection of a specimen.
- Scan the chart for information that supports the possibility that an infection exists, such as: elevated white blood cell count, fever, increased pulse rate, continued need for frequent analgesia, poor dietary intake, and reduced activity.
- Examine the wound. Be alert especially to any signs that the wound is red, warm, and swollen. If purulent exudate is present, it likely contains a mixture of white blood cells and pathogens.
- Inspect around sutures or staples for areas where the wound is failing to close or has reseparated.

SUBJECTIVE DATA

- Ask the client to identify and describe local discomfort.
- Inquire concerning the client's appetite, desire for rest, and response to activity.
- Assess the client's environmental comfort; note if he feels chilled or exceptionally warm.

RELEVANT NURSING DIAGNOSES

The client who has an actual or possible wound infection is likely to have nursing diagnoses, such as:

- *Altered Comfort*
- *Altered Body Temperature*
- *Activity Intolerance*
- *Impaired Skin or Tissue Integrity*

PLANNING

ESTABLISHING PRIORITIES

A wound infection slows healing. Coping with an infection taxes the physiologic reserves which assist in restoring a client's health. Therefore, it is important to confirm or rule out the presence of an infection as soon as possible. To obtain valid results from a culture, the specimen optimally should be collected before any antibiotic therapy has begun. However, it is not unusual to begin administering a broad-spectrum antibiotic while awaiting the results of the culture, thus avoiding a 1- to 2-day delay in treatment.

SETTING GOALS	• The client will understand the procedure and why it is being performed.
	• A sufficient quantity of the specimen is collected and nourished in order to reveal microbial growth.
	• The client is treated with an antibiotic to which the pathogen is sensitive.
PREPARATION OF EQUIPMENT	The nurse will need selected items from the following list:

Sterile culturette tube with enclosed swab (or culture tube with individual swabs)
Sterile gloves
Clean disposable gloves
Plastic bag for soiled dressing
Label for culturette tube
Laboratory requisition with rubber band or plastic bag

Technique for collecting a wound culture

ACTION	RATIONALE
1. Explain the procedure to the client.	An explanation encourages client cooperation and reduces apprehension.
2. Gather equipment.	Organization promotes efficient time management.
3. Wash your hands.	Handwashing deters the spread of microorganisms.
4. Don clean disposable gloves. Remove the dressing and assess wound drainage as described in Procedure III-17, steps 5 through 11.	Using gloves protects the nurse when handling contaminated dressings.
5. Using aseptic technique, don sterile gloves and cleanse the wound. See Procedure III-17, step 15. Remove the gloves when completed.	Cleansing the wound before collecting the culture removes or reduces skin flora that are present but more than likely nonpathogenic.
6. Twist the cap from the culturette tube to loosen the swab or open separate swabs and remove the cap from the culture tube, keeping the inside uncontaminated.	These measures maintain the sterility of the equipment, ensuring that the only source of collected microbes is the wound.
7. Don a new sterile glove if contact with the wound may be necessary.	Use of a culturette does not require any direct contact with the skin or wound. If contact with the wound is necessary to collect a specimen, wearing a glove prevents introducing microbes from the nurse into the wound and protects the nurse from pathogens present in the wound.
8. Carefully insert the swab into the drainage, and roll it gently. Use another swab if collecting a specimen from another site.	It is important to collect a sufficient amount of exudate for optimum analysis. Using separate swabs prevents cross-contamination with microorganisms.
9. Place the swab in the culturette tube, as shown in Fig. III-21-1, being careful not to touch the outside of the container. Twist the cap to secure.	The results of the culture will be invalid if microbes other than those from the wound become transferred onto or within the specimen.
10. If using a culturette tube, crush the ampule of medium at the bottom of the tube, as shown in Fig. III-21-2.	The culture medium surrounds the drainage on the swab and nourishes it so that microbes are more likely to remain viable.
11. Remove gloves from the inside out, and discard them in a bag for collecting wastes.	Containing contaminated supplies prevents the spread of microorganisms.
12. Wash your hands.	Handwashing deters the spread of microorganisms.

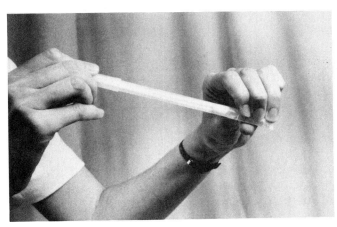

Figure III-21-1 This swab is inserted within its container. The nurse exercises care to avoid touching the swab during removal and replacement.

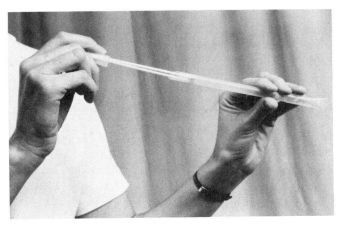

Figure III-21-2 The ampule of medium at the bottom of the culturette tube is crushed. This ensures that the organisms collected for the test will survive until they can be incubated on a culture plate.

13. Apply a clean dressing to the wound. See Procedure III-17, steps 16 through 20.

A dressing absorbs drainage from a wound.

14. Wash your hands. Remove all equipment and make the client comfortable.

Handwashing deters the spread of microorganisms.

15. Label the specimen container appropriately with the client's name, date, time, nature of the specimen. Attach a laboratory requisition slip to the tube with a rubber band or place the tube in a plastic bag with the requisition attached. Send to the laboratory within 20 minutes.

Labeling ensures proper identification of the specimen. Overgrowth of other organisms can interfere with test results if the specimen remains at room temperature for an extended period of time.

16. Record the collection of the specimen, appearance of the wound, and description of drainage in the chart.

A written summary provides accurate documentation of the procedure.

SAMPLE DOCUMENTATION

Date	Time	Nurse's note
3/03	0945	Purulent, foul-smelling drainage coming from lower margin of the incision. Skin is taut and red at the bottom of the wound. Experiences discomfort as wound is cleansed in this area. Feels chilly with oral temp. of 102°F. Aerobic and anerobic culture of wound drainage obtained and sent to lab immediately. Wound redressed. *C. Blaire, RN*

EVALUATION

REASSESSMENT

The nurse can reevaluate the response of the client to therapeutic measures by continuing to assess vital signs every 4 hours or four times a day. The wound should gradually manifest signs associated with healing, such as reduction or change in the characteristics of the drainage. The client's appetite will return, and he is likely to become more active. Monitoring the white blood cell count and data on subsequent wound culture reports can provide additional data on the progress of the client.

EXPECTED OUTCOMES

The culture is collected before any antibiotic drugs are administered.
The culture is obtained under aseptic conditions.
The client experiences minimal discomfort while the specimen is obtained.

The specimen is properly identified and delivered to the laboratory within 20 minutes after it is obtained.

UNEXPECTED OUTCOMES

The specimen was insufficient for producing adequate growth of microorganisms.

The specimen cools or dries, thus inhibiting the continued growth and reproduction of the microorganisms.

Normal flora rather than pathogens are identified in the specimen.

MODIFICATIONS IN SELECTED SITUATIONS

GENERAL VARIATIONS

The nurse may have the independent authority in certain agencies to obtain a wound culture under the institution's infection control policies.

Both aerobic and anerobic cultures may be ordered. Anerobic culture collection kits contain carbon dioxide gas or nitrogen to eliminate the presence of oxygen that may inhibit the viability of anerobic organisms.

The physician may aspirate drainage from the wound for a culture. The nurse may need to premedicate the client with an analgesic at least ½ hour before the procedure. In addition to the listed equipment, the nurse should bring a 5-ml or 10-ml syringe and a large gauge needle for removing drainage which is likely to be thick.

If more than one specimen is obtained, the nurse should take care to identify the area from which each sample was obtained.

If the client is in isolation, the specimen should be double-bagged and labeled, indicating that it came from a client being cared for with infection control measures.

AGE-RELATED VARIATIONS

A parent may hold a child while a culture is obtained or provide verbal support if desired.

HOME-HEALTH VARIATIONS

The specimen should be transported to the laboratory immediately following the home visit.

RELATED HEALTH TEACHING

Explain and demonstrate appropriate handwashing technique to the client and family.

Review the isolation precautions with visitors, and ensure that they comply with the infection control measures.

Explain the need for collecting specimens differently or the rationale for collecting more than one specimen.

Identify the cluster of signs and symptoms that relate to infection. Discuss with the client the indications used as evidence for improvement.

PERFORMANCE CHECKLIST

When obtaining a wound culture, the learner:

C	A	U	
[ ]	[ ]	[ ]	Gathers data from colleagues and the client's record.
[ ]	[ ]	[ ]	Checks the written medical order or reviews the agency's policy concerning infection control.
[ ]	[ ]	[ ]	Selects equipment.
[ ]	[ ]	[ ]	Explains the procedure to the client.
[ ]	[ ]	[ ]	Washes hands.
[ ]	[ ]	[ ]	Dons a clean glove and removes dressing according to principles of medical asepsis.
[ ]	[ ]	[ ]	Washes hands.
[ ]	[ ]	[ ]	Opens dressing supplies for future use.
[ ]	[ ]	[ ]	Cleanses the wound.
[ ]	[ ]	[ ]	Removes the cap from the culture tube.
[ ]	[ ]	[ ]	Swabs drainage from within the wound.
[ ]	[ ]	[ ]	Replaces the swab within the tube without touching the outside of the container.
[ ]	[ ]	[ ]	Maintains the viability of the specimen using the appropriate medium.
[ ]	[ ]	[ ]	Dresses the wound.
[ ]	[ ]	[ ]	Washes hands.
[ ]	[ ]	[ ]	Makes the client comfortable.
[ ]	[ ]	[ ]	Attaches identification and requisition slips to all specimens.
[ ]	[ ]	[ ]	Transports the specimen to the laboratory.
[ ]	[ ]	[ ]	Charts significant information.

Outcome: [ ] Pass   [ ] Fail

C = competent; A = acceptable; U = unsatisfactory

Comments: _____

_____

_____

_____   _____
Student's Signature   Date

_____   _____
Instructor's Signature   Date

RELATED LITERATURE

PROCEDURE III-1
ASSISTING THE
CLIENT WITH
ORAL CARE

Harrison A: Oral hygiene: denture care. Nursing Times 83(19):28–29, May 13–19, 1987

Richardson A: A process standard for oral care. Nursing Times 83(32):38–40, August 12–18, 1987

Shepherd G, Page C, Sammon P: Oral hygiene: the mouth trap. Nursing Times 83(19):24–27, May 13–19, 1987

PROCEDURE III-2
PROVIDING ORAL
CARE FOR THE
DEPENDENT CLIENT

Newman GR: An oral-hygiene program for long-term care facilities. Journal of Long Term Care Administration 15(2):11–14, Summer 1987

Warner LA: Lemon-glycerine swabs should be used for routine oral care . . . little agreement exists. Critical Care Nurse 6(6):82–83, November–December 1986

PROCEDURE III-3
GIVING THE
BED BATH

Lund CA: We made our skin care problems disappear. RN magazine 50(5):18, 20, May 1987

Simpson B: An inexpensive bathseat for handicapped children. Canadian Journal of Occupational Therapy 54(1):28–30, February 1987

Wolf ZR: Nurses' work: the sacred and the profane. Holistic Nursing Practice 1(1):29–35, November 1986

PROCEDURE III-4
SHAMPOOING HAIR

Feldmeier DM, Poole JL: The position adjustable hair dryer. American Journal of Occupational Therapy 41(4):246–247, April 1987

von Nostitz P: Why is my hair falling out? Parents 62(2):167–170, February 1987

Zuker RM: The use of tissue expansion in pediatric scalp burn construction. Journal of Burn Care & Rehabilitation 8(2):103–106, March–April 1987

PROCEDURE III-5
SHAVING FACIAL HAIR

Wagnild G: Personal-care complaints: a descriptive study . . . in nursing homes. Journal of Long Term Care Administration 14(3):27–29, Fall 1986

PROCEDURE III-6
PROVIDING FOOT AND
TOENAIL CARE

Barnett A, Odugbesan O: Foot-care for diabetics. Nursing Times 83(22):24–26, January 3–9, 1987

Footpain: important considerations in the physical examination. Hospital Medicine 22(12): 106–108, 111–113, December 1986

Kpea NT, Scher RK: Nail abnormalities: easily observed signs of systemic diseases. Consultant 27(8):47–50, 52–53, 56, August 1987

Paronychia: classification and treatment. Hospital Medicine 22(10):173, October 1986

Patterson C, Turpie I, Dedes B: The prevalence of common foot disorders in patients admitted to a geriatric assessment unit. Gerontion 2(2):17–19, Summer 1987

Sykes P, Openshaw N, Sutherlund D: Surgical dressing after nail surgery. Nursing Times 83(5):45, February 4–10, 1987

PROCEDURE III-7
GIVING A BACK
MASSAGE

Cohen N: Massage is the message . . . effects on mentally handicapped patients. Nursing Times 83(19):19–20, May 13–19, 1987

Day JA, Mason RR, Chesrown SE: Effect of massage on serum level of B-endorphin and B-lipotropin in healthy adults. Physical Therapy 67(6):926–930, June 1987

D'Urso MA: Massage for the masses. Health 19(4):63–64, 66–67, 89, April 1987

Estabrooks CA: Touch in nursing practice: a historical perspective . . . 1900 to 1920. Journal of Nursing History 2(2):33–49, April 1987

Fakouri C, Jones P: Relaxation RX: slow stroke back rub. Journal of Gerontological Nursing 13(2):32–35, February 1987

Harrison A: Therapeutic touch: getting the massage. Nursing Times 82(48):34–35, November 26–December 2, 1986

Sims S: Slow stroke massage for cancer patients . . . change in symptom distress and mood in female patients. Nursing Times 82(47):47–50, November 19–25, 1986

**PROCEDURE III-8
PROVIDING PERINEAL
CARE**

Conti MT, Eutropius L: Preventing UTIs: what works. American Journal of Nursing 87(3): 307–309, March 1987

Cronck M: Perineal suturing. Nursing Times 83(7):62, February 18–24, 1987

Giroux JA: Bacteriuria in elderly males with spinal cord injury . . . frequency of perineal hygiene. Journal of American Urological Association Allied 7(4):8–11, April–June 1987

Kempster H: Perineal care: "confused, battered and unwanted." Community Outlook 8–10, June 1987

**PROCEDURE III-9
SHAVING THE
SKIN OF THE
PREOPERATIVE CLIENT**

Dale J: Sterile pursuit . . . skin preparations for surgery, some obsolete practices. Nursing Mirror 159:14, December 19–26, 1984

Harvey CK: Future trends in perioperative nursing technology. Nursing Administration Quarterly 11(2):38–41, Winter 1987

Huey FL: Working smart . . . rituals with dropping and why. American Journal of Nursing 86(6):679–684, June 1986

Recommended practices: basic aseptic technique. Journal of American Operating Room Nurses. 45(3):784, 786, 788–789, March 1987

**PROCEDURE III-10
APPLYING BINDERS**

Bridges J: Restorative proctocolectomy to avoid a stoma. Nursing Times 83(4):63, 65–66, January 28–February 3, 1987

Deters GE: Managing complications after abdominal surgery. RN magazine 50(3):27–32, March 1987

Helping your wound heal. Patient Care 21(11):259, June 15, 1987

Lamb C: Suiting the dressing to the wound. Patient Care 21(11):164–166, 168, 173+, June 15, 1987

McCormack A, Itkin J, Cloud C: RN master care plan: if your patient develops peritonitis. RN magazine 50(3):31–32, March 1987

Sieggreen MY: Healing of physical wounds. Nursing Clinics of North America 22(2):439–447, June 1987

Weber BB, Speer M, Swartz D: Irritation and stripping effects of adhesive tapes on skin layers of coronary artery bypass graft patients. Heart & Lung: Journal of Critical Care 16(5):567–572, September 1987

**PROCEDURE III-11
APPLYING A ROLLER
BANDAGE**

Bray TJ, Gould N, Orban DJ: Acute care for ankle sprain. Patient Care 21(2):48–51, 54, 56–58, January 30, 1987

Karlin L: Musculoskeletal trauma. Emergency Care Quarterly 3(1):57–60, May 1987

Kinach I, Peters G, Ritchuck M: Controlling edema of the hand through ace wrapping. Canadian Journal of Occupational Therapy 54(3):139–141, June 1987

Maher AB: Early assessment and management of musculoskeletal injuries. Nursing Clinics of North America 21(4):717–727, December 21, 1986

McPhee SD: Extension block splinting for the proximal interphalangeal joint. American Journal of Occupational Therapy 41(6):389–390, June 1987

Osterman HM, Pinzur MS: Amputation: last resort or new beginning? Geriatric Nursing: American Journal of Care for the Aging 8(5):246–248, September–October 1987

PROCEDURE III-12 APPLYING TRANSDERMAL MEDICATION

Gaska JA: Current angina treatment. Journal of Practical Nursing 37(1):20–27, March 1987

SerVass C: More about estrogen skin patches. Saturday Evening Post 259(1):52–54, 100, 104, January–February 1987

Transdermal estrogen: a promising dosage form. Patient Care 21(2):25, January 30, 1987

PROCEDURE III-13 GIVING A SITZ BATH

Bouis P Jr, Hoffman M, Newton W: Cost analysis of mucoadhesive foam versus conventional treatment for postepisiotomy patients. Hospital Formulary 21(2):1226–1228, December 1986

Ramler D, Roberts J: A comparison of cold and warm sitz baths for relief of postpartum perineal pain. Journal of Obstetric, Gynecologic, and Neonatal Nursing 15(6):471–474, November–December 1986

Zadeh AT, Kirchner B: Outpatient hemorroidectomy: laser treatment and case results. Journal of American Operating Room Nurses 44(6):966–968, 970, 972+, December 1986

PROCEDURE III-14 PREVENTING PRESSURE SORES

Brestow JV, Goldfarb EH, Green M: Clinitron therapy: is it effective? Geriatric Nursing 8(3): 120–124, May–June 1987

Chagares R, Jackson BS: Sitting easy: how six pressure-relieving devices stack up. American Journal of Nursing 87(2):191–193, February 1987

Masoorli ST: Preventing pressure sores is a family affair. RN magazine 50(7):67–68, July 1987

Maklebust J: Pressure ulcers: etiology and prevention. Nursing Clinics of North America 22(2):359–377, June 1987

Messner R: The prevention of pressure sores. Journal of Practical Nursing 37(1):16–17, March 1987

Sebern M: Home-team strategies for treating pressure sores. Nursing 87 17(4):50–53, April 1987

Wienki VK: Pressure sores: prevention is the challenge. Orthopaedic Nursing 6(4):26–30, July–August 1987

PROCEDURE III-15 APPLYING AN EXTERNAL HEATING DEVICE

Airhihenbuwa CO, St Pierre RW, Winchell D: Cold vs heat therapy: a survey of physician's recommendations for first-aid treatment of strain. Emergency 19(1):40–43, January 1987

Burn prevention checklist. Patient Care 21(7):152, April 1987

Grigg B: Warming to the idea: heat research may help hearts, kidneys, and man's best friend. FDS Consumer 21(4):25–27, May 1987

Stackhouse DE: Hypothermia: rewarming and therapy. Physician Assistant 11(2):37–38, 41, 43–46+, February 1987

PROCEDURE III-16 APPLYING WARM STERILE COMPRESSES TO AN OPEN WOUND

Callaham ML, Jordan RC, Macknin ML: Mammalian bite wounds. Patient Care 21(13):157–159, 161, 163–167, August 15, 1987

Helping your wound heal. Patient Care 21(11):259, June 15, 1987

Lemmink JA: Infection control: when a surgical wound becomes infected. RN magazine 50(9):24–28, September 1987

Open soft-tissue wounds: closure and follow-up, *part 2*. Physician Assistant 11(4):37–38, 42–44, 46, April 1987

PROCEDURE III-17 CLEANING A WOUND AND APPLYING A CLEAN DRESSING

Avoid use of hydrogen peroxide and povidone iodine in open wounds. Nurses' Drug Alert 11(6):41, June 1987

DeWitt DE: Conservatism in wound management—or habit? . . . transparent dressings are not being used to the degree one might expect. Emergency Medicine 19(9):3, 16, May 15, 1987

Lamb C: Suiting the dressing to the wound. Patient Care 21(11):164–166, 169, 173+, June 15, 1987

Leaper D, Cameron S, Lancaster J: Wound care: antiseptic solutions. Community Outlook 30, 32, 34, April 1987

Mather DG, Woods LS: A form that makes wound assessment easier. RN magazine 50(6):37–39, June 1987

Moores J: Wound care: tried and tested . . . the Biofilm dressing. Community Outlook 24, 26, April 1987

Neuberger GB, Reckling JB: Wound care: what's clear, what's not. Nursing 87 17(2):34–37, February 1987

Thielman DE: When a dressing won't do the job . . . trying a pouch instead. RN magazine 50(6):35–36, June 1987

Thomlinson D: To clean or not to clean? . . . cleaning discharging surgical wounds. Nursing Times 83(9):71, 73, 75, March 4–10, 1987

PROCEDURE III-18 IRRIGATING A WOUND AND INSERTING PACKING

Ayton M: A healing process. Senior Nurse 6(4):21–23, April 1987

Callaham ML, Jordan RC, Macknin ML: Mammalian bite wounds. Patient Care 21(13):157–159, 161, 163–167, August 15, 1987

Johnson CL: Wound healing and scar formation. Topics in Acute Care and Trauma Rehabilitation 1(4):1–14, April 1987

Sieggreen MY: Healing of physical wounds. Nursing Clinics of North America 22(2):439–447, June 1987

PROCEDURE III-19 REMOVING SUTURES OR STAPLES

Comparative study suggests greater care necessary in selecting absorbable sutures in surgical closings. Canadian Operating Room Nursing Journal 5(2):26, April 1987

Cronk M: Perineal suturing. Nursing Times 83(7):62, February 18–24, 1987

Mather DG, Woods LS: A form that makes wound assessment easier. RN magazine 50(6):37–39, June 1987

Wound closure and infection control. Canadian Operating Room Nursing Journal 5(1):32, 34, February 1987

PROCEDURE III-20 MAINTAINING AND REMOVING A WOUND DRAIN

Birdsall C, Fiore-Lopez N: How do you manage pancreatic sump tubes? American Journal of Nursing 87(6):770–771, June 1987

Carroll PF: The ins and outs of chest drainage systems. Nursing 86 16(12):26–34, December 1986

Clark LK: Discharge instructions for wound catheters . . . your Jackson-Pratt (JP) wound drain. Journal: Society of Otorhinolaryngology Head-Neck 5(1):31, Winter 1987

Fay MF: Drainage systems: their role in wound healing. Journal of American Operating Room Nurses 46(3):442–443, 445, 447+, September 1987

Holloway NM: Tension pyothorax and acute empyema. Critical Care Nurse 6(6):65–72, November–December 1986

Hutchinson M, Himes TM, Davis LE: Preventing multiple body tube mix-ups. Nursing 87 17(4):57, April 1987

Lockhart CG: Thoracic trauma. Critical Care Quarterly 9(3):32–40, December 1986

Simpson G: Assessment and choice . . . wound management. Community Outlook 16–18, July 1987

PROCEDURE III-21 COLLECTING A WOUND CULTURE

DeCrosta T: Nosocomial infections: every patient is a target. Fighting the problem *part 2*. Nursing Life 6(6):44–47, November–December 1986

Stayley T: Care of the uncomplicated burn. Canadian Nurse 83(5):28–30, May 1987

Taylor L, Josse E: Nursing aid: developing infection control. Nursing Times 82(49):32, December 3–9, 1986

Tideiksaar R: Infections in the elderly: diagnosis and treatment, *part 1*. Physician Assistant 11(2):17–24, 28, 31, February 1987

Walsh TJ, Vlahov D, Hansen SL: Prospective microbiologic surveillance in control of nosocomial methicillin-resistant *Staphlococcus aureus*. Infection Control 8(1):7–14, January 1987

IV   *Procedures pertaining to the gastrointestinal tract*

IV-1 — *Administering oral medications*

Most medications are taken through the mouth and eventually are absorbed from the gastrointestinal tract. Oral medications are available in solid or liquid preparations.

PURPOSES OF PROCEDURE

Medications are administered by the oral route to:

1. Treat a client's disease or symptoms chemically.
2. Use a convenient and comfortable method for administering drugs.
3. Ensure safety and efficacy of drug therapy.

ASSESSMENT

OBJECTIVE DATA

- Read the medical order.
- Compare the transcribed information on the medication card or Kardex with the physician's written order.
- Review the action of the drug, side-effects, contraindications, usual dosage, route(s) of administration, and other pertinent information in an appropriate pharmacology reference, if unfamiliar with the medication.
- Determine which medications are better given on an empty stomach and which should be taken with food. Avoid combining foods and drugs that may cause adverse interactions.
- Note the results of pertinent laboratory tests.
- Be aware of any currently scheduled tests that require that the client remain NPO (nothing by mouth).
- Identify the client by checking his admission armband.
- Interview and examine the client to obtain data that are pertinent to the action of the medication and the client's response to taking medication in the past.
- Question the client specifically concerning any allergies or other conditions that would contraindicate taking the prescribed medication.
- Determine the client's ability to swallow.
- Read the medication label at least three times to verify that the right medication and the right dosage for the prescribed route has been supplied for the client.
- Verify that the scheduled routine for the drug's administration complies with the medication order.

SUBJECTIVE DATA

- Ask the client to explain any special measures he uses when taking medications, such as taking one medication at a time.
- Encourage the client to describe symptoms that would otherwise be unknown to the nurse without his cooperation.

RELEVANT NURSING DIAGNOSES

The client who receives oral medication has multiple collaborative problems which may occur as a result of experiencing side-effects or toxic effects of each individual drug. The nurse monitors the client closely and reports the findings to the physician. In addition, the nurse may identify nursing diagnoses, such as:

- *Anxiety*
- *Fear*
- *Potential for Injury*
- *Knowledge Deficit*

PLANNING

ESTABLISHING PRIORITIES

The scheduled time pattern for medication administration should be strictly observed. The nurse should give the medications as closely to the prescribed time as possible. A common principle is that the nurse may safely administer a drug $\frac{1}{2}$ hour before or after the designated time for administration. Any deviation from this span of time, unless the medication is specifically delayed or withheld for good reason, is otherwise considered an error. STAT medications must be given without delay. The primary nurse may need to temporarily delegate less important tasks to other nursing personnel to accommodate changing priorities.

SETTING GOALS

- The client will receive the correct medication in the proper dose, by the intended route, at the scheduled time.
- The drug will achieve its therapeutic effect.
- The client will not manifest undesirable side-effects.

PREPARATION OF EQUIPMENT

The nurse will need the following when administering oral medications:

Medication Kardex, cards, or record form
Medication cart or tray
Medication cups (disposable)
Straw
Water or juice

Technique for administering oral medications

ACTION	RATIONALE
1. Gather equipment. Check each medication order against the original physician's order as per agency policy. Clarify any inconsistencies. Check the client's chart for allergies.	This comparison helps to identify errors that occurred when orders were transcribed. The physician's order is the legal record of medication orders for each agency.
2. Know the actions, special nursing considerations, and side-effects of medications to be administered.	Knowing specific drug information aids the nurse in evaluating the therapeutic effect of the medication in relation to the client's diagnosis.
3. Wash your hands.	Handwashing deters the spread of microorganisms.
4. Move the medication cart to outside the client's room, as the nurse in Fig. IV-1-1 is doing, or prepare for administration in the medication area.	Organizing medication preparation saves time and helps prevent errors.

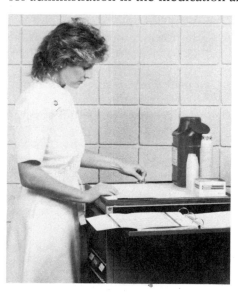

Figure IV-1-1 This mobile cart and the Kardex are taken to the client's room when medications are given. Each client's medications are stored in a separate drawer, numbered according to the client's room. When not in use, the cart is kept locked.

5. Unlock the medication cart or drawer.

Keeping medications locked safeguards each client's medication supply.

6. Prepare medications for one client at a time.

Attention to only one client's drug therapy prevents errors in medication administration.

7. Select the proper medication from the drawer or stock and compare it with the Kardex or order, as the nurse is doing in Fig. IV-1-2. Check the expiration dates, and perform calculations if necessary.

Comparison of medication label with the physician's order reduces medication administration errors. Verify calculations with another nurse if necessary. This is the *first* safety check.

   a. Place unit-dose packaged medications in the disposable cup. *Do not open the wrapper* until at the bedside. Keep narcotics and medications that require special nursing assessments in a separate container.

The label provides an additional safety check. Prerequisites to giving certain medications may include monitoring of certain vital signs.

   b. When removing tablets or capsules from a bottle, pour the necessary number into the bottle cap, and then place the tablets in a medication cup. Break only scored tablets if necessary to obtain the proper dosage.

Pouring tablets or capsules into the nurse's hand is unsanitary.

   c. Hold liquid medication bottles with the label against the palm of the hand. Use the appropriate measuring device when pouring liquids, and read the amount of medication at the bottom of the meniscus at eye level, as shown in Fig. IV-1-3. Wipe the lip of the bottle with a paper towel.

Accuracy is possible when the appropriate measuring device is used and then read accurately. Liquid that may drip onto the label makes the label difficult to read. Fluid in a column has a curved appearance. The level at the center of the curve, observed at eye level, is the best indicator of the volume.

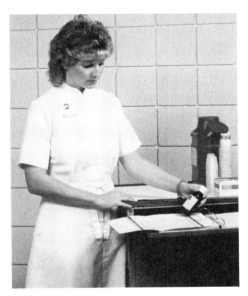

Figure IV-1–2 The nurse carefully checks the medication label with the Kardex. Reading the label at least three times helps to prevent medication errors.

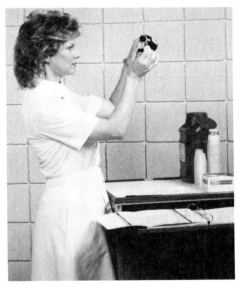

Figure IV-1–3 Holding the calibrated cup at eye level ensures that the volume of medication will be measured at the most accurate point of the meniscus.

8. Recheck each medication package, card, or preparation with the Kardex as it is poured.

This is the *second* check to guard against a medication error.

9. When all medications for one client have been prepared, recheck once again with the medication Kardex before taking them to the client.

This is the *third* check to ensure accuracy and to prevent errors.

10. Transport the medications to the client's bedside carefully, and keep the medications in sight at all times.

Careful handling and close observation prevent accidental or deliberate disarrangement of medications.

11. See that the client receives the medications at the correct time.

Check the agency policy. Most allow for administration within a period of 30 minutes before or 30 minutes after the designated time.

12. Identify the client carefully. There are three correct ways to do this:

The nurse is responsible for identifying the client accurately to guard against error.

    a. Check the name on the identification band, as the nurse in Figure IV-1-4 is doing.

Checking the wristband is the most reliable method for identifying the client.

    b. Ask the client his name.

The client should know his identity, but illness and strange surroundings often cause clients to be confused.

    c. Verify the identity of the client with a staff member who is familiar with the names and faces of individuals. Do not assume that the name on a door or over a bed is necessarily the true identity of the client.

Checking with someone who knows the client well is another way to identify individuals. Confused clients may wander into the room or bed of another person.

13. Complete assessments necessary before the administration of medications. Explain the purpose and action of each medication to the client.

Assessment is a prerequisite to the administration of medications.

14. Assist the client to an upright position or lateral position.

Swallowing is facilitated by proper positioning. Medications can be aspirated by trying to swallow in a supine position.

15. Administer the medications:

The nurse assists the client with taking his medication.

    a. Offer water or other permitted fluids with pills, capsules, tablets, and some liquid medications.

Liquids facilitate swallowing of solid drugs. Some liquid drugs, like cough medications, are intended to adhere to the pharyngeal area, in which case, liquid is not offered with the medication.

    b. Ask the client his preference regarding medications in his hand or a cup, or one at a time or all at once.

Encourage client participation and identification of his medications.

    c. If a capsule or tablet falls on the floor, it must be discarded and a new one administered.

The floor is highly contaminated with dirt and microbes. Discarding soiled articles supports medical asepsis.

    d. Record any fluid intake if the client's intake and output are being measured.

Recording every time fluid is consumed provides accurate documentation and valid data.

16. Remain with the client until each medication is swallowed, as shown in Fig. IV-1-5. Unless the nurse

The client's chart is a legal record. Only with a physician's order can medications be left at the bedside.

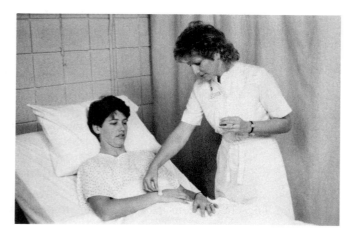

Figure IV-1-4 The nurse checks the medication card with the client's name on the identification bracelet.

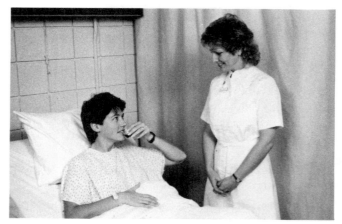

Figure IV-1-5 The nurse is responsible for ensuring that the client swallows the medication. (Photos © Ken Kasper)

has seen the client swallow the drug, it cannot be recorded that the drug was administered.

17. Wash your hands.

Handwashing deters the spread of microorganisms.

18. Record each medication given on the medication Kardex or record using the required format.

Prompt recording avoids the possibility of accidentally repeating the administration of the drug.

a. If the drug was refused or omitted, record an explanation in the appropriate area on the client's record.

Recording verifies why the medication was not administered rather than appearing to have been accidentally missed.

b. In addition to charting on the client's record, record the administration of a narcotic on the narcotic sheet which is used to tabulate the use and count of controlled substances.

Controlled substance laws necessitate careful recording of narcotic use.

19. Check the client within 30 minutes to verify his response to the medication.

Reassessment provides the opportunity for documenting the effect of the medication on each individual client.

SAMPLE DOCUMENTATION

Date	Time	Nurse's note
6/11	0900	NPO for upper GI x-ray. To radiology department per wheelchair. *G. Rooney, RN*
	1015	Zantac 150 mg. p.o. given following return from x-ray. *G. Rooney, RN*

EVALUATION

REASSESSMENT

It is wise to check the client's chart and the medication Kardex for new orders especially after the physician has made rounds. The response of the client to the medication may take at least $\frac{1}{2}$ hour or longer before any effects can be noted.

EXPECTED OUTCOMES

The client swallows the medication without any discomfort.
The client's condition improves, or symptoms are relieved.

UNEXPECTED OUTCOMES

The client has difficulty swallowing the medication.
The client vomits shortly after taking the medication.
The client experiences an allergic reaction or some other type of untoward response.

MODIFICATIONS IN SELECTED SITUATIONS

GENERAL VARIATIONS

If a client questions a medication order or states that the medication is different from usual, *always* recheck and clarify with the original order before proceeding to give the medication.

If a client has an altered level of consciousness or impaired swallowing, check with the physician to clarify the route of administration or alternative forms of medication.

Have a client use a straw to swallow a liquid medication that may have a harmful effect on the teeth or mucous membranes.

For clients who find it difficult to take liquid medication from a cup, the medication can be placed in the mouth directly from an extractor or a syringe. An extractor is an instrument that resembles a syringe and fits tightly into the neck of a bottle.

To assist the client with medications that are large or difficult to swallow, crush oral medications except those that are enteric-coated or sustained-release.

Stimulate swallowing by massaging the laryngeal prominence or the area below the chin for clients who are weak.

Provide the client with a piece of ice to suck for a few minutes before taking unpleasant tasting medications. The ice numbs the taste buds and makes the objectionable flavor less discernable.

Mix crushed or whole medications with soft foods, such as potatoes, cooked cereal, or applesauce, for clients who have difficulty swallowing tablets.

If the client has a nasogastric tube, verify the location of the distal end. Administer crushed and liquid oral medications through the tube. Flush the mixture with 30 ml to 50 ml of water. Clamp a tube used for suction for at least $\frac{1}{2}$ hour after administering medications.

AGE-RELATED VARIATIONS

Expect that dosages will be reduced for pediatric and geriatric clients. Weight is more often the criterion for dosage calculation than age.

Special devices, such as droppers and dosing spoons, are available in a pharmacy to ensure accurate dosage calculations for small children and infants.

HOME-CARE CONSIDERATIONS

Encourage the client to discard outdated prescription medications.

Remind the client or his caregivers to obtain refills of medications.

Discuss safe storage of medications when there are children and pets in the environment.

Check agency policy and the mental status of the client before setting up medications in advance.

Devices are available to help the client remember to take medications as scheduled. These may be simple charts or containers that can be made in the home. An empty egg carton labeled with dates and times for medications can be used. More elaborate devices can be purchased in a pharmacy or from the manufacturer.

Administer medication only to the client admitted to the home health service. Give only medications that have been prescribed for the client. Advise the client not to take medications that have been prescribed for others.

RELATED TEACHING

Explain the purpose and action of each medication to the client.

Explain that enteric-coated tablets should never be chewed or crushed.

Tell the client to never take or give medications that have been prescribed for other persons.

Instruct the client to always take a drug as it has been prescribed. Alterations should never be made until after consulting with the physician.

Advise the client to never use medication from a container that is missing a label. Instruct the client to avoid mixing medications from one container to another.

Teach the client that sublingual drugs are absorbed through superficial blood vessels under the tongue. Therefore, this type of medication should not be swallowed.

PERFORMANCE CHECKLIST

When administering oral medications, the learner:

C	A	U	
[ ]	[ ]	[ ]	Checks the written order.
[ ]	[ ]	[ ]	Compares the written order to the transcribed information on the medication Kardex or card.
[ ]	[ ]	[ ]	Reviews drug-related information, if unknown.
[ ]	[ ]	[ ]	Reads the chart to obtain health information.
[ ]	[ ]	[ ]	Examines the client and asks pertinent questions that have a relationship to the drug.
[ ]	[ ]	[ ]	Reads and compares the drug label with the medication card or Kardex at least three times before administering a medication.
[ ]	[ ]	[ ]	Washes hands.
[ ]	[ ]	[ ]	Prepares the solid drugs, liquids, or unit dose packets.
[ ]	[ ]	[ ]	Checks the identity of the client.
[ ]	[ ]	[ ]	Assists the client to a sitting position.
[ ]	[ ]	[ ]	Fills a glass with fresh water.
[ ]	[ ]	[ ]	Helps the client take the medication.
[ ]	[ ]	[ ]	Washes hands.
[ ]	[ ]	[ ]	Records the volume of fluid consumption and the administration of the medication.
[ ]	[ ]	[ ]	Reassesses the client within 30 minutes.

Outcome: [ ] Pass   [ ] Fail

C = competent; A = acceptable; U = unsatisfactory

Comments: _____
_____
_____

_____   _____
Student's Signature   Date

_____   _____
Instructor's Signature   Date

IV-2 *Inserting a nasogastric tube*

A nasogastric tube is inserted through the nose into the stomach. The path of a nasogastric tube is shown in Fig. IV-2-1. Various types and sizes of tubes are available. Clear instruction and patient support can do much to obtain the client's cooperation during this procedure.

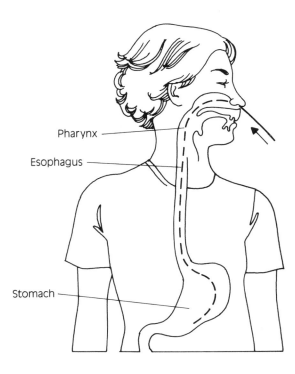

Pharynx

Esophagus

Stomach

Figure IV-2-1 The nasogastric tube passes through several structures along its pathway to the stomach.

PURPOSES OF PROCEDURE

A nasogastric tube may be inserted for any one or several of the following reasons:

1. Instill liquid nourishment.
2. Dilute and remove a consumed poison.
3. Instill iced solution to control gastric bleeding.
4. Obtain a specimen of gastric secretions or stomach contents.
5. Prevent stress on an operative site by decompressing the stomach of secretions and gas.
6. Relieve vomiting and distention.

ASSESSMENT

OBJECTIVE DATA

- Read the physician's written order.
- Read the chart or ask related questions when obtaining an admission history about current and past conditions that increase the risk for upper gastrointestinal problems, such as cancer, depression, and alcohol abuse.
- Examine emesis for volume, color, consistency, and any identifiable substances, like ingested pills or capsules.

- Weigh the client and compare the data with the client's stated weight or weight on previous admissions. Use a nomogram or table for determining the client's ideal weight for his age and height.
- If the client has accidentally or intentionally swallowed a toxic substance, try to discover the name of the substance, the amount, and the time when it was ingested.
- Listen for the presence and activity of bowel sounds in all four quadrants of the abdomen.
- Palpate and percuss the abdomen to assess tympanites. Measure abdominal girth, if appropriate.
- Review laboratory data that may reflect alterations due to nutritional deficiencies, such as red cell count and hemoglobin, blood sugar level, ketones in the urine.
- Inspect the nares observing each for patency, straightness, size, and indications of recent or past trauma. Have the client alternately occlude each nostril and breathe.
- Stimulate the back of the throat to assess that the client's gag reflex is present.

SUBJECTIVE DATA

- Ask the client to describe his nutritional pattern, the types and amounts of food and fluids consumed in a normal 24-hour period.
- Determine if the client has been on a therapeutic diet or a self-imposed diet. Ask the person to describe the types of restrictions he maintains.
- Inquire about recent changes in appetite, dysphagia, and food intolerances. Be alert to information concerning nausea, vomiting, indigestion, belching, distention, flatulence, or diarrhea.
- Ask the client the date of his last bowel movement and to describe its usual characteristics and any recent changes.

RELEVANT NURSING DIAGNOSES

The client who needs a nasogastric tube inserted may have nursing diagnoses, such as:

- *Altered Nutrition: Less than Body Requirements*
- *Altered Comfort*
- *Anxiety*
- *Potential Altered Oral Mucous Membranes*
- *Fluid Volume Deficit*
- *Altered Health Maintenance*
- *Potential for Injury*

PLANNING

ESTABLISHING PRIORITIES

When a nasogastric tube is necessary to treat a life-threatening condition, such as hemorrhage or attempted suicide, the procedure requires highest priority. The nurse should plan to insert a nasogastric tube as soon as possible when the client is experiencing repeated vomiting and acute distention. Other situations that involve nasogastric intubation should be evaluated according to that which threatens the various levels of needs. For instance, depending on the nutritional reserves of a client, the tube may be necessary to meet a client's basic need for nutrition.

SETTING GOALS

- The tube will be inserted gently and safely through the nose, pharynx, esophagus, and will terminate in the stomach.

PREPARATION OF EQUIPMENT

The nurse will need selected items from the following list:

Nasogastric tube of appropriate size
Small basin filled with ice (optional)
Water-soluble lubricant
Tongue blade
Flashlight
Stethoscope
Normal saline (for irrigation only)
Asepto bulb syringe or Toomey syringe (20 ml to 50 ml)

Tape (1 inch wide)
Tissues
Glass of water with straw
Suction apparatus
Bath towel or disposable pad
Safety pin and rubber band
Clamp
Emesis basin

Technique for inserting a nasogastric tube

ACTION	RATIONALE
1. Check the physician's order for inserting a nasogastric tube.	Checking the order clarifies the procedure and type of equipment required.
2. Explain the procedure to the client.	An explanation reduces apprehension and facilitates cooperation.
3. Gather the equipment.	Organization promotes efficient time management.
4. If the nasogastric tube is rubber, place it in a basin with ice for 5 to 10 minutes (optional).	Cold will stiffen the rubber tube making it easier to insert. A plastic tube is usually firm enough, and icing will not be necessary.
5. Assess the client's abdomen.	Baseline data concerning the presence of bowel sounds and the amount of distention will serve for future comparisons.
6. Wash your hands.	Handwashing deters the spread of microorganisms.
7. Assist the client to a high Fowler's position, and drape his chest with a bath towel or disposable pad. Have an emesis basin and tissues handy.	An upright position is more natural for swallowing and protects against aspiration, should the client vomit. Passage of the tube may stimulate gagging and tearing of the eyes.
8. Check the nares for patency by asking the client to occlude one nostril and breathe normally through the other. Select the nostril through which air passes more easily.	The tube will pass more easily through the nostril with the larger opening.
9. Measure the distance to insert the tube by placing the tip of the tube at the client's nostril and extending it to the tip of the earlobe, as shown in Fig. IV-2-2, and	This measurement is called the NEX (nose-earlobe-xiphoid) measurement. It is one method for estimating the length of tubing needed to reach the client's stom-

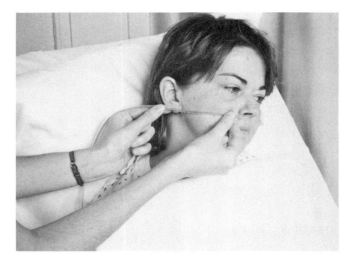

Figure IV-2-2 The nurse measures the distance for inserting the nasogastric tube. The distance from the nose to the earlobe corresponds to the internal distance from the nose to the oropharynx.

then continue to the tip of the xiphoid process, as shown in Fig. IV-2-3. Mark the tube with a piece of tape.

10. Lubricate the first 10 cm to 20 cm (4 inches to 8 inches) of the tube with water-soluble jelly.

11. Ask the client to lift his head, and insert the tube into the nostril while directing the tube downward and backward, as the nurse in Fig. IV-2-4 is doing. Expect that the client may gag when the tube reaches the pharynx.

ach. See the section on modifications for a second method that may be used for measuring the distance for nasogastric tube insertion.

Lubrication reduces friction and facilitates passage of the tube into the stomach. Water-soluble lubricant will not cause pneumonia if the tube accidentally enters the lungs.

Following the normal contour of the nasal passage while inserting the tube reduces irritation and the likelihood of mucosal injury. The gag reflex is readily stimulated by the tube.

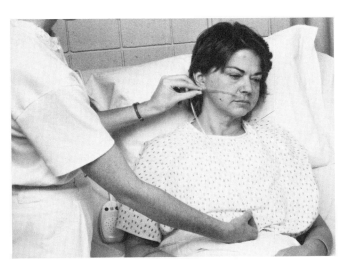
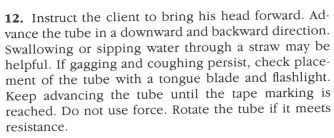

Figure IV-2-3 Adding the distance from the nose to the xiphoid process provides the approximate distance for reaching the stomach.

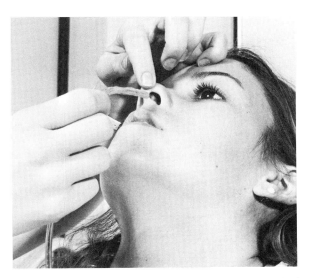

Figure IV-2-4 Note that the end of the tube is lubricated. The nurse is ready to insert the tube after hyperextending the client's neck while in a high Fowler's position.

12. Instruct the client to bring his head forward. Advance the tube in a downward and backward direction. Swallowing or sipping water through a straw may be helpful. If gagging and coughing persist, check placement of the tube with a tongue blade and flashlight. Keep advancing the tube until the tape marking is reached. Do not use force. Rotate the tube if it meets resistance.

13. Discontinue the procedure and remove the tube if there are signs of distress, such as gasping, coughing, cyanosis, and the inability to speak or hum.

14. Determine that the tube is in the client's stomach:

    a. Attach the syringe to the end of the tube and aspirate 10 ml to 20 ml of stomach contents.

    b. Place 10–20 ml of air in a syringe and inject it into the tube while simultaneously auscultating over the left upper quadrant of the client's abdomen with a stethoscope.

Bringing the head forward helps close the trachea and open the esophagus. Swallowing helps advance the tube and causes the epiglottis to cover the opening to the trachea. Excessive coughing and gagging may occur if the tube has curled in the back of the throat. Forcing the tube may injure mucous membranes.

The tube is not in the esophagus if the client shows signs of distress and is unable to speak or hum.

The nurse collects data that indicates anatomical placement.

The tube is in the stomach if its contents can be aspirated.

A whooshing sound can be heard when the air enters the stomach through the tube. If the client belches, the tube is probably in the esophagus.

15. Secure the tube to the client's face with tape. Be careful not to pull the tube too tightly against the nose:

    a. Cut a 4-inch piece of tape and split the bottom 2 inches, as shown in Fig. IV-2-5.

    b. Place the unsplit end over the bridge of the client's nose.

    c. Wrap the split ends around the tubing.

Securing the tube prevents migration or displacement from the stomach. Constant pressure of the tube against the skin and mucous membranes causes tissue injury.

16. Attach the tube to suction or clamp the tube with a screw type clamp according to the physician's orders.

Suction will provide for decompression of stomach and drainage of gastric contents.

17. Secure the tube to the client's gown by using a rubber band or tape and a safety pin, as illustrated in Fig. IV-2-6.

Pinning the tube to the gown prevents tension and tugging on the tube.

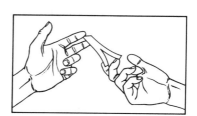

Figure IV-2–5 A piece of tape is prepared for securing a nasogastric tube to the nose by partially splitting one end.

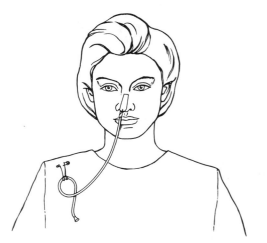

Figure IV-2–6 The nasogastric tube is secured by attaching the tape to the nose and winding the split ends about the tube so there is no pulling on the side of the nostril causing a pressure sore to form. Providing a loop of tubing and pinning it to the gown gives the client some freedom for head movement.

18. Wash hands. Remove all equipment, and make the client comfortable.

Handwashing deters the spread of microorganisms.

19. Record the insertion procedure, type and size of tube, description of gastric contents, and the client's response.

A written record provides accurate documentation of care.

SAMPLE DOCUMENTATION

Date	Time	Nurse's note
2/19	2130	States, "I've been nauseated and vomiting for the past 5 days." Bowel sounds are hypoactive. Oral mucous membranes are pale and sticky. #14 Levin tube inserted. Connected to low intermittent suction. Draining light yellow fluid.
		M. Franz, RN

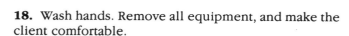

EVALUATION

REASSESSMENT

If a nasogastric tube is being used to withdraw stomach contents, the nurse can observe the progressive increase in volume and characteristics of the drainage to confirm that the tube is patent. The client's girth, percussion of the abdomen, and incidence of nausea and vomiting around the tube may be indications that the tube has become obstructed. Before instilling any liquid through a nasogastric tube, the nurse must assess its location. The nurse is accountable for noting and responding to changes in the nasal, pharyngeal, and oral mucosa due to the presence of the tube and the lack of usual oral intake. Weight changes and electrolyte values may reflect restoration of nutritional balance. Correlating intake volume with output helps determine fluid balance.

EXPECTED OUTCOMES

The nasal mucosa is intact.
The client swallows the tube without incident.
Stomach contents are obtained during aspiration.
Air can be heard over the stomach when instilled through the tube.

UNEXPECTED OUTCOMES

The client is unable to cooperate during insertion.
One or both nares are unsuitable for use.
The tube curls within the pharynx during insertion.
The client gags or vomits during insertion.
The client experiences respiratory distress during insertion.

MODIFICATIONS IN SELECTED SITUATIONS

GENERAL VARIATIONS

If there has been concurrent or recent nasal trauma, such as from an automobile accident, the tube may be inserted through the mouth.

An alternative method for measuring the potential distance to the stomach can be determined by using the following formula:

$$\frac{NEX - 50 \text{ cm } (20 \text{ inches})}{2} + 50 \text{ cm } (20 \text{ inches}) = \text{total insertion length}$$

This measurement seems to be the more accurate method for locating the distal end of the tube in the stomach in most clients.

Hold a rigid plastic tube under warm running water to provide more flexibility and thus reduce the potential for injury.

Table IV-2-1 shows various types of tubes that may be used for gastric intubation. To promote comfort for the client, use the smallest diameter tube that will facilitate the passage of liquid. Most gavage feedings will instill adequately through a size 8 French tube.

Table IV-2–1
Comparisons of gastric tubes

Description	Advantage	Disadvantage
Levin tube: Rubber or plastic single lumen, unvented	Simple, traditional use facilitates a large group who can provide safe care.	Suction can cause the tube to adhere to gastric mucosa and cause injury or obstruction.
Ewald tube: Rubber, large gauge, unvented	Inserted through the mouth usually when lavage is necessary.	Persons who are unfamiliar with the tube may attempt nasal insertion.
Salem sump: Plastic, double lumen, vented	Vent prevents adherence to gastric mucosa.	Vent must not be obstructed or used for irrigation.
Dubbhoff tube: Small bore, very flexible, stylet used during insertion	Easily inserted with minimal trauma. Can be inserted into the stomach or duodenum.	Obstruction occurs more likely due to small diameter. May need x-ray to determine placement.

It may be agency policy that a small, flexible tube, like the Dubbhoff tube, inserted with the assistance of a stylet not be used until an x-ray validates its location in the stomach or duodenum.

Develop a signal before inserting a nasogastric tube that the client may use to indicate distress.

Place the client in a lateral position, never supine, if he cannot be placed in a high Fowler's position.

If the client begins coughing and experiencing difficulty breathing, withdraw the tube to the nasopharynx. By avoiding withdrawing it completely, the nurse can reduce the stress and potential for injury during a subsequent attempt at reinsertion.

Instill a bolus of lubricant within the nostril if lubricating the tip has been insufficient to facilitate its passage.

Stroke the throat of an unconscious client to stimulate a swallowing reflex when passing a nasogastric tube.

Test the *p*H of aspirated secretions with a chem-strip or litmus paper to validate that the tube is located in the stomach. A *p*H of 2 or 3 indicates that the aspirated specimen is acid. Blue litmus paper will turn to red if the specimen is acid.

Place a mark on the tube after it has been secured with tape. This helps in double-checking that the tube has not slipped in or out of its location.

Clean the nose and face daily. Apply new tape as it becomes soiled or loose.

Provide frequent mouth care. Let the client suck limited amounts of ice chips or sour candy, or chew gum to promote salivation.

Alternate nostrils, if possible, when replacing a nasogastric tube.

AGE-RELATED VARIATIONS

A nasogastric tube may be removed and reinserted each time an infant receives a tube feeding.

The diameter of the tube must be correlated with the size of the infant or child. The diameter of the tube should allow the passage of air through the nostril used for insertion.

To determine the approximate distance to the stomach in an infant or newborn, measure the tube from the bridge of the nose to just beyond the tip of the sternum.

HOME-HEALTH VARIATIONS

Use a recliner chair, if available, to assist in placing the client in a Fowler's position while inserting a nasogastric tube.

RELATED TEACHING

Explain the procedure and reason for checking placement.

Instruct the client on how to insert, use, and remove a tube used intermittently while at home. Plan time for the client to practice and demonstrate his proficiency.

PERFORMANCE CHECKLIST

When demonstrating the insertion of a nasogastric tube, the learner:

C	A	U	
[ ]	[ ]	[ ]	Collects a baseline of data related to the function of the gastrointestinal system.
[ ]	[ ]	[ ]	Checks the written order.
[ ]	[ ]	[ ]	Explains the procedure.
[ ]	[ ]	[ ]	Establishes a distress signal.
[ ]	[ ]	[ ]	Assembles the equipment.
[ ]	[ ]	[ ]	Provides privacy.
[ ]	[ ]	[ ]	Washes hands.
[ ]	[ ]	[ ]	Positions the client.
[ ]	[ ]	[ ]	Assesses the nares.
[ ]	[ ]	[ ]	Measures and marks the tube.
[ ]	[ ]	[ ]	Modifies the flexibility of the tube, if necessary.
[ ]	[ ]	[ ]	Lubricates the tip of the tube.
[ ]	[ ]	[ ]	Inserts the tube to the oropharynx.
[ ]	[ ]	[ ]	Instructs the client to lower his chin to his chest and begin swallowing sips of water.
[ ]	[ ]	[ ]	Advances the tube while the client swallows.
[ ]	[ ]	[ ]	Responds to any signals or signs of distress.
[ ]	[ ]	[ ]	Tests for placement location.
[ ]	[ ]	[ ]	Tapes the tube to the client's nose.
[ ]	[ ]	[ ]	Clamps the end of the tube or connects it to suction.
[ ]	[ ]	[ ]	Pins the free end of the tube to the client's gown.
[ ]	[ ]	[ ]	Removes equipment.
[ ]	[ ]	[ ]	Washes hands.
[ ]	[ ]	[ ]	Charts significant information.

Outcome: [ ] Pass   [ ] Fail

C = competent; A = acceptable; U = unsatisfactory

Comments: _____

_____

_____

_____   _____
Student's Signature   Date

_____   _____
Instructor's Signature   Date

IV-3 *Feeding by gastric gavage*

Whenever possible, clients are given oral diets. However, if the client's gastrointestinal tract is functional, but the client is unable or unwilling to consume an adequate oral intake, a tube feeding may be used.

PURPOSES OF PROCEDURE

A gastric gavage feeding is administered to:

1. Provide total or supplemental nutrition.
2. Restore fluid, electrolyte, and acid–base balance.
3. Reduce or eliminate catabolism and negative nitrogen balance.

ASSESSMENT

OBJECTIVE DATA

- Review the results of laboratory tests that indicate the effects of malnourishment, such as red blood cell count, hemoglobin level, serum albumin, lymphocyte count, blood *p*H.
- Weigh the client and compare the weight to the normal range according to the client's height and age.
- Review the trend in intake and output.
- Assess vital signs. Take the blood pressure both lying and sitting to evaluate the presence of postural hypotension.
- Note signs that correlate with poor nutrition, such as dull and brittle hair, pale skin and conjunctiva, lack of energy, absence of subcutaneous fat, impairment in skin integrity, changes in menstrual regularity.
- Consult the chart or client concerning food allergies.
- Auscultate the abdomen to determine the presence and activity of bowel sounds.
- Observe the urine; note its color and odor. Measure and record each voiding.
- Ask the client to identify the date of his last bowel movement and its characteristics.
- Observe the client's response to activity.
- Validate the location of a nasogastric tube, if it is already in place.
- Read the physician's written order concerning gastric feeding.

SUBJECTIVE DATA

- Request that the client describe any food intolerance, changes in taste, smell, appetite, digestion, and elimination.

RELEVANT NURSING DIAGNOSES

The client who requires nourishment by a tube may have nursing diagnoses, such as:

- *Impaired Swallowing*
- *Altered Nutrition: Less than Body Requirements*
- *Fluid Volume Deficit*
- *Altered Health Maintenance*
- *Altered Oral Mucous Membranes*
- *Self-Care Deficit*
- *Hopelessness*

PLANNING

ESTABLISHING PRIORITIES

Eating is a basic need. The well-nourished client can easily withstand deficits that may occur when food is withheld, reduced, or restricted for a short period of time. Clients with increased metabolic requirements or who face a period longer than 2 days without food will require dietary supplementation.

406

SETTING GOALS
- Data will validate that the distal end of the tube is in the stomach.
- The stomach will not become overdistended with formula or air.
- The tubing will remain patent.
- The client will not vomit, aspirate, or experience other adverse effects.

PREPARATION OF EQUIPMENT

The nurse will need selected items from the following list:

Formula at room temperature
Stethoscope
Asepto or Toomey syringe, feeding bag, or prefilled tube feeding set
Clamp (Hoffman or butterfly)
Disposable pad or towel
Water
Gauze square
Rubber band
Enteral feeding pump (if ordered)
IV pole

Technique for feeding by gastric gavage

ACTION	RATIONALE
1. Explain the procedure to the client.	An explanation reduces apprehension and promotes cooperation.
2. Assemble equipment. Check the amount, concentration, type, and frequency of the tube feeding by reading the physician's order or the agency's policy.	Organization promotes efficient time management. Checking ensures the correct feeding will be administered.
3. Wash your hands.	Handwashing deters the spread of microorganisms.
4. Position the client with the head of the bed elevated at least 30 degrees or as near normal position for eating as possible.	Elevating the head minimizes the possibility of aspiration into the trachea.
5. Unpin the tube from the client's gown and check to see that the gastric tube is properly located in the stomach, as described in Procedure IV-2, step 14.	Even when initially positioned correctly, a gastric tube left in place can become dislodged between feedings. The instillation of water or nourishment could lead to serious respiratory problems if a gastric tube is in the trachea or a bronchus, rather than in the stomach.
6. Aspirate all gastric contents with a syringe and measure. Return the aspirated volume through the tube and proceed with the feeding if the amount of residual does not exceed the policy of the agency or the physician's guideline. Disconnect the syringe from the tubing.	Measuring residual provides an indication of gastric emptying time. A residual of more than 50% of the previous intake is significant and must be reported to the physician. Fluid should be returned to the stomach so as not to cause any fluid or electrolyte losses.
7. When using an Asepto or Toomey syringe for feeding:	A syringe is used when the feeding is intermittent.
a. Remove the plunger or bulb from the syringe and attach the syringe to the nasogastric tube which has been pinched with the fingers. Fill the syringe, release the tubing, and introduce the prescribed amount slowly, as the nurse in Fig. IV-3-1 illustrates.	The syringe acts to hold and deliver the nourishment. Introducing the formula slowly gives the stomach time to accommodate to the fluid and decreases gastrointestinal distress.
b. Hold the syringe approximately 12 inches above the stomach. Allow the solution to run in by gravity. Raise the syringe to increase the rate of flow, and lower the syringe to decrease the rate of flow.	Nourishment enters the stomach by gravity when gastric gavage is used. Adjusting the height of the container regulates the speed of the infusion.

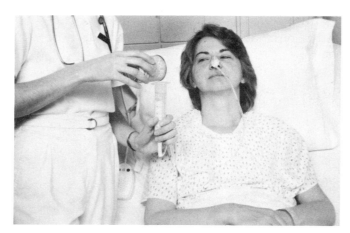

Figure IV-3-1 After checking to see that the tube is in the client's stomach, the nurse removes the bulb from the syringe and pours the formula. The rate at which it flows into the stomach is determined by the height of the syringe.

Figure IV-3-2 Once an intermittent bolus gavage feeding is completed, the nurse flushes the tube with water and clamps it until it will be used again.

c. Do not let the syringe empty while introducing the nourishment.

d. Introduce 30 ml to 60 ml (1 oz to 2 oz) of water into the tube after the nourishment is completely introduced.

e. Clamp the gastric tube when water fills the tubing. Disconnect the syringe and cover the end of the tubing with gauze secured with a rubber band, as shown in Fig. IV-3-2.

8. When using a feeding bag:

a. Hang the bag on an IV pole and adjust to about 12 inches above the stomach. Clamp the tubing, and pour the formula into the bag. Release the clamp enough to allow the formula to run through the tubing, as shown in Fig. IV-3-3. Close the clamp.

Keeping the syringe and the tubing filled prevents air from entering the stomach.

Flushing the gastric tube with water forces the formula remaining in the tube into the stomach and prevents nourishment from adhering to the tube and souring.

Clamping the tube prevents loss of fluid from the tube and air from entering the stomach. The gauze cover deters entry of microorganisms and protects the client and linens from any fluid leakage from the tube.

Formula can infuse through a suspended unit rather than one held by the nurse.

The formula displaces air in the tubing.

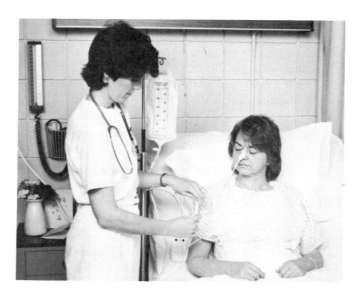

Figure IV-3-3 This client is receiving nourishment through a feeding bag. The formula has been placed in a container suspended on an IV pole. The nurse regulates the rate by adjusting the clamp and counting the drops as they fall into the drip chamber.

b. Attach the tubing to the nasogastric tube, open the clamp, and regulate the drip according to the physician's order.

c. Add 30 ml to 60 ml (1 oz to 2 oz) of water to the feeding bag when the feeding is almost completed, and allow it to run through the tube, as shown in Fig. IV-3-4.

Introducing the formula at a slow, regular rate allows the stomach to adjust to the feeding and decreases gastrointestinal distress.

Water rinses the feeding from the tube and helps to keep it patent.

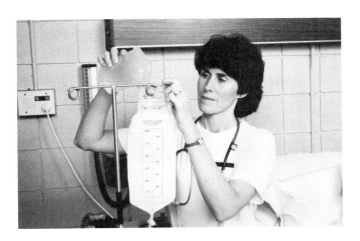

Figure IV-3-4 The nurse adds water to the feeding bag following the instillation of the formula. If residual formula remained within the tubing, it could solidify and obstruct the lumen before the next feeding.

d. Clamp the tubing immediately after the water has been instilled. Disconnect the feeding bag from the nasogastric tube. Clamp the nasogastric tube and cover the end with gauze secured with a rubber band.

9. When using a prefilled tube feeding set-up:

a. Remove the screw-on cap, and attach the administration set-up with the drip chamber and tubing. Hang the set on an IV pole and adjust to about 12 inches above the stomach. Clamp the tubing and squeeze the drip chamber to fill one-third to one-half of capacity. Release the clamp, and run the formula through the tubing. Close the clamp.

b. Follow steps B, C, and D as explained in step 8. A feeding pump may be used with a tube feeding to regulate the drip.

10. Observe the client's response during and after a tube feeding.

11. Have the client remain in an upright position for at least 30 minutes after an intermittent feeding.

12. Wash and clean equipment or replace it according to agency policy. Wash your hands.

13. Record the type and amount of feeding and the client's response. Monitor urine or blood glucose if ordered by the physician.

Clamping the tube prevents air from entering the stomach. Covering the end of the nasogastric tube deters the entry of microorganisms and protects the client and linens from any fluid leakage from the tube.

Manufacturers have produced premixed formulas for the convenience of the nurse and for clients' home use.

The formula displaces the air in the tubing.

A feeding pump uses mechanical pressure to infuse the formula rather than just gravity. A pump may be used when a slow, continuous infusion is desired.

Pain may indicate stomach distention and may lead to vomiting. The nurse is accountable for the client's safety.

This position minimizes risk of backflow and discourages aspiration should any vomiting occur.

Washing and cleaning prevents contamination and deters the spread of microorganisms.

A written summary provides accurate documentation of the procedure. Many feedings contain high levels of carbohydrate.

SAMPLE DOCUMENTATION

Date	Time	Nurse's note
1/20	1700	NG tube aspirated with Asepto. 30 mL of clear, lt. green liquid removed and reinstilled. Sustagen formula hung and regulated to infuse at 100 mL per hr. No distention or diarrhea noted. Bowel sounds are active in all four quads.
		L. Brown, RN

EVALUATION

REASSESSMENT

Always assess the location of the distal end of a nasogastric tube before administering any liquid. To obtain the most valid data for evaluating the client's weight, the nurse should attempt to duplicate the same conditions each time. Use the same scales; dress the client in similar clothing; weigh the client at approximately the same time of day. Malnourished clients often have low levels of albumin which causes fluid to be trapped in tissue. A fuller appearance caused by edema should not be misinterpreted as evidence of improved nutritional status. Monitor changes in baseline data gathered before tube feedings were begun. Assess the blood sugar using a glucometer, or test the urine for glucose several times a day to determine the client's response to the concentration of carbohydrate in the formula.

EXPECTED OUTCOMES

The client does not feel hungry.
The client maintains or gains weight.
The formula infuses at the prescribed rate.
The client's fluid volume and electrolytes remain balanced.
The client's blood sugar remains in normal ranges.

UNEXPECTED OUTCOMES

The client loses weight.
The infusion of the formula speeds or slows.
The client experiences intestinal cramping or diarrhea.
The client's stomach distends, causing fullness or vomiting.
The client manifests hyperglycemia or glycosuria.

MODIFICATIONS IN SELECTED SITUATIONS

GENERAL VARIATIONS

Administer crushed oral medications as a bolus through the tube in fluid separate from the tube feeding. It is preferable to administer medications orally if the client is capable of swallowing. Crushed medications may obstruct the tubing.
Follow agency protocols. Most direct that the formula be diluted when initiating nourishment by tube feeding. The formula may be eventually reconstituted to full strength if the client does not have any adverse symptoms.
Slowly infuse an intermittent bolus tube feeding so that it lasts approximately 15 minutes to 30 minutes or the time it would normally take to eat. A rapidly instilled feeding can cause gastrointestinal distress, such as nausea, cramping, and diarrhea, due to the concentrated content of carbohydrates. Use the time for social interaction which usually accompanies normal eating.
Introduce formula at ambient room temperature. Warming the formula or allowing a large volume to stand for a long period of time can support bacterial growth.
Use 7-Up rather than water to rinse the tubing following an intermittent feeding. The carbonated liquid tends to loosen particles that may cling to the inner surface of the tube.

AGE-RELATED VARIATIONS

The nasogastric tube is inserted and removed with each feeding.
Aspirate the air used to check tube placement to avoid distending the stomach of an infant.
Infants can usually tolerate an infusion rate of 3 ml/min. The tubing can be rinsed with 1 ml to 2 ml of water afterwards.

Place an infant on the right side with the isolette elevated 15 to 30 degrees to promote retention of the formula.

Hold, cuddle, and talk to an infant to simulate the sensory stimulation that accompanies feeding.

During a tube feeding, provide the infant with a pacifier or similar substitute to promote or satisfy his sucking needs and promote the digestive process.

HOME-HEALTH VARIATIONS

If the client's condition permits, encourage him to join family members at the table during meal times.

Portable enteral pumps are available for home use if the client is receiving continuous feedings.

Change small bore tubes, like Entriflex, Keofeed, and Dubbhoff, according to agency policy or manufacturer's recommendations. Most suggest that these tubes not remain in place longer than 4 weeks because tube deterioration is possible from exposure to gastric secretions.

RELATED TEACHING

Explain the purpose and describe the steps in the procedure before they are performed.

Instruct the client to remain sitting for a time following an intermittent tube feeding. This promotes retention of the formula in the stomach, preventing esophageal reflux with possible aspiration.

Inform the client of possible responses to the formula such as fullness, distention, nausea, and diarrhea. Advise the client to report any feelings of discomfort.

(Performance checklist next page)

PERFORMANCE CHECKLIST

When administering gastric gavage, the learner:

C	A	U	
[ ]	[ ]	[ ]	Checks the written order for the volume, type of formula, and rate or frequency of administration.
[ ]	[ ]	[ ]	Explains the procedure to the client.
[ ]	[ ]	[ ]	Assembles equipment.
[ ]	[ ]	[ ]	Washes hands.
[ ]	[ ]	[ ]	Gathers pertinent assessment data.
[ ]	[ ]	[ ]	Places the client in high Fowler's position, or lateral position, if unconscious.
[ ]	[ ]	[ ]	Frees the tube from the client's gown.
[ ]	[ ]	[ ]	Attaches a syringe.
[ ]	[ ]	[ ]	Checks the tube for gastric placement.
[ ]	[ ]	[ ]	Aspirates stomach contents into the syringe.
[ ]	[ ]	[ ]	Measures the stomach's residual contents.
[ ]	[ ]	[ ]	Refeeds aspirated volume.
[ ]	[ ]	[ ]	Instills fresh formula according to the medical order or volume of aspirated residual.
[ ]	[ ]	[ ]	Maintains a constant flow of formula throughout the instillation.
[ ]	[ ]	[ ]	Flushes the tube with water after all the formula has been administered.
[ ]	[ ]	[ ]	Clamps the tube.
[ ]	[ ]	[ ]	Removes the syringe.
[ ]	[ ]	[ ]	Protects the end of the tube with gauze.
[ ]	[ ]	[ ]	Maintains the client's comfort in a sitting position for 30 minutes following the feeding.
[ ]	[ ]	[ ]	Cleans reusable equipment and replaces items in the designated location.
[ ]	[ ]	[ ]	Washes hands.
[ ]	[ ]	[ ]	Charts significant information.

Outcome: [ ] Pass   [ ] Fail

C = competent; A = acceptable; U = unsatisfactory

Comments: _____

_____

_____

_____   _____
          Student's Signature   Date

_____   _____
         Instructor's Signature   Date

IV-4 | *Monitoring a nasogastric tube*

A nasogastric tube can be used for reasons other than administering nourishment. Additional purposes can be reviewed in Procedure IV-2. It is the nurse's responsibility to make pertinent observations of any equipment used in the care of the client.

PURPOSES OF PROCEDURE

A nasogastric tube is monitored to:

1. Maintain the safety of the client.
2. Promote the efficacy of the treatment.
3. Identify malfunctions of the equipment.
4. Assess untoward responses.

ASSESSMENT

OBJECTIVE DATA

- Determine the reason(s) for using a nasogastric tube in each client's case.
- Identify the span of time that the nasogastric tube has been in place.
- Consult the physician's written orders or the agency's policies for directives on the type and amount of suction, if that is being used.
- Review the documentation on the client's chart to determine the pattern of responses that have been unique to this person with a nasogastric tube.

SUBJECTIVE DATA

- Ask the client to identify problems he attributes to the use of the nasogastric tube.

RELEVANT NURSING DIAGNOSES

The client who requires monitoring of a nasogastric tube can have nursing diagnoses, such as:

- *Altered Comfort*
- *Potential for Injury*
- *Potential Impaired Skin Integrity*
- *Diversional Activity Deficit*
- *Fluid Volume Deficit*
- *Potential Impaired Gas Exchange*

Because suctioning removes electrolytes and acid secretions, the client has collaborative problems like:

- *Potential for hypokalemia, hyponatremia, and hypochloremia*
- *Potential for metabolic alkalosis*

PLANNING

ESTABLISHING PRIORITIES

Each nurse is accountable for meeting the agency's standards for care. It is important that the nurse make comprehensive observations of the client and the nasogastric tube early in the shift. Subsequent focus assessments should be obtained every 2 hours.

SETTING GOALS

- The client will remain free of iatrogenic (treatment caused) complications.
- The equipment will continue to function safely and effectively.

PREPARATION OF EQUIPMENT

The following items may be needed when monitoring a nasogastric tube:

Chem-strips for assessing characteristics of the gastric secretions
Graduated pitcher

413

Stethoscope
Syringe (20 ml or larger)
Irrigation solution

Technique for monitoring a nasogastric tube

ACTION	RATIONALE
1. Confirm the physician's order for the nasogastric tube, the type of suction, and the specifications for irrigation.	Checking the medical order ensures the correct implementation of the physician's directives.
2. Observe the drainage from the tube. Check the amount, color, consistency, and odor. Hematest drainage to confirm the presence of blood in the drainage.	Normal color of gastric drainage is light yellow to green in color due to the presence of bile. Bloody drainage may be expected after gastric surgery, but must be monitored closely. The presence of coffee-ground type drainage may indicate bleeding.
3. Inspect the suction apparatus, as shown in Fig. IV-4-1. Check that the setting is correct for the type of suction (continuous or intermittent), range of suction (low, medium, or high), and that movement of drainage through the tubing is taking place.	Checking the mechanical settings ensures that the prescribed settings are correctly adjusted. Loose connections or a kink or blockage in the tube may interfere with the suction.
4. Assess the placement of the nasogastric tube. See Procedure IV-5, Irrigating a Nasogastric Tube, step 6.	A nasogastric tube may be displaced into the trachea through movement or manipulation.
5. Assess the comfort of the client. Check for the presence of nausea and vomiting, feeling of fullness, or pain.	Using objective and subjective assessments can lead to identifying malfunction of nasogastric suction or blockage in the tube.
6. Assess the client's abdomen for distention, as shown in Fig. IV-4-2. Auscultate for the presence of bowel sounds.	Abdominal distention may be related to the accumulation of gas or internal bleeding. The presence of bowel sounds indicates that peristalsis is occurring.

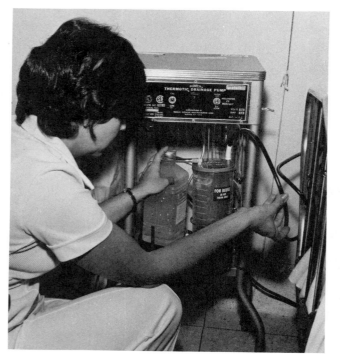

Figure IV-4-1 The nurse is responsible for checking the settings on the suction machine and observing the movement and characteristics of the drainage.

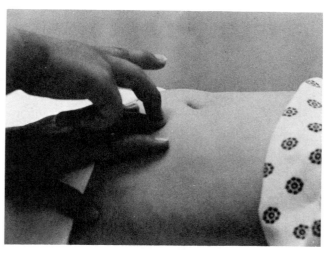

Figure IV-4-2 The nurse uses percussion to detect dull or resonant sounds. Dull sounds indicate solid structures or structures that are filled with solid substances. Resonant or hollow sounds indicate structures that are filled with air.

7. Assess the mobility of the client and his respiratory status.

Turning from side to side in bed and ambulating when permitted prevents cardiopulmonary, vascular, and musculoskeletal complications. Movement facilitates peristalsis and drainage.

8. Observe the condition of the client's nostrils and oral cavity.

Nostrils need cleansing and lubrication with water-soluble lubricant as well as a periodic change of the tape to minimize irritation from the tube. Frequent mouth care, at 2-hour intervals, improves comfort and maintains moisture in the oral mucosa.

9. Monitor the overall safety of the client with a nasogastric tube.

A nasogastric tube that is secured to the client's nose with tape and pinned to the gown, allows easier movement. A call bell within reach allows the client ready access to nursing assistance. Any kinks or obstruction interfere with the patency of a nasogastric tube. A semi-Fowler's position facilitates drainage and minimizes any risk of aspiration.

10. Monitor the nasogastric tube and the suction unit at least every 2 hours. Irrigate the tube at intervals ordered by the physician. (See Procedure IV-5.)

Monitoring promotes safe operation of the system. Any change in the client's condition or type of drainage necessitates more frequent observation and notification of the physician.

11. Measure the irrigation and drainage and record the amounts on the intake and output sheet. Document the description of the drainage and the client's response on the chart.

Irrigations are recorded as intake. Drainage from the nasogastric tube is measured as output every 8 hours. If drainage is copious, more frequent emptying of the collection container will be necessary. Documentation provides an accurate record of the client's response to gastric suctioning.

12. Replenish supplies and maintain equipment according to the agency's policy and the manufacturer's recommendations.

Stocking equipment ensures the availability of necessary supplies. Following maintenance policies provides for safe operation of the equipment and efficient drainage of the client's gastric contents.

SAMPLE DOCUMENTATION

Date	Time	Nurse's note
10/01	0730	Nasogastric tube connected to intermittent, low suction. Gastric drainage is greenish yellow with flecks of brown. Lung sounds are clear throughout. Bowel sounds are present and active in all four quads. Abdomen is soft. Instructed to perform leg exercises and deep breathing q 2°. Oral mucosa is pink and moist. Nose cleaned and K-Y jelly applied to R nostril. Turned from R to L side. Drainage moving freely into collection device. NG irrigation not needed.

B. Friedman, RN

EVALUATION

REASSESSMENT

Focus assessments are generally conducted every 2 hours. The nurse should analyze the balance of intake and output at the end of each shift. Serum electrolytes and arterial blood gases may be monitored as they become available.

EXPECTED OUTCOMES

The suction is regulated according to agency policy or the physician's order.
The nasal and oral mucosa are moist and intact.
The distal end of the tube remains in the stomach.
The tube remains patent.

The drainage appears light yellow to green.
Laboratory data indicate normal values.
Respiratory and bowel function are not altered.

UNEXPECTED OUTCOMES

The suction unit does not function accurately.
The nostril used for tube insertion appears red.
Secretions stop draining through the tube.
The client's abdomen becomes distended.
Secretions are bloody or contain brown granules.
Laboratory values reflect abnormalities associated with nasogastric suctioning.

MODIFICATIONS IN SELECTED SITUATIONS

GENERAL VARIATIONS

Suction may be controlled by wall units or portable suction machines. The pressure settings may differ depending on the type of unit being used.

If the client is receiving oral medications, try to obtain them in liquid form. Give solid oral medications orally. If this is not possible, crush the tablets or open and empty the contents of capsules; mix the medication with water before instilling them into the nasogastric tube. Flush the tube with water to deposit all the medication into the stomach. Clamp the tube for at least $\frac{1}{2}$ hour after administration of medication to avoid removing it with suction. Enteric-coated tablets should never be crushed and administered through a nasogastric tube.

AGE-RELATED VARIATIONS

Avoid setting suction pressure above 25 mm Hg on an unvented nasogastric tube used on children. Vented nasogastric tubes can be set at 30 to 40 mm Hg.

HOME-HEALTH VARIATIONS

If a vented tube is used, remind the family and caregivers not to tie a knot in the vent. If drainage comes through the vent, a gauze square or other absorbent material can be secured around the opening with a rubber band. As another solution, try taping the vented end through the lid and within a plastic prescription container. Make sure that a second hole is made in the lid to allow the escape of air.

If electronic suction is used, remind the family and caregivers that the machine is to be operational even during times of sleep. It should not be turned off.

Oral medication tablets can be crushed by placing them between two souffle cups or paper cups for cupcakes and tapping gently with a hammer.

PERFORMANCE CHECKLIST

When monitoring a nasogastric tube, the learner:

C	A	U	
[ ]	[ ]	[ ]	Checks pertinent written medical orders.
[ ]	[ ]	[ ]	Reviews recorded observations.
[ ]	[ ]	[ ]	Observes the characteristics of the gastric drainage.
[ ]	[ ]	[ ]	Checks the suction settings.
[ ]	[ ]	[ ]	Checks the placement of the tube.
[ ]	[ ]	[ ]	Questions the client to obtain subjective data.
[ ]	[ ]	[ ]	Auscultates lung sounds.
[ ]	[ ]	[ ]	Palpates the abdomen and auscultates bowel sounds.
[ ]	[ ]	[ ]	Promotes exercise and movement.
[ ]	[ ]	[ ]	Inspects and provides preventive care of the nose and oral mucosa.
[ ]	[ ]	[ ]	Examines the tube for obstruction or kinking.
[ ]	[ ]	[ ]	Stabilizes the tube with tape and a safety pin or clip in such a way to limit pulling or displacement.
[ ]	[ ]	[ ]	Irrigates the tube when ordered and necessary.
[ ]	[ ]	[ ]	Measures and records drainage at the end of the shift.
[ ]	[ ]	[ ]	Cleans and replaces treatment supplies.
[ ]	[ ]	[ ]	Charts significant information.

Outcome: [ ] Pass   [ ] Fail

C = competent; A = acceptable; U = unsatisfactory

Comments: _____

_____

_____

_____   _____

Student's Signature   Date

_____   _____

Instructor's Signature   Date

IV-5   *Irrigating a nasogastric tube*

The nurse is responsible for observing and analyzing signs that indicate the patency of the tube. Nasogastric tubes are not routinely irrigated unless the doctor specifies because this dilutes and removes electrolytes. The tube is flushed prophylactically after each tube feeding or administration of crushed medications. However, in the latter situations, there is no attempt to aspirate or siphon the instilled fluid.

PURPOSES OF PROCEDURE

A nasogastric tube is irrigated to:

1. Maintain patency of the tube.
2. Relieve an obstruction due to thick secretions.
3. Relieve pressure from retained secretions and gas.

ASSESSMENT

OBJECTIVE DATA

- Check the medical order for the frequency for irrigation.
- Review agency policy for the recommended volume if not specified in the physician's order.
- Check that the suction equipment is on and cycling according to the prescribed settings.
- Note the movement of drainage through the tubing into the container.
- Observe the characteristics of drainage within the collection container.
- Review the intake and output totals in the previous 8 hours.
- Check that all connections are intact.
- Examine the length of the tubing for kinking or compression.
- Palpate the abdomen and auscultate bowel sounds.

SUBJECTIVE DATA

- Ask the client to indicate if he is experiencing a feeling of fullness, nausea, or the potential for vomiting.

RELEVANT NURSING DIAGNOSES

A client who needs his nasogastric tube irrigated can have nursing diagnoses, such as:

- *Altered Comfort*
- *Potential for Injury*
- *Impaired Gas Exchange*
- *Altered Cardiac Output*

PLANNING

ESTABLISHING PRIORITIES

In certain instances there is a primary need to maintain the function of the nasogastric tube. For instance, a client who has a partial or complete bowel obstruction or one who has had recent gastrointestinal surgery may develop life-threatening complications if pressure from retained fluid and gas becomes excessive. In addition to this, a distended abdomen can reduce tidal volume and affect the client's ability to oxygenate cells adequately. A stomach that enlarges due to the stasis of its contents can interfere with cardiac filling thus limiting the amount of blood it can eject with each beat.

SETTING GOALS

- The nasogastric tube will remain patent.
- The client will remain free of gastrointestinal discomfort.

PREPARATION OF
EQUIPMENT

The nurse will need items from the following list:

Irrigation set (Asepto or Toomey syringe and container for irrigating solution)
Normal saline for irrigation
Stethoscope
Disposable pad or bath towel
Clamp

Technique for irrigating a nasogastric tube

ACTION	RATIONALE
1. Monitor and collect pertinent assessments.	The nurse uses information to identify problems and select appropriate solutions.
2. Check the physician's order for irrigation.	Reading the written order ensures that the procedure will comply with the directives of the physician.
3. Explain the procedure to the client.	An explanation reduces apprehension and promotes the client's cooperation.
4. Assist the client to a semi-Fowler's position unless this is contraindicated.	Gravity promotes the distribution of fluid to the lower levels of the stomach and minimizes the risk of aspiration.
5. Clamp the suction tubing near the connection site. Disconnect the nasogastric tube from the suction unit and lay it on the disposable pad or towel.	Clamping protects the client from leakage of gastric drainage.
6. Check the placement of the nasogastric tube:	Fluid must never be instilled until data support that the tip is located in the stomach.
a. Attach an Asepto or Toomey syringe to the end of the tube, as the nurse in Fig. IV-5-1 is doing, and aspirate gastric contents.	The tube is in the stomach if its contents can be aspirated.
b. Place 10–20 ml of air in the syringe, and inject it through the tube while simultaneously auscultating over the epigastric area with a stethoscope, as shown in Fig. IV-5-2.	A whooshing sound can be heard when the air enters the stomach through the tube. If the client belches, the tip is likely in the esophagus.
c. Ask the client to speak.	If the tube is misplaced in the trachea, the client will not be able to speak.

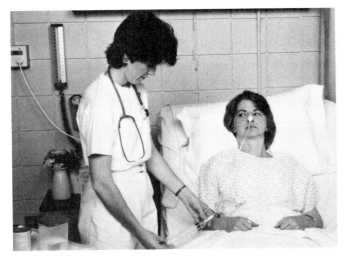

Figure IV-5-1 The nurse prepares to check the distal placement of the nasogastric tube by attaching an Asepto syringe to the proximal end of the tube.

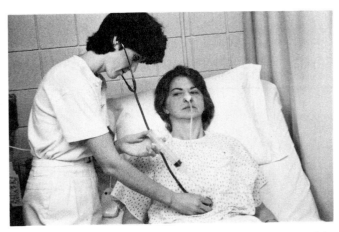

Figure IV-5-2 The nurse listens over the left upper quadrant of the client's abdomen while simultaneously instilling a bolus of air.

7. Pour irrigating solution into a container, as shown in Fig. IV-5-3. Draw up 30 ml of saline (or the amount ordered by the physician) into the syringe.

Measuring the amount ensures that the precise amount is delivered through the tube. Using saline compensates for electrolytes lost through nasogastric drainage.

8. Place the tip of the syringe into the nasogastric tube. Hold the syringe upright, and allow the solution to instill by gravity or gently promote instillation manually, as shown in Fig. IV-5-4. Do not force the solution into the nasogastric tube.

Gravity instillation is less traumatic to the gastric mucosa.

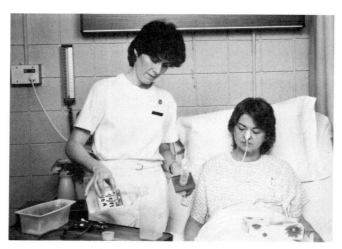

Figure IV-5–3 The nurse is preparing the irrigating solution that will be used to flush the nasogastric tube.

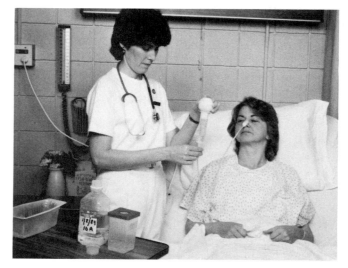

Figure IV-5–4 The nurse is irrigating the nasogastric tube by using gentle pressure to compress the bulb on the syringe.

9. If unable to irrigate the tube, reposition the client and attempt the irrigation again. Check with the physician if repeated attempts to irrigate the tube fail.

The tip of the tube may be positioned against gastric mucosa. Changing the position of the client may free the tip and open the tube for the passage of fluid.

10. Withdraw or aspirate the fluid into the syringe. If no return, instill 20 ml of air and aspirate again.

Instilling air may reposition or clear the tube.

11. Reconnect the nasogastric tube to suction. Observe the movement of the drainage.

Movement indicates patency of the nasogastric tube and the functional operation of the suction device.

12. Measure and record the amount and description of the irrigant and returned solution.

The irrigant placed in the nasogastric tube is considered intake; solution returned is recorded as output.

13. Rinse the equipment if it will be reused.

Rinsing promotes cleanliness and prepares the equipment for the next irrigation.

14. Wash your hands.

Handwashing deters the spread of microorganisms.

15. Record the irrigation procedure, description of the drainage, and the client's response.

A written summary facilitates the documentation of the procedure and provides a record of comprehensive care.

SAMPLE DOCUMENTATION

Date	Time	Nurse's note
4/09	1030	20 ml of air instilled into nasogastric tube and simultaneously auscultated over the stomach. 30 mL of normal saline instilled into NG tube and repeated a second time. 45 mL of dark green, thick drainage aspirated from tube. Reconnected to low, intermittent suction. Drng. moving freely into collection container.

C. Voijtek, RN

EVALUATION

REASSESSMENT

The flow and characteristics of gastric drainage should be assessed every 2 hours. Most nurses observe and analyze data with each client contact.

EXPECTED OUTCOMES

The distal end of the tube remains located within the stomach.
The irrigation solution instills easily without force.
Drainage moves freely into the collection container.
The client does not become distended or nauseous.

UNEXPECTED OUTCOMES

The placement of the tube is uncertain.
The irrigation solution fails to instill.
Instilled solution is not aspirated.
Drainage is slow in moving into the collection reservoir.
The client becomes short of breath, manifests tachycardia, is nauseated, or his abdomen distends.

MODIFICATIONS IN SELECTED SITUATIONS

GENERAL VARIATIONS

Instill air into the vent of a double lumen tube after reconnecting the tube to suction. This breaks any seal between the tip and the gastric mucosa.
Change the client to a side-lying position to facilitate a return of the irrigation solution once the tube is connected back to suction.

AGE-RELATED VARIATIONS

Aspirate any air used to check placement from an infant's nasogastric tube. The air occupies space and could cause distention or regurgitation of fluid. Regurgitation increases the potential for aspiration into the lungs.

HOME-HEALTH VARIATIONS

The client does not necessarily need to return to bed when the nasogastric tube is irrigated.

RELATED TEACHING

Explain the purpose of the procedure and each step as it is performed.
Identify the signs indicating obstruction, and encourage the client to communicate any signs or symptoms that he may experience.

(Performance checklist next page)

PERFORMANCE CHECKLIST

When irrigating a nasogastric tube, the learner:

C	A	U	
[ ]	[ ]	[ ]	Verifies the specifics of the medical order.
[ ]	[ ]	[ ]	Gathers equipment.
[ ]	[ ]	[ ]	Explains the procedure.
[ ]	[ ]	[ ]	Washes hands.
[ ]	[ ]	[ ]	Provides privacy.
[ ]	[ ]	[ ]	Adjusts the height of the bed.
[ ]	[ ]	[ ]	Helps the client to a sitting position.
[ ]	[ ]	[ ]	Protects the bedclothing and linen with a towel or pad.
[ ]	[ ]	[ ]	Disconnects the tube from suction.
[ ]	[ ]	[ ]	Checks placement of the tube.
[ ]	[ ]	[ ]	Instills 30 ml, or the amount specified, of saline.
[ ]	[ ]	[ ]	Aspirates the irrigation solution.
[ ]	[ ]	[ ]	Repeats the instillation if the results are unsatisfactory.
[ ]	[ ]	[ ]	Connects the tube back to suction.
[ ]	[ ]	[ ]	Lowers the bed and helps the client to a position of comfort.
[ ]	[ ]	[ ]	Measures the returned volume.
[ ]	[ ]	[ ]	Records the intake and output of fluid.
[ ]	[ ]	[ ]	Cleans and replaces reusable equipment.
[ ]	[ ]	[ ]	Washes hands.
[ ]	[ ]	[ ]	Charts significant information.

Outcome: [ ] Pass   [ ] Fail

C = competent; A = acceptable; U = unsatisfactory

Comments: _____

_____

_____

_____   _____
        Student's Signature   Date

_____   _____
       Instructor's Signature   Date

IV-6   *Removing a nasogastric tube*

A nasogastric tube is generally a temporary measure. Removal must be performed as carefully and safely as it was inserted.

PURPOSES OF PROCEDURE

A nasogastric tube is removed to:

1. Discontinue gastric decompression.
2. Replace a tube that has been inserted several days.
3. Resume normal eating.
4. Rotate the nostril for insertion when it has become irritated due to pressure.
5. Complete a diagnostic test or emergency treatment.

ASSESSMENT

OBJECTIVE DATA

- Validate that the physician has written an order for removal, if the tube has been in continuous use.
- Review agency policy for recommendations on the length of time the same tube can remain in place.
- Inspect the naris for inflammation and signs of pressure necrosis.

SUBJECTIVE DATA

- Ask the client to describe any discomfort he associates with the nasogastric tube.

RELEVANT NURSING DIAGNOSES

A client who is about to have a nasogastric tube removed can have nursing diagnoses, such as:

- *Altered Comfort*
- *Impaired Skin Integrity*
- *Altered Oral Mucous Membranes*
- *Potential for Injury*
- *Impaired Swallowing*

PLANNING

ESTABLISHING PRIORITIES

A nasogastric tube can cause discomfort and limit a client's activity and ambulation. Once it has been determined that removal is appropriate, the nurse should revise the plan for care in order to attend to performing this procedure.

SETTING GOALS

- The nasogastric tube will be withdrawn without leakage of gastric contents.
- The client will not aspirate gastric secretions.

PREPARATION OF EQUIPMENT

The nurse will need the following items when removing a nasogastric tube:

Tissues
Bath towel or disposable pad
Plastic disposable bag
Clean disposable glove

Technique for removing a nasogastric tube

ACTION	RATIONALE
1. Check the physician's order for removal of the nasogastric tube.	Validating the medical order ensures the correct implementation of the physician directives.
2. Explain the procedure to the client.	An explanation reduces apprehension and facilitates cooperation.
3. Gather equipment.	Organization promotes efficient time management.
4. Wash your hands. Don a clean, disposable glove on the hand that will remove the tube.	Handwashing deters the spread of microorganisms. The glove protects the hand from contact with gastric secretions.
5. Discontinue the suction and separate the tube from suction. Unpin the tube from the client's gown and carefully remove the adhesive tape from the bridge of the nose.	Detaching the tube allows for unrestricted removal of the nasogastric tube.
6. Place the towel or disposable pad across the client's chest. Hand tissues to the client.	The towel or pad protects the client from contact with gastric secretions. Tissues are convenient if the client wishes to blow his nose when the tube is removed.
7. Instruct the client to take a deep breath.	Holding the breath prevents accidental aspiration of any gastric secretions in the tube.
8. Clamp the tube with the fingers. Quickly and carefully remove the tube while the client holds his breath, as the nurse in Fig. IV-6-1 is doing.	Clamping prevents any leakage of gastric contents from the tube. Using care minimizes trauma and discomfort for the client.

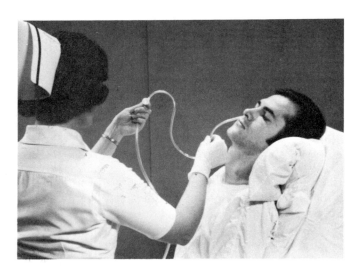

Figure IV-6–1 The nurse removes a nasogastric tube using a clean, disposable glove to protect her hand.

ACTION	RATIONALE
9. Place the tube in a disposable plastic bag. Remove the glove and place it in the bag.	Enclosing soiled items prevents contamination with any microorganisms.
10. Offer mouth care to the client, and make the client comfortable.	Comfort measures are a component of conscientious nursing care.
11. Measure gastric drainage. Remove all equipment and dispose according to agency policy. Wash your hands.	Measuring gastric drainage provides for accurate recording of output. Proper disposal deters the spread of microorganisms.
12. Record the removal of the nasogastric tube, the client's response, and measurement of drainage.	A written summary provides accurate documentation of the care and treatment that the client received.

SAMPLE DOCUMENTATION

Date	Time	Nurse's note
2/23	1110	L naris intact with no signs of pressure. States throat feels "sore" especially when swallowing saliva. Bowel sounds are present and active throughout abdomen. Expelling flatus. Levin tube removed as ordered by Dr. Robbins. Mouth and nose care provided. 100 mL of green drainage disposed. Taking sips of water with no nausea, vomiting, or distention.
		C. Bashur, RN

EVALUATION

REASSESSMENT

It is important to observe the client's response to taking oral liquids and nourishment. The skin around the nasal orifice, mucous membranes of the mouth and pharynx should be assessed daily if they have become irritated while the tube was in use. Bowel sounds and bowel elimination patterns should be noted to evaluate the return of normal gastrointestinal function.

EXPECTED OUTCOMES

The tube is withdrawn easily.
The mucosa of the esophagus, pharynx, or naris is not irritated by gastric secretions.
The client tolerates the procedure without retching or vomiting.

UNEXPECTED OUTCOMES

There is resistance to the effort to remove the tube.
The mucosa of structures above the stomach become irritated from leakage of gastric contents.
The naris is red or ulcerated due to pressure from the gastric tube.
The client becomes nauseated and vomits.

MODIFICATIONS IN SELECTED SITUATIONS

GENERAL VARIATIONS

When a tube is being discontinued after a period of gastric decompression, the nurse may clamp the tube for a while prior to its removal. While the tube is clamped, offer the client sips of clear fluids orally to determine his tolerance to the addition of volume into the stomach. If the client becomes nauseated, becomes distended, or vomits, consult the physician before removing the tube.
Some nurses prefer to hold the tube within a towel while it is being removed so the client does not see it. This may help to prevent gagging, nausea, or vomiting. It also protects the nurse's hands and absorbs any liquid that may leak from the tube.
When normal eating is resumed, gradually progress a client from clear to full liquids; increase the volume according to tolerance, and plan small, frequent feedings rather than the traditional three meals per day.

HOME-HEALTH VARIATIONS

If the client has a tendency to remove tubes, teach the caregivers proper restraint techniques. Include instruction on periodic release of the restraints with proper exercise and skin care for the restrained extremities.
Instruct the caregivers on the steps to follow in the event the client removes the nasogastric tube. Identify the circumstances that warrant immediate notification. Provide information on whom to contact and how soon to call.

RELATED TEACHING

Explain the purpose of the procedure and each step before it is performed.
Explain all dietary or fluid intake restrictions.
Tell the client to inform the nurse or record any fluid volume that is consumed. Remind the client to save voided urine for measurement until intake and output calculation is no longer necessary.
Advise the client to indicate if he begins to feel nauseous.

PERFORMANCE CHECKLIST

When removing a nasogastric tube, the learner:

C	A	U	
[ ]	[ ]	[ ]	Confirms the medical order.
[ ]	[ ]	[ ]	Explains the procedure.
[ ]	[ ]	[ ]	Assembles equipment.
[ ]	[ ]	[ ]	Adjusts the height of the bed.
[ ]	[ ]	[ ]	Helps the client to a sitting position.
[ ]	[ ]	[ ]	Discontinues the suction.
[ ]	[ ]	[ ]	Washes hands.
[ ]	[ ]	[ ]	Frees the tubing from the client's face and gown.
[ ]	[ ]	[ ]	Dons a clean glove.
[ ]	[ ]	[ ]	Protects the client's chest with a towel or pad.
[ ]	[ ]	[ ]	Provides the client with tissues.
[ ]	[ ]	[ ]	Indicates when the client should hold his breath.
[ ]	[ ]	[ ]	Pinches the tube.
[ ]	[ ]	[ ]	Withdraws the tube.
[ ]	[ ]	[ ]	Disposes of the tube, glove, and disposable pad out of the view of the client.
[ ]	[ ]	[ ]	Washes hands.
[ ]	[ ]	[ ]	Provides mouth and nose care.
[ ]	[ ]	[ ]	Lowers the bed.
[ ]	[ ]	[ ]	Removes the suction machine or collector from the wall unit.
[ ]	[ ]	[ ]	Measures the volume before disposal.
[ ]	[ ]	[ ]	Removes and cleans reusable equipment.
[ ]	[ ]	[ ]	Washes hands.
[ ]	[ ]	[ ]	Charts significant information.

Outcome: [ ] Pass [ ] Fail

C = competent; A = acceptable; U = unsatisfactory

Comments: _____

_____

_____

_____ _____
Student's Signature Date

_____ _____
Instructor's Signature Date

IV-7 *Administering a cleansing enema*

An enema is the introduction of a solution into the large intestine. The instilled solution distends the lower bowel, may irritate intestinal mucosa, and thus increases peristalsis.

PURPOSES OF PROCEDURE

A cleansing enema is administered to:

1. Relieve constipation or fecal impaction.
2. Prevent involuntary escape of fecal material during surgical procedures.
3. Promote visualization of the lower intestinal tract when an x-ray or endoscopic examination is performed.
4. Help establish normal bowel function during a bowel retraining program.
5. Remove the contrast media used following upper or lower gastrointestinal x-rays.

ASSESSMENT

OBJECTIVE DATA

- Review the medical order for the type of solution to use.
- Consult agency policy on the recommended volume for administering the prescribed enema.
- Identify the client's bowel elimination pattern, such as regularity, numbers of stools per day, color, consistency, and effort required to expel stool.
- Auscultate bowel sounds in all four quadrants of the abdomen listening for their presence and activity.
- Percuss the abdomen in a systematic clockwise manner; note any changes in resonance.
- Palpate each quadrant, feeling for enlargement while observing the client's effort at muscular resistance or an indication of tenderness.
- Inspect the anus and perineum for excoriation, trauma, or masses.
- Insert a gloved finger and palpate for the presence and characteristics of stool and internal areas of the rectum.

SUBJECTIVE DATA

- Request that the client describe his dietary habits, such as the types of food and the volume of fluids normally consumed.
- Ask the client to indicate his use of laxatives and other bowel aids.
- Explore the client's level of exercise or other risk factors, such as the use of drugs that slow peristalsis.

RELEVANT NURSING DIAGNOSES

The client who requires a cleansing enema is likely to have nursing diagnoses, such as:

- *Altered Bowel Elimination: Constipation*
- *Altered Comfort*
- *Altered Health Maintenance*
- *Knowledge Deficit*
- *Self-Care Deficit: Toileting*

PLANNING

ESTABLISHING PRIORITIES

Bowel elimination is a basic human need. Measures to promote the passage of feces require primary attention when the client's bowel regularity is threatened or when the client is at risk for developing problems with bowel elimination. Despite the client's normal bowel function, certain diagnostic tests and surgical procedures require bowel cleansing before they can be performed.

SETTING GOALS

- The contents of the lower bowel will be expelled.
- The client will have a soft, formed bowel movement naturally every 1 to 3 days without discomfort.
- The client will identify measures that promote bowel elimination.

PREPARATION OF EQUIPMENT

The nurse will need items from the following list when administering a cleansing enema:

Disposable enema set
Water-soluble lubricant
Solution as ordered by the physician
  Temperature:
  For adult = 105°F to 110°F (40°C to 43°C)
  For children = 100°F (37.7°C)
  Amount: Varies depending on the type of solution, age of the person, and the client's ability to retain the solution. An average cleansing enema for an adult may range from 750 ml to 1000 ml.
Necessary additives (soap, salt, and so on)
Bath thermometer
Waterproof pad
Bath blanket
Bedpan and toilet tissue
IV pole
Disposable gloves (optional)
Paper towel
Washcloth, soap, towel, or Handiwipes

Technique for administering a cleansing enema

ACTION	RATIONALE
1. Review the written medical order.	Reading the order ensures that the nurse follows the doctor's directives.
2. Assemble the necessary equipment.	Organization promotes efficient time management.
3. Warm the solution, and check the temperature with a bath thermometer. If tap water is used, adjust the temperature as it flows from the faucet.	The nurse is held accountable for any injury, such as burning. If a bath thermometer is not available, warm the solution to room temperature or slightly higher and test on the inner wrist.
4. Explain the procedure, and plan with the client where he will defecate. Have a bedpan, commode, or nearby bathroom ready for his use.	The client is better able to relax and cooperate if he is familiar with the procedure and knows everything is in readiness when he feels the urge to defecate. Defecation usually occurs within 5 to 15 minutes.
5. Wash your hands.	Handwashing deters the spread of microorganisms.
6. Add enema solution to the container. Release the clamp, and allow the fluid to progress through the tube before reclamping.	Releasing the clamp allows air to be expelled from the tubing. Although permitting air to enter the intestine is not harmful, it may further distend the intestine.
7. Place a waterproof pad under the client.	A waterproof pad protects the bed linen from becoming wet.

8. Provide for the client's privacy. Position and drape the client on his left side in Sim's position with the anus exposed as shown in Fig. IV-7-1, or on his back, as dictated by his comfort and condition.

Ensuring the client's privacy and warmth aids in relaxation. The position of the reclining person has not been found to alter the results of the enema significantly.

9. Put on disposable gloves (if desired).

Gloves protect the nurse from contact with microorganisms in the feces.

10. Elevate the solution so it is 45 cm (18 inches) above the level of the client's anus. Plan to give the solution slowly over a period of 5 to 10 minutes.

Gravity forces the solution to enter the rectum. The amount of pressure will determine the rate of flow and pressure exerted on the intestinal wall. Giving the solution too quickly causes rapid distention and pressure in the intestine, resulting in too rapid expulsion of the solution, poor defecation, or damage to the mucous membrane.

11. Generously lubricate the end of the rectal tube for 5 cm to 7 cm (2 inches to 3 inches), as shown in Fig. IV-7-2. A disposable set may have a prelubricated rectal tube.

Lubrication facilitates the insertion of the rectal tube through the anal sphincter and prevents injury to the mucosa.

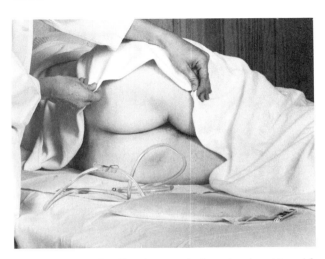

Figure IV-7–1 The client is properly draped and positioned for administering a cleansing enema.

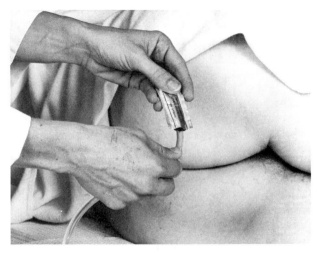

Figure IV-7–2 The nurse lubricates the rectal tube by placing the end of the tube into a single-use package of lubricant. Alternatively, the lubricant can be spread on a paper towel and then spread on the surface of the tip.

12. Lift the client's buttock to expose the anus, as illustrated in Fig. IV-7-3. Slowly and gently insert the rec-

Good visualization of the anus helps prevent injury to tissues. The anal canal is approximately 2.5 cm to 5 cm

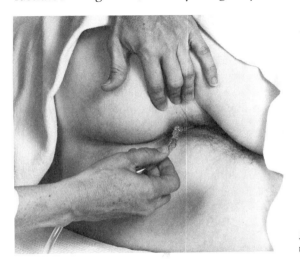

Figure IV-7–3 The nurse has exposed the anus and is about to insert the rectal tube at an angle that points toward the patient's umbilicus.

tal tube 7 cm to 10 cm (3 inches to 4 inches). Direct it at an angle pointing toward the umbilicus, as illustrated in Fig. IV-7-4.

(1 inch to 2 inches) in length. The tube should be inserted past the internal sphincter. Further insertion may damage intestinal mucous membrane. The suggested angle follows the normal intestinal contour. Slow insertion of the tube minimizes spasms of the intestinal wall and sphincters.

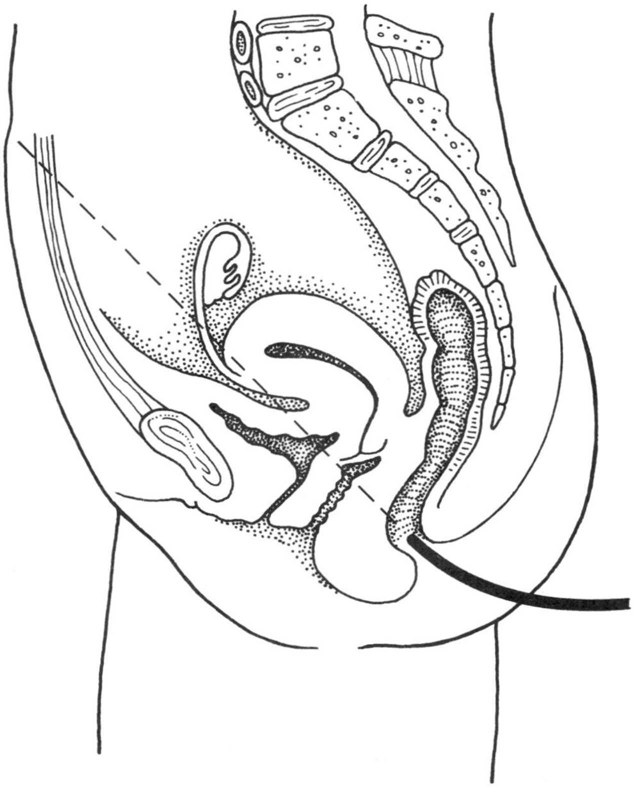

Figure IV-7-4   The tip of the enema tube is shown inserted so that the tip of the tube is directed toward the umbilicus.

13. If the tube meets resistance while you are inserting it, permit a small amount of solution to enter, withdraw the tube slightly, then continue to insert it. Do not force entry of the tube. Ask the client to take several deep breaths.

Resistance may be due to spasms of the intestine or failure of the internal sphincter to open. The solution may help to reduce spasms and relax the sphincter, thus making continued insertion of the tube safe. Forcing a tube may cause injury to the intestinal wall. Taking deep breaths helps relax the anal sphincter.

14. Introduce the solution slowly over a period of 5 to 10 minutes. Hold the tubing all the time that the solution is being instilled, as the nurse in Fig. IV-7-5 is doing. Commercial preparations may be administered by compressing the container with the hands according to package directions, as shown in Fig. IV-7-6.

Introducing the solution slowly helps prevent rapid distention of the intestine and a desire to defecate.

15. Clamp the tubing or lower the container if the client has the desire to defecate or cramping occurs. The client may also be instructed to take small, fast breaths or to pant.

Various techniques can be used to help the client relax muscles and prevent the expulsion of the solution prematurely.

16. After the solution has been given, clamp the tubing and remove the tube. Have a paper towel ready to receive the tube as it is withdrawn. Have the client retain the solution until the urge to defecate becomes strong, usually in about 5 to 15 minutes.

This amount of time usually allows muscular contractions to become sufficient to produce good results.

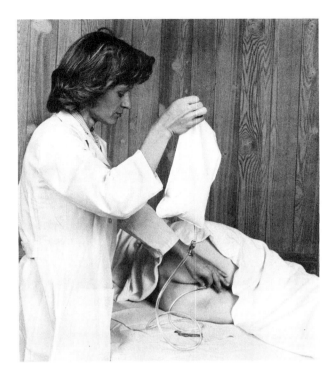

Figure IV-7-5 The nurse holds the enema tube with one hand and holds the bag containing the solution with her other hand approximately 45 cm (18 inches) above the client's anus.

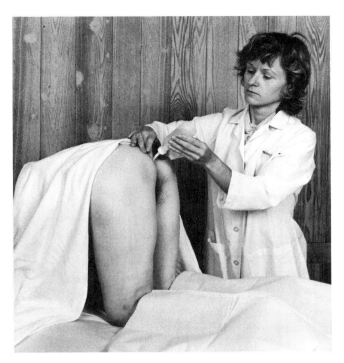

Figure IV-7-6 The nurse is preparing to administer a hypertonic solution enema to the client. The client is in a knee–chest position. Note that the client's body is bent at approximately a 90-degree angle at the hips. The client's arms are resting along side the head.

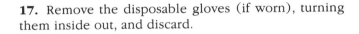

17. Remove the disposable gloves (if worn), turning them inside out, and discard.

The gloves are removed to avoid contact with any microorganisms that may be present on the outside of the gloves.

18. When the client has a strong urge to defecate, place him in a sitting position on a bedpan or assist him to a commode or to the bathroom.

The sitting position is most natural and facilitates the act of defecation.

19. Record the character of the stool and the client's reaction to the enema. Remind the client not to flush the commode before the nurse inspects the results of the enema.

The nurse needs to evaluate and record the client's response to treatment and record the results. Additional enemas may be necessary if the physician has ordered enemas "until clear."

20. Assist the client if necessary with cleansing the anal area. Offer a wash cloth, soap, and water to wash his hands.

Cleansing deters the spread of microorganisms.

21. Leave the client clean and comfortable. Care for the equipment properly.

There is abundant growth of bacteria in the intestine, which can be spread to others when equipment is not properly cared for.

22. Wash your hands.

Handwashing deters the spread of microorganisms.

23. Record the procedure and the results of the enema.

A written summary documents the care provided and the client's response.

SAMPLE DOCUMENTATION

Date	Time	Nurse's note
1/13	2000	1000 mL soap suds enema given. Mod. amt. of hard brown formed stool expelled. Expresses relief at having passed feces.

C. Colberg, RN

EVALUATION
REASSESSMENT

A record of the client's bowel elimination should be kept current. The characteristics of the stool should be assessed if there is some actual or potential alteration. During daily assisted hygiene, the nurse has an ongoing opportunity for inspecting the condition of the anus and perineum. A cleansing enema should only be a temporary measure. The nurse should revise the plan to include measures to restore natural bowel elimination.

EXPECTED OUTCOMES

The client holds and briefly retains the fluid volume that is instilled within the rectum.
The enema solution is expelled along with the formed feces in the lower bowel.
The client's abdomen becomes soft.
The client feels relief having expelled stool and flatus.

UNEXPECTED OUTCOMES

The client is unable to retain the enema solution.
The enema solution is retained but not expelled.
The client expels the solution but no stool.
The client becomes fatigued and distressed during the procedure.

MODIFICATIONS IN SELECTED SITUATIONS

GENERAL VARIATIONS

Adjust the volume of the solution according to the client's ability to tolerate the procedure and the size of the client. The amount of enema solution given to an average adult is usually between 750 ml to 1000 ml.
Give the enema in an area that is as close to the bathroom as possible. If using a bedpan or commode, have them readily accessible.
If the client is incontinent or has difficulty retaining the enema solution, the enema tip may be inserted through a baby bottle nipple with the tip cut off. This substitutes as a sphincter and helps to prevent backward leakage.
Reinsert the enema tubing if there has not been any return of the solution within 1 hour. Assist the client onto his right side and position the solution container lower than his body to promote siphoning the solution from the rectum.
A small volume enema, usually 100 ml to 200 ml of an oil-based mixture designed to be retained totally or temporarily for approximately 30 minutes, may be given to lubricate a mass of feces or its passage. This type of enema should be administered slowly with a smaller gauge tube (between #14 and #20 French) to avoid stimulating peristalsis and an immediate desire to defecate.
Administer an oil retention enema solution at room temperature to minimize the muscular stimulation caused by a warmer or cooler solution.
A premixed disposable enema solution container can be warmed by placing it within a basin or sink and adding warm water around it.

AGE-RELATED VARIATIONS

The volume of an enema can be adjusted according to the body weight of a pediatric client. One recommendation is to prepare 10 ml to 15 ml per kg (2.2 lb) of body weight.
Insert the enema tip only 2 inches to 3 inches when the client is young.
Pad the bed well because an infant or toddler will probably expel the enema solution during the procedure.
Pediatric disposable enemas come already prepared in a reduced volume and shortened insertion tip.

HOME-HEALTH
VARIATIONS

Disposable enemas can be purchased in volumes appropriate for adults or children.

Enema administration equipment can be purchased from drug stores or medical suppliers.

Pad the bed with a large, plastic bag to prevent soiling the linen or mattress during the administration of an enema.

Enema equipment may be reused by the same client if cleansed and stored properly.

If the client can expel the enema solution in the toilet, check with other members of the household to assure that the bathroom will be available. To minimize the time involved in getting to the bathroom, assist the client to put on his slippers and robe before administering the enema.

RELATED TEACHING

Recommend that the client respond to the urge to defecate.

Delaying or ignoring the stimulus causes water to be absorbed from retained feces causing it to become dry, hard, and painful to pass.

Instruct the client on measures that promote natural bowel elimination. Dietary bulk, such as that found in fresh fruits, fresh vegetables, and whole grain breads or cereals, contribute volume to the stool and movement through the intestinal tract. The nurse can also suggest taking hot water or prune juice upon awakening to stimulate mass peristalsis and an urge to defecate.

Advise a constipated client to practice regular daily exercise, such as a brisk walk. A lack of activity can cause poor abdominal muscle tone, anorexia, and sluggish peristalsis which can all contribute to irregular or infrequent bowel movements.

Teach the client to minimize the use of over-the-counter cathartic drugs which may lead to laxative dependence. Refer the client to the physician if other prescribed medication, such as an antacid containing aluminum or narcotic analgesics, could be causing constipation.

Advise a client against overuse of mineral oil as a stool softener. This substance is a petroleum product and interferes with the absorption of fat-soluble vitamins.

PERFORMANCE CHECKLIST

When administering a cleansing enema, the learner:

C	A	U	
[ ]	[ ]	[ ]	Reads the medical order.
[ ]	[ ]	[ ]	Obtains equipment.
[ ]	[ ]	[ ]	Prepares and warms the solution.
[ ]	[ ]	[ ]	Explains the procedure to the client.
[ ]	[ ]	[ ]	Collaborates with the client to determine the location for expelling the enema solution.
[ ]	[ ]	[ ]	Washes hands.
[ ]	[ ]	[ ]	Provides privacy.
[ ]	[ ]	[ ]	Positions the client.
[ ]	[ ]	[ ]	Drapes the client.
[ ]	[ ]	[ ]	Protects the bed linen.
[ ]	[ ]	[ ]	Displaces air from the tubing.
[ ]	[ ]	[ ]	Dons a clean glove.
[ ]	[ ]	[ ]	Lubricates the tip of the tube.
[ ]	[ ]	[ ]	Inserts the tube 3 inches to 4 inches and holds it in place.

C = competent; A = acceptable; U = unsatisfactory

(Continued)

PERFORMANCE CHECKLIST (Continued)

C	A	U	
[ ]	[ ]	[ ]	Releases the clamp.
[ ]	[ ]	[ ]	Infuses the solution slowly by elevating the container 18 inches above the anus.
[ ]	[ ]	[ ]	Slows or stops the infusion if the client experiences cramping or a need to expel the solution.
[ ]	[ ]	[ ]	Resumes instillation once discomfort passes.
[ ]	[ ]	[ ]	Clamps the tubing when an adequate volume of the solution has been administered.
[ ]	[ ]	[ ]	Withdraws the tubing.
[ ]	[ ]	[ ]	Wipes solution and lubricant from the anal area.
[ ]	[ ]	[ ]	Removes the glove, turning it inside out.
[ ]	[ ]	[ ]	Instructs the client to retain the solution 5 to 15 minutes.
[ ]	[ ]	[ ]	Provides the client with a signal device.
[ ]	[ ]	[ ]	Discards disposable equipment.
[ ]	[ ]	[ ]	Cleans and replaces reusable equipment.
[ ]	[ ]	[ ]	Responds to the client's signal for assistance.
[ ]	[ ]	[ ]	Assists the client onto a bedpan, commode, or to the bathroom.
[ ]	[ ]	[ ]	Requests that the client not flush away any expelled stool, if the toilet is used for defecation.
[ ]	[ ]	[ ]	Identifies the location of the alarm signal in the bathroom.
[ ]	[ ]	[ ]	Removes the bedpan, if used.
[ ]	[ ]	[ ]	Helps clean the anus, if assistance is needed.
[ ]	[ ]	[ ]	Removes the absorbent, disposable pad or soiled towel.
[ ]	[ ]	[ ]	Empties or flushes the expelled material after assessing the characteristics of the stool.
[ ]	[ ]	[ ]	Provides the client with the opportunity to wash his hands.
[ ]	[ ]	[ ]	Washes hands.
[ ]	[ ]	[ ]	Charts significant information.

Outcome: [ ] Pass   [ ] Fail

Comments: _____

_____

_____

_____   _____
Student's Signature   Date

_____   _____
Instructor's Signature   Date

RELATED LITERATURE

**PROCEDURE IV-1
ADMINISTERING ORAL
MEDICATIONS**

Caserta JE: It's a jumble—no, it's a maze—no, it's your client's medication shelf . . . medication management in the home. Home Healthcare Nurse 5(1):1, January–February 1987

Cerrato PL: When food and drugs collide. RN Magazine 50(4):85–86, April 1987

Match your meals and medicines. Changing Times 40(11):68–70, 72, November 1986

Osis M: Scheduling drug administration: drug and food interactions. Gerontion 1(5):8–10, November–December 1986

Stillwell S: Ensuring safe, effective drug therapy. Nursing Life 6(6):33–40, November–December 1986

**PROCEDURE IV-2
INSERTING A
NASOGASTRIC TUBE**

Eastwood GL: Upper GI bleeding: differential diagnosis and management, *part 2*. Hospital Medicine 23(3):44, 49–50, 52+, March 1987

Feickert DM: Gastric surgery: your crucial pre- and postop role. RN Magazine 50(1):24–35, January 1987

Ricci JA: Alcohol-induced upper GI hemorrhage: case studies and management. Critical Care Nurse 7(1):56, 58–65, January–February 1987

Roberts A: Senior systems: the stomach and duodenum, *part 8*. Nursing Times 82(47):43–46, November 19–25, 1986

**PROCEDURE IV-3
FEEDING BY GASTRIC
GAVAGE**

Hendler RS, Miranda S: Home nutritional therapy. Nutritional Support Services 7(5):24–25, May 1987

Holmes S: Artificial feeding. Nursing Times 83(31):49, 51, 53–54+, August 5–11, 1987

Horbal-Shuster M, Irwin M: Keeping enteral nutrition on track. American Journal of Nursing 87(4):523–524, April 1987

Krachenfels MM: Home tube feedings: gastrointestinal complications, *part 1*. Home Healthcare Nurse 5(1):41–42, January–February 1987

Krachenfels MM: Update on tube feeding formulas. Home Healthcare Nurse 5(3):47–50, May–June 1987

Moore MC: Do you still believe these myths about tube feeding? RN Magazine 50(5):51–54, May 1987

Weibley TT, Adamson M, Clinkscales N: Gavage tube insertion in the premature infant. American Journal of Maternal Child Nursing 12(1):24–27, January–February 1987

**PROCEDURE IV-4
MONITORING A
NASOGASTRIC TUBE**

Feickert DM: Gastric surgery: your crucial pre- and postop role. RN Magazine 50(1):24–35, January 1987

Flynn KT, Norton LC, Fisher RL: Enteral tube feeding: indications, practices and outcomes. Image: Journal of Nursing Scholarship 19(1):16–19, Spring 1987

Mangieri D: Looking at the tube and we don't mean TV. Nursing 83 13(4):47–49, April 1983

Swift DE: Respiratory complications of nasogastric tubes. The Canadian Journal of Respiratory Therapy 23(3):15–16, July 1987

**PROCEDURE IV-5
IRRIGATING A
NASOGASTRIC TUBE**

Moore MC: Do you still believe these myths about tube feeding? RN Magazine 50(5):51–52, 54, May 1987

Crocker KS, Krey SH, Markovic M: Microbial growth in clinically used enteral delivery systems. American Journal of Infection Control 14(6):250–256, December 1986

**PROCEDURE IV-6
REMOVING A
NASOGASTRIC TUBE**

Creighton H: Legal implications of removal of feeding tubes. Nursing Management 18(3):20, 22, 24, March 1987

Kolpan K: Removing feeding tubes from patients in persistent vegetative state. Journal of Head Trauma Rehabilitation 1(1):83–84, March 1986

**PROCEDURE IV-7
ADMINISTERING A
CLEANSING ENEMA**

Hahn K: Think twice about diarrhea. Nursing 87 17(9):78–80, September 1987

Roberts A: Senior systems: diverticular disease: carcinoma of the colon and rectum, *part 13.* Nursing Times 83(16):53–56, April 22–28, 1987

Roberts A: Senior systems: rectal bleeding, *part 12.* Nursing Times 83(11):47–50, March 18–24, 1987

Sondheimer JM: Resolving chronic constipation in children. Patient Care 21(5):108–112, 114, 116–118, March 15, 1987

Turner J: Some fundamentals of flexible sigmoidoscopy. Emergency Medicine 19(6):79–81, 85–86, 88–89, March 30, 1987

Understanding chronic constipation in your child. Patient Care 21(5):126–127, March 15, 1987

V Procedures pertaining to the cardiovascular system

V-1 — *Applying elastic stockings*

Blood that reaches the veins is not propelled forward by the pulsations from the left ventricle. The alternate contraction and relaxation of skeletal muscles helps to move blood through veins toward the heart. Valves within the veins prevent the blood that has moved forward from slipping back toward the feet under the influence of gravity. When circulation slows, clots are more likely to form. Therefore, elastic stockings are often used for clients who are at risk for developing blood clots, such as those with limited activity or incompetent valves in peripheral veins.

Most elastic stockings are worn from the foot to the knee. Some are available in lengths that extend to the thigh or waist. They are intended for continuous wear but should be removed and reapplied once each shift following hygiene and assessment. A second pair is needed as an alternate when one pair requires laundering.

PURPOSES OF PROCEDURE

Elastic stockings are applied to:

1. Promote the circulation of venous blood from the legs back to the heart.
2. Support valves within peripheral leg veins so that blood is less likely to pool when in a dependent position.
3. Prevent thrombus formation or subsequent embolus.
4. Relieve symptoms such as aching and heaviness in the lower legs.

ASSESSMENT

OBJECTIVE DATA

- Review the client's record to identify conditions that increase the potential for poor circulation or clot formation, such as immobility, vascular disorders, dehydration, or conditions that increase abdominal pressure, like pregnancy or ascites.
- Examine the lower extremities for signs of poor circulation, such as dependent edema, cyanotic feet, thick toenails, feet that feel cool, shiny or taut skin, ulcerated areas that are slow to heal, and tortuous and distended leg veins.
- Identify if the client's occupation or avocations require prolonged standing or sitting thus increasing the potential for blood pooling in the lower areas of the legs.
- Measure the length of the client's leg from the heel to the popliteal space for knee-high stockings or to the gluteal fold for thigh-high stockings; measure the circumference of the calf, and the thigh for longer stockings, at the widest point.

SUBJECTIVE DATA

- Inquire about the client's past history in developing blood clots.
- Ask the client to describe sensations that are experienced in the legs after extended periods of standing or sitting.

RELEVANT NURSING DIAGNOSES

The client who benefits from wearing elastic stockings may have nursing diagnoses, such as:

- *Impaired Physical Mobility*
- *Altered Tissue Perfusion*
- *Altered Comfort*
- *Potential Impaired Skin Integrity*

PLANNING

ESTABLISHING PRIORITIES

Elastic stockings should be applied or changed before a client stands or sits up in the morning. This ensures that blood will not become trapped in the lowest areas of the body as a result of gravity. If the client is sitting or has been up and about, have the client lie down with his feet and legs well elevated for at least 15 minutes before reapplying the stockings. The nurse should avoid massaging the legs if the client manifests signs that a clot has formed, such as pain on dorsiflexion of the foot, referred to as a positive Homan's sign, or a warm, swollen, tender area in the calf. Massage can transform a thrombus to an embolus which is life-threatening.

SETTING GOALS

- The client's venous circulation will be promoted throughout the period of limited or restricted mobility.
- Homan's sign will remain negative.

PREPARATION OF EQUIPMENT

When applying elastic stockings, the nurse will need selected items from the following list:

Measuring tape
Elastic stockings (in correct size)
Talcum powder (optional)
Lotion (optional)

Technique for applying elastic stockings

ACTION	RATIONALE
1. Explain the rationale for the use of elastic stockings to the client.	An explanation relieves apprehension and promotes cooperation.
2. Wash your hands.	Handwashing deters the spread of microorganisms.
3. Assist the client to a supine position.	A dependent position of the legs encourages blood to pool in the veins.
4. Provide privacy. Expose one leg at a time. Powder the legs lightly unless the client has dry skin. If the skin is dry, lotion may be used.	Powder and lotion reduce friction and make application of stockings easier.
5. Fold stocking inside out down to the heel.	Exposing the outside of the stocking facilitates easier application.
6. Ease the foot of the stocking over the client's toes, foot, and heel, as shown in Fig. V-1-1. Check that the stocking is straight and smooth, as the nurse in Fig. V-1-2 is doing.	Wrinkles or improper fit interfere with circulation.

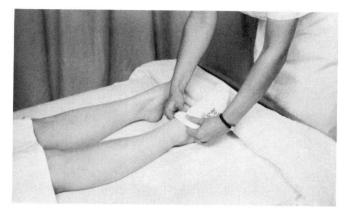

Figure V-1-1 The nurse eases the inverted stocking over the toes and foot.

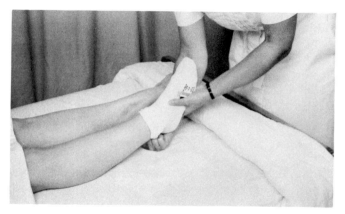

Figure V-1-2 The nurse lifts the leg slightly to continue easing the elastic stocking over the heel.

7. Using fingers and thumbs, grasp the gathered stocking, and ease it gradually to its full length, as shown in Fig. V-1-3. Check that the stocking is straight and smooth. Readjust as necessary. Repeat for the other leg. Caution the client not to roll the stockings partially down.

Easing the stocking carefully into position ensures proper fit of the stocking to the contour of the leg. Rolling stockings may have a constricting effect on the veins.

8. Wash your hands.

Handwashing deters the spread of microorganisms.

9. To remove the stockings: Grasp the top of the stocking with the thumb and fingers and gradually pull the stocking off inside out to the heel, as illustrated in Fig. V-1-4. Support the foot and ease the stocking over it.

Preventing uneven stretching preserves the uniform elasticity and contour of the stocking.

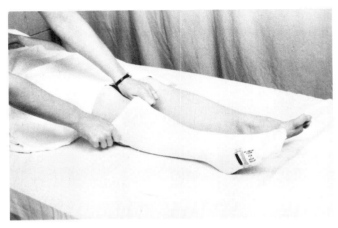

Figure V-1-3   The nurse gradually pulls the stocking up the length of the leg so that no wrinkles form.

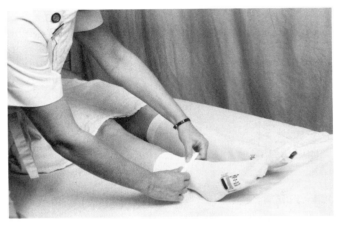

Figure V-1-4   The stockings are being pulled off inside out to prevent bulky pressure from great folds of fabric which could temporarily interfere with circulation.

10. Remove the stockings once every shift for 20 to 30 minutes. Wash and air dry the stockings as necessary (according to the manufacturer's directions).

Removing the stockings for short periodic intervals allows observation of the circulatory status and condition of the skin on the lower extremities.

11. Record the application of elastic stockings as well as the assessment of the circulatory status and skin condition.

A written summary provides accurate documentation of the procedure and the client's response.

SAMPLE DOCUMENTATION

Date	Time	Nurse's note
4/20	0630	Measured for elastic stockings. Calf: $15\frac{1}{2}$″, leg length from heel to back of knee: 14″. Large adult size stockings applied. Toes are warm and pink. *E. Hedges, RN*

EVALUATION

REASSESSMENT

Elastic stockings are made so as to provide access to the toes for periodic assessment of color, temperature, swelling, and mobility. The nurse should inspect that the stockings are uniformly smooth and that the stocking has not rolled on itself forming a tight band. The nurse can inspect the condition of the skin and palpate the quality of peripheral pulses in the leg when they are removed briefly each shift. If Homan's sign remains negative, it is a good indication that the measures used to prevent thrombus formation are effective. Any elevation of temperature should alert the nurse for a possible inflammatory process, such as a thrombophlebitis.

EXPECTED OUTCOMES

The stockings remain in place and wrinkle free.
The client's toes are warm with normal size, color, and mobility.
The client's skin remains intact.
The client does not experience calf pain or tenderness.

UNEXPECTED OUTCOMES

The stockings fit loosely or tightly.
The toes become dusky, swollen, and cold.
Areas of the skin become red or impaired.
The client demonstrates a positive Homan's sign.

MODIFICATIONS IN SELECTED SITUATIONS

GENERAL VARIATIONS

Use elastic roller bandages to wrap extremities of those clients whose measurements are not compatible with manufactured standard sizes. Reassessments should be frequent because roller bandages may loosen or wrinkle more easily over a period of time especially if the client moves about.

Elastic garments, such as waist-high stockings, can be custom made for persons with long-term vascular problems.

Stockings are available with an air chamber which cycles alternately between inflation and deflation. This device simulates the promotion of venous circulation through muscle contraction and relaxation.

HOME-HEALTH VARIATIONS

If the application of elastic stockings is a nursing order or a comfort measure, support pantyhose may be used.

RELATED TEACHING

The client should understand the reason for applying elastic stockings before the legs are in a dependent position or why the legs should be elevated for 15 minutes.

Clients should be instructed on how to measure for elastic stockings, especially if responsible for purchasing replacement pairs.

Teach the client to do isometric and isotonic leg exercises as another prophylactic measure for preventing thrombus formation.

Explain that an adequate fluid intake helps to promote the free movement of blood cells and prevents their congestion in the vascular system.

Advise the client to avoid sitting, standing, or crossing the knees for long periods of time. Recommend that on long trips or during sedentary work that the person take frequent breaks that involve moving and walking.

Discourage the client from wearing tight clothing, such as girdles or belts, which can restrict the movement of venous blood back to the heart.

If the client is taking an anticoagulant, teach the client to observe for skin bruises or other evidence of bleeding, such as from the gums, in emesis, urine, sputum, or stool.

Instruct the client to avoid activity and massaging the legs if pain, tenderness, or local warmth is noted in either leg. Inform the client that the nurse and doctor should be told about these symptoms immediately.

PERFORMANCE CHECKLIST

When applying elastic stockings, the learner:

C	A	U	
[ ]	[ ]	[ ]	Assesses the client's peripheral vascular status and his potential for forming blood clots.
[ ]	[ ]	[ ]	Checks the physician's written order or the agency's protocols for caring for client's with restricted activity.
[ ]	[ ]	[ ]	Explains the purpose for using elastic stockings and the directions for their use.
[ ]	[ ]	[ ]	Washes hands.
[ ]	[ ]	[ ]	Provides privacy.
[ ]	[ ]	[ ]	Takes appropriate measurements.
[ ]	[ ]	[ ]	Maintains the client on bed rest or elevates the legs for at least 15 minutes before applying the stockings.
[ ]	[ ]	[ ]	Inspects the integrity of the skin; applies corn starch, talcum powder, or lotion depending on the condition of the client's skin.
[ ]	[ ]	[ ]	Turns the stockings inside out.
[ ]	[ ]	[ ]	Inserts the client's toes.
[ ]	[ ]	[ ]	Pulls the stocking gradually over the foot and the length of the leg.
[ ]	[ ]	[ ]	Smooths any wrinkles that form.
[ ]	[ ]	[ ]	Palpates the popliteal pulse when knee-high stockings have been applied or the femoral pulse when thigh-high stockings are in place.
[ ]	[ ]	[ ]	Washes hands.
[ ]	[ ]	[ ]	Charts significant information.
[ ]	[ ]	[ ]	Returns within an hour to reassess the neurovascular status of the client's feet and toes.

Outcome: [   ] Pass   [   ] Fail

C = competent; A = acceptable; U = unsatisfactory

Comments: _____
_____
_____

_____   _____
Student's Signature   Date

_____   _____
Instructor's Signature   Date

V-2 *Administering cardiopulmonary resuscitation*

Cardiopulmonary resuscitation (CPR) is the combination of mouth-to-mouth breathing, which supplies oxygen to the lungs, and chest compressions, which circulates blood. This type of life-saving measure is best performed by two rescuers, but one rescuer can perform both activities successfully. The resuscitative methods for each situation are covered in this procedure.

PURPOSES OF PROCEDURE

Cardiopulmonary resuscitation is performed to:

1. Restore breathing.
2. Restore circulation.
3. Maintain perfusion of oxygenated blood to cells.
4. Prevent biological death until advanced cardiac life-support measures can be attempted.

ASSESSMENT

- Identify clients who are at risk for sudden pulmonary or cardiac arrest, such as a client with a recent heart attack, high serum potassium level, a thrombus, unstable pulmonary disease, central nervous system diseases that may affect the muscles for breathing, infants with apneic episodes, and so on.
- Observe the client's color; note pallor or cyanosis.
- Assess the client's level of consciousness when stimulating the client by shaking and shouting.
- Watch for signs that the chest rises and falls.
- Position your face and ear above the client's nose and mouth to detect breathing.
- Open the mouth and inspect for objects or accumulated secretions or food particles.
- Palpate for the carotid pulse.

RELEVANT NURSING DIAGNOSES

The client who receives CPR may have one or all of the following nursing diagnoses:

- *Ineffective Airway Clearance*
- *Impaired Gas Exchange*
- *Actual or Potential Altered Cardiac Output*

PLANNING

ESTABLISHING PRIORITIES

Resuscitation should be started immediately whenever breathing, or breathing and heart beat are absent. The brain is very sensitive to hypoxia and will sustain irreversible damage after 4 to 6 minutes of no oxygen. The faster CPR is initiated, the greater the chance of revival with little or no deficits.

SETTING GOALS

- Adequate pulmonary and circulatory functions will be initiated immediately upon finding the victim.
- The per minute ventilations and compressions will be appropriate for the client's age.
- Resuscitation efforts will continue until the client responds, advanced life support is instituted, or the rescuer(s) become exhausted.

PREPARATION OF EQUIPMENT

The following optional items may be used when administering cardiopulmonary resuscitation:

Back board
AMBU bag and mask
Mouth protector

Technique for administering cardiopulmonary resuscitation

ACTION	RATIONALE

ONE RESCUER

1. Assess the victim's unresponsiveness. Gently shake his shoulder and ask, "Are you okay?" Call for help.

Shaking and shouting may arouse a person and this will indicate that CPR measures are not needed.

2. Position the victim flat on his back on a firm surface. Support the head and neck and turn the person as a unit.

A firm surface provides for maximum compression and proper positioning.

3. Tilt the head backwards by placing a hand on the forehead. Place the fingers of the other hand underneath the jaw and lift it upward and forward, as shown in Fig. V-2-1.

This head-tilt maneuver opens the airway in most persons.

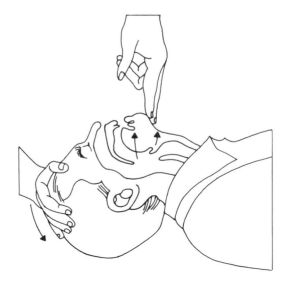

Figure V-2-1 The head tilt opens the victim's airway in most cases.

4. Determine breathlessness by placing an ear over the victim's mouth and observing the chest.

Expired air can be heard and felt on the cheek as well as observed as the chest rises and falls in a breathing victim.

5. Remove dentures if they are loose; if snug, leave them in place.

Loose dentures may block the airway. If they are snug, they help seal the mouth.

6. Keeping the head tilted backwards, pinch the victim's nose shut with a thumb and fingers of the hand that is on the forehead. Seal your lips tightly around the victim's mouth. Ventilate two times at 1 to 1.5 seconds per breath. Observe the chest rise, and lift your face away from the victim between breaths.

Pinching the nose shut allows maximum ventilation with no escape of air through the nostrils. The force of breathing needs to be sufficient so that the chest visibly rises when air is forced into the victim's mouth and falls with the victim's passive exhalation.

7. Determine pulselessness by feeling for the carotid pulse on the near side of the victim for 5 to 10 seconds

The carotid artery is large, centrally located, and ordinarily readily accessible. A 5- to 10-second pause is

while maintaining the head tilt with the other hand, as shown in Fig. V-2-2. Send anyone who responds to the call for help to activate the Emergency Medical System (EMS).

8. Begin chest compressions if the pulse is absent.

   a. Kneel by the victim's shoulders.

   b. Locate the xiphoid process on the sternum by following the lower rib to the notch on the sternum where the rib meets. Measure 4 cm to 5 cm (1½ inches to 2 inches) above the xiphoid process, about the width of two fingers, as shown in Fig. V-2-3.

needed to adequately assess for pulselessness.

Compressing the chest circulates the blood.

Kneeling facilitates proper positioning.

Proper hand position keeps pressure off the xiphoid process and prevents injury to underlying organs and ribs.

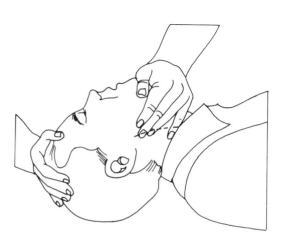

Figure V-2-2 The carotid pulse on the side of the neck is compressed to assess for a heart beat. As long as the heart is beating, only pulmonary resuscitation needs to be continued.

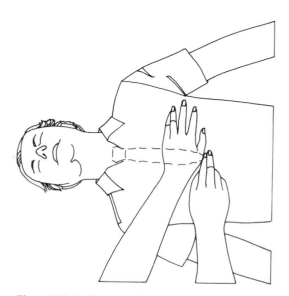

Figure V-2-3 The nurse identifies anatomical landmarks and locates hands in the optimum location for administering cardiac compressions.

   c. Place the heel of one hand on this point and position the heel of the other hand on top of the first hand. Preferably, the fingers should interlock. Bring the shoulders over the hands and keep the elbows locked and the arms straight, as shown in Fig. V-2-4.

   d. Use the body weight to depress the victim's sternum about 4 cm to 5 cm (1½ inches to 2 inches). Relax the pressure immediately, but keep your hands on the sternum during the up stroke.

   e. Compress at the rate of 80 to 100/min or 15 per 9 to 11 seconds.

9. Perform four cycles of 15 compressions and 2 ventilations. Observe the chest rise on ventilations (1 to 1½ sec/inspiration).

10. Reassess cardiopulmonary status. Feel for a carotid pulse for at least 5 seconds.

Interlocking the fingers helps keep them off the victim's ribs, where pressure may cause fractures of the ribs. This position, with the elbows and arms straight, allows for the best exertion of pressure on the sternum over the heart.

The depression of the sternum with pressure causes the heart to be compressed against the vertebral column forcing blood into the aorta and pulmonary arteries. Relaxation of the pressure allows the heart to expand and refill. Keeping the hands in place over the sternum helps administer regular and even compressions.

This compression rate maintains adequate blood pressure and flow to sustain cell integrity.

This rate and frequency provide for maintenance of adequate blood flow and oxygenation for an adult.

Restoration of the pulse indicates that the rescuer can discontinue the compressions.

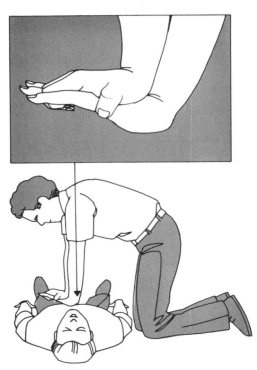

Figure V-2-4   The rescuer has his fingers interlaced, has the heel of his hand on the victim's sternum above the xiphoid process, and has brought his shoulders over his hands. The rescuer is in position to begin external cardiac compressions.

11. If a pulse is absent, continue CPR. Ventilate twice (1 to 1½ sec/inspiration) and then resume compression/ventilation cycles. Feel for the carotid pulse every few minutes.

Continuation of compression/ventilation rate is necessary to sustain life.

Technique for administering cardiopulmonary resuscitation

ACTION	RATIONALE

TWO RESCUERS

1. The rescuer who will ventilate initiates the airway assessments. Continue the sequence for One Rescuer, steps 1 through 6.

Observing for breathlessness is one of the first indications for performing CPR.

2. The first rescuer continues to assess for pulselessness. If none is detected, he states, "No pulse."

By sharing the result of the assessment verbally, the first rescuer indicates clearly to the second to initiate compressions.

3. The rescuer who will be performing compressions gets into position, locates the anatomical landmarks, and begins. The correct ratio of compressions to ventilations is 5:1 with a compression rate of 80 to 100/min. Stop compressing for each ventilation. Continue for a minimum of ten cycles.

The rate of 10 to 15 regularly spaced breaths per minute is considered necessary to supply the victim with sufficient oxygen to sustain cell integrity.

4. Call for a switch with a clear signal, when the person performing compressions becomes fatigued. The compressor completes the fifth compression and the ven-

It is important to carry out CPR without interruption to assure adequate blood flow with oxygenated blood to sustain cell integrity.

tilator completes the ventilation after the fifth compression. Rescuers switch simultaneously. The person who becomes the ventilator does a 5-second pulse check, states, "No pulse" (if pulse is absent), and ventilates once. The person who becomes the compressor then begins compressions at a 5:1 ratio.

SAMPLE DOCUMENTATION

Date	Time	Nurse's note
6/15	0243	Found unconscious. Color ashen. No response to shaking and shouting. No respirations detected. Airway opened with no spontaneous breathing. Two quick breaths given. No pulse noted. Compressions begun at a ratio of 15 to 2 breaths and continued for 5 minutes without any return of a pulse. Code team called and responded.
		H. Fox, RN

EVALUATION

REASSESSMENT

Observe that the chest rises on ventilations to determine if the airway is patent or air may be entering the esophagus and stomach. Palpate for the carotid pulse every few minutes. Note if the client's color improves. The victim is generally given resuscitation until he responds, until advanced life support arrives, or until the rescuer is exhausted. Some persons have been reported to have survived without permanent brain damage even after signs of death were present for as long as an hour or two. This has been found to be the case especially with children involved in cold water drownings and others suffering from hypothermia.

EXPECTED OUTCOMES

CPR is initiated as soon as it is determined that there is no breathing or pulse. The adult client receives approximately 12 breaths per minute.

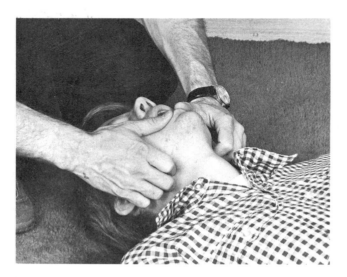

Figure V-2-5 The jaw thrust is an alternate method for opening the airway. The rescuer's fingers are placed behind the victim's jaws, and the jaws are pushed forward with the rescuer's thumbs.

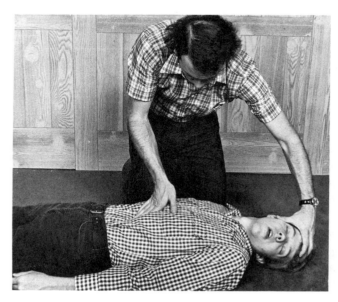

Figure V-2-6 To decompress the stomach when it is distended, the rescuer exerts moderate pressure over the victim's upper abdomen with his fingers. His fingers are between the victim's lower rib margin and the navel. The victim's head is turned to help fluid from the stomach escape from the mouth.

The adult client receives at least 80 compressions per minute.
Breathing and heart beat are restored.

UNEXPECTED OUTCOMES

The client's airway remains obstructed.
The client vomits.
The client does not demonstrate signs of restored breathing or heart beat.
The client's pupils become fixed and dilated for 30 minutes.

MODIFICATIONS IN SELECTED SITUATIONS

GENERAL VARIATIONS

Open the airway using the jaw-thrust technique shown in Fig. V-2-5, as an alternate method if the traditional head-tilt technique is not effective.
Administer CPR through the stoma of a person who has had the larynx removed.
Decompress the stomach, as shown in Fig. V-2-6, if it becomes distended with air.
Use a self-inflating breathing bag and mask, if one is available.
Some persons carry a mouth protector in case a victim requires mouth-to-mouth resuscitation. The protector acts as a barrier against contact with oral secretions which may contain pathogens. Although the HIV viruses causing AIDS are found in all body fluids of infected persons, it has not been proven to spread by other than direct contact with blood or semen.
The nurse may position the client's upper body over a board so that chest compressions may be administered more effectively.

AGE-RELATED VARIATIONS

Table V-2-1 indicates modifications in the administration of CPR when the client is an infant or child.

Table V-2-1
CPR modifications for infants and children*

	Infant to 1 yr	1 to 8 yr
Breaths		
Initial	2 breaths	2 breaths
Subsequent	1 every 3 seconds	1 every 4 seconds
Rate	20/min.	15/min.
Compressions		
Location	In midline, one finger's width below the nipples	Two fingers' width above the tip of the sternum
Hand use	Two fingers, or for neonates, encircle the chest and use both thumbs	Heel of one hand
Rate	At least 100/min	80–100/min.
Depth	$\frac{1}{2}$ inch–1 inch	1 inch–$1\frac{1}{2}$ inch

* Recommendations from the American Heart Association.

Use the brachial artery to check for a pulse on an infant, as shown in Fig. V-2-7. The apical pulse can be felt with the fingers, as the nurse in Fig. V-2-8 is doing, positioned at a point under the nipple line and just to the left of the sternum.

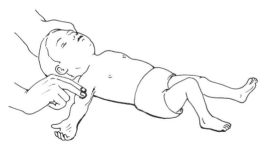

Figure V-2-7 The fingers are shown palpating for a pulse at the site of the brachial artery when administering CPR to an infant.

Tilt the head of an infant or young child backward very gently to open the airway to avoid injury.

If the child is small, cover both the nose and the mouth when administering ventilation. Use puffs of breaths, smaller than those for an adult, but enough to cause the chest to rise.

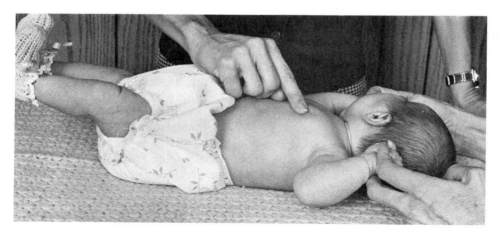

Figure V-2-8 The nurse has placed an index finger under the nipple and to the left of the sternum to feel for the infant's apical pulse.

Use the index and middle fingers, as shown in Fig. V-2-9, or encircle the infant's thorax and exert compressions with thumbs, as shown in Fig. V-2-10, when the victim is an infant.

Follow the same CPR guidelines used on adults when a child is over 8 years of age.

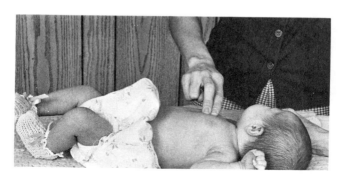

Figure V-2-9 The nurse uses an index and middle finger to deliver cardiac compressions to an infant.

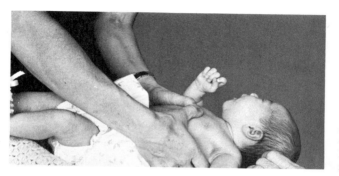

Figure V-2-10 The nurse encircles the infant's thorax with two hands and compresses the infant's midsternum with two thumbs.

HOME-HEALTH
VARIATIONS

Substitute a large tray or table leaf for a backboard.

For high-risk clients, post emergency telephone numbers near all telephones. Frequently review the procedure for administering CPR with caregivers.

Remind caregivers that CPR should be initiated wherever the client is found. Time should not be wasted trying to return the client to his room or bed.

RELATED TEACHING

Recommend and support efforts to teach CPR to lay persons. Community education courses are offered frequently through local hospitals and the American Heart Association or the Red Cross.

Maintain current basic cardiac life support certification for yourself and encourage the same for paraprofessional staff.

Urge all persons to administer CPR quickly and without hesitation when an emergency arises.

Advise persons to post the numbers for emergency assistance near or on the telephone.

Inform a client with a history of cardiac problems if a hot-line number to a cardiac unit of a hospital is available.

PERFORMANCE CHECKLIST

When demonstrating CPR, the learner:

C	A	U	
[ ]	[ ]	[ ]	Makes appropriate assessments.
[ ]	[ ]	[ ]	Places the victim flat on a firm surface.
[ ]	[ ]	[ ]	Opens the airway.
[ ]	[ ]	[ ]	Observes for breathing.
[ ]	[ ]	[ ]	Inspects the mouth for loose material.
[ ]	[ ]	[ ]	Administers two quick breaths.
[ ]	[ ]	[ ]	Checks for a carotid pulse.
[ ]	[ ]	[ ]	Sends someone for help, if possible.
[ ]	[ ]	[ ]	Locates the xiphoid process.
[ ]	[ ]	[ ]	Interlocks hands and places them $1\frac{1}{2}$ inches to 2 inches above the xiphoid process.
[ ]	[ ]	[ ]	Compresses the chest four to five times within 3 to 4 seconds, if assisted, or 15 compressions every 9 to 11 seconds, if alone.
[ ]	[ ]	[ ]	Pauses for second rescuer to administer one breath after each 5 compressions, or gives two ventilations after each 15 compressions.
[ ]	[ ]	[ ]	Continues maintaining appropriate rate and frequency of compressions to respirations in order to equal 80 to 100 compressions and 10 to 15 breaths per minute.
[ ]	[ ]	[ ]	Assesses for a pulse at periodic intervals.

Outcome: [ ] Pass   [ ] Fail

C = competent; A = acceptable; U = unsatisfactory

Comments: _____

_____

_____

_____	_____
Student's Signature	Date

_____	_____
Instructor's Signature	Date

RELATED LITERATURE

**PROCEDURE V-1
APPLYING ELASTIC
STOCKINGS**

Cherry G: Leg ulcers: in support of stockings. Community Outlook 29–31, October 1986

Coon WW, Hirsch J, Rubin LJ: Preventing deep vein thrombosis. Patient Care 21(3):82–86, 89–90, February 15, 1987

McMahan BE: Why deep vein thrombosis is so dangerous. RN Magazine 50(1):20–23, January 1987

Smith K: Preventing postoperative venous thrombosis . . . graduated compression stockings. Nursing Mirror 16:20–30, May 15, 1985

**PROCEDURE V-2
ADMINISTERING
CARDIOPULMONARY
RESUSCITATION**

Andersen E: Home defibrillators for high-risk cardiac patients. Caring 6(2):32–35, February 1987

Birdsall C, Ruggio J: Mouth-to-mouth resuscitation—is there a safe, effective alternative? American Journal of Nursing 87(8):1019, August 1987

Curley MAQ, Vaughn SM: Assessment and resuscitation of the pediatric patient. Critical Care Nurse 7(3):26–27, 30–34, 36, May–June 1987

Dracup K, Breu C: Teaching and retention of cardiopulmonary resuscitation skills for families of high-risk patients with cardiac disease. Focus on Critical Care 14(1):67–72, February 1987

Fracassi J, Moran P: Cardiac arrest: when documentation is critical. Critical Care Nurse 7(3): 90–93, May–June 1987

Hazinski MF: New guidelines for pediatric and neonatal cardiopulmonary resuscitation and advanced life support, *part 2*. Pediatric Nursing 12(6):445–448, November–December 1986

Muscarella SM: Controversies in cardiac resuscitation. Emergency Nursing Reports 1(6):1–8, September 1986

Sanford TM: Where to go from here . . . more people trained in CPR. Emergency 19(1): 35–37, January 1987

Scherer P: ACLS guidelines: what nurses are saying about the drug changes. American Journal of Nursing 86(12):1352–1358, December 1986

Sheehy SB: A quick overview of the new standards and guidelines for cardiopulmonary resuscitation and emergency cardiac care. Journal of Emergency Nursing 13(1):47–49, January–February 1987

VI

Procedures pertaining to the respiratory system

VI-1 *Administering oxygen*

There is approximately 20% oxygen present in atmospheric air. Some clients experience a deficit in the amount they inspire and deliver to cells. The amount of oxygen the client breathes can be increased by providing a supplemental supply at higher percentages than the amount available in ambient air. The amount and method of providing therapeutic oxygen are usually prescribed by the physician. However, the nurse may be called on to administer oxygen independently in emergency situations.

PURPOSES OF PROCEDURE

Oxygen is administered to:

1. Relieve dyspnea.
2. Reduce or prevent hypoxemia and hypoxia.
3. Alleviate the anxiety associated with the struggle to breathe.

ASSESSMENT

OBJECTIVE DATA

- Observe the client's skin color, the color of nailbeds and oral mucous membranes.
- Watch the effort the client uses to breathe; note the desire to sit up rather than recline.
- Observe the contour of the chest and the use of accessory muscles for breathing; note if the chest moves symmetrically with each respiration.
- Count the respiratory rate for a full minute.
- If a cough is present, note if it is productive and examine the characteristics of any raised secretions.
- Inspect the nails, as shown in Fig. VI-1-1, for evidence of changes associated with chronic hypoxia.
- Count the heart rate and note its rhythm. Tachycardia and arrhythmia generally accompany a need for oxygen.

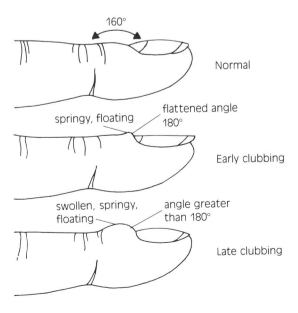

160°

Normal

springy, floating — flattened angle 180°

Early clubbing

swollen, springy, floating — angle greater than 180°

Late clubbing

Figure VI-1-1 Inspecting the nails can yield a great deal of data. Clubbed nails are a sign of long-term oxygen deficits throughout a person's life time.

- Assess blood pressure. Anxiety created by breathlessness can elevate the blood pressure.
- Auscultate breath sounds over the trachea, bronchi, and lungs. Note the movement of air and the location and characteristics of any abnormal sounds, like wheezes, crackles, and gurgles. Determine if any wet sounds clear with voluntary or spontaneous coughing.
- Review the results of chest x-ray, red blood cell and hemoglobin levels, arterial blood gases, and pulmonary function tests, if available.
- Assess the client's level of consciousness, evidence of confusion or disorientation, and restlessness.
- Read the physician's order for the amount, method for providing oxygen, and the duration for its administration.

SUBJECTIVE DATA

- Ask the client, or another who has accompanied the client, to identify past illnesses, allergies, and the smoking history.
- Ask the client to confirm or deny if he is experiencing any chest pain, peripheral tingling, dizziness, or sleeplessness.

RELEVANT NURSING DIAGNOSES

Multiple nursing diagnoses are associated with altered respiratory functioning. The following list indicates a representative list of conditions that may be improved by administering oxygen:

- *Ineffective Breathing Patterns*
- *Impaired Gas Exchange*
- *Activity Intolerance*
- *Anxiety*
- *Altered Comfort*

PLANNING

ESTABLISHING PRIORITIES

Breathing is a basic need. Therefore, maintaining or restoring optimum exchange of oxygen and carbon dioxide represents an immediate nursing priority. When the nurse uses judgment to initiate oxygen administration independently, several factors must be considered. First, oxygen must be humidified to avoid the drying effects to the mucous membranes. Secondly, the rate will vary depending on the condition of the client and the route for its administration. Table VI-1-1 shows the oxygen percentages that can be achieved by various methods at a respective liter flow. The nurse should exercise caution when providing oxygen to clients with chronic lung conditions, such as emphysema. Most can safely tolerate 2 liters of oxygen by nasal cannula. Higher amounts should only be administered after consulting with a physician. Thirdly, the nurse must eliminate any safety hazards that could contribute to fire or explosion when oxygen is used.

Table VI-1-1
Conversion equivalents for oxygen therapy

Method of delivery	Liters/min.	Equivalent percentage
Nasal cannula	2	28%
	4	36%
	6	44%
Simple mask	5	40%
	6–7	50%
	7–8	60%
Mask with reservoir bag	6	60%
	7	70%
	8	80%
	9	90%
	10	95%

SETTING GOALS

- The client's respiratory rate will return to the normal range for his age.
- The client's color and comfort will improve.
- The client's blood *p*H will be restored to 7.35 to 7.45 or show evidence of compensation.

PREPARATION OF EQUIPMENT

The nurse will need selected items from the following list when administering oxygen:

Flowmeter connected to oxygen supply
Humidifier with sterile distilled water
Equipment for administering oxygen (*i.e.,* nasal cannula, mask, tent, and so on)
Gauze to pad potential areas of pressure (optional)
Oxygen analyzer, if humidity tent is used
Ice, if humidity tent is used
Bath blankets and extra gowns when humidity tent is used

Technique for administering oxygen

ACTION	RATIONALE

NASAL CANNULA

1. Explain the procedure to the client and review safety precautions necessary when oxygen is in use. Place "No Smoking" signs.

An explanation relieves apprehension and promotes cooperation. Oxygen supports combustion. The nurse promotes the safety of the client and others by providing pertinent information.

2. Wash your hands.

Handwashing deters the spread of microorganisms.

3. Connect the nasal cannula, as shown in Fig. VI-1-2, to the oxygen set-up with humidification. Adjust the flowmeter, as shown in Fig. VI-1-3.

Oxygen forced through a water reservoir is humidified before it is delivered to the client, thus preventing dehydration of the mucous membranes.

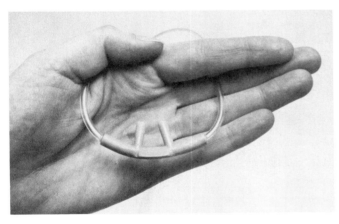

Figure VI-1-2 The prongs of a nasal cannula are inserted into the client's nose. This method of administering oxygen does not interfere with eating. The nurse should observe from time to time that the client is not breathing through his mouth rather than his nose.

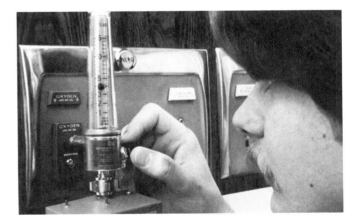

Figure VI-1-3 Oxygen is delivered through a piped-in wall unit. The flowmeter determines the rate at which the oxygen is bubbled through the humidifier bottle.

4. Place the prongs in the client's nostrils (Fig. VI-1-4). Adjust according to the type of equipment:

    a. Over and behind each ear with the adjuster comfortably under the chin, as shown in Fig. VI-1-5, or

    b. Around the client's head.

Correct placement of the prongs and fastener facilitates oxygen administration and comfort for the client.

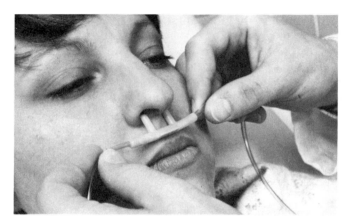

Figure VI-1-4   The nurse inserts the cannula into the client's nose.

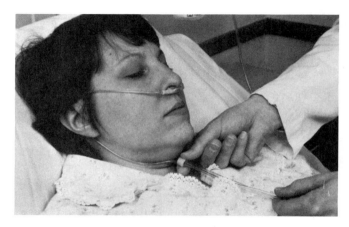

Figure VI-1-5   The tubing is placed around the ears and adjusted beneath the chin.

ACTION	RATIONALE
5. Use gauze pads at the ears beneath the tubing as necessary.	Pads reduce the irritation and pressure and protect the skin.
6. Encourage the client to breathe through his nose with his mouth closed.	Keeping the mouth closed provides optimal delivery of oxygen to the client's lungs.
7. Wash your hands.	Handwashing deters the spread of microorganisms.
8. Assess and chart the client's response to therapy.	The client's respirations, color, and so on indicate the effectiveness of the oxygen therapy.
9. Remove and clean the cannula and nares at least every 8 hours or according to agency recommendations. Check the nares for evidence of irritation or bleeding.	The continued presence of the cannula causes irritation and dryness of the mucous membranes. Humidification counteracts the drying effects of oxygen.

Technique for administering oxygen

ACTION	RATIONALE
MASK	
1. Explain the procedure to the client, review the safety precautions, place signs indicating oxygen precautions in appropriate areas.	An explanation relieves apprehension and promotes the client's cooperation. Oxygen supports combustion. The nurse promotes the safety of the client and others by providing pertinent information.
2. Wash your hands.	Handwashing deters the spread of microorganisms.
3. Attach the face mask to the oxygen set-up with humidification. Start the flow of oxygen at the specified rate.	Oxygen forced through a water reservoir is humidified before it is delivered to the client, thus preventing dehydration of the mucous membranes.
4. Position the face mask over the client's nose and mouth, as shown in Fig. VI-1-6. Adjust it with the elastic strap so that the mask fits snugly but comfortably on the face.	A loose or poorly fitting mask will result in oxygen loss and decreased therapeutic value. Masks may cause a feeling of suffocation, and the client may need frequent attention and reassurance.
5. Use gauze pads to reduce irritation on the client's ears and scalp.	Pads reduce irritation and pressure and protect the skin.
6. Wash your hands.	Handwashing deters the spread of microorganisms.
7. Remove the mask and dry the skin every 2 to 3 hours if the oxygen is running continuously. Do not powder around the mask.	The tight-fitting mask and the moisture from condensation can irritate the skin on the face. There is danger of inhaling powder if it is placed on the mask.

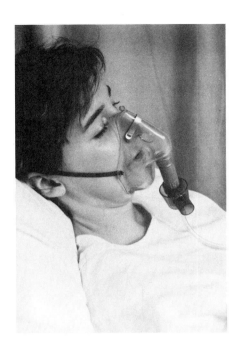

Figure VI-1-6 This client is receiving oxygen through a Venturi mask, a method that allows a high percentage of oxygen to be delivered. Other types of masks are available for administering oxygen.

8. Assess and chart the client's response to therapy.	The client's respiratory rate and pattern, color, and so on, indicate the effectiveness of oxygen therapy.

Technique for administering oxygen

ACTION	RATIONALE
HUMIDITY TENT (CROUPETTE)	
1. Explain the procedure to the client and the family.	An explanation relieves apprehension. Usually pediatric clients receive oxygen by tent.
2. Gather the equipment.	Organization promotes efficient time management.
3. Wash your hands.	Handwashing deters the spread of microorganisms.
4. Use a bath blanket to cover the mattress. Place a second bath blanket over the bottom sheet.	A bath blanket minimizes the potential for static electricity from a plastic mattress. An additional bath blanket is used to provide warmth and absorb moisture.
5. Prepare the tent on the canopy over the bed, as shown in Fig. VI-1-7. Attach the tent to the oxygen source.	The tent allows for oxygen to be delivered in a confined environment.
6. Fill the ice trough or start the refrigeration component.	Body heat can radiate within the tent and raise the temperature above comfort limits. The ice or the refrigeration unit cools the air in the tent.
7. Fill the nebulizer or humidifier to the recommended level with sterile distilled water. Turn on the flowmeter and adjust the oxygen flow to deliver the required amount. Use the oxygen analyzer to obtain a measurement of the concentration of oxygen and recheck it at least every 4 hours.	Humidification of oxygen prevents excessive drying of the respiratory tract. An oxygen analyzer measures the oxygen concentration which is difficult to maintain at a consistent level in the large environment within a tent.
8. Secure the tent below the mattress.	Oxygen is heavier than air. If the tent is not secured, the oxygen content may be decreased.
9. Place the client in the tent after it has been flooded with oxygen for at least 15 minutes. Observe all safety precautions.	It will take approximately 15 minutes to reach adequate therapeutic levels. Oxygen supports combustion.

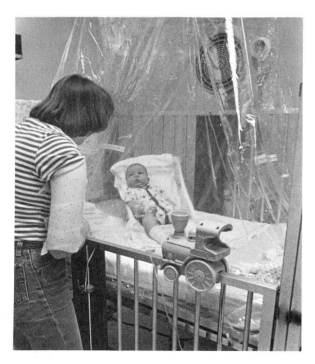

Figure VI-1-7 This infant has been placed in a humidity tent. The clear plastic canopy allows communication and sensory stimulation while enclosing the baby in an oxygen-rich atmosphere.

10. Wash your hands.

Handwashing deters the spread of microorganisms.

11. Open the tent as little as possible by organizing nursing care.

Oxygen escapes each time the tent is opened. Keeping the tent closed maintains the oxygen content.

12. Assess the client at frequent intervals (vital signs, color, response to therapy). Monitor the equipment on a frequent basis.

Oxygen toxicity may develop in response to exposure to a high concentration of oxygen.

13. Change the client's gown and linens as necessary. Edges of tent may be loosened and the tent may be secured with a bath blanket under the client's chin when performing hygienic care or other procedures.

When performing these tasks the nurse demonstrates a conscientious concern for the client's comfort and warmth.

14. Record the type of therapy and the client's response.

A written summary provides an accurate documentation of the care and response of the client to treatment.

SAMPLE DOCUMENTATION

Date	Time	Nurse's note
3/31	0420	Restless during sleep. R-32, P-118, BP 148/92. Color is dusky. Crackles heard in L lower base with no improvement with coughing. Placed in high Fowler's position. O₂ by mask at 4 L/min.
		C. Clark, RN

EVALUATION

REASSESSMENT

The nurse should make periodic focused assessments of the respiratory system and vital signs at 4-hour intervals. The data can be compared with that obtained earlier or with the original baseline information. The most reliable indicators of the client's response to oxygen therapy are the results of arterial blood gases. The nurse should evaluate each test as the report is obtained. When abnormal arterial blood gas values are evident, the nurse should collaborate with the physician on modifications of the current treatment approaches.

Oxygen can be toxic at high concentrations with prolonged use. The nurse should be alert to untoward effects. Indications of oxygen toxicity include: nasal stuffiness, sore throat, nonproductive cough, and substernal pain.

EXPECTED OUTCOMES

The oxygen bubbles through the humidifier at the prescribed liter flow.
The client inhales the oxygen with each respiration.
The client's color and vital signs improve.
The mucous membranes remain moist and intact.
The client feels more comfortable and relaxed while receiving oxygen therapy.

UNEXPECTED OUTCOMES

The oxygen is prevented from maximum delivery due to leaking or efforts made by the client to remove the device used for its administration.
The client becomes apneic and less responsive to stimulation.
Pressure areas are noted under elastic straps.
Mucous membranes appear dry and irritated. The client indicates he has a headache or sinus pain.

MODIFICATIONS IN SELECTED SITUATIONS

GENERAL VARIATIONS

Reduce the liter flow and contact the doctor if the client seems to be developing oxygen toxicity.
Avoid pulling the privacy curtains or otherwise creating a feeling of being closed-in while the client is dyspneic. These actions may psychologically potentiate the feelings of suffocation.
Locate the client near the nursing station and respond promptly to any call for help. Being available relieves anxiety.
If the client who ordinarily receives oxygen by mask becomes dyspneic while it is removed for eating, temporarily substitute oxygen by nasal cannula.

AGE-RELATED VARIATIONS

Place the oxygen analyzer in a humidity tent near the client's face for a more accurate assessment of the oxygen being delivered to the client.
Refill the ice or water reservoir in a humidity tent at least every 8 hours.
A face tent fits more loosely than a mask and is more likely to be tolerated by a child.
Let a child explore a tent before being placed inside. Suggest that the tent is like camping in order to reduce a child's apprehension. Allow the child to have toys that will not spark within the tent.

HOME-HEALTH VARIATIONS

Check that the electric equipment used near the oxygen is grounded and three-pronged plugs are used.
Clients will use oxygen supplied in cylinders, as shown in Fig. VI-1-8. Refilled cylinders and oxygen supplies are delivered to the home on a scheduled basis. Placing the cylinders on a portable tank cart allows a homebound client to move from room to room or outside the home. Extension tubing is also available for improving the client's ability to remain mobile within a greater distance from the source of oxygen.
Note any potential safety hazards, such as oxygen stored or used close to open flames or other flammable substances. If a tent is used, avoid using electrical devices, such as television remote controls and cordless telephones, within the tent.
Post the telephone number of the fire department near the telephone.

RELATED TEACHING

Identify and provide the client with a list, whenever possible, of hazards to avoid when oxygen is in use.
Instruct the client with dyspnea to use pursed lip breathing. Have the client slowly inhale through the nose while counting to three, purse the lips as though preparing to whistle, and exhale while tightening abdominal muscles while counting to seven.
To reduce tachypnea, increase tidal volume, and reduce residual volume, demonstrate deep breathing exercises using the muscles of the abdomen and diaphragm.

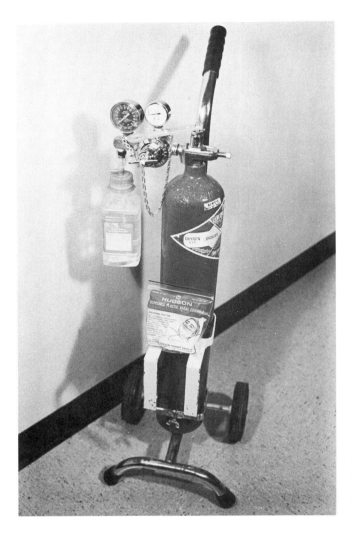

Figure VI-1-8 A small cylinder of oxygen is supported on a mobile stand. The client can roll the container from room to room. The regulator and humidifier are attached and ready for use.

Have the client place one hand on the stomach and the other in the middle of the chest. Instruct the client to breath through his nose while feeling the abdomen protrude as far as possible. Tell the client to exhale slowly through pursed lips.

Explain to the client that coughing is a means of keeping the airway clear unless it is nonproductive. Differentiate between the ingredients and indications for cough suppressants, such as diphenhydramine and dextromethorphan, and expectorants, such as ammonium chloride and ipecac.

Recommend increasing humidification in the home if the client is prone to respiratory infections. Room humidifiers and vaporizers tend to be less expensive than central humidifiers.

Suggest that the client sleep with his head elevated. Some clients sleep better in a recliner chair. An over-the-bed table can be padded so the client can sleep with the upper body supported.

Advise clients with chronic pulmonary diseases to avoid crowds. This increases the risk of acquiring a respiratory infection. Also exposure to environmental pollutants and allergens should be avoided.

Remind the client that discontinuing cigarette smoking is the single most beneficial measure for improving one's health. The American Lung Association, the American Heart Association, and the American Cancer Society sponsor community education programs to help persons eliminate this habit for a healthier life-style.

PERFORMANCE CHECKLIST

When administering oxygen, the learner:

C	A	U	
[ ]	[ ]	[ ]	Washes hands before contact with the client.
[ ]	[ ]	[ ]	Makes pertinent assessments.
[ ]	[ ]	[ ]	Reads the medical orders for directives on the use of oxygen.
[ ]	[ ]	[ ]	Places the client in a semi- or high Fowler's position.
[ ]	[ ]	[ ]	Explains the purpose of the procedure and precautions.
[ ]	[ ]	[ ]	Connects the flowmeter to the source of oxygen.
[ ]	[ ]	[ ]	Attaches and fills the humidifier; fills the ice trough or nebulizer on a humidity tent.
[ ]	[ ]	[ ]	Connects the tubing to the oxygen.
[ ]	[ ]	[ ]	Adjusts the flow to an amount appropriate for the client's condition or the amount prescribed.
[ ]	[ ]	[ ]	Applies the oxygen delivery device to the client, or if a tent is used, tucks the ends under the mattress and floods it with oxygen for 15 minutes.
[ ]	[ ]	[ ]	Adjusts the fit of the cannula or mask for comfort and to avoid leaking.
[ ]	[ ]	[ ]	Posts signs indicating oxygen use and precautions.
[ ]	[ ]	[ ]	Observes the client's immediate response.
[ ]	[ ]	[ ]	Provides the client with a signal device.
[ ]	[ ]	[ ]	Washes hands.
[ ]	[ ]	[ ]	Charts significant information.
[ ]	[ ]	[ ]	Returns to obtain reassessment data.
[ ]	[ ]	[ ]	Refills humidifier and ice trough as needed.

Outcome: [ ] Pass   [ ] Fail

C = competent; A = acceptable; U = unsatisfactory

Comments: _____

_____

_____

_____
Student's Signature

_____
Date

_____
Instructor's Signature

_____
Date

VI-2

Suctioning the nasopharyngeal and oropharyngeal areas

The airway includes the passages through which the air from the atmosphere moves to and from the lungs. Secretions that collect and accumulate narrow the passageways. Reduction of the area through which air moves interferes with optimal ventilation and the transportation of oxygen to the blood and cells of the body. At the same time, carbon dioxide accumulates and can alter acid-base balance. Voluntary coughing may be sufficient to clear the upper airway. However, the client may be too weak to expectorate the raised mucus. Suctioning the upper airway may become necessary.

PURPOSES OF PROCEDURE

Nasopharyngeal or oropharyngeal suctioning may be performed to

1. Remove excess saliva or emesis from the oral cavity
2. Clear the upper airway of mucoid secretions
3. Promote adequate gas exchange
4. Prevent pneumonia and atelectasis
5. Obtain a sputum culture
6. Relieve respiratory distress

ASSESSMENT

OBJECTIVE DATA

- Count the respiratory rate and observe the effort expended to breathe.
- Note the presence of a productive cough and the ability of the client to raise and expectorate the secretions with voluntary coughing.
- Observe the characteristics of any secretions that are raised.
- Auscultate over the trachea, bronchi, and lungs for adventitious sounds.
- Observe the client's skin color and the color of the lips and nailbeds. Be alert to signs of cyanosis.
- Count the heart rate and note the rhythm. Poor oxygenation is likely to cause tachycardia and irregular rhythm.
- Measure the blood pressure. Anxiety can cause mild hypertension in previously normotensive individuals.
- Review the most recent chest x-ray interpretation, if available.
- Survey the chart for conditions that may contribute to excessive production of respiratory secretions, such as chronic obstructive pulmonary disease (COPD), or conditions affecting the ability to raise secretions, such as chronic pain from a thoracic incision, debilitation, or coma.
- Monitor the results of arterial blood gas reports.
- Read the medical orders for a directive to perform suctioning.

SUBJECTIVE DATA

- Ask the client to indicate if he feels the need to cough or is experiencing difficulty breathing.

RELEVANT NURSING DIAGNOSES

The client who needs suctioning may have nursing diagnoses, such as

- *Anxiety*
- *Ineffective Airway Clearance*
- *Impaired Gas Exchange*

- *Potential Altered Cardiac Output*
- *Potential for Infection*
- *Potential for Injury*
- *Potential Altered Oral Mucous Membrane*

PLANNING

ESTABLISHING PRIORITIES

If the airway becomes partially or totally occluded, the client's life is in jeopardy. The nurse may independently take action when this is the case. Some agencies have written protocols that require suction equipment at the bedside in case of an emergency. Examples include the care of the postoperative tonsillectomy client and as part of seizure precautions.

SETTING GOALS

- The client's respirations will be noiseless, effortless, and within the normal rate for his age.
- There will be no adventitious sounds heard in the upper airways.
- The client will maintain adequate gas exchange as evidenced by normal arterial blood gas values.

PREPARATION OF EQUIPMENT

The nurse will need equipment from the following list:

Portable or wall suction unit with tubing
Sterile suction catheter with Y-port
Sterile water or saline
Sterile disposable container
Sterile gloves
Towel or waterproof pad

Technique for suctioning the nasopharyngeal and oropharyngeal areas

ACTION	RATIONALE
1. Explain the procedure to the client.	An explanation provides reassurance and promotes co-operation.
2. Assemble the equipment.	Organization promotes efficient time management.
3. Wash your hands.	Handwashing deters the spread of microorganisms.
4. Adjust the bed to a comfortable working position. Lower the side rail closer to you. Place the client in a semi-Fowler's position if conscious. An unconscious client should be placed in the lateral position facing you.	Having the client in a sitting position helps him to cough and makes breathing easier. Gravity also facilitates the insertion of the catheter. A lateral position prevents the airway from becoming obstructed and promotes drainage of secretions.
5. Place a towel or waterproof pad across the client's chest.	Using absorbent material protects the client's clothing and bed linen.
6. Turn on the suction to the appropriate pressure. Appropriate wall unit pressures are Adult: 110 mm Hg to 150 mm Hg Child: 5 mm Hg to 10 mm Hg Infant: 2 mm Hg to 5 mm Hg	Negative pressure must be at a safe level or alveoli may collapse.
7. Open the sterile suctioning package. Touch only the outside surface and pour sterile saline or water into it.	Sterile normal saline or water is used to lubricate the outside of the catheter, thus minimizing irritation of the mucosa as it is being introduced.
8. Put a sterile glove on the hand that will handle the catheter.	Handling the sterile catheter with the hand wearing a sterile glove helps prevent introducing organisms into the respiratory tract.

9. With the sterile gloved hand, pick up the sterile catheter and connect it to the suction tubing that is held with the unsterile hand, as shown in Figure VI-2-1.

Touching one sterile object with another ensures that surgical asepsis is maintained.

10. Moisten the catheter by dipping it into the container of sterile saline. Occlude the Y-tube to check the suction.

Lubricating the inside of the catheter with saline helps move secretions in the catheter.

11. Estimate the distance from the earlobe to the nostril and place the thumb and forefinger of the gloved hand at that point on the catheter.

Determining the approximate distance for advancing the catheter ensures that it will remain in the pharynx rather than in the trachea.

12. Gently insert the catheter, like the nurse in Figure VI-2-2 is doing, with the suction off by leaving the vent on the Y-connector open. Slip the catheter gently along the floor of an unobstructed nostril toward the pharynx to suction the nasopharynx. Or, insert the catheter along the side of the mouth toward the pharynx to suction the oropharynx. Never apply suction as the catheter is introduced.

Using suction while inserting the catheter can cause trauma to the mucosa and removes oxygen from the respiratory tract. Coughing may occur. This helps the client raise secretions toward the tip of the catheter and upper airway.

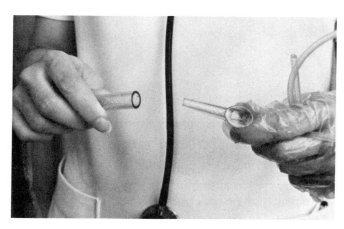

Figure VI-2-1 The sterility of the suction catheter is protected while connecting it to the tubing.

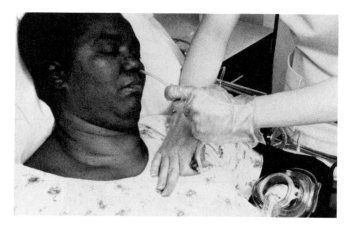

Figure VI-2-2 The nurse prepares to insert the suction catheter into the client's nose.

13. Apply suction, as shown in Figure VI-2-3, by occluding the suctioning port with your thumb and gently rotate the catheter as it is being withdrawn. Do not allow the suctioning to continue for longer than 10 to 15 seconds at a time.

Turning the catheter as it is withdrawn helps clean all surfaces of the respiratory passageways. Suctioning the client for longer than 10 to 15 seconds robs the respiratory tract of oxygen, which may result in hypoxia.

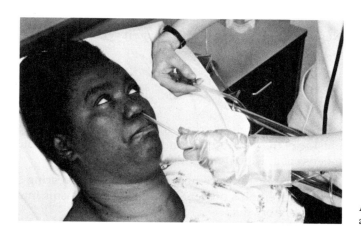

Figure VI-2-3 The nurse occludes the port on the suction catheter and rotates the catheter while it is being withdrawn.

14. Flush the catheter with saline and repeat suctioning as needed and according to the client's toleration of the procedure.

Flushing cleans and clears the catheter and lubricates it for the next insertion.

15. Allow at least a 20-second to 30-second interval if additional suctioning is needed. The nares should be alternated when repeated suctioning is required. Do not force the catheter through the nares. Encourage the client to cough and deep breathe between suctionings.

Normal breathing between suctioning helps compensate for any hypoxia induced by the previous suctioning.

16. When suctioning is completed, remove the sterile glove inside out, as shown in Figure VI-2-4, and dispose of the glove, catheter, and container with solution in the proper receptacle. Wash your hands.

Keeping microorganisms confined supports principles of medical asepsis. Handwashing deters the spread of microorganisms.

17. Use auscultation to listen to the chest to assess the effectiveness of suctioning, as the nurse in Figure VI-2-5 is doing.

Listening to lung sounds helps determine whether the respiratory passageways are clear of secretions.

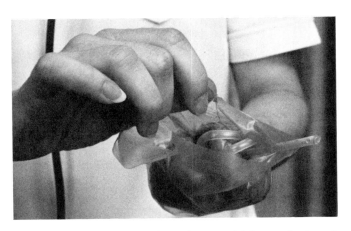

Figure VI-2–4 The nurse reduces the potential for transferring microbes from the client's respiratory tract by enclosing the contaminated catheter within the inverted glove.

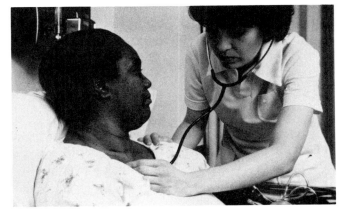

Figure VI-2–5 Auscultation is a method for assessing the effectiveness of suctioning.

18. Record the time of suctioning and the nature and amount of secretions. Also note the character of the client's respirations before and after the suctioning.

A written summary provides an accurate record of the care provided and the client's responses.

19. Offer oral hygiene after suctioning.

Respiratory secretions that are allowed to accumulate in the mouth are irritating to mucous membranes and are unpleasant for the client.

SAMPLE DOCUMENTATION

Date	Time	Nurse's note
7/01	0635	Noisy respirations audible. Wet sounds detected with a stethoscope over trachea and R bronchus. Nasal flaring noted. R-30, P-100 and regular, BP 146/90. Encouraged to breathe deeply, hold, and cough. Secretions not raised with this technique. Positioned to promote postural drainage.

K. Burnham, RN

0650   Able to bring mucus to back of throat. Oropharynx suctioned. Mod. amt.
of white, opaque, thick secretions removed. Deep breathing encouraged.
R-24 and quiet. No abnormal sounds heard. Mouth care provided.

K. Bunham, RN

EVALUATION

REASSESSMENT

The rate and character of respirations should be evaluated after suctioning. The lungs and upper airway may be auscultated for evidence of clearing. Watch the client for diminished restlessness and improved color. Describe the amount and characteristics of the suctioned material for future comparisons. Monitor the client's temperature as an indicator of possible pulmonary infection from retained secretions.

EXPECTED OUTCOMES

The suction catheter is inserted without trauma.
The client's heart beats at a normal rate and rhythm remains regular.
Secretions are removed within 10 to 15 seconds.
Respirations become less labored and noisy.
Arterial blood gases indicate adequate oxygenation.

UNEXPECTED OUTCOMES

The nasal or oral mucosa becomes traumatized.
The client gags when the catheter is inserted into the oropharynx.
The client manifests an irregular pulse during suctioning.
Secretions are blood tinged.
Wet sounds continue to be heard in various locations throughout the respiratory tract.
Arterial blood gases indicate inadequate gas exchange.

MODIFICATIONS IN SELECTED SITUATIONS

GENERAL VARIATIONS

Use gravity to help drain lung secretions to an area where suctioning can remove them. Various positions, illustrated in Figure VI-2-6, drain particular lobes of the lung.
Encourage a 2000-ml to 3000-ml fluid intake per day unless the client must restrict fluids. The added volume will tend to thin secretions and permit spontaneous, independent expectoration.
Use a Yankauer suction tip for oropharyngeal suctioning rather than a flexible catheter. It is easier to control while passing it along the side of the mouth. The nurse is less likely to stimulate the client's gag reflex when the tip is more firm and under control.
Use a separate catheter for the nose and mouth to avoid transferring microbes from one area to another.
If the client requires frequent suctioning, fold a sterile towel forming a pocket. Tape or pin the cloth pocket to the bed. Label the pocket with the date and time and indicate if the catheter is to be used in the nose or mouth. Place the catheter in the sterile pocket for subsequent reuse. Discard and replace the catheter each shift to avoid the risk of infection.
Attach a mucous trap to the suction catheter if a sputum specimen is needed.
Place anyone who has difficulty clearing the airway on the abdomen or in a lateral position to avoid potential aspiration.
Change the client's position at least every 2 hours to prevent pooling of secretions that could occlude small airways.
Empty the suction container at least each shift.

AGE-RELATED VARIATIONS

Use a hand-held bulb syringe to remove secretions from a newborn's nose or mouth.
A DeLee mucous trap can be used for removing secretions in the pharynx of a neonate. This device requires that the nurse create suction by sucking through a catheter that has been inserted into the infant's pharynx. The trap collects secretions before they could reach the nurse's mouth.

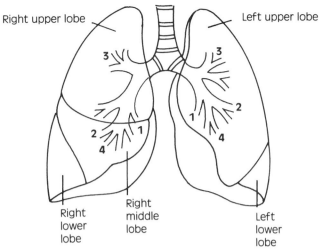

Figure VI-2-6 These are four positions that utilize gravity to assist the drainage of secretions from the smaller bronchial airways into the main bronchi and trachea.

Lower lobes, superior segments

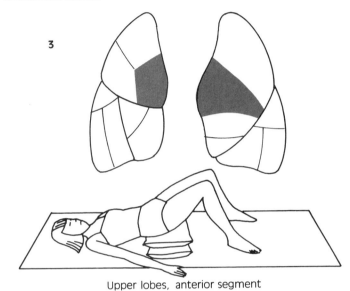

Upper lobes, anterior segment

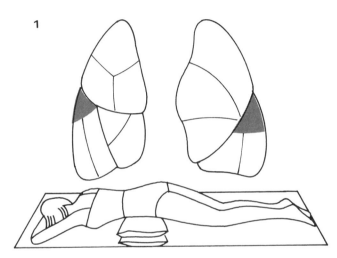

Lower lobes, anterior basal segment

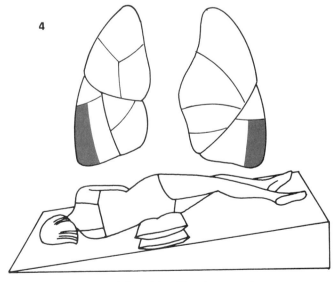

Lower lobes, lateral basal segment

To determine the approximate depth for inserting an oropharyngeal catheter on an infant or child, measure the distance from the tragus, the cartilage beside the entrance to the ear, to the naris.

Use the following scale when selecting the size of a suction catheter:

Newborns and infants: 5 to 8 French

Children: 8 to 12 French

Older children and adults: 12 to 18 French

When suctioning a child, limit the time to 5 to 10 seconds since a child has less oxygen reserve and residual capacity.

HOME-HEALTH VARIATIONS

Advise individuals who require suctioning at home to use a room humidifier or vaporizer to thin secretions.

Recommend damp dusting, low-cut carpet, and other measures that will reduce the amount of inhaled irritants.

RELATED TEACHING

Demonstrate and practice voluntary coughing to promote the movement and expectoration of thick secretions.

PERFORMANCE CHECKLIST

When suctioning nasopharyngeal or oropharyngeal areas, the learner:

C	A	U	
[ ]	[ ]	[ ]	Washes hands before direct contact with the client
[ ]	[ ]	[ ]	Obtains appropriate assessments
[ ]	[ ]	[ ]	Utilizes approaches other than suctioning to clear the airway
[ ]	[ ]	[ ]	Explains the purpose and sequence of steps for suctioning
[ ]	[ ]	[ ]	Gathers and assembles equipment
[ ]	[ ]	[ ]	Positions the client in a semi-Fowler's position
[ ]	[ ]	[ ]	Applies a sterile glove
[ ]	[ ]	[ ]	Attaches the catheter to the suction source
[ ]	[ ]	[ ]	Wets the catheter tip and tests the suction
[ ]	[ ]	[ ]	Inserts the catheter into the nose or mouth and into the pharynx
[ ]	[ ]	[ ]	Occludes the vent when the catheter is in place
[ ]	[ ]	[ ]	Rotates the catheter during withdrawal
[ ]	[ ]	[ ]	Rinses the catheter
[ ]	[ ]	[ ]	Allows the client to rest and recover before passing the catheter another time
[ ]	[ ]	[ ]	Pulls the glove off over the catheter
[ ]	[ ]	[ ]	Discards the soiled equipment
[ ]	[ ]	[ ]	Washes hands
[ ]	[ ]	[ ]	Reassesses the effectiveness of the procedure
[ ]	[ ]	[ ]	Assists with mouth care and other comfort measures
[ ]	[ ]	[ ]	Charts significant information

Outcome: [ ] Pass   [ ] Fail

C = competent; A = acceptable; U = unsatisfactory

Comments: _____
_____
_____

_____   _____
Student's Signature   Date

_____   _____
Instructor's Signature   Date

VI-3 *Clearing an obstructed airway*

Various situations can cause a sudden occlusion of the airway, such as aspirating food or solid nonfood objects. Quick action on the part of the nurse can reverse a life-threatening situation.

PURPOSES OF PROCEDURE

Efforts to clear an obstructed airway are implemented to

1. Remove an object from the airway
2. Promote air exchange
3. Prevent pulmonary and cardiac arrest

ASSESSMENT

OBJECTIVE DATA

- Observe if the client demonstrates the universal distress signal, that is, clutching at the throat with both hands.
- Assess the situation and circumstances of respiratory distress; note if the person has been eating or if broken toys or other small objects are in the area.
- Note if the client can cough or speak.
- Observe skin color and any chest movement.
- Determine if air is moving in or out of the nose or mouth.

SUBJECTIVE DATA

- If the client is conscious, ask if he is choking and note his response.

RELEVANT NURSING DIAGNOSES

The individual who has an obstructed airway may have nursing diagnoses, such as

- *Ineffective Airway Clearance*
- *Ineffective Breathing Pattern*
- *Impaired Gas Exchange*
- *Fear*
- *Potential Altered Cardiac Output*

PLANNING

ESTABLISHING PRIORITIES

In a partial airway obstruction with good air exchange, the client can cough forcefully. The person should be allowed and encouraged to cough and breathe spontaneously. If adequate air exchange progresses to inadequate or absent respiration, immediate action is necessary or the client will become hypoxic and death may ensue.

SETTING GOALS

- The airway obstruction will be relieved.
- There will be no injury to the ribs or abdominal organs.

Technique for clearing an obstructed airway

ACTION	RATIONALE
CONSCIOUS ADULT	
1. Assess the victim. Ask, "Are you choking?" Determine if he can speak or cough.	The inability to speak or cough indicates that the airway is obstructed.

2. If the victim is obstructed, initiate abdominal thrusts (Heimlich maneuver):

    a. Stand behind the victim.

    b. Wrap your arms around the victim's waist.

    c. Make a fist with one hand with the thumb outside of the fist. Place the thumb side of the fist against the victim's abdomen above the navel and well below the xiphoid process, as shown in Figure VI-3-1.

    d. Grasp the fist with the other hand and press upward with quick, firm thrusts.

    e. Continue distinct thrusts until the foreign body is expelled or the victim becomes unconscious.

Firm abdominal thrusts force exhalation of air through the victim's airway and aid in dislodging the obstructed object.

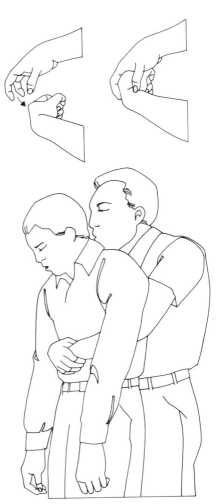

Figure VI-3-1 The rescuer has positioned himself behind this victim. The thumb side of one fist is located below the xiphoid process while the other hand is used to grasp it.

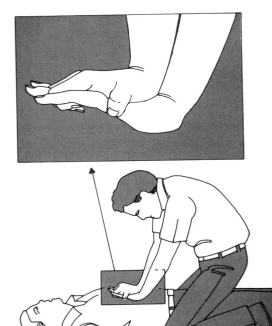

Figure VI-3-2 With the hands in position, the rescuer presses upward to move air that is trapped in the lungs with enough force to dislodge the obstructed object.

UNCONSCIOUS ADULT

1. Assess the victim's unresponsiveness. Gently shake his shoulder and ask, "Are you okay?" Call for help.

Unresponsiveness indicates a potential need for cardiopulmonary resuscitation (CPR).

2. Position the victim on his back on a flat, firm surface. Support the victim's head and neck and turn as a unit.

A firm surface provides for the maximum effect from abdominal thrusts. Supporting the head and neck while turning prevents injury.

3. Tilt the head backward by placing one hand on the victim's forehead. Place the fingers of the other hand underneath the victim's jaw and lift upward and forward.

This motion opens the airway and may be all that is necessary for spontaneous breathing to begin.

4. Determine if the victim is breathless by placing an ear over the victim's mouth and observing the chest.

Expired air can be heard and felt on the cheek as well as observed as the chest rises and falls if the victim is breathing.

5. Attempt ventilation if breathless. Seal the victim's mouth and nose properly. If resistance is met, reposition the victim's head and attempt to ventilate again. If anyone responds to the call for help, send them to activate the emergency medical system (EMS).

If the airway is not positioned properly or is obstructed, resistance will be felt when ventilating. Air will not enter the lungs and the chest will not rise.

6. Initiate abdominal thrusts (Heimlich maneuver) as shown in Figure VI-3-2:

Firm abdominal thrusts force exhalation of air through the victim's airway and aid in dislodging the obstructed object.

    a. Straddle the victim's thighs.

    b. Place the heel of one hand against the victim's abdomen above the navel and well below the xiphoid process.

    c. Place the second hand directly on top of the first hand.

    d. Press upward with quick, firm thrusts.

    e. Perform 6 to 10 distinct abdominal thrusts.

7. Perform a finger sweep using the jaw lift to open the victim's mouth.

The finger sweep detects an expelled foreign body and facilitates its removal, thus preventing it from being forced back into the airway.

8. Attempt ventilation again using the maneuver described in Step 5. If unable to ventilate, repeat the sequence of thrusts, finger sweep, and ventilations until successful.

Forceful ventilation in an unconscious victim may bypass the obstruction and enable aeration of the lungs.

9. If successful in ventilation, continue with further required resuscitation efforts: check the pulse, administer chest compressions if pulseless, and continue artificial breathing.

Once the airway is open, the need for continued intervention must be established if the victim does not respond spontaneously.

SAMPLE DOCUMENTATION

Date	Time	Nurse's note
2/06	1745	Observed choking while eating. Not able to speak, cough, or breathe. Dusky color. 5 abdominal thrusts administered. Lg. piece of meat expelled from mouth. Deep, rapid respirations followed episode. P-98; color improved. O at 10 L adm. per mask for 15 minutes. Breathing without distress.

S. Barton, RN

EVALUATION

REASSESSMENT

Analyze if a partial obstruction is becoming worse. Indications include a forceful cough that becomes weak and ineffective, high-pitched noises while inhaling, increased breathing difficulties, cyanosis, and loss of consciousness. After delivering successive abdominal thrusts without restoration of breathing, provide artificial ventilation to reassess if the airway has been cleared.

EXPECTED OUTCOMES

The client breathes spontaneously.
The client expels the foreign object.
The client ventilates adequately.

UNEXPECTED OUTCOMES

A partial obstruction progresses to full obstruction.
The foreign object is retained.
The client's heart stops beating.

MODIFICATIONS IN SELECTED SITUATIONS

GENERAL VARIATIONS

Use chest thrusts rather than abdominal thrusts on a pregnant or very obese victim. Place the fist on the middle portion of the sternum and thrust backward.
Restaurants may have a "choke-saver" instrument for retrieving food from the mouth or throat of a victim. However, the victim's life can be saved without any instrumentation and time should not be lost by frantically searching for one. Furthermore, use by an excited and unprepared employee can cause additional trauma.

AGE-RELATED VARIATIONS

Note a child's ability to cry if too young to speak as a method for assessing air exchange.
Position the head of an infant under the age of 1 year lower than the rest of the body to administer four back blows with the heel of the hand between the shoulder blades, as shown in Figure VI-3-3, as a first step to clearing the airway.

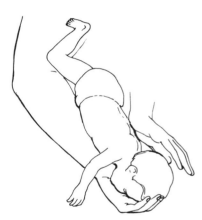

Figure VI-3-3 Back blows are being administered to this infant under the age of 1 year. Lowering the head utilizes gravity in removing the obstructed object.

Place a child who has aspirated an object crosswise over the rescuer's thighs with the head lower than the rest of the body. Having the head lower permits gravity to assist in removing an object from the respiratory tract.
Avoid using abdominal thrusts in infants and children because of the danger of injuring internal organs. Use chest thrusts instead. Administer chest thrusts to the middle of an infant's sternum at the level of the nipples, well away from the lower end of the sternum with two fingers, as shown in Figure VI-3-4.

HOME-HEALTH VARIATIONS

For high-risk clients, such as those with Parkinson's disease or stroke, ensure that caregivers are competent in recognizing and clearing an obstructed airway. Periodically review the procedure with the caregivers. Practice hand placement.
Post emergency numbers near all telephones.

RELATED TEACHING

Encourage all individuals to learn to perform the Heimlich maneuver and basic cardiac life support (CPR).

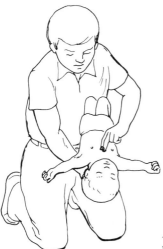

Figure VI-3-4   Chest thrusts are delivered to an infant who has aspirated an object.

Instruct others on ways to prevent choking, such as
  Do not talk or laugh with food in the mouth.
  Cut food into small pieces and chew it well.
  Make sure dentures fit well.
  Do not drink alcoholic beverages in excess while eating.
  Avoid purchasing toys with small objects that can be removed.
  Do not give small children popcorn, peanuts, or pieces of hard candy that can be
    aspirated.

PERFORMANCE CHECKLIST

When clearing an obstructed airway, the learner:

C	A	U	
[ ]	[ ]	[ ]	Makes appropriate assessments
[ ]	[ ]	[ ]	Positions self behind or over the victim
[ ]	[ ]	[ ]	Forms a fist
[ ]	[ ]	[ ]	Locates hands below the xiphoid process if the victim is not pregnant and not obese
[ ]	[ ]	[ ]	Administers 6 to 10 abdominal thrusts
[ ]	[ ]	[ ]	Evaluates the success of the efforts
[ ]	[ ]	[ ]	Repeats the series of abdominal thrusts until the victim responds or becomes unconscious
[ ]	[ ]	[ ]	Administers artificial ventilation if the client remains breathless and unconscious
[ ]	[ ]	[ ]	Sends someone for help, if possible
[ ]	[ ]	[ ]	Performs CPR if the airway is opened but the victim is pulseless and unresponsive

Outcome: [ ] Pass   [ ] Fail

C = competent; A = acceptable; U = unsatisfactory

Comments: _____
_____
_____

_____   _____
Student's Signature   Date

_____   _____
Instructor's Signature   Date

VI-4   *Suctioning the tracheostomy*

A tracheostomy is an artificial opening made into the trachea. A curved metal or plastic tube is inserted into the opening. It is essential to maintain the patency of the airway. The client may be able to cough and clear both the natural and artificial airway. When this is not possible, the nurse must be prepared to provide suctioning.

PURPOSES OF PROCEDURE

A tracheostomy is suctioned to

1. Clear the airway of secretions
2. Relieve respiratory distress
3. Reduce or prevent hypoxia
4. Allay anxiety

ASSESSMENT

OBJECTIVE DATA

- Examine the client for signs of alteration in adequate respiration, such as tachypnea, abnormal breath sounds, and presence and characteristics of a cough.
- Analyze the client's color, especially the skin around the lips and nailbeds.
- Count the heart rate and note its rhythm.
- Monitor the most recent arterial blood gas report, if available.
- Note the efforts made by the client to breathe and cough.
- Observe the amount and characteristics of secretions that are expelled onto the tracheostomy dressing.
- Examine the condition of the skin about the stoma.
- Check that oxygen and humidification equipment is functioning properly.

SUBJECTIVE DATA

- Ask the client questions to which he can respond by shaking his head, or provide a magic slate or some other means for communicating since the ability to speak is impaired when a tracheostomy tube is in place.
- Ask the client if he feels the need for suctioning.

RELEVANT NURSING DIAGNOSES

The client with a tracheostomy is likely to have nursing diagnoses, such as

- *Anxiety*
- *Ineffective Airway Clearance*
- *Impaired Gas Exchange*
- *Potential for Infection*
- *Impaired Verbal Communication*
- *Potential for Injury*
- *Potential Altered Oral Mucous Membrane*

PLANNING

ESTABLISHING PRIORITIES

The frequency of suctioning varies with the amount of secretions present, but it should be done often enough to keep ventilation effective and as effortless as possible. Suctioning is irritating to the mucosa and removes oxygen from the respiratory tract. Thus, it is necessary that the client be hyperoxygenated prior to suctioning. The suctioning catheter should be small enough not to occlude the airway but large enough to remove secretions. Principles of surgical asepsis must be followed to protect the client from infection. If the client experiences cardiopulmonary distress, such as an arrhythmia or bronchospasm, suctioning should be discontinued and restorative measures, such as ventilation with oxygen, instituted.

SETTING GOALS
- The client's airway will remain patent.
- Accumulating secretions will be cleared as they begin to interfere with adequate ventilation.
- The client's gas exchange will remain adequate.

PREPARATION OF EQUIPMENT
The nurse will need items from the following list:

Portable or wall suction device with connecting tubing
Sterile suction kit or the following separate items:
    Sterile suction catheter of appropriate size with Y-port
        Infants: 6 to 8 French
        Children: 8 to 10 French
        Adults: 12 to 16 French
    Sterile container
    Sterile glove
Sterile normal saline
Clean towel or sterile drape (optional)

Technique for suctioning the tracheostomy

ACTION	RATIONALE
1. Obtain focus assessments of cardiopulmonary function.	An immediate baseline serves as an index for needing suctioning as well as a basis for evaluating its effectiveness.
2. Explain the procedure to the client and reassure him that you will interrupt the procedure if he indicates respiratory difficulty.	An explanation relieves apprehension and facilitates cooperation. Any procedure that compromises respiration is frightening for the client.
3. Gather equipment and provide privacy for the client.	Organization promotes efficient time management.
4. Wash your hands.	Handwashing deters the spread of microorganisms.
5. Assist the client to a semi-Fowler's or Fowler's position if conscious. An unconscious client should be placed in the lateral position facing you.	A sitting position helps the client to cough and breathe more easily. This position also uses gravity to aid in the insertion of the catheter. A lateral position prevents the airway from becoming obstructed and promotes drainage of secretions.
6. Turn the suction on to the appropriate pressure:	Negative pressure must be at a safe level or damage to the tracheal mucosa may occur.

a. Wall unit

Adult: 110 mm Hg to 150 mm Hg
Child: 95 mm Hg to 110 mm Hg
Infant: 50 mm Hg to 95 mm Hg

b. Portable unit

Adult: 10 mm Hg to 15 mm Hg
Child: 5 mm Hg to 10 mm Hg
Infant: 2 mm Hg to 5 mm Hg

7. Place a clean towel, if one is being used, across the client's chest.	Absorbent material protects the client and bed linens.

8. Open the sterile suction kit, as shown in Figure VI-4-1, or arrange sterile equipment in preparation for suctioning.

An artificial airway compromises the client's natural defenses. Using sterile equipment reduces the risk of infection.

a. Place a sterile drape, if available, across the client's chest.

A sterile drape provides an area that is free of microorganisms.

b. Open the sterile container and place it on the bedside table or overbed table without contaminating the inner surface. Pour sterile saline into it.

The chambers within the container maintain the sterility of items that will be in direct contact with the client's airway.

c. Preoxygenate the client for 1 to 2 minutes.

Providing increased percentages of oxygen prevents hypoxia during suctioning.

d. Don a sterile glove on the dominant hand and pick up the folded sterile suction catheter. Remove the wrapper around the catheter with the nondominant unsterile hand and discard.

Using the sterile hand to hold the catheter maintains its sterility.

e. Connect the sterile suction catheter, shown in Figure VI-4-2, to the suction tubing that is held with the unsterile hand.

Sterile technique prevents introducing organisms into the respiratory tract.

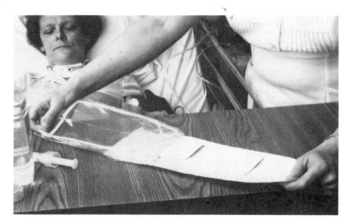

Figure VI-4–1   The nurse peels the protective cover from the sterile suction kit. Use of sterile disposable equipment provides an organized and convenient method for performing tracheostomy suctioning.

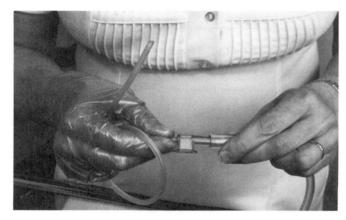

Figure VI-4–2   The sterile suction catheter is connected to the suction tubing. The tubing provides extra length with which to reach from the source of suction to the client.

9. Moisten the catheter by dipping it into the container of sterile saline. Occlude the port to check suction.

Lubricating the inside of the catheter with saline helps move secretions through the catheter.

10. Remove the oxygen administration equipment with the unsterile hand, as the nurse in Figure VI-4-3 is doing.

Removing the oxygen allows access to the tracheostomy tube.

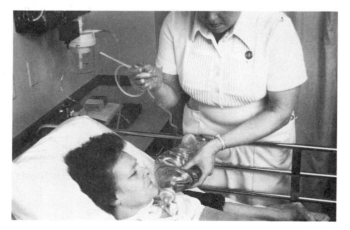

Figure VI-4–3   The nurse has finished preoxygenating the client and is removing the oxygen in order to insert the suction catheter.

11. Using the sterile hand, gently insert the catheter into the trachea, as illustrated in Figure VI-4-4. Advance the catheter to 12.5 cm (4 inches to 5 inches) or until the client coughs. *Do not occlude the Y-port when inserting the catheter.*

12. Apply suction by occluding the Y-port with the thumb of the unsterile hand. Gently rotate the catheter with the thumb and index finger of the gloved hand as it is being withdrawn. Try to limit suctioning to no longer than 10 seconds. Encourage the client to cough during suctioning.

13. Flush the catheter with saline and assess the need to repeat suctioning. Allow the client to rest at least 1 minute between suctionings. Readminister oxygen between suctioning efforts and when suctioning is completed.

14. When the procedure is completed, turn off the suction and disconnect the catheter from the suction tubing. Remove the sterile glove inside out, as shown in Figure VI-4-5, and dispose of the glove, catheter, and container in a waste receptacle. Wash hands.

Using the suction when inserting the catheter can cause trauma to the mucosa and removes oxygen from the respiratory tract.

Turning the catheter while withdrawing it helps clean the surfaces of the respiratory tract and prevents injury to tracheal mucosa. Suctioning for longer than 10 seconds increases the potential for hypoxia. Coughing helps loosen and move secretions to the area of the catheter.

Flushing cleans and clears the catheter and lubricates it for the next insertion. Allowing a time interval and replacing the oxygen help compensate for hypoxia induced by the previous suctioning.

Keeping contaminated articles confined to certain areas limits the transmission of microorganisms. Handwashing deters the spread of microorganisms by direct contact.

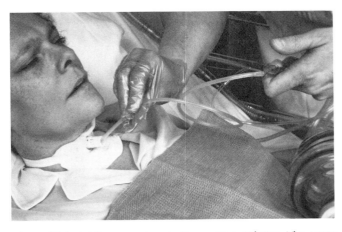

Figure VI-4-4 The nurse inserts the suction catheter. The nurse waits to occlude the Y-port until the catheter has been fully inserted and the nurse is ready to begin its withdrawal.

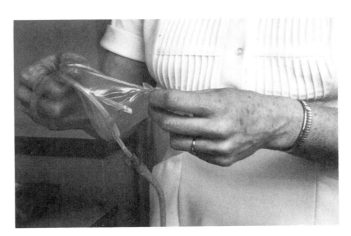

Figure VI-4-5 The nurse pulls the glove off over the catheter to contain microorganisms within a confined area.

15. Adjust the client's position. Auscultate the chest to evaluate breath sounds.

16. Record the time of the suctioning and the nature and amount of secretions. Also note the character of the client's respirations before and after suctioning.

Reassessment helps evaluate the effect suctioning has had in clearing the respiratory passageways of secretions.

A written summary provides accurate documentation of comprehensive care.

SAMPLE DOCUMENTATION

Date	Time	Nurse's note
1/25	1245	Shallow, noisy respirations @ 32 per min. Accessory muscles used while sitting in upright position. Lips are dark. Perspiring and looks anxious. P-108 and regular. Preoxygenated with 100% O_2 through T-piece for 2 minutes. Tracheostomy suctioned. Sm. amt. of thick opaque secretions removed. Reoxygenated @ 100% O_2 for 1 minute then reduced to 40%. R-28, P-100 within 10 minutes after suctioning. No abnormal breath sounds noted at this time.

B. Marzietti, RN

EVALUATION

REASSESSMENT

If the client's cardiac status is being monitored, observe the heart rate and rhythm on the screen. After the client has received supplemental oxygen, compare the respiratory rate and lung sounds to the previous findings. Avoid obtaining arterial blood gases shortly after suctioning because the results will likely be abnormal due to the temporary deficit in oxygenation.

EXPECTED OUTCOMES

The client's respirations are improved as evidenced by reduced rate and effort. Audible or auscultated wet sounds disappear or are reduced after suctioning. The client appears relaxed and is oriented and alert.

UNEXPECTED OUTCOMES

The client experiences respiratory distress or cardiac arrhythmia. Adventitious sounds continue to be evident despite suctioning. The trend in the client's arterial blood gases worsens. The client's level of consciousness becomes obtunded.

MODIFICATIONS IN SELECTED SITUATIONS

GENERAL VARIATIONS

Monitor the airway and respiratory status closely immediately after the tracheostomy has been performed. Expect that secretions will be blood tinged because of the trauma of the incision.

Instill 4 ml to 5 ml of sterile normal saline into the tracheostomy tube with a syringe before suctioning. Adding moisture will dilute sticky, thick mucus or loosen crusty dried secretions.

Have the client turn his head to the right when there is a need to suction the left bronchus and *vice versa* for reaching the right bronchus.

Use a room humidifier to help keep respiratory secretions thinned.

Also ensure that the client's parenteral fluid intake is adequate.

AGE-RELATED VARIATIONS

Expect that an endotracheal tube will be used in children or adults rather than a tracheostomy if the airway assistance will likely be of short duration.

Reassure a child and child's parents who are naturally fearful about the seriousness of the medical condition. Their fears may be heightened by the fact that the tracheostomy tube prevents speech and the ability to make sounds while crying.

Apply restraints to prevent a child from removing the tracheostomy tube. Maintain duplicate equipment in readiness in case extubation occurs.

A child may be placed in a croupette to keep the environmental air saturated with oxygen and moisture.

Children under 5 years of age are not likely to have a double-cannula tracheostomy tube. Cuffed tracheostomy tubes are seldom used with children.

HOME-HEALTH VARIATIONS

Encourage arranging occasional respite care so that family caregivers can have relief from the constant responsibility for care.

RELEVANT TEACHING

The client may be taught to perform suctioning independently. Provide a mirror and step-by-step instructions. Practice with the client. When the client demonstrates competency, encourage self-care.

Teach the client to perform deep breathing exercises.

Advise family and friends with respiratory infections to maintain a distance of several feet when visiting the client. Wearing a mask may also be beneficial. Instruct individuals with colds to use a fresh tissue to cover the nose and mouth when coughing or sneezing, to dispose of it properly, and to perform frequent hand-washing to control transmitting the infection.

(Performance checklist next page)

PERFORMANCE CHECKLIST

When suctioning a tracheostomy, the learner:

C	A	U	
[ ]	[ ]	[ ]	Washes hands before contact with the client
[ ]	[ ]	[ ]	Provides privacy
[ ]	[ ]	[ ]	Makes pertinent assessments
[ ]	[ ]	[ ]	Assembles the suction equipment
[ ]	[ ]	[ ]	Positions the client either in semi-Fowler's or Fowler's position; alternatively utilizes a lateral position for an unconscious client
[ ]	[ ]	[ ]	Preoxygenates the client
[ ]	[ ]	[ ]	Drapes the client
[ ]	[ ]	[ ]	Tests the function of the suction equipment
[ ]	[ ]	[ ]	Opens the suction kit or separate equipment
[ ]	[ ]	[ ]	Adds rinsing solution to a sterile container
[ ]	[ ]	[ ]	Dons at least one sterile glove on the dominant hand
[ ]	[ ]	[ ]	Connects the sterile catheter to the tubing
[ ]	[ ]	[ ]	Lubricates or moistens the catheter tip
[ ]	[ ]	[ ]	Removes the oxygen equipment
[ ]	[ ]	[ ]	Inserts the suction catheter gently to the depth desired
[ ]	[ ]	[ ]	Occludes the vent when fully inserted
[ ]	[ ]	[ ]	Rotates the catheter while removing it over a 10-second period
[ ]	[ ]	[ ]	Rinses the catheter
[ ]	[ ]	[ ]	Readministers oxygen
[ ]	[ ]	[ ]	Evaluates the efficacy of the treatment and the client's recovery
[ ]	[ ]	[ ]	Repeats suctioning, if necessary
[ ]	[ ]	[ ]	Turns off the source of suction
[ ]	[ ]	[ ]	Disconnects the catheter from the tubing
[ ]	[ ]	[ ]	Removes the glove over the catheter
[ ]	[ ]	[ ]	Washes hands
[ ]	[ ]	[ ]	Attends to the client's comfort
[ ]	[ ]	[ ]	Gathers repeat focus assessments
[ ]	[ ]	[ ]	Washes hands
[ ]	[ ]	[ ]	Charts significant information

Outcome: [ ] Pass   [ ] Fail

C = competent; A = acceptable; U = unsatisfactory

Comments: _____

_____

_____

_____   _____
Student's Signature   Date

_____   _____
Instructor's Signature   Date

RELATED LITERATURE

PROCEDURE VI-1 ADMINISTERING OXYGEN

Ahrens TS: Concepts in the assessment of oxygenation. Focus on Critical Care 14(1):36–44, February 1987

Chatburn RL, Primiano FP Jr: A rational basis for humidity therapy. Respiratory Care 32(4): 249–254, April 1987

D'Epiro P: Prescribing home oxygen therapy. Patient Care 21(9):91–93, 96, May 15, 1987

D'Epiro P: When the patient needs oxygen—stat. Patient Care 21(9):83–86, 89, May 15, 1987

Herman JC: New oxygen delivery systems. Respiratory Management 17(3):30–32, 34+, May–June, 1987

Jenkinson SG: Oxygen toxicity: Part 1. Current Reviews for Respiratory and Critical Care 9(14):111–116, April 9, 1987

Jenkinson SG: Oxygen toxicity: Part 2. Current Reviews for Respiratory and Critical Care 9(15):118–124, April 23, 1987

Mims BC: The risks of oxygen therapy. RN 50(7):20–26, July 1987

Petty TL: New developments in home oxygen therapy. Respiratory Management 17(3):24, 27, 29, May–June 1987

Questions and answers about oxygen therapy. Patient Care 21(9):174, 177, May 15, 1987

Tiep BL: New portable oxygen devices. Respiratory Care 32(2):106–112, February 1987

Transtracheal oxygen: The nose knows the difference. Am J Nurs 87(4):421–422, April 1987

PROCEDURE VI-2 SUCTIONING THE NASOPHARYNGEAL AND OROPHARYNGEAL AREAS

Hoffman LA, Maszkiewicz RC: Airway management for the critically ill patient. Am J Nurs 87(1):39–53, January 1987

Ritz R, Scott LR, Coyle MB: Contamination of a multiple-use suction catheter in a closed circuit system compared to contamination of a disposable, single-use suction catheter. Respiratory Care 31(11):1086–1091, November 1986

Shekleton ME, Nield M: Ineffective airway clearance related to artificial airway. Nurs Clin North Am 22(1):167–178, March 1987

PROCEDURE VI-3 CLEARING AN OBSTRUCTED AIRWAY

Castleman M: What should you do? . . . the Heimlich maneuver. Medical SelfCare 39:19, March–April 1987

Decker SJ: The patient with an obstructed airway. Topics in Emergency Medicine 8(4):1–12, January 1987

DeVito AJ, Kleven M: Dyspnea: Finding the cause. Treating the symptoms. RN 50(6):40–46, June 1987

Eggler D: The Heimlich maneuver: Mandatory for nursing home employees. Geriatric Nursing 8(1):26–27, January–February 1987

First aid for a choking child. Patient Care 21(13):222–224, August 15, 1987

Walkenstein MD: Upper airway obstruction: An often overlooked cause of respiratory failure. Emergency Medicine 19(13):133–134, 136–138, July, 1987

**PROCEDURE VI-4
SUCTIONING THE
TRACHEOSTOMY**

Bostick J, Wendelgass ST: Normal saline instillation as part of the suctioning procedure: Effects on PaO_2 and amount of secretions. Heart & Lung: Journal of Critical Care 16(5): 532–537, September 1987

Chulay M: Hyperinflation/hyperoxygenation prevent endotracheal suctioning complications. Critical Care Nurse 7(2):100–102, March–April 1987

Feinstein D: What to teach the patient who's had a total laryngectomy. RN 50(4):53–54, April 1987

Hanley MV, Tyler ML: Ineffective airway clearance related to airway infection. Nurs Clin North Am 22(1):135–150, March, 1987

Hoffman LA: Ineffective airway clearance related to neuromuscular dysfunction. Nurs Clin North Am 22(1):151–166, March, 1987

Lockhart JS, Griffin C: Action STAT! Occluded trach tube. Nursing '87 17(4):33, April 1987

Pierce JB, Piazza DE: Differences in postsuctioning arterial blood oxygen concentration values using two postoxygenation methods. Heart & Lung: Journal of Critical Care 16(1):34–38, January 1987

Walsh CM, Bada HS, Korones SB: Controlled supplemental oxygenation during tracheobronchial hygiene. Nurs Res 36(4):211–215, July–August 1987

VII Procedures pertaining to urinary elimination

VII-1

Offering and removing a bedpan or urinal

Optimal elimination occurs when a client can use a toilet. People in Western cultures have been conditioned to feel more comfortable when eliminating in private. However, there are varying circumstances that require hospitalized clients to use a bedpan or urinal for elimination. The sensitive nurse understands that this situation is less than desirable.

PURPOSES OF PROCEDURE

A bedpan or urinal is offered and removed to

1. Facilitate bowel and bladder elimination when the client's level of activity is restricted
2. Collect specimens
3. Promote continence during bowel and bladder retraining

ASSESSMENT

OBJECTIVE DATA

- Read the client's record to determine past or present illnesses, such as diverticulosis, that may affect the processes of elimination.
- Refer to the client's record of bowel and urinary elimination to determine the pattern since admission to the agency.
- Review the list of current medications, such as narcotic analgesics or diuretic drugs, and diagnostic tests, such as an earlier upper gastrointestinal x-ray study, that can affect elimination.
- Observe the contour of the abdomen for distention. A protruding abdomen may indicate weak abdominal muscles that could affect the effort for expelling stool or urine.
- Auscultate bowel sounds throughout all quadrants.
- Note the client's strength and ability to lift and turn his body.
- Determine if the client can sit with his head elevated or stand at the bedside.

SUBJECTIVE DATA

- Ask the client to indicate when he last moved his bowels and emptied his bladder.
- Question the client on his usual patterns for elimination, such as frequency, time of day, description of the usual characteristics of his stool and urine.
- Encourage the client to discuss any problems with elimination or recent changes in usual patterns.
- Inquire about any aids the client has used to facilitate elimination.

RELEVANT NURSING DIAGNOSES

The client who uses a bedpan or urinal may have nursing diagnoses, such as

- *Altered Bowel Elimination*
- *Altered Patterns of Urinary Elimination*
- *Anxiety*
- *Self-Care Deficit: Toileting*
- *Potential Impaired Skin Integrity*
- *Disturbance in Self-Concept*

PLANNING

ESTABLISHING PRIORITIES

Elimination of waste products is a natural process critical to human functioning. Many clients feel uncomfortable about using a bedpan or urinal for elimination. The nurse can communicate to all clients that postponing the urge to eliminate can lead to more severe problems. Offering the use of a bedpan or urinal before and after meals and at bedtime may relieve the client's embarrassment or self-consciousness.

SETTING GOALS

- The client will use the bedpan or urinal for bladder or bowel elimination.
- The client's privacy will be maintained during the use of the bedpan or urinal.

PREPARATION OF EQUIPMENT

The nurse will need selected items from the following list when offering and removing a bedpan or urinal:

Bedpan or urinal
Toilet tissue
Handwashing supplies
Cover for the bedpan or urinal (cloth or disposable pad)

Technique for offering and removing a bedpan or urinal

ACTION	RATIONALE
1. Make appropriate assessments.	The nurse uses information as a basis for planning care.
2. Bring the bedpan or urinal and equipment to the bedside.	Having the equipment on hand saves time by avoiding unnecessary trips to the storage area.
3. Warm the bedpan, if it is made of metal, by rinsing it with warm water.	A cold bedpan feels uncomfortable and may make it difficult for the client to void. Plastic bedpans do not require warming.
4. Place an adjustable bed in the high position.	Having the bed in the high position reduces strain on the nurse's back when assisting the client onto the bedpan.
5. Place the bedpan or urinal on the chair next to the bed or on the foot of the bed. Fold the top linen back just enough to allow for placement of the bedpan or urinal.	Folding back the linen in this manner prevents unnecessary exposure while still allowing the nurse to place the bedpan or urinal.
6. If the client needs assistance to move onto the bedpan, have him bend his knees and rest some of his weight on his heels. Lift the client by placing one hand under his lower back, and slip the bedpan into place with the other hand, as shown in Figure VII-1-1.	The client uses less energy as the nurse assists by lifting him onto the bedpan. The nurse uses less energy when the client can assist by placing some of his weight on his heels.
7. Two people may be required to lift an entirely helpless client onto the bedpan. Or, the client may be placed on his side, the bedpan is placed against his buttocks, and the client is rolled back onto the bedpan, as Figure VII-1-2 illustrates.	Having two people lift a helpless client causes less strain on the nurse's back. Rolling the client takes less energy than lifting the client onto a bedpan.
8. When the bedpan is in the proper place, the client's buttocks rest on the rounded shelf of the bedpan, as Figure VII-1-3 illustrates. The urinal is properly placed between slightly spread legs, with the penis positioned in it, and with the urinal resting on the bed, as shown in Figure VII-1-4.	Having the bedpan or urinal in the proper place prevents spilling contents onto the bed and prevents injury to the skin from a misplaced bedpan.
9. If permitted, raise the head of the bed as near to the sitting position as tolerated.	This position generally makes it easier for the client to void or defecate, avoids strain on the client's back, and allows gravity to aid in elimination.

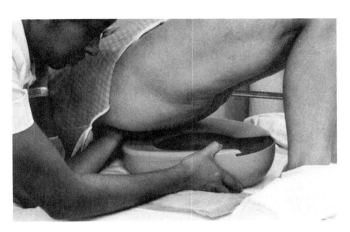

Figure VII-1-1 The nurse places the bedpan under the client's buttocks. The client is able to help lift his own weight from the bed.

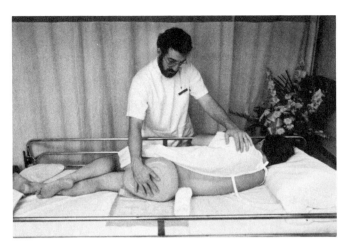

Figure VII-1-2 This client is not strong enough to lift his own weight. Rather than risk back strain trying to lift the client, the nurse turns the client to the side and places the bedpan against the buttocks.

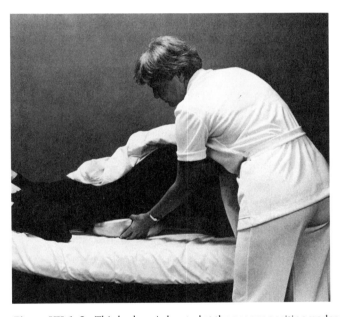

Figure VII-1-3 This bedpan is located at the proper position under the client's buttocks.

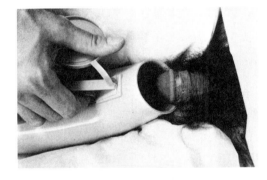

Figure VII-1-4 The nurse helps position the penis within the urinal.

10. Place the call device and toilet tissue within easy reach. Leave the client if it is safe to do so. Use side rails appropriately.

11. Remove the bedpan in the same manner in which it was offered, being careful to hold it steady. If it is necessary to assist the client, wrap tissue around the hand several times, and wipe the client clean, using one stroke from the pubic area toward the anal area. Discard the tissue, and use more until the client is clean. Place the client on his side, and spread the buttocks to clean the anal area. Cover the bedpan.

12. Do not place the toilet tissue in the bedpan if a specimen is required or if measurement of urine elim-

Falls can be prevented when the client does not have to reach for needed items. Side rails are an additional safety precaution. Leaving the client alone, if possible, promotes self-esteem and respects privacy.

Holding the bedpan steady prevents spilling its contents. Cleaning the area from front to back minimizes fecal contamination of the vagina and urinary meatus. Cleaning the client after he has used the bedpan prevents offensive odors and irritation to the skin.

Toilet tissue mixed with a specimen makes laboratory examination more difficult and also interferes with ac-

ination is required. Have a receptacle handy for discarding the tissue.

13. Offer the client supplies to wash and dry his hands, assisting him as necessary.

14. Collect the specimen as necessary, following agency procedure. Empty and clean the bedpan and urinal. Record according to agency policy.

curate output measurement.

Washing hands after using the bedpan or urinal helps prevent the spread of organisms.

Following protocols ensures accuracy and uniformity within an agency.

SAMPLE DOCUMENTATION

Date	Time	Nurse's note
12/14	2120	Lg. amt. of brown formed stool expelled in bedpan 15 min. p̄ adm. of suppository.
		G. Farr, RN

EVALUATION

REASSESSMENT

Continue to record and evaluate the frequency of elimination. Note the characteristics of stool and urine. Irregular elimination is likely to cause the stool to be drier and more difficult to pass. Urine may appear dark in color and emit a strong odor. Inspect the perineum and perianal area for proper wiping and cleansing. Note the appearance of hemorrhoids or fresh bleeding when the client experiences constipation. Examine the skin over the coccyx for signs of breakdown from pressure caused by sitting or lying on the hard surface of the bedpan.

EXPECTED OUTCOMES

The client uses the bedpan or urinal when necessary.
The skin remains intact.
Handwashing and hygiene follow elimination.

UNEXPECTED OUTCOMES

The client resists using the bedpan or urinal by delaying elimination.
The client develops complications from retaining stool or urine, such as retention with overflow, constipation, and so on.
Skin over the coccyx breaks down.
Handwashing is ignored following elimination.

MODIFICATIONS IN SELECTED SITUATIONS

GENERAL VARIATIONS

Request that visitors in the room leave when the client has the need to use the bedpan or urinal.
Answer the call light as soon as the signal is noted. Use an air freshener to control odors.
Attach an overbed trapeze to the bed so that the client can assist with lifting when being placed on a bedpan.
A fracture pan, shown in Figure VII-1-5, may be substituted when it is difficult or uncomfortable to use a regular bedpan.

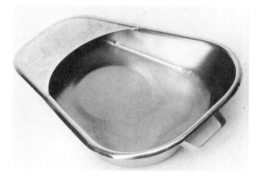

Figure VII-1-5 A fracture bedpan is tapered in the area on which the buttocks rest. It is used primarily by individuals with orthopedic injuries.

Place a disposable, absorbent pad beneath a fracture bedpan so that if the contents overflow, the linen will not have to be changed completely.

If it is difficult to slide a client onto the bedpan, powder may be used on the resting surfaces of the pan to eliminate friction. Powder should not be used if a specimen is required because contamination could result.

Roll one or two towels into the form of a tube and place them in the lumbar curve when a client cannot be raised to a sitting position on the bedpan.

Use a urinal holder that attaches to the bed for easy access by the client rather than leaving the urinal rest on the bedside stand or overbed table.

Protect the anal area of a plaster hip spica cast before placing the client on a fracture bedpan. Use kitchen plastic wrap and tuck one end inside the cast. The cellophane acts as a barrier to moisture from urine and stool. The plastic wrap can be discarded in a lined waste receptacle after each use of the bedpan. A cast that becomes saturated with urine or stool can emit an offensive odor. The soiled cast material may disintegrate and lead to skin breakdown.

Help male clients to stand at the bedside when using a urinal whenever this is possible. Standing to void is the most natural position for men.

AGE-RELATED VARIATIONS

Use a smaller-sized bedpan for pediatric clients.

A U-bag, a self-adhesive collection bag, can be placed over a male infant's penis and scrotum when collecting a specimen. It may also be used for females, but not as satisfactorily.

HOME-HEALTH VARIATIONS

Clients who are capable of lifting themselves onto the bedpan may prefer to keep the bedpan beside them concealed with a cover.

If the bedpan or urinal does not fit under the lavatory faucet for rinsing, use liquid detergent bottles filled with soapy solution to rinse the bedpan.

Recommend cleaning a bedpan or urinal with diluted bleach and cool soapy water. Odors in plastic bedpans or urinals may be reduced by soaking the equipment in a white vinegar solution.

RELATED TEACHING

Explain that squatting or sitting slightly forward with the thighs flexed is the optimal position for bowel elimination. Toddlers who are being toilet-trained do better with a miniature commode that permits them to push their feet against a firm surface, like the floor.

Tell the client who is concerned about incontinence to avoid sitting for prolonged periods on the bedpan. Pressure and shearing force can lead to impairment in skin integrity.

Advise home-care clients that in order to reduce the transmission of organisms, the bedpan in current use should be stored in an area at the bedside separate from other equipment, such as a drinking glass, wash basin, and so on.

Female clients often need to be taught the proper technique for perineal care after urination. Wiping of the perineal area should be from the urethra toward the rectum. The reverse direction can result in fecal organisms being introduced into the urethra or vagina. This type of contamination is a common cause of urinary tract and vaginal infections.

(Performance checklist next page)

PERFORMANCE CHECKLIST

When offering and removing a bedpan or urinal, the learner:

C	A	U	
[ ]	[ ]	[ ]	Pulls the curtain to provide privacy
[ ]	[ ]	[ ]	Removes the bedpan or urinal from its stored area
[ ]	[ ]	[ ]	Warms a metal container
[ ]	[ ]	[ ]	Raises the height of the bed
[ ]	[ ]	[ ]	Folds back the linen for proper placement
[ ]	[ ]	[ ]	Instructs the client to raise the buttocks, if possible
[ ]	[ ]	[ ]	Places the bedpan beneath the buttocks
[ ]	[ ]	[ ]	Raises the head of the bed
[ ]	[ ]	[ ]	Provides toilet tissue and the signal cord
[ ]	[ ]	[ ]	Raises the side rail
[ ]	[ ]	[ ]	Leaves the room and shuts the door
[ ]	[ ]	[ ]	Washes hands
[ ]	[ ]	[ ]	Watches and returns to the client when signaled
[ ]	[ ]	[ ]	Removes the bedpan
[ ]	[ ]	[ ]	Assists with cleaning the rectum or urethra
[ ]	[ ]	[ ]	Covers the bedpan
[ ]	[ ]	[ ]	Measures the volume of urine, if the client's intake and output are being assessed
[ ]	[ ]	[ ]	Empties the contents of the bedpan or urinal, noting the characteristics of the stool and urine
[ ]	[ ]	[ ]	Rinses and cleans the inner areas of the equipment
[ ]	[ ]	[ ]	Replaces the bedpan or urinal in the appropriate location
[ ]	[ ]	[ ]	Provides soap, washcloth, and basin of water for handwashing or offers the client a disposable wipe
[ ]	[ ]	[ ]	Washes own hands
[ ]	[ ]	[ ]	Uses air freshener, if necessary
[ ]	[ ]	[ ]	Makes client comfortable
[ ]	[ ]	[ ]	Charts significant information

Outcome: [ ] Pass   [ ] Fail

C = competent; A = acceptable; U = unsatisfactory

Comments: _____

_____

_____

_____   _____
Student's Signature   Date

_____   _____
Instructor's Signature   Date

VII-2 *Catheterizing the female and male urinary bladder*

Urinary catheterization is the introduction of a catheter through the urethra into the bladder. A catheter is a tube used for instilling or removing fluids. Because catheterization increases the client's risk for acquiring a urinary tract infection, it is only used as a last resort when other measures for promoting continence and urinary elimination are less than adequate.

PURPOSES OF PROCEDURE

Catheterization is performed to

1. Control urinary incontinence
2. Relieve urinary retention
3. Obtain a sterile urine specimen
4. Measure the residual urine remaining in the bladder after voiding
5. Maintain an empty bladder during surgery
6. Provide access for instilling medication into the bladder
7. Monitor hourly urine production in seriously ill clients

ASSESSMENT

OBJECTIVE DATA

- Note the ability of the client to control urine voluntarily within the bladder and the ability to void spontaneously. Note any involuntary escape of urine or the inability to void.
- Measure the quantity of urine. The adult bladder holds 400 ml to 500 ml but can accommodate up to 1000 ml to 1800 ml. Usually the urge to void occurs when stretch receptors in the bladder are stimulated by the presence of 200 ml to 300 ml of urine. This would mean that an adult with normal fluid intake would void approximately 5 to 8 times a day.
- Check the trends in the client's intake and output, if these data are available.
- Palpate the bladder above the symphysis pubis. It ought not to be identifiable unless distended with urine.
- Percuss over the lower abdomen. A dull sound indicates that the bladder contains urine.
- Observe the gross characteristics of voided urine. Note its color, transparency, and odor.
- Use a dipstick to test for abnormal components in urine, such as blood, albumin, sugar, ketones, and bilirubin.
- Use a urinometer, hydrometer or spectrometer to test the specific gravity.
- Monitor the laboratory urinalysis results.
- Review the conclusions of x-ray studies and other diagnostic tests involving kidney function.
- Scan the list of medications for those that can alter urinary elimination, such as diuretics, nephrotoxic antibiotics, and cholinergic and anticholinergic drugs.
- Note medical conditions that influence urinary elimination, such as an enlarged prostate gland, diabetes mellitus or diabetes insipidus, paraplegia or hemiplegia, and so on.

- Inspect the urinary meatus. Look for signs of inflammation and the odor of urine or ammonia that may be present on the surrounding skin. Note if a male is circumcised or uncircumcised.
- Observe the integrity of the skin in the perineal area.
- Check the written medical order indicating the directives for inserting a catheter.

SUBJECTIVE DATA

- Ask the client to describe his usual patterns of urinary elimination. Specifically ask about nocturia, the ability to initiate urination, and any change in the force of the stream.
- Determine the client's usual daily intake of fluids.
- Ask the client to indicate if he or she experiences frequency, urgency, burning, or back or flank pain.
- Inquire as to the female client's practice of using hygiene products such as bubble bath or perineal sprays.

RELEVANT NURSING DIAGNOSES

Depending on the cluster of data obtained, the nurse may identify nursing diagnoses, such as

- *Altered Patterns of Urinary Elimination, such as Reflex Incontinence, Total Incontinence, or Urinary Retention*
- *Anxiety*
- *Altered Comfort*
- *Potential for Infection*
- *Impaired Skin Integrity*
- *Sleep Pattern Disturbance*
- *Self-Care Deficit: Toileting*
- *Disturbance in Self-Concept*
- *Knowledge Deficit*

PLANNING

ESTABLISHING PRIORITIES

The nurse should plan to relieve a distended bladder as soon as possible. Filling beyond the bladder's normal capacity can lead to serious consequences, such as hydronephrosis. The nurse should also be prepared to act quickly when there is a need to measure residual urine. The volume of residual urine remaining in the bladder should be measured immediately after voiding to obtain valid data because urine is produced continuously. Other circumstances also require that the planning of care be adapted to accommodate catheterization, such as when the procedure is part of the client's preoperative preparation.

SETTING GOALS

- The catheter will be inserted within the bladder.
- Urine will drain from the catheter.
- The catheter will remain patent throughout its use.
- The client will remain free of urinary tract infection.

PREPARATION OF EQUIPMENT

The nurse will need the following when preparing to catheterize a female or male client:

Sterile catheterization kit containing
    Sterile gloves
    Sterile drapes (one of which is fenestrated)
    Antiseptic solution
    Lubricant
    Cotton balls or gauze squares
    Forceps
    Prefilled syringe
    Basin (base of kit usually serves as this)
    Specimen container
Straight or indwelling catheter
Flashlight or lamp

Urine collection bag and drainage tubing (may be connected to a sterile indwelling catheter if a closed drainage system is used)
Velcro leg strap or tape
Disposal bag (outside wrapper of kit can be used)
Waterproof pad

Technique for female catheterization of the urinary bladder (straight and indwelling)

ACTION	RATIONALE
1. Assemble equipment. Wash your hands. Explain the procedure and its purpose to the client.	Organization promotes efficient time management. Handwashing deters the spread of microorganisms. An explanation reduces apprehension and encourages co-operation.
2. Provide for good light. Artificial light is recommended (use of a flashlight requires an assistant to hold and position it).	Good lighting is necessary to see the meatus clearly.
3. Provide for privacy by closing curtains and door.	The client has the right to be protected from being seen by others.
4. Assist the client to the dorsal recumbent position with the knees flexed and the feet about 2 feet apart, and drape the client. Slide a waterproof pad under the client.	Good visualization of the meatus is important. Embarrassment, chilliness, and feeling tense can interfere with introducing the catheter. The comfort of the client will promote relaxation. A waterproof pad protects the bed linens from moisture.
5. Cleanse the genital and perineal area with warm soap and water if the area is noticeably soiled. Rinse and dry. Wash your hands again.	Cleansing the area with soap decreases the possibility of introducing organisms into the bladder.
6. Prepare the urine drainage tubing and bag if an indwelling catheter is to be inserted.	Extended tubing facilitates connecting the catheter to the drainage system.
7. Open the sterile catheterization tray on the overbed table using sterile technique.	Placement of the equipment near the work site increases efficiency. Sterile technique protects the client and prevents the spread of microorganisms.
8. Put on sterile gloves. Grasp the upper corners of the drape and unfold it without touching unsterile areas. Fold back a cuff over the gloved hands. Ask the client to lift the buttocks and slide the sterile drape underneath with gloves protected by the cuff, as shown in Figure VII-2-1.	A drape provides a sterile field below the area where the equipment and hands will be located. Covering the gloved hands helps keep the gloves sterile while placing the drape.

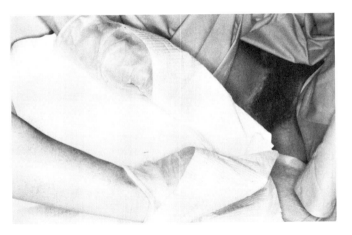

Figure VII-2-1 This nurse maintains the sterility of the gloves by forming a protective cuff while placing a drape beneath the client.

9. Place the fenestrated drape over the perineal area, exposing the labia.

10. Place the sterile tray on the drape between the client's thighs.

11. Open the contents within the tray.

   a. *If the catheter is to be indwelling,* test the catheter balloon, shown in Figure VII-2-2. Remove the protective cap on the tip of the syringe and attach the syringe prefilled with sterile water to the injection port. Instill the appropriate amount of fluid. If the balloon inflates properly, withdraw the fluid.

   b. Pour antiseptic solution over cotton balls or gauze. Open the specimen container if a specimen is to be obtained.

   c. Lubricate 1 inch to 2 inches of the catheter tip.

12. Pick up a moistened cotton ball using forceps. Wipe the labia majora on one side from the upper area toward the lower. Discard the cotton ball. Repeat on the opposite side.

13. With the thumb and one finger of your nondominant hand, spread the labia and identify the meatus, as

Exposing just the labia expands the sterile field. Some practitioners feel the use of a fenestrated drape limits visualization and is therefore considered optional.

Positioning the tray on the client's bed provides easy access to supplies.

Once a hand is used to separate the labia it cannot be used to touch the sterile contents in the kit.

A balloon that does not inflate or that leaks needs to be replaced prior to insertion in the client.

Opening containers with one hand would be awkward and likely to result in contamination.

Lubrication facilitates the insertion of the catheter and reduces trauma to the tissues.

Outer anatomical structures are cleansed first.

Separating the labia helps expose the meatus so its location is visible. Allowing the labia to drop back into

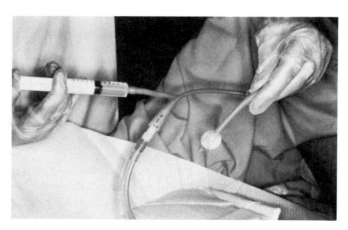

Figure VII-2-2 The nurse pretests the balloon by instilling fluid and observing if it inflates and remains intact.

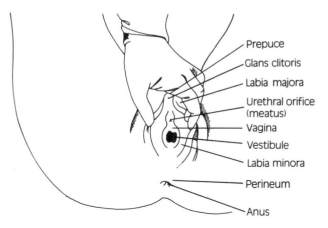

Figure VII-2-3 The nurse uses the nondominant hand to separate the labia majora and labia minora to expose the urinary meatus.

shown in Figure VII-2-3. Be prepared to maintain separation of the labia with that hand until urine is flowing well and continuously.

14. Using separate cotton balls held with forceps, cleanse the inner labial folds and then directly over the meatus, as shown in Figure VII-2-4. Move the cotton ball from above the meatus down toward the rectum. Discard each cotton ball after one downward stroke.

15. With the uncontaminated gloved hand, place the drainage end of the catheter in the basin. For inserting an indwelling catheter that is *preattached* to sterile tubing and a drainage container (closed drainage system), position the catheter and the bag within easy reach on the sterile field.

position may contaminate the area around the meatus, as well as the catheter. Your nondominant hand is contaminated when the labia is separated.

Cleansing the meatus last helps reduce the possibility of introducing organisms into the bladder.

Placing the catheter as described facilitates collecting the draining urine and minimizes the risk of contaminating sterile equipment.

16. Insert the catheter tip into the meatus, shown in Figure VII-2-5, 5 cm to 7.5 cm (2 inches to 3 inches) or until urine flows. Do not use force to push the catheter through the urethra into the bladder. Ask the client to breathe deeply, and rotate the catheter gently if slight resistance is met as the catheter reaches the sphincter. *For an indwelling catheter,* once urine drains, advance the catheter another ½ inch to 1 inch.

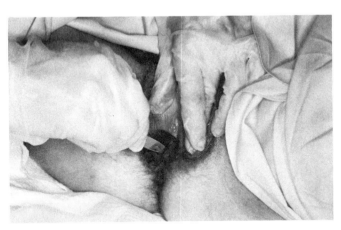

Figure VII-2-4 The labia and the meatus are cleansed with cotton balls that are saturated with antiseptic. Each cotton ball is used for one stroke starting at the upper portion of the vulva and moving toward the perineum. The meatus is the last area cleansed since it is the area that should be kept the cleanest.

17. Hold the catheter securely with your nondominant hand while the bladder empties. Collect a specimen, if required. Continue drainage according to agency policy.

18. Remove the catheter smoothly and slowly, if a straight catheterization was ordered.

19. If the catheter is to be indwelling

    a. Inflate the balloon, as the nurse in Figure VII-2-6 is doing, according to the manufacturer's recommendations.

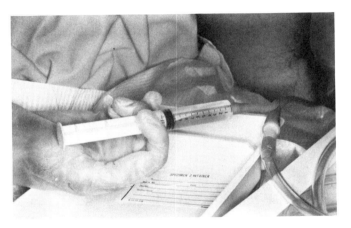

The female urethra is about 3.7 cm to 6.2 cm (1½ inches to 2½ inches) long. Applying force on the catheter is likely to injure mucous membranes. The sphincter relaxes and the catheter can enter the bladder easily when the client relaxes. Advancing an indwelling catheter an additional ½ inch to 1 inch ensures placement within the bladder and facilitates inflation of the balloon without damaging the urethra.

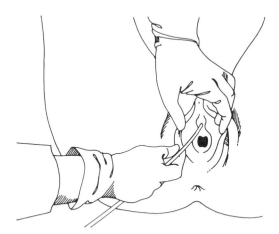

Figure VII-2-5 The labia are kept separated while the catheter tip is inserted into the meatus.

Movement, even though it is slight, increases the risk of introducing organisms within the urethra. In general, no more than 750 ml of urine should be removed at one time. Pelvic floor blood vessels may become engorged from the sudden release of pressure, leading to a possible hypotensive episode.

The catheter is only needed to drain urine presently in the bladder and is not intended for continuous use.

To drain continuously, the catheter will need to be retained within the bladder.

The balloon anchors the catheter so it cannot slip from the bladder. Sterile water is used as a precaution in case the balloon ruptures within the bladder.

Figure VII-2-6 The balloon is inflated with sterile water.

b. Tug gently on the catheter after the balloon is inflated to feel resistance, as shown in Figure VII-2-7.

Improper inflation can cause discomfort or displacement of the catheter.

c. Attach the catheter to the drainage system if necessary.

A drainage system collects urine so that it can be measured and assessed.

d. Secure the catheter to the upper thigh with a Velcro leg strap or tape. Leave some slack in the catheter to allow for leg movement.

Proper attachment prevents trauma to the urethra and meatus from tension on the tubing.

e. Hang the drainage collector from the bed frame, shown in Figure VII-2-8. Check that the drainage tubing is not kinked and that movement of the side rails does not interfere with the catheter or drainage bag.

Preventing obstruction facilitates drainage of urine and prevents stasis within the bladder or back flow to the ureters and kidneys.

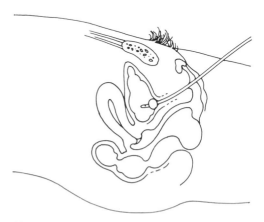

Figure VII-2–7 Applying gentle traction on the catheter is a method for assessing the inflated balloon's effectiveness in retaining the catheter within the bladder.

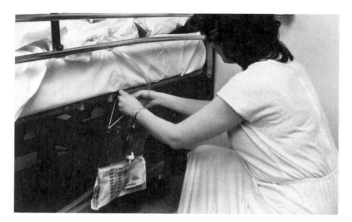

Figure VII-2–8 The catheter drainage tubing should hang straight from the bed into the bag. It should be secured in such a way that parts of the bed will not obstruct the flow of urine.

20. Remove the equipment and make the client comfortable in bed. Cleanse and dry the perineal area, if necessary. Care for the equipment according to agency policy. Send urine specimen to the laboratory promptly or refrigerate it.

Urine kept at room temperature may cause organisms, if present, to grow and distort laboratory findings.

21. Wash your hands.

Handwashing deters the spread of microorganisms.

22. Record the time of the catheterization, the amount of the urine removed, a description of the urine, the client's reaction to the procedure, and your name.

A careful record is important for documenting data that affect the client's care.

Technique for male catheterization of the urinary bladder (straight and indwelling)

ACTION

RATIONALE

1. Assemble the equipment and follow Steps 1 through 3 for female catheterization, above.

2. Position the male client on his back with the legs extended and the thighs slightly apart. Drape the client so that only the area around the penis is exposed.

The male urethra is readily accessible without flexing the hips or knees. Draping demonstrates respect for the client's modesty and prevents unnecessary exposure.

3. Follow steps 5 through 7 of the technique for female catheterization.

4. Put on sterile gloves. Open the sterile drape and place it on the client's thighs. Place the fenestrated drape with the opening over the penis.

Sterile gloves and drapes maintain surgical asepsis, thus reducing the risk of introducing microorganisms during the procedure.

5. Place the catheterization tray on the sterile drape that covers the client's legs.

The sterile tray can be placed without fear of contamination on the drape where it will be convenient for the nurse.

6. Open all supplies:

The nurse will need two hands to manipulate and prepare the contents of the kit. Once the nurse touches the client's penis, one hand is contaminated.

a. *If the catheter is to be indwelling,* test the catheter balloon. Remove the protective cap on the tip of the prefilled syringe and attach it to the injection port. Instill the appropriate amount of fluid. If the balloon inflates properly, withdraw the fluid.

A balloon that does not inflate or that leaks needs to be replaced prior to insertion in the client.

b. Pour antiseptic solution over the cotton balls. Open the specimen container if a specimen is to be obtained.

It is necessary to open all supplies while both hands are sterile.

7. *Generously* lubricate the catheter for about 15 cm to 18 cm (6 inches to 7 inches).

Generous lubrication is especially important because of the length and tortuousness of the male urethra. The lubricant decreases friction.

8. Lift the penis with your nondominant hand, which is then considered contaminated. Retract the foreskin in the uncircumcised male. Cleanse the area at the meatus, as the nurse in Figure VII-2-9 is doing, with a cotton ball held with the forceps. Use a circular motion; move from the meatus toward the base of the penis for three cleansings.

When a sterile object comes in contact with one that is nonsterile, it becomes contaminated with microorganisms. Cleansing the area around the meatus and under the foreskin in the uncircumcised male helps prevent infection. Moving from the meatus toward the base of the penis prevents bringing organisms to the meatus.

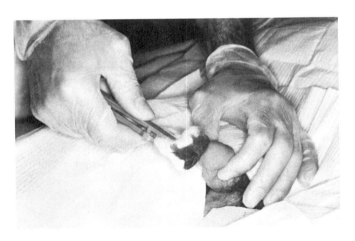

Figure VII-2–9 The meatus of the male is cleansed in a circular manner. Each cotton ball is used for only one complete rotation about the penis. The nurse cleanses from the tip of the penis outward from the meatus.

9. Hold the penis with slight upward tension and perpendicular to the body. Ask the client to bear down as if voiding. With your dominant hand, place the drainage end of the catheter in a compartment of the tray. For insertion of an indwelling catheter that is *preattached* to sterile tubing and drainage container (closed drainage system), position the system within easy reach on the sterile field.

Holding the penis up with slight tension helps straighten the urethra. Bearing down relaxes the external sphincter and may facilitate insertion. Placing the distal end of the catheter in the tray provides a means of collecting the urine without wetting the bed. A closed drainage system will provide immediate collection of urine in the drainage bag.

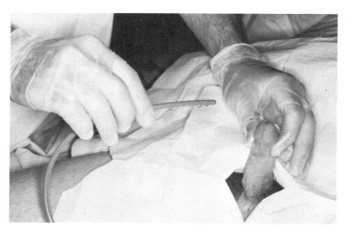

Figure VII-2-10 The nurse lubricates the catheter and inserts it into the meatus while holding the penis upward to straighten the urethra.

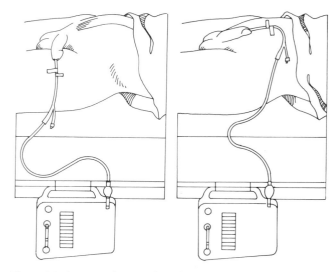

Figure VII-2-11 Utilizing either of these two anchoring methods is a safe manner for securing the catheter for a male.

10. Insert the tip of the catheter into the meatus, as shown in Figure VII-2-10. Advance the catheter 15 cm to 20 cm (6 inches to 8 inches) or until urine flows. Do not use force to introduce the catheter. If the catheter resists entry, ask the client to breathe deeply, and rotate the catheter slightly. *For an indwelling catheter,* once urine drains, advance the catheter another ½ inch to 1 inch. Lower the penis.

11. Follow Steps 16 through 21 for female catheterization, except that the catheter may be secured to the upper thigh or lower abdomen, as shown in Figure VII-2-11. Slack should be left in the catheter to prevent tension.

The male urethra is about 20 cm long. Deep breaths or slight twisting of the catheter may ease the catheter past the resistance of the sphincters. Advancing an indwelling catheter an additional ½ inch to 1 inch ensures placement in the bladder and facilitates inflation of the balloon without damaging the urethra.

Stabilizing the catheter in either of these two positions prevents irritation at the angle of the penis and the scrotum.

SAMPLE DOCUMENTATION

Date	Time	Nurse's note
8/22	1830	No urine elimination since before vaginal delivery @ 0900 today. Bladder can be felt to extend 2 inches above the symphysis pubis. Unsuccessful in efforts to urinate following sitz bath. #14 Foley catheter inserted. 750 ml of clear light amber urine obtained. Balloon inflated and catheter clamped. To be released and clamped at 2-hr intervals and removed in AM.

W. Smietanski, RN

EVALUATION

REASSESSMENT

The nurse should observe and record the volume of urine at 8-hour intervals. The appearance of abnormal characteristics warrants notifying the physician. The client's temperature, pulse, and subjective symptoms can indicate the presence of infection. Though agencies generally have written protocols indicating the frequency for changing indwelling catheters, the nurse can individually evaluate the need by noting patency of the catheter and the collection of crystallized sediment within the rubber tubing. Inspect the appearance of the meatus during daily hygiene.

EXPECTED OUTCOMES

The catheter is inserted without difficulty and drains urine immediately.
The purpose for catheterization is achieved.

UNEXPECTED OUTCOMES

The meatus is not identifiable due to anatomic abnormality.
Resistance is apparent and cannot be overcome during insertion.
No urine drains from the catheter.

MODIFICATIONS IN SELECTED SITUATIONS

GENERAL VARIATIONS

A female who cannot bend her hips or knees may be placed in a lateral or Sims' position during catheterization. Place the buttocks near the edge of the bed with the shoulders at the opposite edge and the knees drawn toward the chest, as shown in Figure VII-2-12.

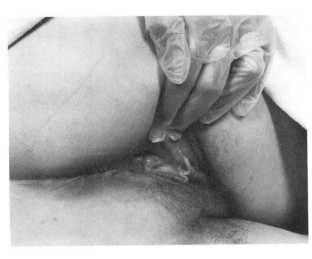

Figure VII-2-12 This female client has been placed in a side-lying position to expose the urinary meatus. The traditional dorsal recumbent position can be painful or impossible for some clients to assume.

When a catheter is inadvertently placed in the vagina, leave it there temporarily. Reattempt to locate the urinary meatus. Eliminate the orifice originally used. Remove the incorrectly placed catheter when the procedure is completed.

Use Teflon-coated or silicone-coated catheters when the client will require long-term use. These are less likely to collect sediment and will not need changing as frequently. Each time a catheter is changed, there is an increase in the risk of infection.

Support the female client's buttocks on a firm cushion if the mattress is soft. A soft mattress lowers the pelvic structures and makes visualization of the meatus difficult.

Proceed with extreme care when catheterizing a woman following a vaginal delivery. A good light is essential because the meatus may be difficult to find due to local swelling. Gentle retraction of the labia and insertion of the catheter help avoid additional perineal discomfort.

Replace the retracted foreskin of an uncircumcised male following catheterization. If left retracted, it could act as a tourniquet about the lower end of the penis.

AGE-RELATED VARIATIONS

Perform a catheterization on an infant or child in a manner similar to an adult. Differences include the size of the catheter that is used and the length to which it is inserted.

Obtain assistance from a parent or other staff person to immobilize the hands or body of a child who must be catheterized. The nurse will be limited in controlling a child while maintaining sterile technique. A papoose board may be used if no other alternative is possible.

Catheterization may seem similar to sexual assault to a young child. It is helpful to have a parent present during the explanation and performance of the procedure.

With children who can cooperate, have them practice deep breathing exercises before catheterization. Deep breathing helps promote relaxation and provides the child with some feeling of control during the procedure.

HOME-HEALTH VARIATIONS

Adults and children can be taught to perform intermittent self-catheterization using clean rather than sterile technique. The bladder's natural resistance to microorganisms normally found in the home makes sterile technique unnecessary. Rubber catheters must be washed thoroughly before boiling for 20 minutes. Dry and store them properly for the next use.

Store dry, sterile catheters in sterile baby food jars.

Teach the client or caregivers that when collecting a urine specimen from a catheter, the catheter should be clamped for a half hour. The tubing is disconnected and urine is collected from the proximal end of the catheter, not the urine collection bag.

RELATED TEACHING

Prior to catheterization, the client should be given an adequate explanation of the procedure and the reason for it. It should be explained that the client can expect to feel pressure and some discomfort when the catheter is inserted.

Instruct catheterized clients to drink sufficient fluids as a means of diluting the urine and promoting drainage. Drinking 8 to 10 (8-oz) glasses of liquid per day is an appropriate goal.

Suggest methods of acidifying the urine, such as drinking cranberry juice or beverages high in ascorbic acid, as a means of reducing the risk of infection.

Explain the concept of measuring intake and output. Provide the client with supplies for recording the fluid he consumes from his carafe of water. Instruct the client to remind whomever removes his dietary tray to record the liquids he has consumed.

Tell the client to avoid lying on the tubing to maintain continuous drainage. Explain that the drainage collection bag should always remain lower than bladder level.

PERFORMANCE CHECKLIST

When catheterizing a client, the learner:

C	A	U	
[ ]	[ ]	[ ]	Obtains appropriate assessment data
[ ]	[ ]	[ ]	Reads the written medical order
[ ]	[ ]	[ ]	Assembles equipment
[ ]	[ ]	[ ]	Explains the procedure to the client
[ ]	[ ]	[ ]	Provides privacy
[ ]	[ ]	[ ]	Raises the bed
[ ]	[ ]	[ ]	Covers the client with a cotton bath blanket
[ ]	[ ]	[ ]	Folds down the top covers
[ ]	[ ]	[ ]	Secures adequate lighting
[ ]	[ ]	[ ]	Positions the client appropriately
[ ]	[ ]	[ ]	Washes hands
[ ]	[ ]	[ ]	Opens the sterile catheterization kit
[ ]	[ ]	[ ]	Dons sterile gloves
[ ]	[ ]	[ ]	Places sterile drape(s)
[ ]	[ ]	[ ]	Opens and prepares equipment on the catheterization tray

C = competent; A = acceptable; U = unsatisfactory

(Continued)

PERFORMANCE CHECKLIST (*Continued*)

C	A	U	
[ ]	[ ]	[ ]	Tests the balloon of an indwelling catheter
[ ]	[ ]	[ ]	Lubricates the tip of the catheter
[ ]	[ ]	[ ]	Pours antiseptic over the cotton balls
[ ]	[ ]	[ ]	Cleanses the area according to the principles of medical asepsis
[ ]	[ ]	[ ]	Inserts the catheter the appropriate distance for a female or male
[ ]	[ ]	[ ]	Observes for urine draining from the catheter
[ ]	[ ]	[ ]	Drains the bladder or collects the specimen if the catheter is not intended for continuous drainage
[ ]	[ ]	[ ]	Advances the catheter slightly further and inflates the balloon if the catheter will remain indwelling
[ ]	[ ]	[ ]	Tests that the balloon holds the catheter in place
[ ]	[ ]	[ ]	Attaches the end of the catheter to the drainage collector
[ ]	[ ]	[ ]	Removes gloves
[ ]	[ ]	[ ]	Secures the catheter to the client's body
[ ]	[ ]	[ ]	Attaches the drainage bag to the bed frame
[ ]	[ ]	[ ]	Stabilizes the tubing in a straight line to the drainage bag
[ ]	[ ]	[ ]	Removes supplies from the bed
[ ]	[ ]	[ ]	Lowers the bed
[ ]	[ ]	[ ]	Makes the client comfortable
[ ]	[ ]	[ ]	Raises the side rail
[ ]	[ ]	[ ]	Measures the urine and notes its characteristics
[ ]	[ ]	[ ]	Removes soiled equipment from the room
[ ]	[ ]	[ ]	Washes hands
[ ]	[ ]	[ ]	Charts significant information
[ ]	[ ]	[ ]	Returns to reassess the client

Outcome: [ ] Pass   [ ] Fail

Comments: _____
_____
_____

_____   _____
         Student's Signature   Date

_____   _____
        Instructor's Signature   Date

VII-3 *Applying a condom catheter*

A condom catheter, shown in Figure VII-3-1, is a device made of soft pliable plastic or rubberized material that is applied over the penis. It is an alternative to an indwelling catheter. It can be connected to a leg bag during the day and a drainage bag at night.

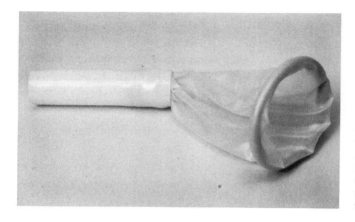

Figure VII-3–1 An example of one of the various types of external catheters available from medical-supply stores. Since these come in various sizes and methods for maintaining their attachment, it may be wise to try several before determining which product is most satisfactory for the individual.

PURPOSES OF PROCEDURE

An external catheter is used to

1. Keep an incontinent male client dry
2. Simplify home care for an incontinent client
3. Reduce the risk of an ascending urinary tract infection

ASSESSMENT

OBJECTIVE DATA

In addition to the information provided in Procedure VII-2, include the following:

• Inspect the skin of the penis for integrity.

RELEVANT NURSING DIAGNOSES

The client who is a candidate for using a condom catheter may have nursing diagnoses, such as

• *Altered Pattern of Urinary Elimination: Functional Incontinence, Reflex Incontinence, or Urge Incontinence*
• *Potential Impaired Skin Integrity*
• *Self-Care Deficit: Toileting*
• *Disturbance in Self-Concept*

PLANNING

ESTABLISHING PRIORITIES

The inability to control urination is embarrassing to most individuals. It is likely to interfere with social relationships and public activities. The holistic nurse makes an attempt to assist the individual regain self-esteem and dignity. Using a condom catheter provides a means by which incontinence is not obvious to others.

SETTING GOALS

• The client's clothing and bed linen will remain dry.
• Urine will drain freely into the leg bag or gravity drainage bag.

• The skin of the penis will remain intact.
• The circulation in the penis will remain adequate.

PREPARATION OF
EQUIPMENT

The nurse will need selected items from the following list:

Condom sheath in appropriate size
Basin of warm water and soap
Washcloth and towel
Bath blanket
Disposable gloves (optional)
Elastic strip or Velcro strap
Reusable leg bag with drainage tubing or gravity drainage bag and tubing

---

Technique for applying a condom catheter

ACTION	RATIONALE
1. Explain the procedure to the client.	An explanation relieves apprehension and promotes cooperation.
2. Assemble the equipment. Prepare the gravity drainage bag and tubing or leg bag for attachment to the condom sheath.	Organization promotes efficient time management.
3. Wash your hands.	Handwashing deters the spread of microorganisms.
4. Assist the client to a supine position. Close the curtain or door. Use a bath blanket and sheet to expose only the genital area.	The nurse respects the client's modesty and protects him from being exposed to others.
5. Don disposable gloves, if desired. Wash the genital area with soap and water, rinse, and dry thoroughly.	The gloves act as a barrier from contact with genital secretions. Washing removes urine, secretions, and microorganisms. The penis must be clean and dry to minimize skin irritation.
6. Roll the condom sheath outward on itself. Grasp the penis firmly with your nondominant hand. Apply the condom sheath by rolling it onto the penis with your dominant hand. Leave 2.5 cm to 5 cm (1 inch to 2 inches) space between the tip of the penis and the end of the condom sheath, as shown in Figure VII-3-2.	Rolling the condom sheath outward allows for easier application. Leaving a space prevents irritation to the tip of the penis and allows for free drainage of urine.
7. Apply an elastic strip or Velcro strap, shown in Figure VII-3-3, in a snug but not tight manner. Do not allow the elastic or Velcro to come in contact with the skin.	An elastic strip or Velcro strap should secure the condom sheath but not interfere with blood circulation to the penis.

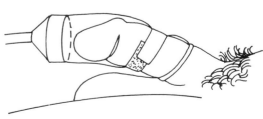

Figure VII-3-2 The nurse should check the space at the end of the condom sheath frequently. The flexible area can twist with movement and position changes, causing urine to collect around the tip of the penis rather than drain freely into the collection bag.

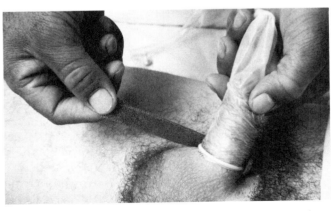

Figure VII-3-3 This Velcro strap is one means of securing the catheter in place. One of the disadvantages of a condom catheter is that it often slips from its original location.

8. Connect the condom sheath to the drainage device. Avoid kinking or twisting the drainage tubing.

Connecting the catheter to a drainage receptacle helps collect the urine, keeping the client dry. Kinked tubing causes backflow of urine.

9. Remove the equipment. Place the client in a comfortable, safe position. Wash your hands.

Removing soiled equipment supports principles of medical asepsis.

10. Assess the client's response and record observations on the chart.

A written record provides documentation of the care of the client.

SAMPLE DOCUMENTATION

Date	Time	Nurse's note
10/07	1030	Repeatedly incontinent. Partial bath given with special care to the genital area and buttocks. Condom catheter applied and secured to penis. Connected to gravity drainage. Urine collecting in reservoir. Color of penis is pink. No penile swelling.

C. Vanderbosch, RN

EVALUATION

REASSESSMENT

The nurse is accountable for frequent inspection to maintain adequate drainage, skin integrity, and circulation. Removing the condom catheter daily while washing and drying the penis provides an opportunity for reassessment of the skin of the penis. Skin that is wet either from moist body heat that cannot evaporate or with urine that has refluxed into the catheter is likely to become excoriated or break down.

EXPECTED OUTCOMES

No leakage occurs.
The skin of the penis is intact.
The penis remains of normal color, temperature, size, and sensation.

UNEXPECTED OUTCOMES

The catheter leaks or no urine drains.
The skin of the penis is irritated.
The penis becomes pale, discolored, swollen, painful, or numb.

MODIFICATIONS IN SELECTED SITUATIONS

GENERAL VARIATIONS

Use some other temporary means of collecting urine, such as keeping a urinal in place, if there are signs of skin or circulatory impairment.
Trim pubic hair that may become pulled while the catheter is attached or during the time of its removal.
Use preparations on the penis that promote adhesion between the skin and the catheter, such as tincture of benzoin or plasticized skin spray.
Wrap the adhesive strips supplied with some commercially manufactured condom catheters in a spiral about the penis to avoid a tourniquet effect.

HOME-HEALTH VARIATIONS

Teach the client and his caregivers never to use a rubberband to secure the condom.

RELATED TEACHING

Instruct the client to avoid using adhesive tape to secure the catheter. Tape will not expand and is more apt to cause circulatory problems.
Teach a client or family how to construct a home-made version of a condom catheter if they have limited funds for purchasing manufactured products. Use the following as a guide:
Insert a flexible drainage tube within the closed end of an unlubricated condom, as shown in Figure VII-3-4.
Secure the tube within the bottom of the condom by wrapping the two with a rubberband or dental floss, as shown in Figure VII-3-5.

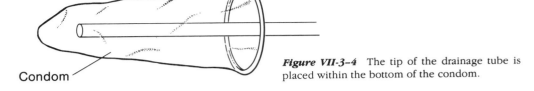

Figure VII-3-4 The tip of the drainage tube is placed within the bottom of the condom.

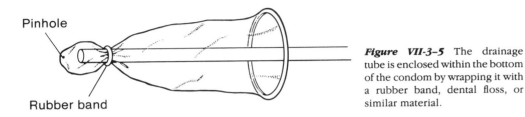

Figure VII-3-5 The drainage tube is enclosed within the bottom of the condom by wrapping it with a rubber band, dental floss, or similar material.

Perforate or slit a small opening in the tip of the condom through which urine can drain.

Reverse the condom over the tubing so the gathered connection is inside the condom, as shown in Figure VII-3-6.

Wrap the connection area once again, if desired, to make doubly sure it will not come apart.

Unwind the rolled condom the length of the penis, as shown in Figure VII-3-7.

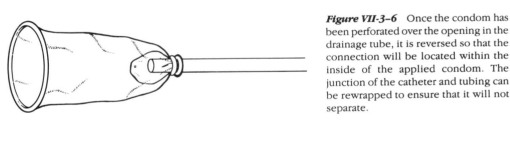

Figure VII-3-6 Once the condom has been perforated over the opening in the drainage tube, it is reversed so that the connection will be located within the inside of the applied condom. The junction of the catheter and tubing can be rewrapped to ensure that it will not separate.

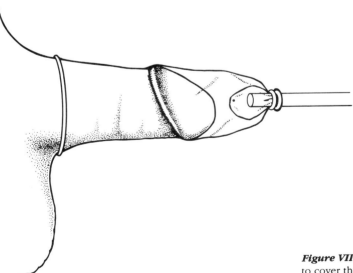

Figure VII-3-7 The condom is unrolled to cover the shaft of the penis.

(Performance checklist next page)

PERFORMANCE CHECKLIST

When applying a condom catheter, the learner:

C	A	U	
[ ]	[ ]	[ ]	Obtains appropriate assessment data
[ ]	[ ]	[ ]	Explains the procedure to the client
[ ]	[ ]	[ ]	Provides privacy
[ ]	[ ]	[ ]	Obtains a condom catheter and other necessary equipment
[ ]	[ ]	[ ]	Washes hands
[ ]	[ ]	[ ]	Dons disposable clean gloves, if desired
[ ]	[ ]	[ ]	Washes and dries the penis
[ ]	[ ]	[ ]	Applies an adhesive spray or liquid to the penis, if necessary
[ ]	[ ]	[ ]	Applies the condom catheter to the penis, leaving a space between the tip of the penis and the end of the catheter
[ ]	[ ]	[ ]	Secures the catheter to the penis with an elastic strip or Velcro strap
[ ]	[ ]	[ ]	Attaches a gravity drainage device or leg bag if the client will dress and ambulate
[ ]	[ ]	[ ]	Removes equipment
[ ]	[ ]	[ ]	Washes hands
[ ]	[ ]	[ ]	Charts significant information
[ ]	[ ]	[ ]	Reassesses the progress of urine collection and the condition of the penis

Outcome: [ ] Pass   [ ] Fail

C = competent; A = acceptable; U = unsatisfactory

Comments: _____

_____

_____

_____   _____
Student's Signature   Date

_____   _____
Instructor's Signature   Date

VII-4 *Giving a continuous bladder irrigation*

Catheters are used in certain situations where it is known that solid particles will drain through the catheter lumen with urine. For example, following a transurethral prostatectomy (TUR), blood cells and tissue add to the volume that collects within the bladder. A continuous bladder irrigation, illustrated in Figure VII-4-1, may be used. This procedure is best performed utilizing a triple-lumen, or three-way, catheter, shown in Figure VII-4-2. This type of catheter is designed so that there are separate openings for the infusion of irrigant, for inflation of the balloon anchoring the catheter within the bladder, and for drainage of the bladder contents.

PURPOSES OF PROCEDURE

A continuous bladder irrigation is given to

1. Maintain patency of the catheter
2. Dilute solid particles present in the bladder with additional fluid volume
3. Prevent bladder distention and discomfort from obstructed drainage
4. Prevent infection from opening the catheter system
5. Instill medication for a local effect

ASSESSMENT

OBJECTIVE DATA

- Observe the gross characteristics of draining urine. Note especially the color, transparency, and consistency. Frank blood is indicative of fresh or recent bleeding. The urine should become lighter with time until it is yellow and transparent.
- Palpate and percuss the bladder to determine the extent or absence of distention.
- Check the length of drainage tubing to validate that it is not kinked or obstructed in any other way.
- Determine that the drainage tubing hangs straight from the bed into the collection bag.
- Assess the pulse and blood pressure to evaluate the significance of blood loss on the circulatory status of the client. A hypotensive and tachycardic client may be losing an excessive volume of blood.
- Note the client's skin color and temperature. As the blood volume becomes depleted, the peripheral blood supply may become compromised.
- Determine the client's level of consciousness. Loss of blood may produce lethargy from which it is more and more difficult to arouse the client.
- Monitor intravenous fluid and blood replacement therapy. The physician may anticipate a potential fluid loss by ordering a compensatory volume by intravenous (IV) infusion.
- Note the written medical order for the irrigating solution and the rate of its administration.

SUBJECTIVE DATA

- Ask the client to describe any discomfort in the bladder or urethral area. Feeling the need to void or attempts to pass urine around the catheter may indicate obstruction.

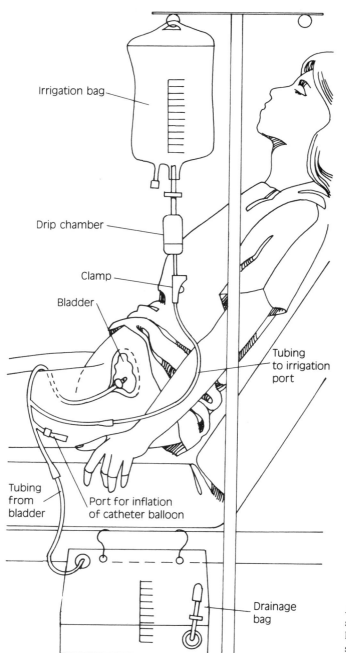

Irrigation bag

Drip chamber

Clamp

Bladder

Tubing
to irrigation
port

Tubing
from
bladder

Port for inflation
of catheter balloon

Drainage
bag

Figure VII-4-1 The irrigation
solution infuses from the bag that
hangs from the IV pole while fluid
simultaneously drains from a port
in the catheter.

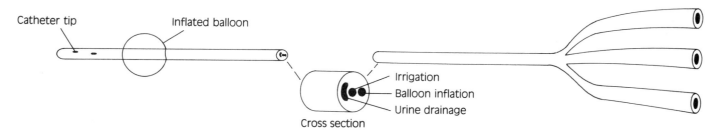

Catheter tip

Inflated balloon

Cross section

Irrigation

Balloon inflation

Urine drainage

Figure VII-4-2 A three-way catheter is constructed so there are three distinct passages through the middle
of the tubing.

RELATED NURSING DIAGNOSES

The client who receives a continuous bladder irrigation may have nursing diagnoses, such as

- *Altered Comfort*
- *Potential Altered Patterns of Urinary Elimination*
- *Potential for Infection*

PLANNING

ESTABLISHING PRIORITIES

Maintaining a patent drainage system is a priority. An obstruction is likely to contribute to bladder spasms. Being free of pain and discomfort is a basic biologic need. If the bladder expands with fluid, the stretching can stimulate the urge to void and cause more bleeding than would otherwise occur.

SETTING GOALS

- The catheter will remain patent.
- The specified solution will infuse at the prescribed rate.
- There will be no evidence of urinary infection.
- The client's comfort will be maintained.

PREPARATION OF EQUIPMENT

The nurse will need items from the following list:

Sterile irrigating solution (usually 2000-ml bags at room temperature or warmed to body temperature)
Sterile tubing with a drip chamber and clamp
IV pole
Three-way Foley catheter in place in client's bladder
Gravity drainage bag and tubing
Bath blanket

Technique for giving a continuous bladder irrigation

ACTION	RATIONALE
1. Explain the procedure and its purpose to the client.	An explanation reduces apprehension and facilitates cooperation.
2. Assemble the equipment.	Organization promotes efficient time management.
3. Wash your hands.	Handwashing deters the spread of microorganisms.
4. Provide for privacy by closing the curtains or door and draping the client with a bath blanket.	The nurse respects the client's modesty and protects the client from being seen by others.
5. Prepare the sterile irrigation solution. Secure the clamp and attach sterile tubing with a drip chamber to the container, as shown in Figure VII-4-3. Hang the so-	Clamped tubing allows the nurse to control filling the drip chamber and tubing. Elevating the container facilitates the flow of solution by gravity. Displacing air from

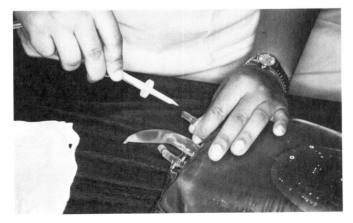

Figure VII-4-3 The nurse inserts the spike from the infusion tubing into the sterile port of the solution container.

lution from an IV pole 2½ to 3 feet above the level of the bladder. Release the clamp and remove the protective cover on the end of the tubing without contaminating it. Allow the solution to flush the air from the tubing, as shown in Figure VII-4-4. Reclamp the tubing.

the tubing ensures that only solution will enter the bladder.

6. Using sterile technique, attach the irrigation tubing to the irrigation port of the three-way catheter.

Using sterile equipment and taking care to avoid contact with sources of pathogens prevent spreading microorganisms into the bladder.

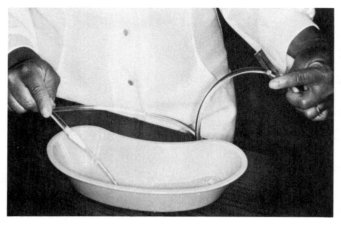

Figure VII-4-4 The nurse releases the clamp and displaces air from the tubing. The basin collects the small amount of solution that may be lost.

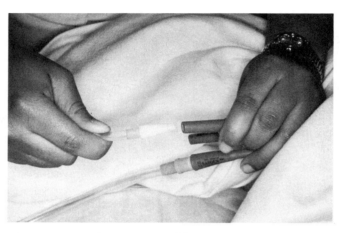

Figure VII-4-5 The nurse is careful to maintain the sterility of the tip of the irrigation tubing while connecting it to the catheter.

7. Release the clamp on the irrigation tubing and regulate the flow according to the physician's order.

The continuous flow of irrigating solution dilutes the contents within the bladder and keeps the catheter patent.

8. As volume of solution becomes low, clamp the tubing. Do not allow the drip chamber to become empty. Disconnect the empty bag and attach a full one. Continue as ordered by the physician.

Keeping fluid within the tubing avoids the need to separate the tubing from the catheter to clear the air. Opening a drainage system increases the risk for introducing microorganisms.

9. Assess the characteristics of the urinary drainage and the client's response to the procedure. Document the observations on the client's chart.

A written summary provides documentation of the care and treatment of the client.

10. Record the amount of irrigant used on the intake section of the intake and output (I & O) flow sheet. Empty and record the amount of drainage from the catheter.

Recording at periodic intervals helps ensure accurate assessment data.

11. Wash your hands.

Handwashing deters the spread of microorganisms.

SAMPLE DOCUMENTATION

Date	Time	Nurse's note
6/15	1550	2000 ml of sterile normal saline hung as a continuous bladder irrigation. Infusing at 75 ml per hour. Catheter is patent and draining. Urine is dark red. Belladonna & opium suppository administered for bladder spasms.
		V. Przyocki, RN

EVALUATION

REASSESSMENT

Check that the irrigation is infusing at the intended rate at hourly intervals. A urine collection device that contains an attached minicollector can be used to observe the volume and characteristics of urine at hourly intervals throughout the day. This helps validate the status of urine drainage. Analyze the ratio of the volume of infused irrigant to the volume collected in the drainage bag to determine the amount of actual urine. Use periodic contacts with the client to assess the patency of the catheter and the need to empty the drainage receptacle. Always suspect catheter obstruction if the client develops lower abdominal discomfort and the urge to void.

EXPECTED OUTCOMES

The irrigation solution infuses according to schedule.
There is continuous drainage from the catheter.
The urine becomes lighter and more transparent.
No signs of infection develop.
The client's discomfort is within an expected and tolerable level.

UNEXPECTED OUTCOMES

The rate of the infusion speeds, slows, or stops.
Drainage from the catheter slows or stops.
The client experiences bladder spasms and attempts to void around the catheter.
The client develops an elevated temperature and elevated white blood cell count; urinalysis shows bacteria present in the urine.

MODIFICATIONS IN SELECTED SITUATIONS

GENERAL VARIATIONS

If the catheter must be replaced due to obstruction, select one with a large lumen, such as a #20 French, and a large-sized balloon, such as 30 ml. The larger lumen provides more room through which solid particles move. The large balloon helps exert pressure on bleeding sites in the area of a prostatectomy.

A Y-connector can be inserted into a two-way catheter to adapt it for a bladder irrigation. This modification allows fluid from an irrigation container to instill into the catheter while the drainage tubing is clamped. When the solution has instilled, the drainage tubing clamp can be released.

Consult with the physician if the catheter has slight traction for controlling bleeding. Prolonged traction can create damage to the sphincter. There should be some schedule for releasing and reapplying the traction.

Before being removed, the physician may modify the irrigation order from one that is continuous to one that is intermittent.

RELATED TEACHING

Clients with indwelling catheters and irrigation systems should be taught how the equipment functions.

Explain that taking liberal amounts of oral fluids acts as a natural irrigant.

Explain that the client should avoid straining to have a bowel movement because this increases intra-abdominal pressure and can potentiate more bleeding. The stool can be kept soft through dietary measures or by requesting a stool softener.

Tell the client there may be a slight burning sensation when voiding for the first time or two after the catheter is removed.

When the catheter is removed, teach the client to perform exercises that increase the tone of urinary sphincter muscles and reduce the potential for incontinence. The client should be taught to contract and relax the buttocks muscles alternately 10 to 20 times per hour while awake.

(Performance checklist next page)

PERFORMANCE CHECKLIST

When giving a continuous bladder irrigation, the learner:

C	A	U	
[ ]	[ ]	[ ]	Obtains appropriate assessment data
[ ]	[ ]	[ ]	Reads the written medical orders
[ ]	[ ]	[ ]	Obtains necessary supplies
[ ]	[ ]	[ ]	Explains the procedure to the client
[ ]	[ ]	[ ]	Empties the current urine drainage in the collection bag and records the amount
[ ]	[ ]	[ ]	Attaches the IV pole to the bed
[ ]	[ ]	[ ]	Washes hands
[ ]	[ ]	[ ]	Provides privacy
[ ]	[ ]	[ ]	Clamps the irrigation tubing
[ ]	[ ]	[ ]	Inserts the tubing spike into the solution container
[ ]	[ ]	[ ]	Hangs the solution from the IV pole
[ ]	[ ]	[ ]	Fills the drip chamber
[ ]	[ ]	[ ]	Flushes air from the tubing without contaminating the free end
[ ]	[ ]	[ ]	Reclamps the tubing
[ ]	[ ]	[ ]	Connects the irrigation tubing to the catheter in a sterile manner
[ ]	[ ]	[ ]	Releases the clamp
[ ]	[ ]	[ ]	Regulates the infusion rate
[ ]	[ ]	[ ]	Labels the solution with the date and time it was hung and adds own initials
[ ]	[ ]	[ ]	Checks the movement of urine through the catheter drainage tubing
[ ]	[ ]	[ ]	Removes supplies
[ ]	[ ]	[ ]	Washes hands
[ ]	[ ]	[ ]	Charts significant information
[ ]	[ ]	[ ]	Reassesses the client, the catheter drainage, and the progress of the infusion in 30 minutes and then hourly

Outcome: [ ] Pass   [ ] Fail

C = competent; A = acceptable; U = unsatisfactory

Comments: _____

_____

_____

_____	_____
Student's Signature	Date
_____	_____
Instructor's Signature	Date

VII-5 *Irrigating a catheter using a closed or open system*

The flushing of a tube, canal, or area with solution is called *irrigation*. Occasionally, irrigations are ordered when debris threatens to block the catheter. In the past, the procedure was done routinely for almost all indwelling catheters. Because this is a potential means of introducing pathogens, it is now recommended that an irrigation should be done only when there is a demonstrated need. "Natural" irrigation of the catheter through an increased fluid intake is the preferred technique.

Most indwelling catheters have a double lumen, as shown in Figure VII-5-1; one lumen leads to the balloon and the other drains urine. One type of catheter drainage tubing commonly in use has a special port so that the catheter need not be separated from the drainage tubing. This is referred to as a *closed system*. It reduces the risk of infection. The other type of catheter drainage tubing must be separated, or opened, from the drainage tubing while performing an irrigation.

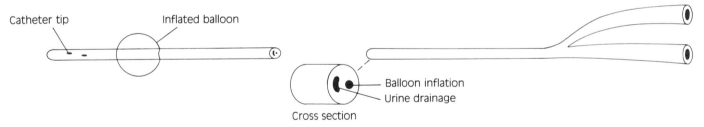

Figure VII-5-1 This two-way catheter has a separate channel that leads to the balloon and another that provides a pathway for urine drainage or irrigation.

PURPOSES OF PROCEDURE

An indwelling catheter is irrigated to

1. Maintain an open drainage pathway through the catheter
2. Dislodge mucus shreds and other debris collecting within the catheter
3. Prevent the need to remove and replace an indwelling catheter

ASSESSMENT

OBJECTIVE DATA

- Observe the gross characteristics of the draining urine, especially the presence of solid particles within the urine.
- Determine the length of time the current catheter has been indwelling.
- Analyze the trend in intake and output measurements; compare the volumes to norms for fluid balance.
- Review the client's record for circumstances that may concentrate the urine or change its characteristics, such as low fluid intake, crystallization from gout or sulfonamide therapy, renal disease, or urinary tract infection.
- Rub the lumen of the catheter within the thumb and index finger, noting the sensation of grit within the lumen.
- Read the physician's written order for irrigating the catheter.
- Inspect the catheter to determine if it contains a self-sealing access port or if it must be separated for irrigation.

SUBJECTIVE DATA

- Ask the client to describe any fullness or discomfort he experiences in the urethra, lower abdomen, or flank areas.

RELEVANT NURSING DIAGNOSES

The client with an indwelling catheter that requires irrigation may have nursing diagnoses, such as

- *Altered Comfort*
- *Potential for Infection*

PLANNING

ESTABLISHING PRIORITIES

Each nurse caring for a catheterized client should make daily pertinent focus assessments that relate to the potential or actual obstruction in drainage through the catheter. Any cessation in the flow of urine should receive immediate attention by the nurse. Milking the tubing in the direction of the urine collection bag may promote limited drainage temporarily.

SETTING GOALS

- The catheter will remain patent.
- Solid particles in the urine will move freely through the catheter.
- The client will remain free of a urinary tract infection.

PREPARATION OF EQUIPMENT FOR CLOSED SYSTEM

The nurse will need selected items from the following list when irrigating the catheter using a closed system:

Sterile basin or container
Gauze squares or cotton balls with disinfectant, or alcohol swabs
Absorbent pad
30-ml to 50-ml syringe with 18-gauge or 19-gauge needle
Sterile irrigating solution (at room temperature or warmed to body temperature)
Bath blanket

Technique for irrigating a catheter using a closed system

ACTION	RATIONALE
1. Assemble equipment. Wash your hands. Explain the procedure and its purpose to the client.	Organization promotes efficient time management. Handwashing deters the spread of microorganisms. An explanation reduces apprehension and facilitates cooperation.
2. Provide for privacy by closing the curtains and door and draping the client with the bath blanket.	The nurse respects the client's modesty and prevents the client from being seen by others.
3. Assist the client to a comfortable position and expose the access port on the catheter drainage tubing. Place the absorbent pad under the catheter and access port.	Uncovering the catheter where it is joined to the drainage tubing provides for adequate visualization. The pad protects the client and the bed from leakage.
4. Open the sterile supplies. Pour sterile solution into the sterile basin. Aspirate 30 ml to 50 ml of irrigant into the sterile syringe through the attached sterile needle.	Using sterile equipment and supplies prevents introducing microorganisms into the urinary tract.
5. Cleanse the access port with an alcohol swab or moistened gauze square.	Cleansing the point of entry removes microorganisms from the area.
6. Clamp or fold the catheter tubing distal to the port.	Temporarily obstructing the tubing below the port allows the instilled solution to flow up the catheter toward the bladder.
7. Insert the needle into the port. Gently instill the solution into the catheter.	Gentle instillation is less traumatic when particles are being flushed from the catheter.

8. Remove the needle from the port. Unclamp the tubing and allow the irrigant and urine to drain. Repeat the procedure as necessary.

Gravity promotes drainage of urine and irrigant from the catheter.

9. Assess the client's response to the procedure and the quality of the drainage. Document observations on the client's chart.

A written summary provides accurate documentation of the client's care and treatment.

10. Record the amount of irrigant used on the intake and output record.

The volume of irrigation solution should not be included as urine output.

11. Remove the equipment and discard the uncapped needle and syringe in an appropriate receptacle. Wash your hands. Make the client comfortable.

Caring for soiled equipment and handwashing deter the spread of microorganisms. Leaving the needle uncapped prevents accidental injury to the nurse.

PREPARATION OF EQUIPMENT FOR OPEN SYSTEM

The nurse will need items from the following list when irrigating a catheter using an open system:

Sterile irrigation tray with
  Sterile container and basin
  Sterile Asepto syringe or irrigation syringe with an adaptor tip
Gauze squares or cotton balls with disinfectant, or alcohol swabs
Absorbent pad
Sterile irrigating solution (at room temperature or warmed to body temperature)
Bath blanket
Sterile cover for the tip of the drainage tubing

Technique for irrigating a catheter using an open system

ACTION

RATIONALE

1. Assemble equipment. Wash your hands. Explain the procedure and its purpose to the client.

Organization promotes efficient time management. Handwashing deters the spread of microorganisms. An explanation reduces apprehension and facilitates co-operation.

2. Provide for privacy by closing the curtain and door and draping the client with the bath blanket.

The nurse respects the client's modesty and prevents the client from being seen by others.

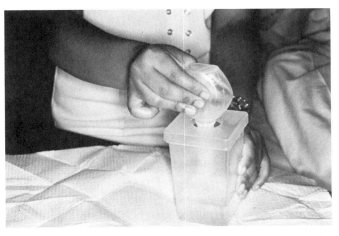

Figure VII-5-2 By squeezing the bulb on this Asepto syringe the nurse aspirates sterile solution for an irrigation.

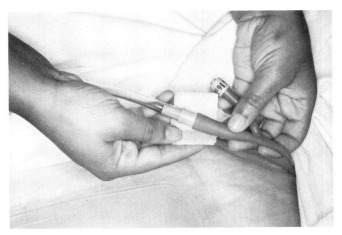

Figure VII-5-3 The nurse cleanses the area where the catheter and drainage tubing connect.

3. Assist the client to a comfortable position and expose the connection between the catheter and drainage tubing. Position the absorbent pad under the catheter where it connects with the drainage tubing.

Uncovering the catheter where it is joined to the drainage tubing provides for adequate visualization. The pad protects the client and the bed from leakage.

4. Open the sterile supplies. Pour the sterile solution into the sterile container. Remove the tip from the syringe and aspirate 30 ml of irrigant into the syringe, as the nurse in Figure VII-5-2 is doing.

Using sterile equipment and supplies prevents introducing microorganisms into the urinary tract.

5. Cleanse the catheter junction with a moistened gauze square or an alcohol swab, as shown in Figure VII-5-3.

Cleansing the point of entry removes organisms from the area.

6. Disconnect the catheter and drainage tube. Place the sterile cover over the tip of the drainage tube, as shown in Figure VII-5-4, and secure the drainage tubing on the bed. Hold the catheter tubing 2.5 cm (1 inch) from its open end.

Capping the tip of the disconnected drainage tube avoids contaminating it with microorganisms. Holding the catheter above the area that was cleansed keeps microorganisms from the opening.

7. Position the sterile basin beneath the catheter. Insert the tip of the syringe into the catheter, as shown in Figure VII-5-5, and gently instill the solution.

Gentle instillation is less traumatic when particles are being flushed from the catheter.

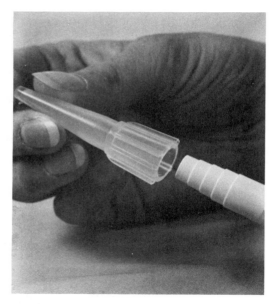

Figure VII-5-4 The nurse places a sterile cap on the end of the drainage tubing to protect it from contamination while irrigating the catheter.

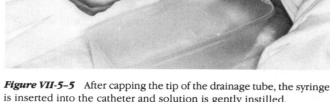

Figure VII-5-5 After capping the tip of the drainage tube, the syringe is inserted into the catheter and solution is gently instilled.

8. Remove the syringe, keeping the bulb compressed, and allow the drainage to return via gravity flow into the basin, as shown in Figure VII-5-6. If there is no return, gently aspirate the solution from the catheter. Continue with irrigation as ordered by the physician.

Gravity aids drainage of urine and irrigant from the catheter. Irrigation maintains patency of the urinary drainage system.

9. Reattach the drainage tube to the catheter, being careful not to contaminate the system. Resecure the catheter with tape or Velcro strap.

Avoiding touching the connection areas of the catheter and drainage tubing prevents entry of microorganisms. Tape or a Velcro strap avoids pulling on the catheter and possible separation.

10. Document the client's response to the procedure and the quality and amount of drainage.

A written summary provides accurate documentation of the client's care and treatment.

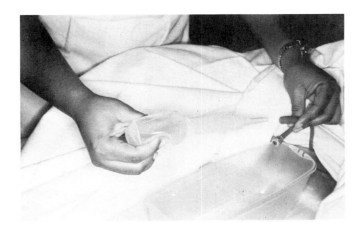

Figure VII-5-6 After the irrigation solution has been instilled, the nurse removes the syringe and waits while the solution drains by gravity into the basin.

11. Subtract the amount of solution instilled from the amount of drainage. Record the difference as urine volume on the output area of the I & O sheet.

Accurate measurements facilitate valid data for assessing fluid balance.

12. Remove the equipment and make the client comfortable. Wash your hands.

Removing and caring for soiled equipment and handwashing deter the spread of microorganisms.

SAMPLE DOCUMENTATION

Date	Time	Nurse's note
9/02	1650	No output through catheter since emptied at 1400. States "I feel like I need to urinate." Slight distention of bladder. Milking is not successful. 60 ml of sterile normal saline instilled into catheter. Solution returned with large-sized clumps of mucus. Catheter draining again.
		C. Maier, RN

EVALUATION

REASSESSMENT

The patency of the catheter and characteristics of the urine require frequent inspection. In long-term care facilities, it may be beneficial for quick reference to record the date on the Kardex that a catheter has been inserted. Keep in mind that the frequency for irrigating a catheter depends on analyzing the data on each individual's urine and drainage function.

EXPECTED OUTCOMES

The irrigating solution instills without resistance.
The instilled solution drains freely by gravity.
Urine drains continuously from the catheter.
The client's fluid volume continues to be balanced.

UNEXPECTED OUTCOMES

Resistance can be felt when attempting instillation of the irrigating solution.
The instilled solution fails to drain through the catheter.
The bladder distends and causes discomfort.
The client excretes significantly less in an 8-hour period than the amount he has consumed.

MODIFICATIONS IN SELECTED SITUATIONS

GENERAL VARIATIONS

A larger volume of solution, for example 100 ml to 200 ml, can be instilled when the intent is to irrigate the bladder. In this case the lumen leading to the drainage tubing is clamped during the instillation. The solution is allowed to dwell within the bladder for a brief time, such as 20 to 30 minutes. The clamp is then released and the irrigation, which may contain medication or chemicals, is allowed to drain.

Use gloves and goggles when a bladder irrigation solution contains a toxic drug or chemical that may be absorbed through the skin or mucous membranes through accidental direct contact. Check protocols for disposing of the drained urine.

Try having the client turn on his side, cough voluntarily, or perform the Valsalva maneuver to promote the return of instilled solution that is sluggish in draining.

Date and initial the irrigating solution kept at the bedside.

Consult agency policies for the maximum time that an opened and resealed container of solution is considered sterile. Most recommend that the solution be considered sterile for only 24 hours once it has been opened.

AGE-RELATED VARIATIONS

Expect that a smaller volume of irrigating solution will be used for infants and children.

HOME-HEALTH VARIATIONS

Help the client and caregivers understand the procedure by using a catheter cut in half to show the cross-section of lumens.

RELATED TEACHING

Always explain the purpose of the equipment and the sequence of steps throughout a procedure.

Instruct the client who is not required to restrict fluid intake to drink a liberal volume of fluid throughout the day to keep the urine dilute. An intake of 2000 ml to 3000 ml is usually sufficient.

Describe the signs and symptoms of a urinary tract infection, such as burning and irritation at the meatus, cloudy urine, strong smelling urine, and fever and chills. Ask the client to inform the nurse if any of these are noted.

PERFORMANCE CHECKLIST

When irrigating a catheter, the learner:

C	A	U	
[ ]	[ ]	[ ]	Acquires appropriate data
[ ]	[ ]	[ ]	Reads the medical order
[ ]	[ ]	[ ]	Assembles the necessary equipment depending on whether a closed or open system will be used
[ ]	[ ]	[ ]	Explains the procedure
[ ]	[ ]	[ ]	Provides privacy
[ ]	[ ]	[ ]	Positions the client comfortably
[ ]	[ ]	[ ]	Protects the bed in the area of the catheter
[ ]	[ ]	[ ]	Opens the sterile supplies without contamination
[ ]	[ ]	[ ]	Fills the irrigation syringe
[ ]	[ ]	[ ]	Cleans the port or area where the catheter will be separated
[ ]	[ ]	[ ]	Caps the separated end of the drainage tube, if an open system is used
[ ]	[ ]	[ ]	Clamps or pinches the catheter when using a closed system
[ ]	[ ]	[ ]	Instills the appropriate amount of irrigating solution slowly without force
[ ]	[ ]	[ ]	Removes the syringe and allows the solution to drain by gravity
[ ]	[ ]	[ ]	Applies gentle aspiration if drainage is sluggish
[ ]	[ ]	[ ]	Reconnects the catheter and tubing if the system was opened
[ ]	[ ]	[ ]	Makes the client comfortable
[ ]	[ ]	[ ]	Measures the volume of drained solution if an open system is used
[ ]	[ ]	[ ]	Records intake and output measurements
[ ]	[ ]	[ ]	Removes soiled equipment from the room
[ ]	[ ]	[ ]	Washes hands
[ ]	[ ]	[ ]	Charts significant information

Outcome: [ ] Pass   [ ] Fail

C = competent; A = acceptable; U = unsatisfactory

Comments: _____

_____

_____

_____   _____
Student's Signature   Date

_____   _____
Instructor's Signature   Date

VII-6 *Changing a stoma appliance on an ileal conduit*

Congenital anomalies, irreversible obstructions, or malignancies in the urinary tract may require some individuals to have the urinary flow diverted surgically. An opening, called a *stoma,* is created on the abdomen. Some surgeons use a separated piece from the ileum, shown in Figure VII-6-1, for this purpose. The reconstructed anatomic parts are collectively referred to as an *ileal conduit.* Since the ileum is not actually a replacement for the bladder, but rather only a passageway for urine, and the stoma does not contain a sphincter, urine drains continuously from the new opening. An appliance, or bag, is worn on the skin over the stoma to collect the urine.

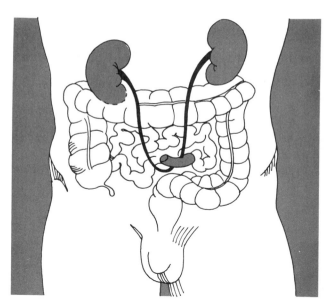

Figure VII-6-1 The ureters are brought to the ileum of the small intestine and a stoma is made where the urine is excreted.

PURPOSES OF PROCEDURE

A stomal appliance is changed to

1. Maintain skin integrity
2. Control odors
3. Care for the stoma

ASSESSMENT

OBJECTIVE DATA

- Inspect the appliance currently in use. Note the state of its adherence to the skin, the design of the appliance, and how it is secured to the skin
- Observe the characteristics of the urine within the appliance, especially the color, odor, and consistency
- Examine the stoma. Normally the stoma is moist, red or bright pink, and protrudes slightly from the skin.
- Note the characteristics of any abdominal incision, if this is a recent procedure.
- If abdominal surgery has been recent, listen for bowel sounds.

SUBJECTIVE DATA

- Ask the client to indicate the sensations he notes in the area around the stoma. Burning is likely to be associated with skin irritation.

RELEVANT NURSING DIAGNOSES

The client with an ileal conduit may have nursing diagnoses, such as

- *Altered Comfort*
- *Potential Altered Skin Integrity*
- *Anxiety or Fear*
- *Self-Care Deficit*
- *Knowledge Deficit*
- *Disturbance in Self-Concept: Body Image*
- *Potential Altered Tissue Perfusion*

PLANNING

ESTABLISHING PRIORITIES

The appliance can be worn indefinitely. The primary criteria for changing it are loosening, impairment of skin integrity, or impairment in the circulation to the stoma. Therefore, inspecting the area is of utmost importance. Leaking urine can irritate the skin. The skin must remain intact since it is directly related to the ability to secure an appliance. If the viability of the tissue in the stoma is jeopardized, necrosis and sloughing can occur. The nurse caring for the client must demonstrate genuine acceptance for the client. The attitudes of others often influence the adjustment of the client to the new change in body image. It is important that the nurse convey interest in the client as an individual rather than be concerned only with the function of the ileal conduit.

SETTING GOALS

- The appliance will adhere securely to the skin.
- The stoma will appear pink and moist.
- The skin around the stoma will remain intact.
- The client will assume self-care of the stomal appliance.

PREPARATION OF EQUIPMENT

The nurse will need selected items from the following list:

Basin with warm water, soap, towel, and washcloth or cotton balls
Graduated container
Skin protectant or barrier
Sterile 2 × 2 gauze squares
Ostomy bag cut to the correct stomal size
Ostomy belt (optional)
Adhesive cement (optional for reusable appliances)

Technique for changing a stoma appliance on an ileal conduit

ACTION	RATIONALE
1. Explain the procedure and encourage the client to observe or participate if possible. Provide for privacy.	An explanation reduces apprehension and facilitates cooperation. Observing or assisting encourages acceptance and competency in self-care. Providing privacy prevents the client from being seen by others.
2. Assemble equipment.	Organization promotes efficient time management.
3. Wash your hands.	Handwashing deters the spread of microorganisms.
4. Have the client sit or stand if he can assist with the procedure or assume a supine position in bed.	These positions result in less abdominal folds and facilitate removal and application of the appliance.
5. Empty the appliance being worn into a graduated container (before removing if it is reusable and not attached to straight drainage).	Having the appliance empty before handling it reduces the likelihood of spilling the urine. The physician may have ordered recording of the intake and output.

6. Remove the appliance faceplate from the skin very gently.

The seal between the surface of the faceplate and the skin must be broken before the faceplate can be removed. Harsh handling of the appliance can cause damage to the skin and impair the development of a secure seal in the future.

7. Discard the appliance appropriately if disposable or wash a reusable appliance in lukewarm soap and water and allow to air dry.

Thorough cleansing and airing of the appliance reduce odor and deterioration. For aesthetic and infection-control purposes, used appliances should be discarded appropriately.

8. Cleanse the skin around the stoma with soap and water or a commercial cleaner using a washcloth or cotton balls. Make sure that you remove all of the old adhesive from the skin.

Cleaning the skin removes urine and old adhesive and skin protectant. Urine or a build-up of other substances can cause irritation and damage to the skin.

9. Pat dry gently. Make sure the skin around the stoma is thoroughly dry. Assess the stoma and condition of the surrounding skin.

Careful drying prevents trauma to the skin and stoma. An intact, properly applied urinary collection device protects skin integrity. Any change in color and size of the stoma may indicate circulatory problems.

10. Place one or two gauze squares over the stoma opening.

Continuous drainage or urine must be absorbed to keep the skin dry during the appliance change.

11. Apply a skin protectant to a 2-inch radius around the stoma and allow it to dry completely, which takes about 30 seconds.

The skin needs protection from the excoriating effect of the urine and adhesive. Allowing the protectant to dry completely enhances its effectiveness.

12. If necessary, enlarge the size of the faceplate opening to fit the stoma.

The appliance should fit snugly around the stoma, with only $\frac{1}{16}$ to $\frac{1}{8}$ inch of skin visible around the opening. A faceplate opening that is too small can cause trauma to the stoma. Exposed skin will be irritated by urine if the opening is too large.

13. Apply adhesive to the faceplate or remove the protective covering from the disposable faceplate, as shown in Figure VII-6-3. Remove the gauze squares from the stoma. Carefully position the appliance and press it in place, moving from the center outward, as shown in Figure VII-6-3.

The appliance is effective only if it is properly positioned and securely adhered.

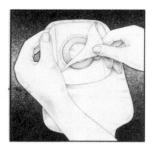

Figure VII-6–2 The adhesive backing is smoothed to avoid wrinkles and air pockets. The strips covering the side edges of the adhesive can be removed once the inner area is in place. (Courtesy of Hollister Incorporated, Libertyville, IL)

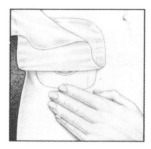

Figure VII-6–3 This type of appliance has a protective cover over the adhesive backing. The side strips allow the appliance to be handled while positioning the opening over the stoma. (Courtesy of Hollister Incorporated, Libertyville, IL)

14. Secure the optional belt to the appliance and around the client.

An elasticized belt helps support the appliance for some persons.

15. Remove or discard equipment and assess the client's response to the procedure. Wash your hands.

Care of soiled articles and handwashing deter the spread of microorganisms. The client's response indicates his level of acceptance and readiness for teaching.

16. Record the appearance of the stoma and surrounding skin as well as the client's reaction to the procedure.

A written summary provides accurate documentation of the client's care and treatment.

SAMPLE DOCUMENTATION

Date	Time	Nurse's note
5/07	1845	Faceplate over stoma is wet and loose. Urine apparent on hospital gown and linen. Appliance removed from skin. Stoma and peristomal skin washed with soap and water. Stoma is bright red and contains a film of mucus. Skin is intact and similar in color to other areas of the abdomen. No burning experienced by client. Area dried. Karaya paste applied to skin. New appliance secured over stoma. Urine collecting within the appliance. No leaking noted following change. Client watched procedure and asked pertinent questions.

F. Martinez, RN

EVALUATION

REASSESSMENT

The stoma and appliance should be inspected at hourly intervals immediately after surgery. This is the time when circulation is most likely to be affected. Once the client's condition has stabilized, a focus assessment is necessary during each shift.

EXPECTED OUTCOMES

The faceplate does not have any wrinkles or loose areas.
The stoma is the normal color and appearance.
The skin is smooth and free of discomfort.
The appliance fits comfortably.

UNEXPECTED OUTCOMES

Small air pockets or loose areas are apparent in the faceplate.
The appliance pinches or pulls on the skin.
The stoma looks dark blue and swollen.
A wide skin margin is exposed around the stoma.
The skin looks pink, feels warm, and burns.

MODIFICATIONS IN SELECTED SITUATIONS

GENERAL VARIATIONS

Try placing a tampon within the stoma rather than the gauze squares. The tampon is sterile and has a large absorbent capacity. It will allow ample time for drying the surrounding skin and applying the skin protectant and adhesive.

Use a measuring card of various circular sizes to determine the appropriate diameter for the opening of the stoma. Allow $\frac{1}{16}$ to $\frac{1}{8}$ inch more in addition to the actual size of the stoma.

Empty the collecting bag when it is one-third to one-half full. This reduces the weight within the appliance and hence relieves the pull and stress on the skin.

HOME-HEALTH VARIATIONS

After cleansing, use a hair dryer on a low to medium setting to dry the skin around the stoma.

Use a hair dryer to dry the inside of a reusable appliance before storing it for future use.

RELATED TEACHING

Be sure the client understands how his reconstructed anatomy functions and what care it needs. Eventually the client can be expected to care for the stoma and appliance himself. Local self-help ostomy groups or referral to an enterostomal therapist may assist the client with questions or problems after discharge.

Instruct the client to maintain a generous fluid intake, at least 2000 ml or more daily. This helps keep urine dilute and free-flowing. It removes organisms and debris that may accumulate in the urine or around the stoma.

Explain suggestions for dietary adjustments. Asparagus is discouraged because it causes the urine to have a strong odor. Advise the client to inform the physician immediately if the stoma becomes dark blue or black, the skin becomes excoriated, or urine ceases to drain.

Explain that an ileal conduit should not affect sexual functioning. Suggest to the client that the appliance can be emptied and then disguised with a fabric cover before intercourse. Some clients choose to modify their underwear so that it opens in the crotch, but continues to cover the appliance from view. Pregnancy may temporarily change the size of the stoma. The client may need to modify or experiment with various types of appliances as the pregnancy progresses.

PERFORMANCE CHECKLIST

When changing a stoma appliance on an ileal conduit, the learner:

C	A	U	
[ ]	[ ]	[ ]	Makes appropriate assessments
[ ]	[ ]	[ ]	Explains the procedure to the client
[ ]	[ ]	[ ]	Gathers equipment
[ ]	[ ]	[ ]	Provides privacy
[ ]	[ ]	[ ]	Washes hands
[ ]	[ ]	[ ]	Raises the bed and lowers the side rail
[ ]	[ ]	[ ]	Assists the client to a convenient position
[ ]	[ ]	[ ]	Drains the appliance
[ ]	[ ]	[ ]	Removes the faceplate
[ ]	[ ]	[ ]	Cleans the skin and the stoma
[ ]	[ ]	[ ]	Controls dripping urine while drying the skin
[ ]	[ ]	[ ]	Applies skin protectant and adhesive, if needed
[ ]	[ ]	[ ]	Presses the faceplate over the stoma and smooths it uniformly into place
[ ]	[ ]	[ ]	Secures the appliance with a belt, if indicated
[ ]	[ ]	[ ]	Removes the equipment
[ ]	[ ]	[ ]	Washes hands
[ ]	[ ]	[ ]	Records pertinent information

Outcome: [ ] Pass   [ ] Fail

C = competent; A = acceptable; U = unsatisfactory

Comments: _____

_____

_____

_____   _____
Student's Signature   Date

_____   _____
Instructor's Signature   Date

RELATED LITERATURE

**PROCEDURE VII-1
OFFERING AND
REMOVING A BEDPAN
OR URINAL**

Mather MLS: The secret to life in a spica. Am J Nurs 87(1):56–58, January 1987

Wells DL, Saltmarche A: Voiding dysfunction in geriatric patients with hip fracture: Prevalence rate and tentative nursing interventions. Orthopaedic Nursing 5(6):25–28, November–December 1986

**PROCEDURE VII-2
CATHETERIZING THE
FEMALE AND MALE
URINARY BLADDER**

Barnes SH: The development of a comprehensive instructional package for teaching intermittent self-catheterization. Journal of Enterostomal Therapy 13(6):238–241, November–December 1986

Blannin J: Managing supplies . . . control for disposable incontinence goods. Nursing Times 83(15):76, April 15–21, 1987

Cefalu CA: Management of the bedridden patient with irreversible urinary incontinence. Hospital Medicine 23(6):183–187, June 1987

Cunha BA: Nosocomial urinary tract infections. Physician Assistant 11(7):51–53, 56–57, July 1987

Fader M: Assessing incontinence in the elderly. Geriatric Nursing Home Care 7(1):10–12, January 1987

Glenister H: The passage of infection . . . emptying catheter bags. Nursing Times 83(22): 68, 71, 73, June 3–9, 1987

Resnick NM: Urinary incontinence in the elderly. Hospital Practice 21(11):80C–80H, 80K–80L, 80Q, November 15, 1986

Whitman S, Kursh ED: Curbing incontinence. Journal of Gerontological Nursing 13(4): 35–40, April 1987

**PROCEDURE VII-3
APPLYING A CONDOM
CATHETER**

McKean C: Chris's story. Community Outlook 23–24, February 1987

Norton C: Maintaining continence. Geriatric Nursing Home Care 7(7):25–27, July 1987

Seth C: Male incontinence. Community Outlook 20–21, February 1987

**PROCEDURE VII-4
GIVING A CONTINUOUS
BLADDER IRRIGATION**

Birdsall C, Brassil D: How do you use renal irrigations? Am J Nurs 87(7):909–910, July 1987

**PROCEDURE VII-5
IRRIGATING A
CATHETER USING A
CLOSED OR OPEN
SYSTEM**

Burgener S: Justification of closed intermittent urinary catheter irrigation/instillation: A review of current research and practice. J Adv Nurs 12(2):229–234, March 1987

Roe B, Chapman R, Crow R: Checking catheter care. Nursing Times 82(48):61, 63, November 26–December 2, 1986

**PROCEDURE VII-6
CHANGING A STOMA
APPLIANCE ON AN
ILEAL CONDUIT**

Adams DA, Selekof JL: Children with ostomies: Comprehensive care planning. Pediatric Nursing 12(6):429–433, November–December 1986

Against all odds: The story of an amazing appliance and an even more amazing relationship. Nursing '87 17(8):52–55, August 1987

Black P: Stoma care: The appliance of science. Community Outlook 27–28, 30, May 1987

Erickson PJ: Ostomies: The art of pouching. Nurs Clin North Am 22(2):311–320, June 1987

Jeffries E: Down to basics. Nursing Times 83(4):59, 61–63, January 28–February 3, 1987

North K: Stoma care: preparing for life after a stoma. Nursing Times 83(18):32, May 6–12, 1987

Theilman DE: When a dressing won't do the job . . . trying a pouch instead. RN 50(6):35–36, June 1987

Watt RC: Nursing management of a patient with a urinary diversion. Seminars in Oncology Nursing 2(4):265–269, November 1986

VIII Procedures pertaining to the musculoskeletal system

VIII-1 *Turning a client in bed*

Most human activities depend on the individual's ability to move. People who lack the capacity even to turn independently in bed are at high risk for serious health problems. The nurse becomes the guardian of their safety and activity.

PURPOSES OF PROCEDURE

The nurse assists the client to turn in bed to

1. Meet the basic human need for movement
2. Facilitate protective body alignment
3. Maintain skin integrity
4. Promote circulation
5. Provide sensory stimulation
6. Improve ventilation

ASSESSMENT

OBJECTIVE DATA

- Note conditions that impair activity, such as stroke, head or spinal trauma, skeletal injury, or immobilizing devices like casts.
- Stimulate the client to ascertain his highest level of consciousness.
- Observe the client's body alignment.
- Watch the client for independent, purposeful movement.
- Inspect muscles for mass, strength, and coordination.
- Put each joint through its range of motion and note any deficits.
- Measure baseline vital signs during rest.
- Read the medical orders for restrictions in activity or if certain positions are contraindicated.
- Inspect to ensure that all tubes are secure and provide ample length to accommodate turning.

SUBJECTIVE DATA

- Ask the client to describe his overall comfort level and indicate specific areas of the body that may be painful, tingle, sensitive to heat or pressure, or numb.
- Determine if the client requires analgesia.

RELATED NURSING DIAGNOSES

Since immobility literally affects all body systems, the client who is assisted with turning in bed may have numerous nursing diagnoses. Each client's nursing diagnoses will depend on a comprehensive assessment of the individual. Therefore, the following may be considered a partial list:

- *Altered Comfort*
- *Impaired Physical Mobility*
- *Self-Care Deficit*
- *Potential for Injury*
- *Powerlessness*
- *Disturbance in Self-Concept*
- *Social Isolation*
- *Altered Tissue Perfusion*

PLANNING

ESTABLISHING
PRIORITIES

The client's safety is a prime factor in planning. The nurse should check the status of mechanical equipment, remove positioning equipment in the bed, enlist the assistance of others, if needed, and have a plan for accomplishing the task.

Activity and exercise must take place regularly. Therefore, the nurse must plan a routine for turning a client at least every 2 hours. More frequent turning and changes in position may be necessary if there is an inability to maintain body alignment or other complications of immobility are developing. This continuous schedule of care provides the opportunity to attend to other basic needs and activities of daily living that the helpless client cannot do independently. Examples include bathing, taking fluids and nourishment, elimination, sensory stimulation, and diversional activity.

SETTING GOALS

• The client will change positions every 2 hours.
• The body will be maintained in alignment.
• Joints will maintain the potential for function.

PREPARATION OF
EQUIPMENT

Assuming the client is already in an adjustable hospital bed with side rails, the nurse may choose to use items from the following list when turning a client:

Trapeze
Bedboard
Turning sheet
Pillows
Towels and washcloths for hand rolls
Footboard
Cradle
Sandbags
Trochanter rolls
Hand splints

Technique for turning a client in bed

ACTION	RATIONALE
1. Explain the procedure to the client.	An explanation reduces apprehension and facilitates cooperation.
2. Wash your hands.	Handwashing deters the spread of microorganisms.

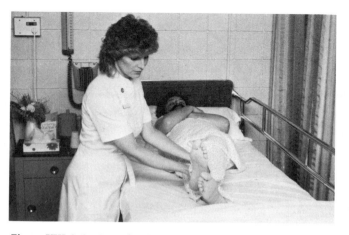

Figure VIII-1-1 Once the client has been positioned to the far side of the bed, the nurse positions the client's arms and legs.

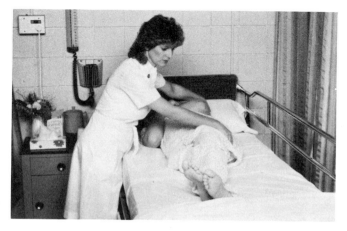

Figure VIII-1-2 This nurse centers herself next to the greatest mass of the client's body and will use her large muscles to move the weight of the client.

3. Raise the bed to your waist level. Adjust the bed to a flat position or as low as the client can tolerate. Lower the side rail nearest you and make sure the side rail on the opposite side is raised.

Adjusting the bed facilitates the turning maneuver and minimizes the strain on the nurse, yet keeps the client safe.

4. Position the client on the side of the bed in the supine position.

Moving the client close to the edge on one side ensures that the client will be in the center of the bed after the turning is accomplished.

5. Place the client's arms across the chest and cross the far leg over the near one, as shown in Figure VIII-1-1.

Positioning the extremities as described facilitates the turning motion and protects the client's arms during the turn.

6. Stand next to the middle of the client's body as the nurse in Figure VIII-1-2 is doing. Spread your feet with one foot ahead of the other. Tighten the gluteal and abdominal muscles and flex your knees.

This locates the nurse opposite the center of the client's body mass. The nurse is in a stable position with good body alignment and is prepared to use large muscles to turn the client.

7. Position your hands on the client's far shoulder and hip and roll him toward you, as shown in Figure VIII-1-3.

This maneuver supports the client's body and makes use of the nurse's weight to assist with turning.

8. Make the client comfortable and positioned in proper alignment, as shown in Figure VIII-1-4.

The nurse supports the structures of the skeletal system to maintain their functional use.

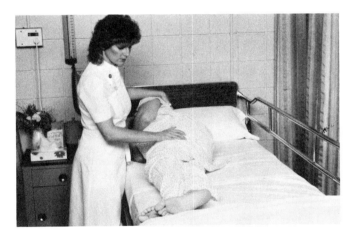

Figure VIII-1-3 The client has been turned toward the nurse and is in a side-lying position.

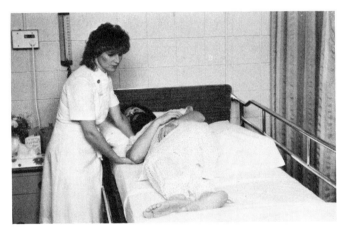

Figure VIII-1-4 The nurse uses pillows to support the client's head and spine. Other positioning devices can be used to support and maintain joint positions.

9. Readjust the bed height and position and raise the side rail.

Lowering the bed and raising side rails protect the client's safety.

10. Wash your hands.

Handwashing deters the spread of microorganisms.

SAMPLE DOCUMENTATION

Date	Time	Nurse's note
3/18	0630	Responds by opening eyes when touched and name is spoken. Turned from supine position to left lateral position. Back and buttocks bathed and massaged. R arm supported on pillows. L foot positioned against footboard to maintain dorsiflexion. Mouth hygiene performed in side-lying position.

E. Nicani, RN

EVALUATION

REASSESSMENT

Each time the client is turned, the nurse should examine alignment and the support of joints. Focus assessments of the skin, circulation, and breathing help to indicate if complications of immobility are being prevented. Joint mobility reflects the potential for future functional use.

EXPECTED OUTCOMES

No injuries occur.
The spine is straight.
Joints are supported in a functional or neutral position.
Chest expansion is unrestricted.
Pressure is relieved over bony prominences.

UNEXPECTED OUTCOMES

The client experiences pain.
The spine is flexed.
Joints are in potentially dysfunctional positions.
Chest expansion is limited.
Dependent edema is present in unsupported arms or legs.

MODIFICATIONS IN SELECTED SITUATIONS

GENERAL VARIATIONS

The nurse should schedule alternative positional changes. Possibilities include Fowler's position, Figure VIII-1-5; supine position, Figure VIII-1-6; lateral position, Figure VIII-1-7; Sims' position, Figure VIII-1-8; and prone position, Figure VIII-1-9. Try to arrange utilization of Fowler's position for times when the client is eating or receiving a tube feeding.

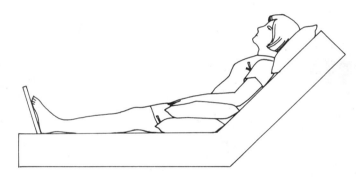

Figure VIII-1-5 The semisitting position is called *Fowler's position.* The head of the bed is elevated from 45 degrees to 60 degrees, although it can be raised as high as 90 degrees and lowered to 30 degrees. The arms are supported to avoid pulling on the shoulder joint. A footboard is used to prevent footdrop.

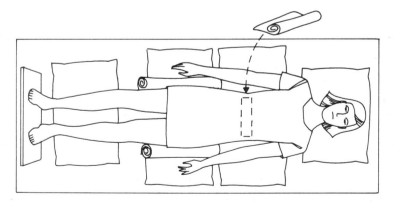

Figure VIII-1-6 In a supine position the client lies flat with the head and shoulders slightly elevated with a pillow. The arms and hands are supported. The feet are maintained in dorsiflexion by using a footboard.

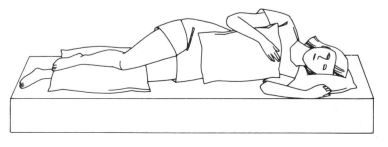

Figure VIII-1-7 A lateral or side-lying position places the client on the side with the main weight of the body borne by the scapula and ilium. Pillows are used to support the upper arm and leg.

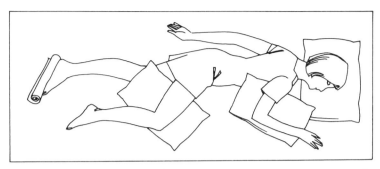

Figure VIII-1–8 The Sims' position is a variation of the lateral position. The client lies on the side but the lower arm is behind the client and the upper arm is flexed at both the elbow and shoulder.

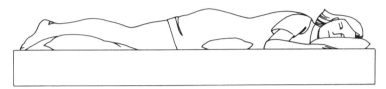

Figure VIII-1–9 In the prone position the client lies on the abdomen with the head turned to the side. A small pillow can be used to support the head and lower leg.

If available, the nurse may requisition one of the specialized beds, such as rocking bed, chair bed, circular bed, or Stryker frame, as an option to the standard adjustable hospital bed.

Provide strengthening and flexibility exercises to restore or maintain musculoskeletal function. For example, while in a supine position or Fowler's position, a rope can be looped over the trapeze for active or assisted arm and shoulder movement.

A client confined to bed may wear canvas sneakers to help in preventing footdrop.

Pad side rails if the client has involuntary muscle spasms.

When a client has a hip spica cast, avoid pulling on the abduction bar while turning the client.

To help a client in a hip spica cast lie on his side, suspend the abducted leg in a sling attached to an overbed frame. This helps the client have a change of position without losing his balance or causing stress on the cast material.

AGE-RELATED VARIATIONS

Provide visual stimuli, such as a mobile or wind-up toys that move about, when a young child's position is changed. Vary the toys and make substitutions frequently to avoid boredom. Move the child's bed or crib to a location where he can observe the activity of others.

HOME-HEALTH VARIATIONS

Hospital beds and equipment may be rented from various medical-supply firms.

Cardboard boxes are very versatile. The base of a box can substitute for a footboard. Cutting the center on two sides of a box can create a cradle.

A sagging mattress can be made more supportive by placing a plywood board between the mattress and box springs.

Zip-lock bags filled with kitty litter or other substance, covered with a towel, can function like sandbags or trochanter rolls.

Post a turning schedule for the caregivers.

RELATED TEACHING

The client should be told the reasons for turning. He may participate, if able, in planning the schedule and choice of position as long as the same position is not overused.

Before turning, the sequence of steps should be described to the client and any assistants.

Demonstrate isometric and isotonic exercises and encourage the client's maximum participation. Assist or supervise range-of-motion exercises of joints that are unused. Advise the client to limit exercise if pain is experienced and to rest when feeling fatigued. Establish realistic goals for specific movements.

PERFORMANCE CHECKLIST

When turning a client in bed, the learner:

C	A	U	
[ ]	[ ]	[ ]	Assesses the client's ability to assist
[ ]	[ ]	[ ]	Provides analgesia, if needed
[ ]	[ ]	[ ]	Complies with the time schedule and selects an appropriate alternative position
[ ]	[ ]	[ ]	Explains the procedure
[ ]	[ ]	[ ]	Washes hands
[ ]	[ ]	[ ]	Provides privacy
[ ]	[ ]	[ ]	Raises the bed, flattens the mattress, and lowers the side rail
[ ]	[ ]	[ ]	Removes positioning devices, such as pillows, trochanter rolls, and so on
[ ]	[ ]	[ ]	Pulls bed clothing down to protect the client from exposure
[ ]	[ ]	[ ]	Folds the top linens to the bottom of the bed
[ ]	[ ]	[ ]	Uses good body mechanics to place the client in supine position
[ ]	[ ]	[ ]	Moves the client close to the side of the bed opposite to where he will be turned
[ ]	[ ]	[ ]	Raises side rail and moves to the opposite side of the bed
[ ]	[ ]	[ ]	Crosses the client's arms over the chest and places one leg forward of the other
[ ]	[ ]	[ ]	Spreads feet, bends knees, and places a hand on the far shoulder and the other on the client's hip
[ ]	[ ]	[ ]	Pulls the client over
[ ]	[ ]	[ ]	Completes repositioning in lateral, Sims', or prone position
[ ]	[ ]	[ ]	Inspects the skin and provides special care
[ ]	[ ]	[ ]	Replaces supportive devices
[ ]	[ ]	[ ]	Covers the client with bed linens
[ ]	[ ]	[ ]	Raises the side rail and lowers the bed
[ ]	[ ]	[ ]	Returns the signal device within reach
[ ]	[ ]	[ ]	Washes hands
[ ]	[ ]	[ ]	Records pertinent information

Outcome: [ ] Pass   [ ] Fail

C = competent; A = acceptable; U = unsatisfactory

Comments: _____
_____
_____

_____   _____
Student's Signature   Date

_____   _____
Instructor's Signature   Date

VIII-2   *Moving a client up in bed*

Clients may slip to the bottom of the bed for a variety of reasons, such as gravity pull, restless movement, and so on. The nurse is often required to move the client up in bed.

PURPOSES OF PROCEDURE

A client is moved up in bed to

1. Prevent injury
2. Promote comfort
3. Restore body alignment

ASSESSMENT

OBJECTIVE DATA

- Observe the client's position in bed and related body alignment.
- Note the client's level of activity.
- Identify the client's level of consciousness and capacity for following directions.
- Determine the client's strength and ability to assist with moving.
- Estimate the effort required to move the client in relation to his size, body weight, or treatment devices.
- Determine if there are any restrictions in the client's activity.
- Inspect the bed for assistive equipment, such as a trapeze or lift sheet.

SUBJECTIVE DATA

- Ask the client to describe his level of comfort and need for analgesia.

RELEVANT NURSING DIAGNOSES

The client who needs assistance moving up in bed may have nursing diagnoses, such as

- *Altered Comfort*
- *Potential for Injury*
- *Potential Altered Skin Integrity*
- *Impaired Physical Mobility*
- *Self-Care Deficit*
- *Sensory Perceptual Alteration: Kinesthetic*

PLANNING

ESTABLISHING PRIORITIES

The nurse is ultimately accountable for the client's safety. Therefore, the client should be assisted in moving up in bed when the nurse first assesses the need. It is best to realistically determine the need for help, especially if the client is obese or combative.

SETTING GOALS

- The client will be moved upward in bed without injury.
- The client's body will be in proper alignment.
- The client will experience improved comfort.

PREPARATION OF EQUIPMENT

When the client is already in an adjustable hospital bed, the nurse may utilize selected items from the following list for moving the client:

Trapeze
Lift sheet

Technique for moving a client up in bed

ACTION	RATIONALE
1. Explain the procedure to the client.	An explanation reduces apprehension and facilitates cooperation.
2. Wash your hands.	Handwashing deters the spread of microorganisms.
3. Raise the bed to a comfortable position for you. Adjust the bed to a flat position if the client can tolerate it. Lower the side rail nearest you.	Adjusting the bed facilitates moving the client upward and minimizes strain on the nurse.
4. Remove the pillow and place it at the head of the bed.	Moving the pillow clears the bed of an obstacle that could interfere with upward movement and protects the client's head from striking the top of the bed.
5. If the client is able to assist, have him flex his knees with the feet flat on the bed, as shown in Figure VIII-2-1.	This position prepares the client for pushing upward using major muscle groups.
6. Assist the client to grasp the overhead trapeze bar, or if the client is unable to assist, fold the client's arms across the chest.	Using the trapeze promotes the client's help and reduces friction on the skin while moving upward.
7. Instruct the client to flex his neck with the chin on the chest.	Flexion prevents hyperextension of the neck while moving.
8. Stand opposite the center of the client's body with your feet spread and turned toward the head of the bed. Position one foot slightly forward, as the nurse in Figure VIII-2-2 is doing.	This position places the nurse at the center of the client's body mass. Spreading the feet provides a wide base of support and improves balance.

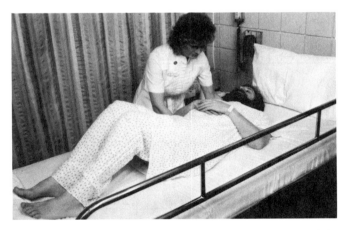

Figure VIII-2-1 The nurse has moved the pillow and instructed the client to bend his knees. If the client can use the large muscles of his legs it will help the nurse move him upward in bed.

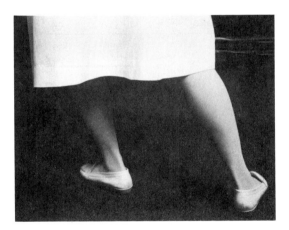

Figure VIII-2-2 Spreading the legs provides a wide base of support.

9. Flex your knees and hips. Place one arm under the client's neck and shoulders, grasping the far shoulder with the hand. Place the other arm under the upper thighs. Pull the client closer to your side of the bed. Move the client's head and legs into alignment.	Positioning in this manner prepares the nurse to use the large muscles of the body to do the work of lifting. Placing the arms under the shoulders and thighs supports and evenly distributes the weight of the client.
10. Tighten your abdominal and gluteal muscles.	These muscles stabilize the pelvis prior to the lifting maneuver.

11. Review the plan for movement with the client. Shift your weight back and forth from the back leg to the front leg. On the count of three, move the client upward in bed, as shown in Figure VIII-2-3. If possible, the client should push with his legs and assist moving upward by grasping the trapeze. Repeat if necessary.

A rocking motion uses the nurse's weight to counter the client's weight when moving him up in bed. If the client assists, less effort is required by the nurse.

12. Assist the client to a comfortable position in the center of the bed, as shown in Figure VIII-2-4. Reposition the pillow. Raise the side rail and adjust the bed position, if necessary.

Lowering the bed and raising the side rail protect the client's safety.

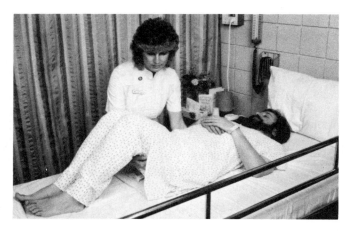

Figure VIII-2-3 The nurse counts out a cadence while rocking. When the signal is given, both the nurse and the client use their combined strength to move upward.

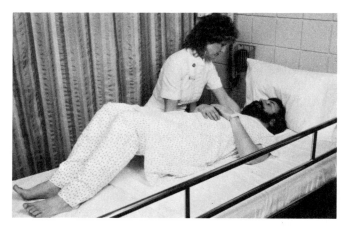

Figure VIII-2-4 Once the client has been moved upward, the nurse can reposition the pillow and provide other supportive measures for making him more comfortable.

13. Wash your hands.

Handwashing deters the spread of microorganisms.

SAMPLE DOCUMENTATION

Date	Time	Nurse's note
7/02	1600	Observed slipping toward bottom of bed. States, ''I have to fix supper.'' Reoriented to person, place, and date. Assisted to move up in bed. Remaining in bed presently.
		P. Lacey, RN

EVALUATION

REASSESSMENT

Determine the client's comfort, position, and alignment after moving the client up in bed. Note the integrity of the skin. Friction and shearing force can lead to skin abrasion and breakdown. A confused client bears close watching. If restlessness and disorientation continue, the nurse may request a room transfer closer to where others can observe the client. A volunteer may stay with the client temporarily until someone from the family arrives. Share concerns for the client's safety with the physician, who may then order the temporary use of a vest restraint.

EXPECTED OUTCOMES

The client is repositioned to the center, upper area of the bed.
The skin remains intact.
The client's posture and alignment are improved.

UNEXPECTED OUTCOMES

The client resists movement.

The client continues to slip to the bottom of the bed.

The skin over the client's back is reddened and fails to blanch when pressure is relieved.

MODIFICATIONS IN SELECTED SITUATIONS

GENERAL VARIATIONS

Use a lift sheet beneath the client. With the help of a second nurse, roll the sheet closely to the client's trunk. While on opposite sides of the body, with knees and hips flexed, coordinate moving the client toward the head of the bed.

Two nurses may opt to interlock arms under the client's shoulders and thighs. Working in unison, the nurses use their combined strength and rocking momentum to move a client up in bed.

Requisition a longer bed if the client is tall and moving does not appreciably improve his comfort and alignment.

Slightly elevate (not gatch) the foot of the bed higher than the upper portion, if this is not contraindicated. The slight incline may overcome the tendency to gravitate toward the lower end of the bed.

HOME-HEALTH VARIATIONS

Hydraulic, mechanical lifts that can be operated by one person can be rented for home care.

RELATED TEACHING

Explain each step while preparing to move the client.

Instruct the client on the use of the trapeze or side rails when moving in bed.

Demonstrate and explain proper body mechanics to family members who help care for the client.

Identify methods for supporting joints and maintaining muscle strength and joint flexibility.

(Performance checklist next page)

PERFORMANCE CHECKLIST

When moving a client up in bed, the learner:

C	A	U	
[ ]	[ ]	[ ]	Gathers appropriate data
[ ]	[ ]	[ ]	Seeks the assistance of other personnel, if needed
[ ]	[ ]	[ ]	Explains the procedure
[ ]	[ ]	[ ]	Washes hands
[ ]	[ ]	[ ]	Provides privacy
[ ]	[ ]	[ ]	Raises the bed and lowers the side rail
[ ]	[ ]	[ ]	Moves the pillow upward so it pads the headboard
[ ]	[ ]	[ ]	Helps the client flex knees and feet
[ ]	[ ]	[ ]	Instructs the client to grasp the trapeze or folds the client's arms across the chest
[ ]	[ ]	[ ]	Tells the client to bend his neck
[ ]	[ ]	[ ]	Uses good body mechanics by assuming a wide base of support at the center of the client's body
[ ]	[ ]	[ ]	Places an arm under the client's neck and shoulders and the other under the upper thighs
[ ]	[ ]	[ ]	Moves the client close to the nurse's center of gravity
[ ]	[ ]	[ ]	Indicates the signal on which the client should push with his legs and pull, if able, on the trapeze
[ ]	[ ]	[ ]	Bends knees and hips
[ ]	[ ]	[ ]	Rocks back and forth to gain momentum
[ ]	[ ]	[ ]	Pulls the client while he pushes at the agreed signal
[ ]	[ ]	[ ]	Replaces the pillow
[ ]	[ ]	[ ]	Realigns the client in a position of comfort
[ ]	[ ]	[ ]	Lowers the bed and raises the side rail
[ ]	[ ]	[ ]	Washes hands
[ ]	[ ]	[ ]	Charts significant information

Outcome: [ ] **Pass**   [ ] **Fail**

C = competent; A = acceptable; U = unsatisfactory

Comments: _____

_____

_____

_____   _____
Student's Signature   Date

_____   _____
Instructor's Signature   Date

VIII-3 *Transferring a client from bed to a stretcher*

Considerable strength, coordination, and care must be utilized when moving a client from a bed to a stretcher. More than one nurse is needed when the client is unconscious or helpless.

PURPOSES OF PROCEDURE

A client is transferred from a bed to a stretcher to

1. Move the client to another department of the agency for diagnostic testing, physical therapy, or surgery
2. Provide diversion through a temporary change in the client's environment
3. Relocate the client to another room or agency

ASSESSMENT

OBJECTIVE DATA

- Note any scheduled tests or procedures that will require moving the client from his room.
- Determine the necessity for using a stretcher as opposed to other alternatives for transport.
- Observe the client's level of consciousness and cognitive abilities. Note the administration of any medications that affect thought processes and coordination, such as narcotic analgesia.
- Identify treatment devices, such as a nasogastric tube, oxygen, intravenous lines, indwelling catheter, and so on, that will require modification during a transfer.
- Determine the client's muscle strength and coordination in bilateral upper and lower extremities.

SUBJECTIVE DATA

- Inquire concerning the need to urinate or move his bowels.
- Ask the client to describe his comfort level and need for pain relief.

RELEVANT NURSING DIAGNOSES

The client who is transferred from bed to a stretcher may have nursing diagnoses, such as

- *Potential for Injury*
- *Impaired Physical Mobility*

PLANNING

ESTABLISHING PRIORITIES

If the client requires analgesia, it should be administered at least a half hour before the expected time for transferring the client. This will provide sufficient time for the drug to achieve its effect. The client should be provided with the opportunity for elimination prior to transfer onto the stretcher. Disconnect or unfasten tubes attached to the bed. Lock the wheels of the stretcher and bed to prevent harming the client. Check that current treatments and medications have been administered before the client leaves the unit. Change any low intravenous solutions that may run dry while the client is absent from the unit. Complete all transfer forms if the client is being transported to another agency.

SETTING GOALS

- The client will move from the bed to the stretcher without injury or discomfort.

PREPARATION OF EQUIPMENT

Items from the following list may be selected when transferring a client from a bed to a stretcher:

Sheet for lifting and pulling
Stretcher with safety belts or side rails
Top sheet, bath blanket, or bed blanket
Portable IV pole (optional)
Oxygen tank (optional)
Catheter clamp (optional)
Clamp for nasogastric tube (optional)

Technique for transferring a client from bed to a stretcher

ACTION	RATIONALE
1. Explain the procedure to the client.	An explanation reduces apprehension and facilitates cooperation.
2. Wash your hands.	Handwashing deters the spread of microorganisms.
3. Move the bed and equipment in the room to accommodate the stretcher. Make sure that assistants are available. Close the door or curtain.	Arranging the room and having adequate help facilitate the activities involved in the transfer. Closing the door or curtain shows respect for the client's modesty and protects him from being seen by others.
4. Raise the bed to the same height as the stretcher and adjust the head of the bed to a flat position if the client can tolerate it. Lower the side rails.	Pushing and pulling require less effort than lifting. This position facilitates moving the client.
5. Place a draw sheet under the client if one is not already there. Use the draw sheet to move the client to the side of the bed, as shown in Figure VIII-3-1, where the stretcher will be placed.	A lift sheet facilitates moving the client and reduces the potential for friction and skin abrasion.

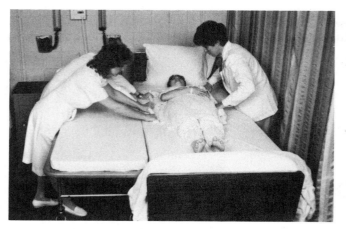

Figure VIII-3–1 These nurses use the draw sheet to move the client to the edge of the bed close to the stretcher.

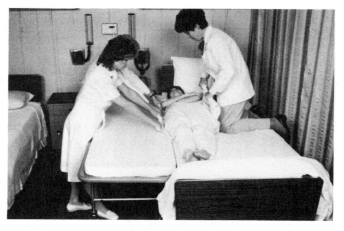

Figure VIII-3–2 In order to locate the mass of the client close to the nurse's center of gravity, one nurse is positioned on the bed next to the client. The flexed knees, hips, and elbows help to utilize major muscle groups in performing the work involved.

6. Position the stretcher next to the bed and parallel to it. Lock the wheels on the stretcher and bed. Remove the pillow from the bed and place it on the stretcher.	Positioning the stretcher and locking the wheels facilitate the safe transfer of the client.
7. To move the client	Moving requires the coordinated effort of the team.

a. The first nurse should kneel on the far side of the bed away from the stretcher. Position one knee at the upper torso closer to the client than the other knee. Grasp the draw sheet securely.

The nurse uses major muscle groups to assist in movement. The nurse's flexed hips help to avoid a back injury.

b. The second nurse should reach across the stretcher and grasp the draw sheet at the head and chest area.

Using the sheet allows the nurse to support the client's head and upper body for a safe transfer.

c. The third nurse should reach across the stretcher and grasp the draw sheet at the waist and thigh area. Ask the client to fold his arms across the chest.

Using the sheet helps support the lower part of the body for a safe transfer.

d. At a signal given by the first nurse, the second and third nurses pull while the first nurse lifts the client from the bed to the stretcher, as the nurses in Figure VIII-3-2 are doing.

Working in unison distributes the work of moving the client and facilitates the transfer.

8. Secure the client on the stretcher until the side rails are raised. Cover the client and assist him to a comfortable position. Leave the lift sheet in place for transferring the client back to bed when he returns.

These measures ensure the client's comfort and safety.

9. Wash your hands.

Handwashing deters the spread of microorganisms.

Technique for transferring the client from bed to stretcher using a three-carrier lift

ACTION	RATIONALE
1. Explain the procedure to the client.	An explanation reduces apprehension and facilitates cooperation.
2. Wash your hands.	Handwashing deters the spread of microorganisms.
3. Place the stretcher at a right angle to the foot of the bed. Lock the wheels of the bed and the wheels of the stretcher. Raise the bed to the height of the stretcher.	The stretcher will be in position for the carriers after they pivot away from the bed.
4. Decide on each person's responsibility during the lift. Each person must support one section of the body:	Opinions differ about how the weight of the client should be distributed among the nurses. Commonly, the strongest helper should support the heaviest body area or the tallest person with the longest reach should support the client's head and shoulders.
a. Head, shoulders, and chest	
b. Hips	
c. Thighs and legs	
5. In preparation for the lift, flex the knees and separate the feet with the foot closest to the bed slightly flexed.	A broad-based stance improves balance and lowers the lifter's center of gravity.
6. Slide the arms under the client as far as possible, and, on signal, all helpers should simultaneously roll the client toward their chests, as shown in Figure VIII-3-3.	"Logrolling" the client onto the carrier brings the mass of the client over each person's center of gravity, thereby increasing the stability of the group and reducing strain on the carriers.
7. On signal, the helpers stand and steady the client securely against their chests, as in Figure VIII-3-4.	Flexed knees allow workers to lift with strong leg muscles.

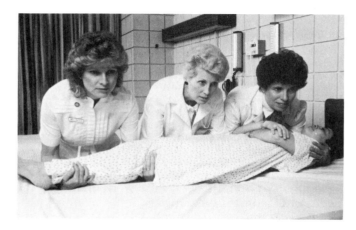

Figure VIII-3–3 These nurses stand elbow to elbow and move the client to the edge of the bed.

8. The helpers should step back together, pivot around to the stretcher, shown in Figure VIII-3-5. On signal, the client is lowered onto the stretcher, shown in Figure VIII-3-6.

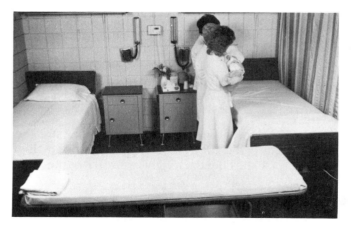

Figure VIII-3–4 On a given signal these nurses simultaneously stand while lifting the client from the bed.

This lets the large leg and arm muscles do the work of lowering the client.

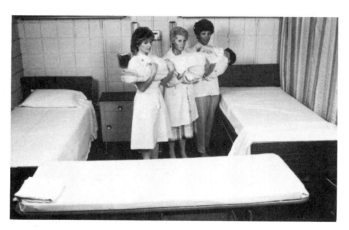

Figure VIII-3–5 While pivoting together, the nurses face the stretcher and begin to move toward it with the client.

9. The client should be covered with a sheet or blanket and positioned as necessary. The stretcher side rails should be raised.

10. Wash your hands.

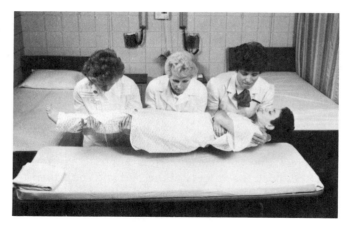

Figure VIII-3–6 The nurses spread their legs with one foot forward of the other, flex their knees, and lower the client to the stretcher.

These measures promote the comfort and safety of the client.

Handwashing deters the spread of microorganisms.

SAMPLE DOCUMENTATION

Date	Time	Nurse's note
8/14	1130	Transferred to stretcher with assistance of two others. Transported to x-ray department.

B. Fortunato, RN

EVALUATION

REASSESSMENT

The client's alignment and comfort should be evaluated once the transfer has been completed. Additional pillows may be used to support parts of the body. Extra blankets can be provided for warmth. Side rails or safety straps should be secured before moving the client. Intravenous sites as well as infusion rates should be reassessed to determine that fluid therapy has not become altered.

EXPECTED OUTCOMES

The client is supported and lifted without injury.
The client's comfort level remains similar to that prior to the transfer.

UNEXPECTED OUTCOMES

The client is frightened and protests the transfer.
Three people are unable to transfer the client.
The client experiences discomfort during the transfer.

MODIFICATIONS IN SELECTED SITUATIONS

GENERAL VARIATIONS

A mechanical lift may be used if the client is extremely heavy or weak, or there is not sufficient personnel available for assistance.
If the client has a spinal injury or surgery, apply a back brace or log roll the client when transferring from bed to stretcher.

HOME-HEALTH VARIATIONS

If a hallway, stairwell, or corners will not accommodate a stretcher, use a backboard or sheet to lift and transfer the client.

RELATED TEACHING

Explain the plan for transferring the client to the stretcher. Before attempting each step, reinstruct the client on what is about to be done and how he can best assist.
(Performance checklist next page)

PERFORMANCE CHECKLIST

When transferring a client from bed to a stretcher, the learner:

C	A	U	
[ ]	[ ]	[ ]	Makes appropriate assessments
[ ]	[ ]	[ ]	Explains the procedure
[ ]	[ ]	[ ]	Provides the opportunity for elimination or other necessities, like pain relief
[ ]	[ ]	[ ]	Clears the room
[ ]	[ ]	[ ]	Positions the stretcher
[ ]	[ ]	[ ]	Enlists assistants
[ ]	[ ]	[ ]	Locks the wheels of the bed and stretcher
[ ]	[ ]	[ ]	Raises the bed and lowers the side rails
[ ]	[ ]	[ ]	Removes pillows, repositions IV solutions, unfastens catheter drainage tube
[ ]	[ ]	[ ]	Positions assistants appropriately
[ ]	[ ]	[ ]	Provides directions to helpers
[ ]	[ ]	[ ]	Moves the client to the side of the bed
[ ]	[ ]	[ ]	Transfers the client from the bed to the stretcher
[ ]	[ ]	[ ]	Positions the client in good alignment
[ ]	[ ]	[ ]	Returns pillow(s) and covers the client with a sheet or blanket(s)
[ ]	[ ]	[ ]	Raises the side rails on the stretcher or fastens safety straps around the client's arms and chest, waist, and legs
[ ]	[ ]	[ ]	Checks all tubes and attached equipment
[ ]	[ ]	[ ]	Helps move the stretcher from the room
[ ]	[ ]	[ ]	Straightens or remakes the hospital bed
[ ]	[ ]	[ ]	Washes hands
[ ]	[ ]	[ ]	Charts pertinent information

Outcome: [ ] Pass   [ ] Fail

C = competent; A = acceptable; U = unsatisfactory

Comments: _____
_____
_____

_____	_____
Student's Signature	Date
_____	_____
Instructor's Signature	Date

VIII-4 *Assisting a client from bed to a chair*

Bed rest can be confining and boring. Eventually the client may be strong enough to sit up in a chair. One person can transfer a helpless client from a bed; using two people reduces the effort required.

PURPOSES OF PROCEDURE

A client is transferred from bed to a chair to

1. Improve comfort
2. Increase his activity level
3. Provide a means of moving the client from the room

ASSESSMENT

OBJECTIVE DATA

- Verify the change in activity by reading the written medical order.
- Identify deficits that may affect the transfer, such as hemiplegia or other types of paralysis, obesity, reduced levels of consciousness, applied casts, orthopedic surgery, arthritis, contractures, and so on.
- Review the recent responses of the client to activity, such as being turned or moved, by reading the nurse's notes or conferring with colleagues.
- Assess vital signs; be especially aware of the respiratory rate and effort, and the pulse rate at rest.
- Measure the blood pressure while the client is lying flat and being elevated to a sitting position. Note any significant drop in blood pressure when the upper body is raised.
- Assess arm strength and coordination.
- Determine the client's ability to follow directions and cooperate during the transfer.
- Inspect the equipment being utilized by the client, such as an intravenous infusion, nasogastric tube and suction, indwelling catheter, and so on.
- Check that elastic stockings are being worn, if so ordered.

SUBJECTIVE DATA

- Ask the client to describe his comfort level and need for pain relief.
- Inquire as to whether the client feels dizzy, nauseous, or weak, or desires to use the bedpan or urinal.

RELEVANT NURSING DIAGNOSES

The client who will transfer from bed to a chair may have nursing diagnoses, such as

- *Potential for Activity Intolerance*
- *Anxiety or Fear*
- *Altered Comfort*
- *Potential for Injury*
- *Impaired Physical Mobility*
- *Self-Care Deficit*
- *Unilateral Neglect*

PLANNING ESTABLISHING PRIORITIES	The nurse must analyze assessment data to determine the safest plan for transfer. It is better to anticipate needing assistance than to endanger the client. Good planning includes adapting or repositioning tubes and machines so as to avoid their displacement or malfunction. The chair and bed must be locked and positioned so the potential for injury is reduced. The nurse should allow ample time for the relief of pain before transferring the client. Hand, back, or leg braces and supportive devices should be applied properly before proceeding with moving the client. The nurse may collaborate with the client to determine the preferred time for sitting in the chair. Some may choose that it coincide with a visit from the family, at mealtime, or while the bed linen is changed. When there are no extenuating circumstances, the conscientious nurse complies with the client's wishes.
SETTING GOALS	• The client will transfer from the bed to a chair without injury. • The client will tolerate the procedure without experiencing ill effects.
PREPARATION OF EQUIPMENT	The nurse may select pertinent items from the following list: Wheelchair or heavy stable room chair, preferably with armrests Slippers Bathrobe

Technique for one nurse assisting a client to transfer from bed to chair

ACTION	RATIONALE
1. Explain the procedure to the client.	An explanation reduces apprehension and facilitates cooperation.
2. Wash your hands.	Handwashing deters the spread of microorganisms.
3. Assess the client's ability to assist with the transfer. Move equipment as necessary to make room for the chair. Close the door or curtain.	Rearranging the room ensures the client's safety and facilitates the transfer. Closing the door or curtain shows respect for the client's modesty and prevents him from being seen by others.
4. Place the bed in low position.	A low bed helps the client to stand and pivot with more safety.
5. Assist the client to put on a robe and slippers.	A bathrobe provides warmth. Slippers protect the feet and provide stability when standing.
6. Position the chair at the bedside.	Until the client's strength is adequate, the nurse restricts the client from walking.

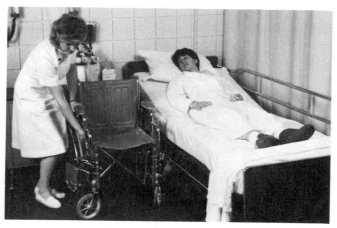

Figure VIII-4-1 The nurse has moved the furnishings to make room for placing the chair beside the bed.

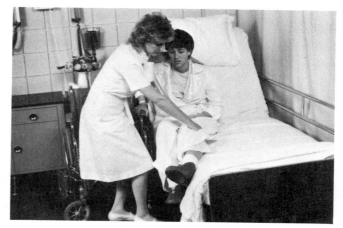

Figure VIII-4-2 The nurse has raised the head of the bed to help the client adjust to an upright position.

a. *For the client with unimpaired mobility:* Bring the chair close to the bedside facing the foot of the bed and, if possible, brace the back of the chair against the bedside table, as shown in Figure VIII-4-1.

Bracing the chair increases its stability and ensures safety during the transfer.

b. *For the client with impaired mobility:* Position the chair facing the head or foot of the bed. When sitting on the side of the bed, the client should be able to steady himself by using the hand on the unaffected side to grasp the arm of the chair.

The position selected should ensure that the stronger side can be used to provide balance and stability during the transfer.

7. Lock the wheels on the chair and bed, if appropriate.

Locking the wheels promotes the client's safety.

8. Raise the head of the bed to the highest position, as shown in Figure VIII-4-2.

Moving from a sitting to a standing position requires less energy. If the client will experience faintness, it is safer to still be in bed.

9. Assist the client to sit on the side of the bed by supporting the head and neck while moving the legs off the bed to dangle, as the nurse in Figure VIII-4-3 is doing. Steady the client in that position for a few minutes.

A sitting position facilitates transferring to the chair and allows the circulatory system to adjust to the change in position.

10. Assist the client to a standing position.

Standing is preferable to lifting the client.

a. *For the client with unimpaired mobility:* Face the client and brace your feet and knees against the client. Place your hands around the client's waist while the client places his arms around your shoulders. Help the client to rise to a standing position.

Bracing the client provides stability and use of major muscle groups to facilitate movement.

b. *For the client with impaired mobility:* Face the client and brace your feet and knees against the client, especially his affected extremity, as shown in Figure VIII-4-4.

Bracing the affected extremity acts as a splint, providing additional stability in order to use the impaired leg and facilitate movement.

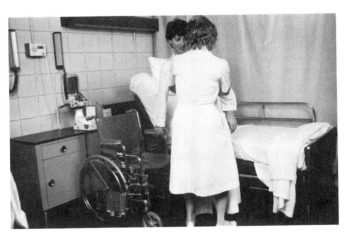

Figure VIII-4-3 The client is steadied as the legs are moved off the bed.

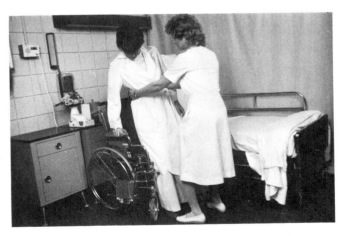

Figure VIII-4-4 The nurse braces the client's knees and supports the upper body while the client raises her body from the bed to assume a standing position.

11. Pivot the client (on the unaffected limb, if applicable) into position in front of the chair with the back of the knees against the seat of the chair.

When the backs of the knees are in contact with the chair, the client is in a safe position for sitting.

12. Encourage the client to place one arm (unaffected limb, if applicable) on the chair and steady himself

Using an arm provides more stability. Using flexed knees and hips helps to utilize major muscle groups for mov-

while slowly lowering to a sitting position. The nurse continues to brace the client's knees while flexing hips and knees when seating him.

ing the client and reducing strain on the back.

13. Adjust the client's position using pillows where necessary. Cover the client and use a restraint if necessary. Position the call bell so it is available for use.

Using pillows helps to support joints and promotes proper body alignment. Access to the signal device provides for comfort and safety.

14. Wash your hands.

Handwashing deters the spread of microorganisms.

15. Observe and document the client's tolerance of the procedure and the length of time in the chair.

Reassessing the client and communicating observations in writing helps provide continuity in care and note progress toward meeting goals.

Technique for two nurses transferring a dependent client from bed to chair

ACTION	RATIONALE
1. Explain the procedure to the client.	An explanation reduces apprehension and facilitates cooperation.
2. Wash your hands.	Handwashing deters the spread of microorganisms.
3. Move equipment as necessary to make room for the chair. Close the door or curtain.	Rearranging the room ensures the client's safety and facilitates an area that is adequate for the transfer. Closing the door or curtain shows respect for the client's modesty and prevents him from being seen by others.
4. Move the client to the near side of the bed and cross his arms across the chest, if possible, as shown in Figure VIII-4-5. Lock the wheels of the bed.	Locating the mass to the nurse's center of gravity requires less effort when moving the client. Locked wheels prevent slipping when the client is moved from the bed.
5. Position the chair next to the bed near the upper end and with the back of the chair parallel to the head of the bed. (If using a wheelchair, remove the armrest closer to the bed, if possible.) Lock the wheels on the wheelchair.	Positioning the chair next to the bed facilitates easier movement into the chair. The armrest is a potential obstacle when moving; removal promotes a smooth transfer. Locking the wheels promotes safety.
6. Adjust the bed to a comfortable level for the nurse. If the armrest cannot be removed, place the bed level with the top of the armrest.	Decreasing the distance from the bed to the chair will reduce the muscle strain on the nurses. Having the bed even with the armrest provides clearance when lowering the client.
7. Prepare to lift the client from the bed to the chair:	Two people can more easily lift the dependent client because the weight is divided, which decreases the effort needed for the transfer.
a. The first nurse should stand behind the chair and slip the arms under the client's axillae and grasp his wrists securely.	One nurse supports the weight of the upper body. This placement of the arms supports the joints rather than pulling on them.
b. The second nurse faces the wheelchair and supports the client's knees by placing the arms under them, as shown in Figure VIII-4-6.	The second nurse lifts the weight of the lower body without pulling on joints.
c. On a predetermined signal, both nurses flex hips and knees and simultaneously lift the client gently into the chair.	Flexing hips and knees uses major muscle groups in order to perform the maximum work more efficiently.

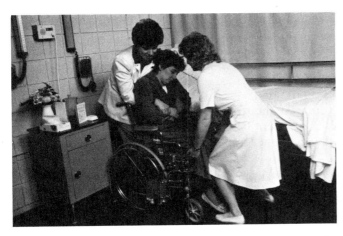

Figure VIII-4-5 The nurse crosses the client's arms to position the bulk of the body weight in one area.

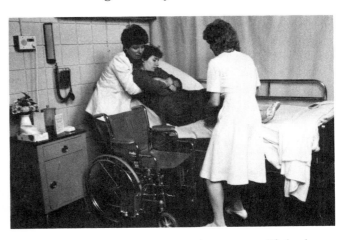

Figure VIII-4-6 These two nurses work as a team to lift the dependent client from bed into the chair. Both nurses bend from the knees and hips to prevent strain on the lower back while lowering the client into the chair.

8. Assist the client to put on a robe and slippers.

Covering the body provides insulation and prevents loss of body heat.

9. Adjust the client's position by using pillows where necessary. Cover the client and use a restraint if necessary.

Using pillows helps support joints and promotes proper body alignment. Covering the client conserves body heat. A restraint protects the dependent client from falling from the chair.

10. Wash your hands.

Handwashing deters the spread of microorganisms.

11. Observe and document the client's tolerance of the procedure and the length of time the client remained in the chair.

Reassessing the client and communicating observations in writing helps provide continuity in care and note progress toward meeting goals.

SAMPLE DOCUMENTATION

Date	Time	Nurse's note
3/31	1000	P-82, R-16 and regular, BP 138/76/72 lying down. Dangled at bedside. BP 134/74/70 while sitting. No dizziness experienced. Helped to a standing position with no weight bearing on R leg. Pivoted and lowered to sitting position in wheelchair. Remained in chair 20 minutes. Remained comfortable and alert while up. States, "Getting up has been the best medicine yet." *M. Coronado, RN*

EVALUATION

REASSESSMENT

The nurse should remain in the room or nearby the first time the client is out of bed. Always provide the client with access to the signal device in case assistance is needed. Observe the client's response to the effort of moving and the positional change. Once the client is seated, recheck the functioning of attached equipment. Adjust the client's clothing and lap covers to accommodate the client's comfort. Apply a vest restraint to prevent injury if the client is confused, disoriented, or weak.

EXPECTED OUTCOMES

The client is transferred easily and comfortably from the bed to the chair.

No harm occurs to the client.

The client manifests stable blood pressure and level of consciousness; respirations and pulse return to preactivity baseline after 5 minutes in the chair.

UNEXPECTED OUTCOMES

The client resists transferring from the bed.

The client experiences pain during the transfer.

The client's blood pressure falls; the client faints.

The client experiences sustained tachypnea and tachycardia.

The client feels excessively fatigued and weak.

MODIFICATIONS IN SELECTED SITUATIONS

GENERAL VARIATIONS

A mechanical lift may be used if the client is extremely heavy or weak, or there is not sufficient personnel for assistance.

Use a sliding board from the bed to the chair when the client has strong upper body strength.

AGE-RELATED VARIATIONS

Use a pediatric-sized wheelchair when the client is a child.

HOME-HEALTH VARIATIONS

Place crutch tips on a straight-leg chair to minimize sliding.

A wheelchair can be maneuvered onto a thick rubber or foam rug to minimize inadvertent rolling.

RELATED TEACHING

Explain the procedure fully before attempting to transfer the client. Emphasize any special instructions, such as "Don't put any weight on your right (or left) leg." Repeat short instructions throughout the transfer as each step is about to be performed.

PERFORMANCE CHECKLIST

When transferring a client from the bed to a chair, the learner:

C	A	U	
[ ]	[ ]	[ ]	Gathers pertinent data
[ ]	[ ]	[ ]	Explains the procedure
[ ]	[ ]	[ ]	Attends to basic needs, such as toileting
[ ]	[ ]	[ ]	Washes hands
[ ]	[ ]	[ ]	Provides privacy
[ ]	[ ]	[ ]	Lowers the bed
[ ]	[ ]	[ ]	Assists with bathrobe and slippers
[ ]	[ ]	[ ]	Positions and locks the chair and bed
[ ]	[ ]	[ ]	Raises the head of the bed
[ ]	[ ]	[ ]	Dangles the client
[ ]	[ ]	[ ]	Helps the client to stand
[ ]	[ ]	[ ]	Pivots so that the posteriors of the knees touch the chair seat
[ ]	[ ]	[ ]	Braces the client's knees
[ ]	[ ]	[ ]	Assists the client to sit
[ ]	[ ]	[ ]	Adjusts the client's position
[ ]	[ ]	[ ]	Covers the client's legs
[ ]	[ ]	[ ]	Provides for safety by providing the signal device and vest restraint, if needed
[ ]	[ ]	[ ]	Notes response of client
[ ]	[ ]	[ ]	Washes hands
[ ]	[ ]	[ ]	Charts significant information

Outcome: [ ] Pass   [ ] Fail

C = competent; A = acceptable; U = unsatisfactory

Comments: _____

_____

_____

_____   _____
Student's Signature   Date

_____   _____
Instructor's Signature   Date

RELATED LITERATURE

**PROCEDURE VIII-1
TURNING A CLIENT
IN BED**

Keating D, Bolyard K, Eichler E: Effects of sidelying positions on pulmonary artery pressures. Heart & Lung: Journal of Critical Care 15(6):605–610, November 1986

Lloyd P: Handle with care . . . back pain in staff . . . role of the manager. Nursing Times 82(47):33–35, November 19–25, 1986

Miner D: Patient positioning: Applying the nursing process. Journal of American Operating Room Nurses 45(5):1117–1120, 1122–1123+, May 1987

Mitchell PH: Intracranial hypertension: Influence of nursing care activities. Nurs Clin North Am 21(4):563–576, December 1986

Shaw R: Persistent vegetative state: Principles and techniques for seating and positioning. Journal of Head Trauma Rehabilitation 1(1):31–37, March 1986

**PROCEDURE VIII-2
MOVING A CLIENT
UP IN BED**

Harvey J: Back to the drawing board . . . training in correct lifting techniques may even increase the amount of back injury. Nursing Times 83(7):47–48, February 18–24, 1987

Mather D, Bennet B: How to move patients the easy way and save your back. Nursing '87 17(3):55–57, March 1987

Viquesney JS: H.O.B. up or H.O.B. down? A guide to postop positioning of neurosurgical patients. Nursing '87 17(4):47–49, April 1987

Wilson M: Lifting patients: Mind your backs . . . community nurses. Community Outlook 11–12, 14, October 1986

**PROCEDURE VIII-3
TRANSFERRING A
CLIENT FROM BED
TO STRETCHER**

Farmer P: Mechanical aids . . . easyslide lifting aid. Nursing Times 83(28):36–37, July 15–21, 1987

Uhl JE, Wilkinson WE, Wilkinson CS: Aching backs? A glimpse into the hazards of nursing. Journal of American Operating Room Nurses 35(1):13–17, January 1987

Wightwick S: Canadian padded transfer board. Physiotherapy 73(6):309–310, June 10, 1987

**PROCEDURE VIII-4
ASSISTING A CLIENT
FROM BED TO CHAIR**

Grunewald J: Wheelchair selection from a nursing perspective. Rehabilitation Nursing 11(6):31–32, November–December 1986

Settle CM: Seating and pressure sores. Physiotherapy 73(9):455–457, September 10, 1987

Steene A, Downs J: Adaptive seating: A wooden insert. Physiotherapy 73(1):49–50, January 1987

Walsh M: Half-lapboard for hemiplegic patients. Am J Occup Ther 41(8):533–535, August 1987

Index

Page numbers followed by *f* indicate figures; numbers followed by *t* indicate tabular material.

ILLUSTRATION CREDITS